ALLIED HEALTHCARE IN PRACTICE

An Introduction to Integrated Patient Care

ALLIED HEALTHCARE IN PRACTICE

An Introduction to Integrated Patient Care

Sally Lukose, PhD
Karuna Singh, PhD
Editors

APPLE ACADEMIC PRESS

First edition published 2026

Apple Academic Press Inc.
1265 Goldenrod Circle, NE,
Palm Bay, FL 32905 USA

760 Laurentian Drive, Unit 19,
Burlington, ON L7N 0A4, Canada

CRC Press
2385 NW Executive Center Drive,
Suite 320, Boca Raton FL 33431

4 Park Square, Milton Park,
Abingdon, Oxon, OX14 4RN, UK

Library and Archives Canada Cataloguing in Publication

CIP data on file with Canada Library and Archives

Library of Congress Cataloging-in-Publication Data

CIP data on file with US Library of Congress

ISBN: 978-1-998511-02-0 (hbk)
ISBN: 978-1-998511-03-7 (ebk)
DOI: 10.1201/9781998511037

About the Editors

Sally Lukose, PhD
Professor (Forensic Science), Sharda School of Allied Science and Director, Ranking, Sharda University, Greater Noida, India

Sally Lukose, PhD, is a Professor (Forensic Science) and Dean of the School of Allied Health Sciences at Sharda University, Greater Noida, India. With more than 19 years of research and teaching experience in the field of Forensic Science, Prof. (Dr.) Sally Lukose is credited with initiating undergraduate (UG) and postgraduate (PG) Forensic Science programs at Amity University (Noida and Dubai campuses), Galgotias University, the College of Traffic Management–IRTE (affiliated with Maharshi Dayanand University, Rohtak), and Sharda University. She has served as Dean of Allied Health Sciences for three years. She has more than 45 research publications in national and international journals, three books, and seven published patents to her credit. Her research publication was recognized as one of the most-read and top-downloaded papers by Wiley in 2018–2019 and 2019–2020. She has supervised numerous master's projects and PhD dissertations. Dr. Lukose has been associated with projects for the Bureau of Police Research and Development (BPR&D), Delhi, and the National Highway Traffic Safety Administration, USA. She also served as Course Director (Forensic Science) for e-PG Pathshala, a project under National Law University, Delhi. Dr. Lukose has imparted training to police officers in more than 15 states on road accident investigation, including at the North Eastern Police Academy. She has been a member of the University Grants Commission (UGC) committee for UGC-NET examinations. Her research work has been widely recognized, earning her multiple awards, including the Forensic Science Forum Award from the Indian Science Congress Association (ISCA) in 2001, the Meritorious Service Award from the South Asian Congress of Forensic Medicine, Forensic Science & Toxicology in 2008, and the prestigious Excellence Award from the Indian Congress of Forensic Medicine & Toxicology in 2010, presented by Shri Veerappa Moily, then Law Minister of India.

Karuna Singh, PhD
Professor (Nutrition and Dietetics) and Dean, School of Allied Health Sciences, Sharda University, Greater Noida, India

Karuna Singh, PhD, is currently a Professor (Nutrition and Dietetics) and Dean in the School of Allied Health Sciences at Sharda University. She is an alumna of Banasthali Vidyapeeth, Rajasthan, and has 20 years of teaching experience. She specializes in functional and therapeutic nutrition, maternal nutrition, and pediatric nutrition. Dr. Singh has supervised five PhD scholars, with six more currently pursuing research in various areas of health and nutrition. She has also guided one MPhil dissertation and more than 40 MSc (Food and Nutrition), MTech (Food Technology), and BTech (Food Technology) theses. She has authored over 50 research papers in reputed national and international journals, contributed 12 book chapters, and published two books. Apart from her academic contributions, she holds patents and copyrights and serves as an editorial board member for various journals. She has managed projects awarded by government agencies such as the Department of Science and Technology (DST) and the Biotechnology Industry Research Assistance Council (BIRAC) and has also worked on various industrial consultancy projects. She has extensive experience in organizing Faculty Development Programs (FDPs), conferences, workshops, and seminars. Dr. Singh is a life member of several professional bodies, including the National Institute of Nutrition (NIN), the Mushroom Society of India, and the Indian Science Congress Association. Her academic excellence has been recognized with multiple awards, including a Gold Medal for MSc, a Gold Medal for Best Dissertation (MSc), the Best Faculty Award, the Best Presenter Award, and the Best Speaker Award (2021).

Contents

Contributors

Krishna Prasad Acharaya
University of Cambridge, UK

Anisha Adya
Department of Nutrition and Dietetics, Sharda School of Allied Health Sciences, Sharda University, Greater Noida, Uttar Pradesh, India

Prashant Agrawal
Department of Forensic Science, School of Allied Health Sciences, Sharda University, Greater Noida, Uttar Pradesh, India

Akansha
Department of Nutrition and Dietetics, Sharda School of Allied Health Sciences, Sharda University, Greater Noida, Uttar Pradesh, India

Md. Sayeed Akhtar
Department of Clinical Pharmacy, King Khalid University, Gurager, Saudi Arabia

Das Anamika
Department of Forensic Science, School of Allied Health Sciences, Sharda University, Greater Noida, Uttar Pradesh, India

Shasta Arzoo
Department of Nutrition, King Khalid University, Saudi Arabia

Ishika Bhardwaj
Department of Forensic Science, Sharda School of Allied Health Sciences, Sharda University, Greater Noida, Uttar Pradesh, India

Sumeet Bharti
Kessler Rehabilitation Center, Weehawken, New Jersey, USA

Muskan Chadha
Department of Nutrition and Dietetics, Sharda School of Allied Health Sciences, Sharda University, Greater Noida, Uttar Pradesh, India

Lalit Chandravanshi
Department of Forensic Science, School of Allied Health Sciences, Sharda University, Greater Noida, Uttar Pradesh, India

Amit Pratap Singh Chouhan
Department of Radiology, School of Allied Health Sciences, Galgotias University, Greater Noida, Uttar Pradesh, India

Pragya Dutt
Select Rehabilitation Nursing Home, Southwood Heights Drive, Jamesville, New York, USA

Jane Ogochukwu Ezeagagwo
Department of Clinical Research, Sharda School of Allied Health Sciences, Sharda University, Greater Noida, Uttar Pradesh, India

Hiba Ahmad
Sharda School of Allied Health Sciences, Sharda University, Greater Noida, Uttar Pradesh, India

Ritika Indoria
Consultant Physiotherapist , Shakti Physiotherapy Centre NOIDA, Uttar Pradesh

Zoobiya Islam
Department of Food and Nutrition, Jamia Hamdard University, New Delhi, India

Sana Kanwal
Department of Radiology, Sharda School of Allied Health Sciences, Sharda University, Greater Noida, Uttar Pradesh, India

Gaurav Kaushik
School of Allied Health Sciences, Sharda University, Greater Noida, Uttar Pradesh, India

Pratishtha Kesarwani
Department of Nutrition and Dietetics, Sharda School of Allied Health Sciences, Sharda University, Greater Noida, Uttar Pradesh, India

Bushra Khan
Department of Radiology, Sharda School of Allied Health Sciences, Sharda University, Greater Noida, Uttar Pradesh, India

Archana Khanna
Department of Physiotherapy, Sharda School of Allied Health Sciences, Sharda University, Greater Noida, Uttar Pradesh, India

Vaishali Kumar
Department of Forensic Science, Sharda School of Allied Health Sciences, Sharda University, Greater Noida, Uttar Pradesh, India

Sally Lukose
Professor (Forensic Science), Sharda School of Allied Science and Director, Ranking, Sharda University, Greater Noida, India

Anjali Malik
Department of Forensic Science, Sharda School of Allied Health Sciences, Sharda University, Greater Noida, Uttar Pradesh, India

Hamid Raza Moqaddasi
Department of Pharmacology, Sharda School of Allied Health Sciences, Sharda University, Greater Noida, Uttar Pradesh, India

Rahamatun Nisha
Sharda School of Allied Health Sciences, Sharda University, Greater Noida, Uttar Pradesh, India

Preeti Pal
Department of Physiotherapy, Sharda School of Allied Health Sciences, Sharda University, Greater Noida, Uttar Pradesh, India

Vandana Prasad
Assistant Professor, School of Forensic Sciences, The West Bengal National University of Juridical Sciences, Kolkata, West Bengal, India

Sumedha Rabra
Department of Physiotherapy, Sharda School of Allied Health Sciences, Sharda University, Greater Noida, Uttar Pradesh, India

Rachna
Associate Professor, Department of Medical Laboratory Technology, Nims college of Allied and health care Sciences, NIIMS University, Jaipur, Rajasthan, India

Tannu Rana
Masters in Nutrition and Dietetics, Sharda School of Allied Health Sciences, Sharda University, Greater Noida, Uttar Pradesh, India

Mayuri Rastogi
Sharda School of Allied Health Sciences, Sharda University, Greater Noida, Uttar Pradesh, India

Anjali Rawat
Department of Optometry, Sharda School of Allied Health Sciences, Sharda University, Noida, Uttar Pradesh, India

Aditi Rikhari
Department of Nutrition and Dietetics, Sharda School of Allied Health Sciences, Sharda University, Greater Noida, Uttar Pradesh, India

Harsh Sable
Department of Forensic Science, Sharda School of Allied Health Sciences, Sharda University, Greater Noida, Uttar Pradesh, India

Kriti Sachan
Department of Physiotherapy, Sharda School of Allied Health Sciences, Sharda University, Greater Noida, Uttar Pradesh, India

Manish Kumar Sah
Department of Optometry, SSAHS, Sharda University, Greater Noida, Uttar Pradesh, India

Ruchika Sah
Department of Optometry, Ramlal Golchha Eye Hospital Foundation, Biratnagar, Nepal

Najmus Saquib
Department of Allied Health Sciences, Sharda University, Greater Noida, Uttar Pradesh, India

Rahul Saxena
Department of Biochemistry, Sharda School of Allied Health Sciences, Sharda University, Greater Noida, Uttar Pradesh, India

Suyash Saxena
Department of Biochemistry, Sharda School of Allied Health Sciences, Sharda University, Greater Noida, Uttar Pradesh, India

Bushra Shaida
Department of Food Technology, Jamia Hamdard, New Delhi

Komal Sharma
Department of Optometry, School of Allied Health Sciences, Noida International University, Gautam Buddha Nagar, Greater Noida, Uttar Pradesh, India

Mayank Shukla
Department of Physiotherapy, Sharda School of Allied Health Sciences, Sharda University, Greater Noida, Uttar Pradesh, India

Ajit Pal Singh
Assistant Professor, Medical Lab Technology, Sharda School of Allied Health Sciences, Sharda University, Greater Noida (UP)

Gaurav Singh
Sharda School of Allied Health Sciences, Sharda University, Greater Noida, Uttar Pradesh, India

Karuna Singh
Sharda School of Allied Health Sciences, Sharda University, Greater Noida, Uttar Pradesh, India

Vandana Singh
Department of Microbiology, Sharda School of Allied Health Sciences, Sharda University, Greater Noida, Uttar Pradesh, India

Rohit Kumar Tiwari
Department of Clinical Research, Sharda School of Allied Health Sciences, Sharda University, Greater Noida, Uttar Pradesh, India

Shalvika Tripathi
Department of Nutrition and Dietetics, Sharda School of Allied Health Sciences, Sharda University, Greater Noida, Uttar Pradesh, India

Richa Vashishtha
Department of Medicine, All India Institute of Medical Sciences, New Delhi, India

Ankush Verma
Department of Radiology, Sharda School of Allied Health Sciences, Sharda University, Greater Noida, Uttar Pradesh, India

Chaitenya Verma
Department of Pathology, The Ohio State University Wexner Medical Center, Columbus, OH, USA

Harshitha Verma
Department of Biochemistry, Manasagangothri, University of Mysuru, Mysuru, Karnataka, India

Meenakshi Verma
Department of Physiotherapy, Sharda School of Allied Health Sciences, Sharda University, Greater Noida, Uttar Pradesh, India

Wesleyan Wende
Department of Clinical Research, Sharda School of Allied Health Sciences, Sharda University, Greater Noida, Uttar Pradesh, India

Rajesh Yadav
Sharda School of Allied Health Sciences, Sharda University, Greater Noida, Uttar Pradesh, India

Abbreviations

μg	microgram
AAFS	American Academy of Forensic Sciences
AAPI	American Association of Physicians of Indian Origin
ACA	Affordable Care Act
ADH	antidiuretic hormone
ADL	activities of daily living
AE	adverse event
AERB	Atomic Energy Regulatory Board
AHP	allied health professional
AHS	allied health science
AI	artificial intelligence
AIIMS	all india institute of medical sciences
ALARA	as low as reasonably achievable
ALPS	aphasia language performance scales
AMP	adenosine monophosphate
AMR	antimicrobial resistance
ANM	auxiliary nurse and midwife
AQ	aphasia quotient
AQP	aquaporins
ARF	acute renal failure
ARMD	age related macular degeneration
ASCLD	American Society of Crime Laboratory Directors
ASCP	American Society for Clinical Pathology
ASPEN	American Society for Parenteral and Enteral Nutrition
ATP	adenosine triphosphate
BAT	brown adipose tissue
BBB	blood brain barrier
BDNF	brain-derived neurotrophic factor
BMI	body mass index
CAD	computer-assisted diagnosis
CAD	coronary artery disease
CADL	communicative abilities in daily L
CBR	community based rehabilitation
CCK	cholecystokinin
CDE	certified diabetes educator
CDSCO	Central Drugs Standard Control Organization

CHD	coronary heart disease
CI	confidence interval
CIMT	constraint-induced movement therapy
CNS	central nervous system
COPD	chronic obstructive pulmonary disease
CRF	chronic renal failure
CRSWD	circadian rhythm sleep–wake disorders
CS	coronary sinus
CSF	cerebrospinal fluid
CSN	cold-sensitive neurons
CSR	corporate social responsibility
CSSD	certified specialist in sports dietetics
CT	computed tomography
CTCAE	common terminology criteria for adverse events
CVD	cardiovascular diseases
CVIC	computer aided visual communication
DASH	disabilities of the arm, shoulder and hand
DCT	distal convoluted tubule
DEXA	dual-energy X-ray absorptiometry
DFIR	digital forensics and incident response
DHA	docosahexaenoic acid
DHHS	Department of Health and Human Services
DNA	deoxyribonucleic acid
DRI	dietary reference intake
DRL	diagnostic reference level
DTI	diffusion tensor imaging
EC	ethics committees
ECCE	extracapsular cataracts retraction
ECF	extracellular fluid
ECG	electrocardiogram
ECG	electrocardiography
ECL Cell	enterochromaffin-like cells
EEC	electroencephalographic
EF	ejection fraction
EHR	electronic health record
EIB	exercise-induced bronchoconstriction
EMR	electronic medical record
EPA	eicosapentaenoic acid
EPCS	evidence-based practice centers
EPS	electrophysiology study
ERC	Ethical Review Committees
ESCAP	Economic and Social Commission for Asia and the Pacific

FCP	functional communication profile
FEC	forced expiratory volume
FFP	filtering face piece
FGF21	fibroblast growth factor 21
FICCI	Federation of Indian Chambers of Commerce and Industry
fMRI	functional magnetic resonance imaging
FVC	forced vital capacity
GBS	guillain-barré syndrome
GDPR	general data protection regulation
GFR	glomerular filtration rate
G	gram
GI	glycemic index
GINA	Genetic Information Non-discrimination Act
GIT	gastrointestinal tract
GLUT	glucose transporter
GoI	Government of India
GP	general practitioner
HA	health assessment
HAI	hospital-acquired infections
HCAIs	healthcare-associated infections
HCL	hydrochloric acid
HCPC	Health and Care Professionals Council
HCW	health care worker
HH	hand hygiene
HIPAA	Health Insurance Portability and Accountability Act
HIS	bundle of his
HPSC	hematopoietic stem cell
HRA	high right atria
HSSC	Healthcare Sector Skill Council
HTML	hypertext markup language
IAP	Indian Academy of Pediatrics
IAPM	Indian Association of Pathologists and Microbiologists
ICCE	intracapsular lens extraction
ICM	infection control manual
ICMR	Indian Council of Medical Research
ICN	infection control nurse
ICO	infection control officer
ICRP	International Commission on Radiological Protection
ICT	infection control team
ICU	intensive care unit
IDFPM	integrated digital forensic process model

IFCC	International Federation of Clinical Chemistry and Laboratory Medicine
INC	inner hair cell
INN	international non-proprietary name
IOP	intraocular pressure
IPC	infection prevention and control
IPC	intra professional collaboration
IPE	interprofessional education
IPHS	Indian Public Health Standards
IPTF	Indian Preventive Task Force
IRB	institutional review boards
ISCR	Indian Society of Clinical Research
ISFG	International Society for Forensic Genetics
IU	international unit
Kcal	kilocalories
Kg	kilogram
LASER	light amplification by stimulated emission of radiation
LASIK	laser *in situ* keratomileusis
LBP	lipopolysaccharide binding protein
LDL	low density lipoprotein
LMICs	low- and middle-income countries
LV	lens vault
MCI	Medical Council of India
MCT	medium chain triglyceride
MDRO	multidrug-resistant organism
Mg	milligram
MHz	megahertz
MLE	mandatory log events
ml	milliliters
MLPs	mid-level practitioners
MLS	medical laboratory scientist
MLT	medical laboratory technology
mmHg	millimeters of mercury
MoHFW	Ministry of Health and Family Welfare
MRI	magnetic resonance imaging
MRR	medical record review
MRSA	methicillin-resistant *staphylococcus aureus*
MSv	millisieverts
MUC	mucin
MUFA	monounsaturated fatty acid
NABL	national accreditation board for testing and calibration laboratories

NAGs	natural apophyseal glides
NCD	non-communicable disease
NCI	National Cancer Institute
NEBs	neuroepithelial bodies
NIMHANS	National Institute of Mental Health and Neurosciences
NMC	National Medical Commission
NREM	non-rapid eye movement sleep
OHC	outer hair cell
OR	odds ratio
OT PT	occupational therapy and physiotherapy
OT	operation theatre
OTC	over-the-counter
PACS	picture archiving and communication systems
PCOS	polycystic ovarian syndrome
PCT	proximal convoluted tubule
PET	positron emission tomography
PHC	primary health care
PHSC	pluripotent hematopoietic stem cells
PICC	peripherally inserted central catheter
PICO	problem, intervention or exposure, comparison, and outcome
PNF	proprioceptive neuromuscular facilitation
POCT	point-of-care testing
PPC	postoperative pulmonary complication
PPE	personal protective equipment
PQ	performance quotient
PREFLEX	presbyopic lens exchange
PRK	photorefractive keratectomy
PRO-CTCAE	patient reported outcomes version of the common terminology criteria for adverse events
PT	physiotherapy
PUFA	polyunsaturated fatty acid
RA	rheumatoid arthritis
RBAC	role-based access control
RBC	red blood cell
RCT	randomized controlled clinical trials
RDA	recommended dietary allowances
RDBMS	Relational Database Management Systems
RDN	registered dietitian nutritionist
REM	rapid eye movement
RLE	refractive lens exchange
RNA	ribonucleic acid
RR	relative risk

RV	right ventricle
SAE	serious adverse event
SARS-CoV-2	severe acute respiratory syndrome coronavirus 2
SCN	suprachiasmatic nucleus
SLP	speech-language pathologist
SNAGs	sustained natural apophyseal glides
SOP	standard operating procedure
SPECT	single-photon emission computed tomography
TA cell	transit-amplifying cell
TB	tuberculosis
TCM	traditional chinese medicine
TENS	transcutaneous electrical nerve stimulation
TFR	total fertility rates
TMT	treadmill test
TRPV1	transient receptor potential vanilloid type 1
TRPV4	transient receptor potential vanilloid type 4
Ucp1	uncoupling protein
UGC	University Grants Commission
URL	uniform resource locator
USG	ultrasound
UV	ultra violet
VAD	vitamin A deficiency
VIC	visual communication therapy
VR	virtual reality
VRE	vancomycin-resistant *enterococcus*
WAB	western aphasia battery
WAT	white adipose tissue
WBC	white blood cell
WHO	World Health Organization
WSN	warm-sensitive neurons

Acknowledgment

Allied Healthcare in Practice: An Introduction to Integrated Patient Care offers a comprehensive exploration of the diverse skills and knowledge essential for allied health professionals. This book delves into the integrated approaches necessary for delivering holistic patient care.

We express our profound gratitude to the Honorable Chancellor of Sharda University and Chairman of SGI, Mr. P. K. Gupta, for his blessings and unwavering encouragement.

Our heartfelt appreciation extends to Mr. Y. K. Gupta, Hon'ble Pro-Chancellor of Sharda University and Vice Chairman of SGI, whose steadfast support was instrumental in overcoming challenges throughout this endeavor.

We also extend our sincere thanks to Prof. (Dr.) Sibaram Khara, Vice Chancellor of Sharda University, for his continuous motivation and support at every stage of this project.

Special recognition is due to the faculty members of the Sharda School of Allied Health Sciences, who generously contributed chapters and shared their valuable expertise in the field of allied health sciences. Their dedication and efforts were indispensable in bringing this volume to fruition.

We would also like to express our sincere appreciation to Apple Academic Press for their unwavering support and cooperation during the publication process.

Finally, we extend our deepest gratitude to our family members, whose unwavering support and encouragement have been invaluable throughout this journey.

Preface

In a world intricately connected through the exchange of ideas, technologies, and innovations, the pursuit of healthcare excellence knows no bounds. While medical sciences have always been at the forefront, allied healthcare—through its diversity and multidisciplinary approach—has carved out a niche, enhancing and adding value to the well-being of individuals and communities. This book, *Allied Healthcare in Practice: An Introduction to Integrated Patient Care,* explores the evolving landscape of the healthcare industry, bringing together insights and experiences from experts across diverse allied health fields.

This book is not merely a compilation of practices; rather, it is a testament to the collective commitment that transcends boundaries in pursuit of integrated patient care. It highlights the importance of collaboration among professionals from different specializations, all working toward a shared goal: the well-being of humanity.

A comparative analysis of global benchmarks reveals that Allied Health Professionals (AHPs) in countries such as the United Kingdom, Thailand, and Singapore have been a focal point of governmental attention for several years. This recognition has led to their inclusion under formal government supervision and licensing. Similarly, India has made notable strides in formalizing its allied healthcare workforce. The Government of India introduced the National Commission for Allied and Healthcare Professionals Bill, 2020, in the Rajya Sabha after its passage in the Lok Sabha on March 24, 2021. This bill aims to regulate allied healthcare professions, acknowledging their critical role within the medical field.

The allied healthcare workforce comprises various technicians working in both clinical and non-clinical capacities, supporting doctors and nursing professionals. In Western countries, AHPs play a crucial role throughout the healthcare service delivery value chain. For instance, in the United States, AHPs constitute 60% of the total healthcare workforce. A report commissioned by the Ministry of Health and Family Welfare (MOHFW) highlights a substantial demand for allied healthcare workers, which exceeds the available supply. Assuming a consistent demand for allied healthcare workers per 1,000 people, India is projected to require between 6,000,000 and 7,000,000 AHPs by the year 2024.

This book comprehensively explores the dynamic and evolving field of allied healthcare, offering readers a foundational understanding of the principles, practices, and challenges associated with integrated patient care. The chapters have been structured to be informative, insightful, and, above all, actionable. Whether you are a healthcare practitioner seeking to expand your expertise or a student taking your first steps into the world of allied healthcare, this book serves as a comprehensive guide toward a holistic understanding of integrated patient care. Through a multidisciplinary approach, it addresses the interplay of various allied health disciplines while also covering essential topics such as communication, ethics, and legal considerations in achieving optimal patient outcomes.

This book provides a detailed overview of allied healthcare professionals and their roles and is divided into four major parts with **36 chapters,** covering topics such as roles, challenges, career prospects, advancements, various specializations, essential skills, and patient care management. All chapters have been written by faculty members and scientists with diverse backgrounds in industry, research and development (**R&D**), and academia.

- **Part I: Introduction to Allied Health Sciences and Career Opportunities** – This section, consisting of four chapters, provides an overview of allied health sciences, career opportunities, and the education and certifications required for professional growth in the field.

- **Part II: Basic Knowledge and Skills for Allied Health Professionals** – Comprising eight chapters, this section covers essential topics such as anatomy, physiology, interrelationships between body systems and organs, health assessment, diagnosis, pharmacology, infection prevention, and control—fundamental knowledge for allied health professionals.

- **Part III: Allied Health Programs: Knowledge and Skills in Medical Imaging and Radiology** – This section, with 14 chapters, explores various allied health specializations such as rehabilitation and therapy, nutrition and dietetics, medical imaging and radiology, and community ophthalmology. It provides insights into the specific skills required in each specialization.

- **Part IV: Safety, Quality, and Patient Care: Patient Safety and Quality Improvement** – The final section consists of 10 chapters focusing on patient safety, quality parameters in patient care, forensic aspects, interprofessional collaboration, and ethical and legal issues.

We hope this book serves as a catalyst for a deeper appreciation of the interconnected nature of allied healthcare disciplines and inspires readers to contribute to the ongoing evolution of patient-centered, integrated healthcare practices.

—Sally Lukose, PhD
Karuna Singh, PhD
Greater Noida, Uttar Pradesh, India

PART I

Introduction to Allied Health Sciences and Career Opportunities

CHAPTER 1

Overview of Allied Health Sciences: Role, Scope, and Challenges

SALLY LUKOSE[1*] and KARUNA SINGH[2]

Sharda School of Allied Science and Director, Ranking, Sharda University, Greater Noida, India

Sharda School of Allied Health Sciences, Sharda University, Greater Noida, Uttar Pradesh, India

*Corresponding author

ABSTRACT

According to the World Health Organization (WHO), health is termed as a holistic state of well-being, where health workers are classified as professionals involved in supporting and enhancing patient care. Allied Health Sciences (AHS) is a broad field that helps in fostering and supporting overall patient care and the healthcare system. They are essential to the worldwide healthcare system because they offer a variety of therapeutic, behavioral, supportive, and diagnostic services. In India, there is a gradual expansion of allied health professionals (AHPs) tracing their roots from traditional medicine to its present-day evolution. It has been observed that there is a dire need for a centralized regulatory authority to harmonize AHS in India and bridge the gap between disparate professional organizations. It urges legislative efforts to promote knowledge about the vital efforts made by AHPs and stresses the value of making educational and training investments to guarantee high-quality healthcare. In conclusion, AHS professionals are portrayed as key stakeholders who improve outcomes, efficacy, and the overall healthcare system. Moreover, this chapter provides an extensive overview of AHS, including its historical development, Indian and global significance, and the need for further development and support.

Allied Healthcare in Practice: An Introduction to Integrated Patient Care. Sally Lukose, Karuna Singh (Eds.)

DOI: 10.1201/9781998511037-2

1.1 INTRODUCTION

World Health Organization (WHO) termed "Health" as an overall condition of complete well-being, which includes mental, physical, and social welfare, rather than only the non-existence of disease. As per the terminology, "health workers" refer to anyone who is involved in the preservation, promotion, or enhancement of the general public's health (Dal Poz et al., 2007). Allied Health Sciences (AHS) is a broad field that encompasses a variety of vital healthcare professions that are crucial to supporting and improving the overall standard of patient care. These professionals, often distinct from physicians and nurses, contribute expertise in areas such as diagnostic technology, therapeutic interventions, rehabilitation, and patient education. These experts provide knowledge in fields including diagnostic technologies, therapeutic approaches, rehabilitation, and patient education, and are frequently separate from doctors and nurses (Sheehan et al., 2021). A range of healthcare professions that were different from medicine, dentistry, and nursing were originally referred to as "allied health" in the 1940s. These professions were regarded as "allied" because they collaborated with doctors and nurses to assist and take care of patients (Institute of Medicine Committee to Study the Role of Allied Health, 1989). Allied Health Professionals (AHP) are described by the U.S. Department of Health and Human Services (DHHS) as qualified professionals in a variety of therapeutic, diagnostic, and preventive measures. These experts are top in their level and combination of clinical and technological skills (Foster, 2021). AHPs work encompasses a broad range of specialties, including speech pathology, occupational therapy, physical therapy, radiography, dietetics, and clinical laboratory science. The idea of AHSs emphasizes the multidisciplinary aspect of healthcare and places a focus on cooperation, specialized knowledge, and a dedication to enhancing both individual and societal health outcomes. According to estimates, up to 60% of the workforce in the healthcare industry is made up of people who work in allied health professions (Konlan et al., 2022).

India has a large and diverse pool of health human resources. They range from a variety of community- and household-based remedies to highly trained biomedical professionals. The negative reputation of AHSs is a result of the broad disparity in perceptions about the idea of an AHP, most commonly referred to as a "paramedic." Despite the enormous need for services from this industry, the AHSs domain is very fragmented.

AHPs and courses are currently separated into smaller groupings and appear to be "regulated" by independent professional organizations at the national and state levels as a result of the lack of a centralized regulatory body for AHPs and courses (Gaur, 2018).

Medical professionals are seen as the main stakeholders in regard to issues of recommendation, enrollment, and discharge in traditional models of health service. These models are often governed by the requirements and skills of different disciplines. Especially for patients who could benefit from initial allied health input, the lack of expert resources frequently results in a lengthy wait for services. As a result, it has been determined that AHPs have the essential clinical competencies and capacity to close the service need imbalance and serve as the patient's initial point of contact during their journey through the healthcare system (Saxon et al., 2014). Variability in terms of use was discovered in a systematic review published in 2006, which concentrated on offering an operational description of broadened scope of practice with regard to improvement and replacement. Additionally, this review showed there was evidence supporting the introduction of these roles; however, the vast majority of papers at the time concentrated on lowering waiting times and reducing the strain on healthcare professionals, with only a small number of papers covering the effect on outcomes for patients, affordability, prerequisites for training, specialist identification, or sustainable development (McPherson et al., 2006).

These professional associations must be united by a single authority in order for the allied health care to develop within the healthcare system. This will enable AHPs to flourish as a family rather than as distinct categories within the community of the healthcare system. Therefore, it is essential to set up a task force that would be instrumental in raising awareness and enhancing public opinion of AHS. This task force should promote the significant role that AHPs play as well as the benefits of all the non-intrusive and preliminary work that they perform. In the context of AHSs education, it is imperative that all education governing bodies, like the University Grants Commission (UGC) in India, adhere to global standards to ensure comprehensive alignment with international benchmarks and elevate the quality of education in the field (Gaur, 2018).

This chapter emphasizes reviewing the major landscape of the different roles, trends, scope, and challenges in allied health services, which are essential to address as they directly impact patient care and the healthcare system.

1.2 SCOPE OF ALLIED HEALTH SCIENCES (AHS) IN INDIA

The major skill shortage in India's AHP is highlighted in recent research by NATHEALTH in partnership with the Boston Consulting Group. This study underlines the urgent need to close this gap and provide new possibilities in the industry. In comparison to other countries, India's AHP capacity is still much below average, leaving a significant 30–40% unmet demand. The research emphasizes that 36 radiology imaging procedures per 1000 individuals would be performed in India by 2022, which is the current penetration rate. By 2027, this figure is expected to increase to 69 per 1000 people.

According to the research, there is a severe scarcity in this area, and it is predicted that it will become worse because demand has already quadrupled in the last 10 years and is only likely to increase. The AHP in India is faced with significant obstacles that need immediate attention, including a lack of personnel and a quickly expanding demand. While earnings for these experts are noticeably low, the supply of competent workers is continuing to expand slowly. Only 6% of the target population is aware of potential careers in Allied Healthcare, which is a worrying result. The survey also emphasizes facilities for AHP. The quality of these training programs, however, frequently falls short of expectations. When it comes to the abilities that qualified students should possess, 77% of institutions alarmingly fall short of the quality threshold (Standard, 2023).

Today, the AHP field includes more than 200 diverse professions, each ranging from skills and expertise in patient care. AHPs can be classified into four main categories: diagnostic and therapeutic services, support services, behavioral health services, and healthcare management. The diagnostic and therapeutic services include professions like occupational, physical, speech, and radiology therapy. They work directly to analyze and provide diagnostic features to patients, which is helpful in improving a wide range of medical conditions and diseases. In parallel, support services comprise medical laboratory technicians, medical assistants, and respiratory therapists. These dedicated professionals work behind the scenes, fostering the efforts of physicians and nurses by undertaking essential tasks such as the collection and analysis of lab samples and the administration of respiratory treatments. Behavioral health services involve professions like social workers, mental health counselors, and marriage and family therapists. These professions collaborate closely with patients, addressing emotional and mental health and supporting patient families. Beyond the clinical facets, healthcare management plays a pivotal role in ensuring the efficient functioning of healthcare systems. It includes professions like health information management, healthcare administration, and healthcare policy, which operate in administrative and managerial capacities. They oversee the operations of the overall healthcare system and are committed to providing high-quality care to patients (Gaur, 2018; Rawekar et al., 2020).

Since 1949, the private healthcare industry has risen rapidly, accounting for 85% of doctors and 93% of hospitals. Therefore, it is vital to regulate these professions by establishing councils like those for nursing, pharmacy, and other professions. The Indian Government suggested creating separate councils in 2007 for AHP for the first time. These councils are in charge of maintaining uniform educational standards in the relevant fields and registering competent individuals to practice the skills (PHFI, 2012).

1.3 HISTORICAL BACKGROUND OF ALLIED HEALTH SCIENCES (AHS)

The first professional training school for nurses was founded in London by Florence Nightingale in 1860, which marks the beginning of the history of AHSs. The rise of nursing as a profession opened the door for the formation of other healthcare specialties, and thus marked the beginning of the contemporary healthcare system. In the United States, the idea of allied health professions first evolved in the early 20th century when doctors realized how crucial it was to collaborate with other healthcare providers in order to offer full patient care (Chadwick et al., 2020; Donini-Lenhoff, 2008).

The Ayurvedic, Yoga, and Naturopathic systems of traditional Indian medicine are the origins of the AHSs discipline in India. Up until the 1950s, the only allied health occupations in India were nursing and midwifery. In India, AHSs have also developed throughout time in various fields including speech and language therapy, audiology, ophthalmology, clinical nutrition, and medical social work (PHFI, 2012).

1.3.1 EVOLUTION OF ALLIED HEALTH SCIENCES (AHS) IN INDIA

The 1950s saw the emergence of various new healthcare fields as distinct professions, which marked the beginning of the development of AHS in India. A number of allied health fields were covered in 1952 by the establishment of the All India Institute of Medical Sciences (AIIMS) (Ruddock, 2021).

Speech therapy and audiology courses were made available by the National Institute of Mental Health and Neurosciences (NIMHANS), which was founded in 1959 (Reddy and Gopalakrishna, 1986).

The growth of AHSs education in India has been significantly aided by the Indian government. The Indian Nursing Council was created in 1949 to regulate the nursing industry. The council oversees nursing practice, education, and training across the nation. The Indian Medical Council was created in 1952 to regulate medical training and practice in the nation. To regulate the teaching and use of AHS in India, numerous regulatory organizations have been established over the years.

There are currently more than a thousand institutions in India that provide AHSs degrees at different levels. To advance AHS education in the nation, the government has launched a number of projects. The National Health Stack, an initiative of the Ministry of Health and Family Welfare to develop a national digital health ecosystem, was introduced in 2018 (NITI Aayog, 2018). To support AHS research and teaching, the government has also established a number of institutions of national significance, including the National Institute of Speech and Hearing (NISH) (NISH, 2023) and the National Institute of Allied Health Sciences (NIAHS) (PHFI, 2012).

The Minister of Health and Family Welfare introduced the National Commission for Allied and Healthcare Professions Bill, 2020 into the Rajya Sabha. The Bill aims to control and harmonize the training and employment of AHP. The key features of the Bill are (Research, 2021):

1. An associate, technician, or technologist who has received training to support the diagnosis and treatment of any ailment, disease, injury, or impairment is referred to as an "allied health professional" in the Bill. According to this Bill, such a professional ought to have earned a diploma or degree. The degree or diploma should take between two and four years and at least 2000 hours to complete.
2. A scientist, therapist, or any other professional who studies, counsels, conducts research, oversees, or offers preventive, curative, rehabilitative, therapeutic, or promotional health services is referred to as a "healthcare professional." According to this Bill, such a professional ought to have earned a degree. The degree should take three to six years to complete, or at least 3600 hours.
3. The Bill designates a number of AHP as recognized categories. Professionals in the fields of life sciences, burn and trauma care,

surgical, and anesthesia-related technologies, physiotherapy (PT), and nutrition science are among those specified in the Schedule to the Bill. After consulting with the National Commission for AHP, the national government may change this Schedule (Research, 2021).

The Indian government's policy think tank, NITI Aayog, has acknowledged the crucial function of AHP in the country's healthcare system. Its report placed a strong emphasis on the requirement for the nation's allied health workforce to be expanded and strengthened. The lack of AHPs in India and the difficulties in finding and keeping them are also highlighted in the report. It states that there is a need to develop a supporting ecosystem that can entice and keep AHPs by providing competitive pay packages, opportunities for professional advancement, and a welcoming work atmosphere. The need to enhance the quality and applicability of allied health education and training in India is also emphasized in the report. It demands the creation of accreditation systems for educational and training institutions, the development of competency-based curricula that are standardized, and the support of opportunities for AHPs for their education and careers is needed. NITI Aayog is aware that attaining the objective of universal health coverage in India will depend on the growth of the allied health workforce. It mentions that the provision of primary care services, enhancing accessibility to healthcare in underserved areas, and tackling the burden of non-communicable diseases in the nation may all be accomplished with the help of AHP (Aayog, 2018).

There is limited data available about the lack of AHPs in India, although various studies indicate that there is a serious shortage of AHPs there. In order to address the healthcare needs of the country's population, India will require over 6.4 million AHPs by 2022–23, according to research released by the Healthcare Sector Skill Council (HSSC) in 2018 (Council, 2023). With just 1.5 million AHPs currently employed in the healthcare industry, the research also emphasizes the lack of skilled AHPs in the nation. AHPs are in great demand in India, particularly in rural regions, according to a new report from the Federation of Indian Chambers of Commerce and Industry (FICCI) in 2020. It also suggests that the nation requires over 3.5 million AHPs to provide basic healthcare to the people, but the number of AHPs already employed can only meet 20% of the demand (PHFI, 2012). The National Health Policy of 2017 also notes the dearth of AHPs in India, stating that more AHPs are needed there in order to raise the quality of healthcare provided. The strategy places a strong emphasis on the need to create and implement policies and programs that will help the healthcare industry attract and retain skilled AHPs (Welfare, 2017).

1.3.2 EVOLUTION OF ALLIED HEALTH SCIENCES FIELD GLOBALLY

The number of occupations in the AHS sector, as well as the range of their specializations, have increased dramatically over time. When careers like physical therapy, occupational therapy, and speech-language pathology first emerged in the United States around the turn of the 20th century, this discipline also originated. In AHS, several other careers, such as radiography, respiratory therapy, audiology, and medical laboratory science, have developed over time. The field of AHS has experienced tremendous expansion in recent years, with the emergence of new careers in genetic counseling, health informatics, and clinical research, among others. New AHPs, including telehealth, digital health, and telemedicine, have emerged as a result of the expanding use of technology in healthcare (Chadwick et al., 2020).

Due to a number of variables, including population expansion, aging populations, and the rising prevalence of chronic diseases, there is an increase in the demand for healthcare services on a global scale. By offering top-notch, patient-centered care, AHPs play a crucial part in overcoming these difficulties (Seaton et al., 2021). The WHO has recommended the creation of national policies and initiatives to strengthen the AHP, acknowledging their significance in achieving universal health coverage. In many countries, including the United States, Canada, Australia, and the United Kingdom, AHPs are regulated and licensed by professional bodies. These bodies set standards for education, training, and practice, and ensure that they meet these standards before they can practice (WHO, 2010).

The need for healthcare services is growing globally, and AHPs are essential in meeting these demands as a result of the field's rapid expansion and the emergence of new professions in response to the evolving healthcare environment. For patients to receive high-quality, patient-centered care, national policies and efforts to enhance the allied health workforce are essential. The need for AHPs is developing quickly as a result of a number of causes, such as an aging population, rising chronic disease rates, and a growing focus on preventative treatment. The Bureau of Labor Statistics projects that employment in the AHS sector will increase by 18% between 2016 and 2026, which is substantially faster than the average for all occupations (Statistics, 2022).

The growing understanding of the significance of the role AHPs play in healthcare is one factor contributing to this growth. The demand for specialized skills and expertise has grown as healthcare gets more complex. A more thorough and efficient approach to patient care is made possible by the special set of abilities and knowledge that AHPs offer to the healthcare team.

The growing focus on preventative care is another element promoting the development of the AHS industry. Prevention is essential for lowering the burden of disease and containing healthcare expenditures, and this understanding is rising as healthcare expenses continue to climb. In promoting and providing preventative care services, including health education, wellness initiatives, and disease screenings, allied health workers are essential (Turnbull et al., 2009).

AHPs are in high demand, and there are numerous prospects for career progression within the industry. Numerous allied health professions provide opportunities for advanced degrees and specialized training, enabling workers to gain knowledge in a particular field of healthcare and assume leadership positions within their organizations. The AHS industry is currently evolving into a vibrant and dynamic field that offers numerous chances for both personal and professional advancement due to strong job growth estimates and an increasing emphasis on preventative care (Elwood, 2021).

1.4 CHALLENGES FACED BY ALLIED HEALTH PROFESSIONALS (AHP)

There are several universal problems that arise in many regions of the world when it comes to attracting and keeping AHPs. Among the principal challenges are:

1. **Education and Training:** One of the major obstacles to hiring AHPs is the dearth of suitable education and training programs in many nations; it can also result in a lack of qualified workers.

2. **Financial Constraints:** Many AHPs are employed in sectors like the public health system that receive little financing. They might consequently have insufficient supplies and tools, which could hinder their capacity to deliver high-quality care. Additionally, this may result in inadequate compensation for their services, which may make it challenging to recruit and retain qualified specialists.

3. **Poor Working Conditions:** Poor working conditions are common among AHPs, which can make the workplace unpleasant and have an impact on job satisfaction.

4. **Limited Opportunities for Job Progression:** AHPs also confront a lack of opportunities for job progression. However, they might not have the same prospects for career advancement as doctors or nurses, despite the fact that many of these professions are highly trained and experienced. Burnout and frustration can result from this, and it might be challenging to attract and keep skilled professionals in the field.

5. **Job Insecurity:** Since many AHPs are employed on a contract or temporary basis, it can be challenging to retain qualified personnel.

6. **Lack of Recognition:** One of the main problems AHPs confront is that their contributions and roles in the healthcare system are not widely understood or appreciated. Despite playing a crucial part in providing specialized treatment and improving patient outcomes, they frequently go unappreciated and unrecognized. It may be difficult for them to deliver high-quality care if their profession is not supported and given the resources it needs as a result of this lack of recognition (PHFI, 2012).

In order to overcome this challenge, advocacy work is required to highlight the value of AHPs to the healthcare sector. To raise awareness of the important role performed by AHPs and to advance the policies and programs that support their work, allied health organizations, professional groups, and individual professionals can collaborate. Additionally, initiatives can be launched to inform the public, employers, and patients. There is also a dire need to emphasize better education and training for these professionals to provide high-quality healthcare (Rawekar et al., 2020).

1.5 CONCLUSION

Professionals in the AHS field offer specialized treatment, enhance patient satisfaction, deliver efficient care, address shortcomings in healthcare, and engage in technological advancement and research. These specialists collaborate with other healthcare professionals to deliver complete care that is tailored to each patient's specific needs, and they play a crucial role in the healthcare system. The efficacy of treatment and outcomes for patients can be enhanced by AHPs by utilizing their expertise and working together with other healthcare experts. Investment in education and training programs, competitive pay, improved working conditions, clear career progression prospects, and job security are necessary to overcome the challenges associated with AHPs globally. To foster a more supportive work environment for these professionals, it is also necessary to increase recognition and respect for AHPs. To guarantee a steady supply of skilled professionals in the future, the gender and age disparities in the AHP workforce must also be addressed.

KEYWORDS

- **allied health professional**
- **evolution**
- **genetic counseling**
- **healthcare shortcomings**
- **respiratory therapy**
- **skills and expertise**
- **speech-language pathology**
- **telemedicine**

REFERENCES

Aayog, N. (2018). *Health Systems for a New India: Building Blocks–Potential Pathways to Reforms.* NITI Aayog, Government of India.

Business Standard. (2023). 30–40% unmet demand for allied health professionals: NATHEALTH-BCG study. *Business Standard.* https://www.business-standard.com/india-news/30-40-unfulfilled-demand-for-allied-health-professionals-report-123063000448_1.html (accessed on 14 March 2025).

Chadwick, M., Larmer, P., & Smythe, L. (2020). The history of allied health: An international perspective. *Journal of Allied Health, 49*(4), 285–289.

Council, H. S. S. (2023). *Healthcare Sector Skill Council: Skilling Today, for Healthier Tomorrow*. https://www.healthcare-ssc.in/ (accessed on 14 March 2025).

Dal Poz, M. R., Kinfu, Y., Dräger, S., & Kunjumen, T. (2007). *Counting Health Workers: Definitions, Data, Methods and Global Results.* World Health Organization.

Donini-Lenhoff, F. G. (2008). Coming together, moving apart: A history of the term allied health in education, accreditation, and practice. *Journal of Allied Health, 37*(1), 45–52.

Elwood, T. W. (2021). Allied health workforce: A web of complexities. *Journal of Allied Health, 50*(2), 95–95.

Foster, C. (2021). *Employee Experiences Towards Workplace Health and Wellness Programs: A Phenomenological Study* (Doctoral dissertation). University of Arizona Global Campus.

Gaur, V. (2018). An overview of redefining paradigm: India's allied health professional. *International Journal of Biochemistry & Biomedical Research, 1*(1), 20–34.

Institute of Medicine Committee to Study the Role of Allied Health. (1989). *Allied Health Services: Avoiding Crises.* National Academies Press (US).

Konlan, K. D., Asampong, E., Dako-Gyeke, P., & Glozah, F. N. (2022). Burnout syndrome among healthcare workers during COVID-19 pandemic in Accra, Ghana. *PLoS One, 17*(6), e0268404.

McPherson, K., Kersten, P., George, S., Lattimer, V., Breton, A., Ellis, B., Kaur, D., & Frampton, G. (2006). A systematic review of evidence about extended roles for allied health professionals. *Journal of Health Services Research & Policy, 11*(4), 240–247.

Ministry of Health and Family Welfare, Government of India. (2017). *National Health Policy.*

National Academy of Sciences. (1989). *Enhancing the Postdoctoral Experience for Scientists and Engineers: A Guide for Postdoctoral Scholars, Advisers, Institutions, Funding Organizations, and Disciplinary Societies.* National Academy of Sciences.

NISH. (2023). *Welcome to NISH.* https://www.nish.ac.in/welcome-to-nish

NITI Aayog. (2018). *National Health Stack: Strategy and Approach.* National Institute for Transforming India, Government of India.

PRS Legislative Research. (2023). *The National Commission for Allied and Healthcare Professions Bill, 2020.* https://prsindia.org/billtrack/the-national-commission-for-allied-and-healthcare-professions-bill-2020 (accessed on 14 March 2025).

Public Health Foundation of India. (2012). *From Paramedics to Allied Health Professionals: Landscaping the Journey and Way Forward.*

Rawekar, A., Gotarkar, S., Patond, S., & Dakhode, S. (2020). Challenges of allied healthcare professionals in India—Establishing the council is need of the hour. *Indian Journal of Forensic Medicine & Toxicology, 14*(4).

Reddy, G., & Gopalakrishna, N. (1986). *A Decade of NIMHANS (1975–1985).*

Ruddock, A. (2021). *Special Treatment: Student Doctors at the All India Institute of Medical Sciences.* Stanford University Press.

Saxon, R. L., Gray, M. A., & Oprescu, F. I. (2014). Extended roles for allied health professionals: An updated systematic review of the evidence. *Journal of Multidisciplinary Healthcare, 7,* 479–488.

Seaton, J., Jones, A., Johnston, C., & Francis, K. (2021). Allied health professionals' perceptions of interprofessional collaboration in primary health care: An integrative review. *Journal of Interprofessional Care, 35*(2), 217–228.

Sheehan, J., Laver, K., Bhopti, A., Rahja, M., Usherwood, T., Clemson, L., & Lannin, N. A. (2021). Methods and effectiveness of communication between hospital allied health and primary care practitioners: A systematic narrative review. *Journal of Multidisciplinary Healthcare, 14,* 493–511.

Turnbull, C., Grimmer-Somers, K., Kumar, S., May, E., Law, D., & Ashworth, E. (2009). Allied, scientific and complementary health professionals: A new model for Australian allied health. *Australian Health Review, 33*(1), 27–37.

U.S. Bureau of Labor Statistics. (2024). *Occupational Outlook Handbook.* https://www.bls.gov/ooh/healthcare/home.htm (accessed on 14 March 2025).

World Health Organization. (2010). *Framework for Action on Interprofessional Education and Collaborative Practice.*

CHAPTER 2

Importance and Relevance of Allied Health Sciences in Healthcare

KARUNA SINGH,[1,*] SALLY LUKOSE[2], and GAURAV SINGH[1]

[1]*Sharda School of Allied Health Sciences, Sharda University, Greater Noida, Uttar Pradesh, India*

[2]*Professor (Forensic Science), Sharda School of Allied Science and Director, Ranking, Sharda University, Greater Noida, India*

*Corresponding author

ABSTRACT

Allied health sciences (AHS) play a pivotal role in modern healthcare systems, contributing to the holistic care and well-being of patients. This review chapter explores the importance and relevance of allied health sciences in healthcare, emphasizing their critical functions, impact on patient outcomes, and their growing significance in an evolving healthcare landscape. Allied health professionals (AHPs) work collaboratively with physicians, nurses, and other healthcare providers to address various aspects of patient care. They offer specialized expertise that complements medical and nursing interventions, ensuring holistic care.

2.1 INTRODUCTION

Healthcare delivery in India has historically tended to be "doctor-focused," with less emphasis placed on specialization in allied health sciences (AHS). Never before in history has investing in allied health professionals (AHPs) been more important for reforms in the public health system. The objective of healthcare reforms in India still includes bridging demand and supply

Allied Healthcare in Practice: An Introduction to Integrated Patient Care. Sally Lukose, Karuna Singh (Eds.)

DOI: 10.1201/9781998511037-3

gaps to guarantee continuous availability of allied health professionals for future generations. Lack of human resources—both in terms of numbers and skills—will be a significant obstacle to India's healthcare sector reforms as the country struggles with a high disease burden, the emergence of noncommunicable diseases, and the urgency of achieving the Millennium Development Goals. It is crucial that we take steps to address both the size and caliber of our health workforce in order to overcome these (Modi, 2014).

In the intricate ecosystem that is the healthcare sector, a range of experts collaborate to assure the delivery of high-quality patient care. A huge workforce of AHPs supports and enhances healthcare services, despite the fact that doctors and nurses receive most of the attention. AHPs are employed in all facets of social and public healthcare. They frequently offer the cross-border fusion required to supply streamlined care to patients and their caregivers, erecting a social solidarity paradigm. AHPs provide quick responses to patient demands in therapeutic domains where obtaining the services of a general practitioner (GP) or consultant always takes longer, thanks to some locations where they provide open access to their services (Bhola and Kumari, 2008).

AHPs are the experts having experience in therapeutic, diagnostic, curative, preventative, and rehabilitative interventions. The main aim of these health professionals is to promote, safeguard, treat, and/or manage a person's physical, mental, social, emotional, and environmental health, as well as their overall well-being, as they collaborate with medical professionals, nurses, and public health authorities in interdisciplinary health teams (Gaur, 2018).

The healthcare workers are classified based on the "International Standard Classification of Occupations (ISCO, 2008 revision)" according to WHO. Following are the five broad categories of healthcare professionals based on their occupation:

1. **Health Professionals:** It comprises all medical, nursing, or physiotherapy (PT) practitioners, which include paramedical practitioners, dieticians and nutritionists, audiologists and speech therapists, optometrists, and ophthalmic opticians.

2. **Health Associate Professionals:** Comprised of medical imaging and therapeutic equipment technicians, medical and pathology laboratory technicians, pharmaceutical technicians and assistants, medical, and dental prosthetic technicians, dental assistants and therapists, medical records and health information technicians,

community health workers, dispensing opticians, medical assistants, environmental, and occupational health inspectors and associates, and ambulance workers.

3. **Personal Care Workers in Health Services:** Comprise health care assistants, home-based personal care workers, and personal care workers in health services not elsewhere classified.
4. **Health Management and Support Personnel:** Consists of medical secretaries, health service managers, health management staff not otherwise classified, life science professionals, social work and counselling professionals, life science technicians, and a group of non-health professionals not otherwise categorized.
5. **Other health service providers not elsewhere classified:** Includes armed forces occupations.

2.2 RECOMMENDED TERMINOLOGIES

It is important to reorganize the different categories of AHPs based on educational levels and specialist degrees to emphasize the value of AHPs as key team members and align with international terminology in the healthcare delivery system. Clarity is required regarding how these health professionals will interact with other professions such as medicine, nursing, and so forth., inside the system (Parry, 2008) (Table 2.1).

TABLE 2.1 Categories of Allied Health Professionals (AHPs) Based on the Specialist Degrees

Educational Level	Categories of Allied Health Professionals
Degree holders	Allied health professionals
Diploma holders	Allied health providers
Certificate holders	Allied health workers

There are two classes of APHs, that is, technicians (assistants) and technologists. The education span of a technician is less than two years, and they are specialized in carrying out laboratory procedures and handling laboratory instruments. Physical therapy assistants, medical laboratory technicians, radiographic technicians, occupational therapy assistants, recreation therapy assistants, and respiratory therapy technicians are among those who operate under the direction of technologists or therapists (Nancarrow et al., 2012).

On the other hand, therapists or technologists learn to evaluate patients, diagnose illnesses, establish appropriate treatment plans while considering potential side effects, determine therapy responses, and make pertinent decisions regarding the continuation or change of treatment (Nancarrow et al., 2012).

The formalization of the allied healthcare workforce has advanced significantly in India. After being approved by the Lok Sabha on March 24, 2021, the National Commission for Allied and Healthcare Professionals Bill, 2020, was presented by the Indian government to the Rajya Sabha. Since allied healthcare professionals are an important component of the medical profession, the law seeks to regulate them.

In 2018, the Government of India (GoI) classified healthcare workers into 15 groups. As seen in Table 2.2, these 15 categories are further divided into 53 subcategories.

TABLE 2.2 Fifteen Categories of Health Care Professions

Sl. No	Categories of Allied Health Professionals
1	Life Science Professional
2	Trauma and Burn Care Professional
3	Physiotherapy Professional
4	Nutrition Science Professional
5	Ophthalmic Sciences Professional
6	Health and Information Management Professional
7	Medical laboratory Sciences Professional
8	Physician Associate or Assistant
9	Occupational Therapy Profession
10	Behavioral Health Sciences Professional
11	Primary, Community and Miscellaneous Care Professional
12	Medical Radiology, Imaging, and Therapeutic Technology Professional
13	Cardiovascular, Neurosciences, and Pulmonary Technology Professional
14	Renal Technology Professional
15	Surgical and Anesthesia-related Technology Professional

The foundational members of the healthcare team are AHPs. They contribute significantly to the provision of healthcare or associated services. To encourage recovery and guarantee the provision of high-quality healthcare services, they collaborate in interdisciplinary healthcare teams with doctors and other specialists (Angus et al., 2022). Details of categories and subcategories of allied health professions are depicted in Figure 2.1.

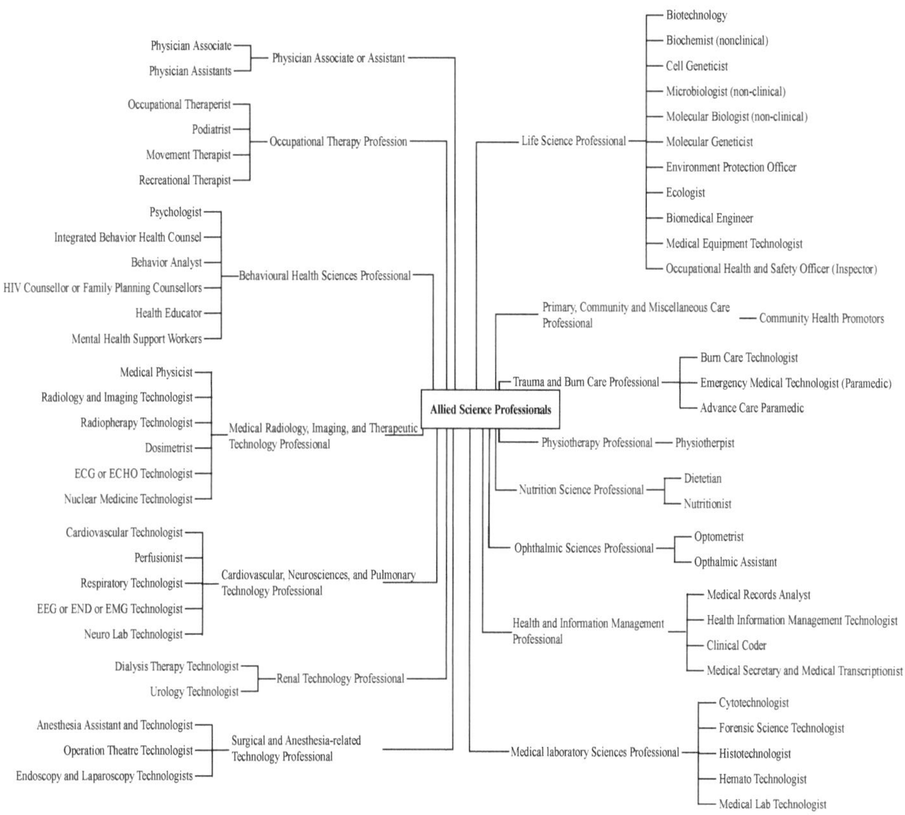

FIGURE 2.1 Categories and subcategories of allied health professionals.

2.3 IMPORTANCE AND RELEVANCE OF ALLIED HEALTH SCIENCES IN HEALTHCARE

The delivery of healthcare and AHSs is a vital aspect of the healthcare system. The following succinctly expresses the value and relevance of AHSs in healthcare (Paul et al., 2017).

2.3.1 PATIENT OUTCOME IMPROVEMENT

Professionals in AHSs collaborate with other healthcare providers to deliver holistic treatment that enhances patient outcomes. Following an illness or accident, occupational therapists (OTs), for instance, can assist patients in regaining their independence and enhancing their quality of life. They can collaborate with patients to create adaptations for daily tasks, provide aids, or offer sensory-motor training to enhance movement and coordination. Dietitians can assist patients with managing chronic illnesses like diabetes and heart disease by creating individualized nutrition plans and educating them on appropriate eating practices. In order to identify and track illnesses, radiographers and medical laboratory scientists (MLS) use imaging and laboratory testing. This can result in earlier discovery and more efficient treatment, improving patient outcomes.

2.3.2 PROVIDING AFFORDABLE PATIENT CARE

By working in the community and encouraging self-management of health issues, experts in the AHSs can deliver care that is both efficient and affordable. Community health workers may give patients information and support to help them manage chronic diseases, which will cut down on the number of hospital admissions and pricey treatments. Inpatient rehabilitation programs are not always necessary because physiotherapists can offer rehabilitation treatments in the community. Additionally, by recognizing and addressing social determinants of health, such as a lack of access to safe housing or good food, which can have a substantial impact on health outcomes, allied health workers can contribute to cost reduction.

2.3.3 OVERCOMING SHORTAGE OF PRIMARY CARE PHYSICIANS

Professionals in the AHSs are essential in filling in the gaps in the healthcare system. In regions where primary care physicians are in limited supply, physician assistants and nurse practitioners can provide primary care services, ensuring that patients have access to the treatment they require. Patients who might not have access to a specialist now have better access to care thanks to audiologists' ability to deliver hearing services in isolated locations. The provision of culturally competent care and the customization of their services to fit the particular requirements of each patient are further ways that AHPs can help reduce healthcare disparities.

2.3.4 ADDRESSING SPECIAL ISSUES

Professionals in the AHSs offer specialized care in disciplines including clinical psychology, occupational therapy, and audiology that can enhance patient outcomes and quality of life. Music therapists can assist patients with mental health concerns, while speech and language therapists can assist patients with communication issues. Patients will receive high-quality care due to the intensive training and education these specialists receive in their fields of expertise. Aside from that, allied health specialists can cooperate with other medical specialists to deliver multidisciplinary care, guaranteeing that patients receive thorough, coordinated care that meets all of their demands.

2.3.5 INNOVATIVE RESEARCH

The advancement of the healthcare system is facilitated by the involvement of specialists in AHSs in research and innovation. While MLSs are active in developing novel laboratory tests that can increase the precision of diagnosis and therapy, radiation therapists are involved in developing new treatments for cancer patients. New technologies and rehabilitation procedures are being developed by physical therapists to aid patients in recovering from illnesses and injuries more quickly. The implementation of evidence-based therapies and the promotion of best practices in their respective sectors are further ways that AHPs can aid in the translation of research into practice.

2.4 FUNCTIONS OF ALLIED HEALTH PROFESSIONALS

A variety of tasks are performed by AHPs, including those in early intervention, health promotion, and assistance for people with chronic diseases, disabilities, and palliative care. The provision of safe, beneficial, responsible, and competent healthcare that is responsive to individual, group, and community needs, as well as the professional situation, within a context of justice and respect for people's rights and dignity, is a responsibility and obligation of AHPs to their patients as well as the larger community. Although allied health practitioners have duties and obligations to their employers, patients, and their profession as a whole, those duties and obligations will always come second (Figure 2.2).

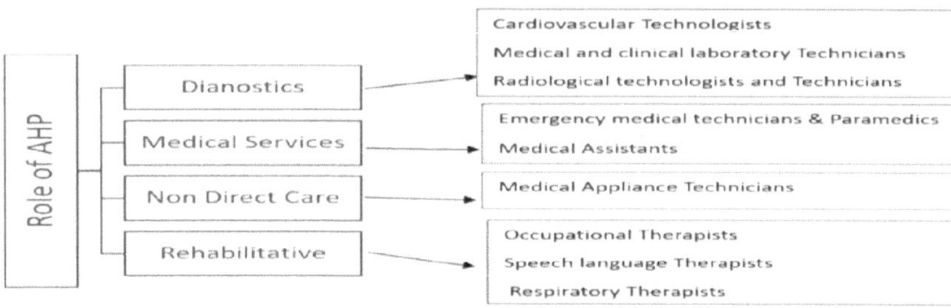

FIGURE 2.2 Role of allied health professionals (AHP).

2.5 MEDICAL CARE

In order to prevent, identify, evaluate, and cure diseases, as well as to manage and prevent patient disabilities and disorders, the healthcare sector must collaborate. A variety of facets of healthcare create a demand for AHPs. AHPs work to improve patients' quality of life. Medical practitioners receive help from allied healthcare experts in the early detection and identification of patients' concerns. Their knowledge, combined with accountable direct patient care, greatly benefits the healthcare team.

2.6 MEDICAL ASSISTANCE

The medical team is assisted by allied health workers in providing clinical support in the wards, outside, and in laboratories. To help the patients, they provide preventive and rehabilitation programs. Allied health workers provide critical care support in ICUs and hospice institutions as part of their services. In addition, allied health cadres assist the medical team in technical areas to relieve the workload of the occupied medical professionals. For example, medical coders and transcriptionists support the management of vital data in the healthcare sector to provide seamless patient care. The medical personnel are supported by the allied health cadres, who also help to enhance overall public health outcomes.

Health on a social, psychological, and environmental level: Beyond physical medicine, AHPs do other duties. Among the variety of services provided by AHPs, a stronger emphasis is placed on those that enhance patients' wellness and quality of life. The cognitive, social, and emotional requirements of patients are met with the assistance of AHPs, who also significantly contribute to quality-of-life improvement. For example, social service providers in the healthcare industry offer patients and their families the much-needed emotional/social support and direction through counseling, referring them for rehabilitation, medical treatment, and specialized counseling services, as needed. Similarly, recreational therapists, who are also members of the AHP group, assess patients, particularly children, to ascertain the kind of recreational activity that would be most appropriate for them.

Allied health workers possess distinct qualities compared to other employees in the healthcare industry. The following are the qualities of healthcare professionals:

1. A basic responsibility of care (duty of care) towards the client.
2. A responsibility to operate in the client's best interests (client independence).
3. A need to act in the client's best interest (principles of benevolence and non-maleficence).
4. Practice is built on a corpus of information and certain abilities.
5. A dedication of continued professional growth and sustaining competency.
6. Reflective practice.
7. Taking decisions based on information at hand and possible outcomes.

2.7 CONCLUSION

Allied health sciences are essential to healthcare because they provide specialized knowledge, all-encompassing care, and a dedication to bettering patient outcomes. An important component of healthcare teams around the world, allied health workers will only become more significant and relevant as healthcare continues to develop. Their efforts have an impact on numerous people's lives and general well-being far beyond the confines of the lab or the treatment room. For healthcare systems to keep improving, it is essential to acknowledge and value their contribution.

KEYWORDS

- **allied health sciences**
- **allied health workers**
- **clinical support**
- **critical care support**
- **health care knowledge**
- **hospice institutions**
- **medical coders**
- **rehabilitation programs**

REFERENCES

Angus, R. L., Hattingh, H. L., & Weir, K. A. (2022). Experiences of hospital allied health professionals in collaborative student research projects: A qualitative study. *BMC Health Services Research, 22*, 729.

Bhola, N., & Kumari, R. (n.d.). Utilization of the health care delivery system in a district of North India. *East African Journal of Public Health, 5*, 147–153.

Gaur, V. (2018). An overview of redefining paradigm: India's allied health professional.

Modi, I. (2014). Health care delivery system: India. In *The Wiley Blackwell Encyclopedia of Health, Illness, Behavior, and Society* (pp. 816–823). John Wiley & Sons.

Nancarrow, S., Moran, A., & Boyce, R. (2012). Evaluation of a system of monitoring allied health service provision, quality, and outcomes. *GSTF Journal of BioSciences, 2*(1).

Parry, R. (2008). Are interventions to enhance communication performance in allied health professionals effective, and how should they be delivered? Direct and indirect evidence. *Patient Education and Counseling, 73*, 186–195.

Paul, P., Bhimali, A., & Aithal, P. S. (2017). Allied medical and health science and advanced telecommunications: Emerging utilizations and its need in the Indian healthcare system. *Current Trends in Biotechnology and Chemical Research, 7*(1, 2), 27–30.

CHAPTER 3

Allied Health Sciences: Navigating Careers in Patient-Centric Professions

MEENAKSHI VERMA,[1] RITIKA INDORIA,[2,*] and SUMEDHA RABRA[1]

[1]*Department of Physiotherapy, Sharda School of Allied Health Sciences, Sharda University, Greater Noida, Uttar Pradesh, India*

[2]*Consultant Physiotherapist, Shakti Physiotherapy Centre NOIDA, Uttar Pradesh, India*

*Corresponding author

ABSTRACT

Allied Health Sciences (AHS) is a growing field that encompasses a range of professions that provide critical support to medical practitioners. This field offers a plethora of career opportunities that allow individuals to contribute to the healthcare industry in various ways. This abstract highlights the career opportunities available in the AHSs, including clinical laboratory science, medical imaging, physical therapy, occupational therapy, respiratory therapy, and speech-language pathology. The demand for professionals in these fields is increasing rapidly, and the scope for growth and development is immense. AHSs professionals play a vital role in patient care and work collaboratively with other healthcare professionals to improve patient outcomes. The abstract also discusses the education and training requirements for these professions and the job outlook for AHSs professionals. Overall, this chapter emphasizes the importance of AHSs in the healthcare industry and the diverse career opportunities available for individuals interested in pursuing a career in this field.

Allied Healthcare in Practice: An Introduction to Integrated Patient Care. Sally Lukose, Karuna Singh (Eds.)

DOI: 10.1201/9781998511037-4

3.1 INTRODUCTION

Allied health sciences (AHS) offer a vast array of career opportunities in the healthcare industry. With a focus on the identification, evaluation, and prevention of diseases and disorders, dietary, and nutrition services, and rehabilitation and health systems management, AHPs play a crucial role in delivering quality healthcare. The World Health Organization (WHO) has long argued that in order to enhance patient outcomes, health professionals must be competent at collaborating in multidisciplinary teams. According to Frenk et al. (2010), "Patient management requires coordinated care across time and space, demanding unprecedented teamwork as well as professionals have to integrate the rapid advancement of knowledge and technologies while struggling with developing functions" in a Lancet Commission review. Interprofessional teams are encouraged to "optimize the skills of their members, share case management, and provide better health services to patients and the community" in this more complicated workplace (Snell et al., 2020; WHO, 2010).

According to Oandasan and Reeves (2005), the capacity to practice collaboratively is defined as "an interprofessional process of communication and decision making that enables the separate and shared knowledge and skills of healthcare providers to synergistically influence the patient care provided." Recognizing the connection between health and education, it is suggested that professional education be changed to generate graduates who can offer healthcare effectively as team members (Frenk et al., 2010; Snell et al., 2020).

With everyday advancements in the medical field, there is a tendency towards living longer, chronic illness rates, and an older population globally. Limited resources are required to run healthcare services. Increases in funding-focused trends are often regarded as unsustainable. An international study of eight industrialized nations revealed challenges for each of the various healthcare systems in terms of cost per patient and patient outcomes. The poll concentrated on individuals with chronic illnesses since this age group receives a higher percentage of health spending. According to this study, there are problems with patient self-management, access, coordination of treatment, and efficiency (such as duplication and patient views of wasted care). According to its conclusions, several of the participating nations transferred resources from managing conventional acute care to more extensive chronic care that was necessary due to the shifting population demography (Saxon et al., 2014).

Numerous areas for improvement have been identified in the literature, including standardization of transition and discharge procedures, technology advancements and their relationship to the quality of healthcare, and expanded responsibilities for non-medical practitioners (Saxon et al., 2014). Medical professionals are seen as the primary decision-makers regarding issues of referral, admission, and discharge in traditional models of health delivery. These models are often governed around the requirements and skills of different disciplines. Even for patients who could benefit from early allied health input, the lack of expert resources frequently results in a lengthy wait for services for patients. Therefore, it has been determined that AHPs have the essential clinical competencies and capacity to close this service demand gap and serve as the patient's initial point of contact during their journey through the healthcare system (Saxon et al., 2014).

In essence, new extended allied health jobs are under consideration, with clinicians accessing specialized training outside of the standard area of their profession in order to increase patient access to timely healthcare. This could entail specific duties that have historically been performed by medical, nursing, physiotherapy (PT), occupational therapy, speech pathology, or other health professionals.

A systematic review that was published in 2006 discovered terminology variation and concentrated on offering a working definition of extended scope of practice in terms of enhancement and substitution (expanding job breadth by working across professional boundaries and deepening job scope by adding skills within a profession) was the main focus of the review (Saxon et al., 2014).

AHPs (AHPs) are an important part of the health and care service system. Within the United Kingdom (UK), the Health and Care Professionals Council (HCPC) regulates AHPs from 14 different professional groups. There were 252,269 AHPs in the HCPC register as of March 2023. The Allied Health Professions Strategy recognizes the need for positive action to examine recruitment and career progression strategies (Atwal et al., 2013).

3.2 PROFESSIONS UNDER ALLIED HEALTH SCIENCES

There are many streams that come under AHSs. This chapter will discuss the career prospects in the following programs of AHSs. Furthermore, professionals can pursue higher studies in these fields.

- Physiotherapy.
- Cardio vascular technology.
- Forensic science.
- Radiological imaging techniques (Radiology/CT/MRI).
- Optometry.
- Nutrition and dietetics.
- Operation theatre technology.
- Medical laboratory technology.

3.2.1 CAREER IN PHYSIOTHERAPY

Action is required on a global scale to maintain a sufficient healthcare workforce that can fulfill the demand for healthcare services (WHO, 2022). The aging and expanding populations are expected to continue this need, which is accompanied by an increase in the prevalence of chronic diseases (Liu et al., 2017; Prince et al., 2015). Despite the critical role that physiotherapists play in the management and rehabilitation of patients with chronic illnesses, clinical shortages have been documented globally (Chartered Society of Physiotherapy, 2018; Childs et al., 2022; Paynter, 2023; Rodés et al., 2021).

Physical therapy, also known as physiotherapy or PT, is a conservative science that uses physical methods such as radiation, heat, cold, exercise, current, waves, manipulation, mobilization, and others to treat and manage diseases after clinical examinations, assessments, and diagnoses in order to restore neuro-musculoskeletal and cardiopulmonary efficiencies, manage pain, and treat some integumentary disorders (Sharma, 2012).

Many organizations have provided their own definitions of PT. Below are a few definitions: According to the American Physiotherapy Association, PT is "clinical applications in the restoration, maintenance, and promotion of optimal physical function" (Sharma, 2012).

Physiotherapy is described as "a branch of medical science that includes examination, assessment, interpretation, physical diagnosis, planning, and execution of treatment, and advice to any person for the purpose of preventing, correcting, alleviating, and limiting dysfunction, acute and chronic bodily malfunction including life-saving measures via chest PT in the intensive care units, curing physical disorders or disability," by the Maharashtra Occupational Therapy and Physiotherapy (OT PT) Council, India. This is a field that is required for each and every person who is experiencing any abnormality or discomfort during the activities of daily living (ADL). The primary aim of a physiotherapist is to rehabilitate the person so that they can be physically and mentally healthy to fulfill their basic life requirements.

In the past, PT was only utilized when a patient was in pain and only on the recommendation of a doctor or orthopedician. The function of PT in several sectors has been demonstrated to be advantageous due to the field's ongoing evolution and the breakthroughs in treatment that are being researched at numerous institutions and research centers. The population suffering from musculoskeletal disorders, cardiorespiratory conditions, obstetrical and gynecological conditions, pediatric conditions, psychiatric conditions, and in sports has seen an exponential surge in demand for PT.

3.2.1.1 SPECIALIZATIONS WITHIN PHYSIOTHERAPY (AMERICAN BOARD OF PHYSICAL THERAPY, 2023)

1. **Orthopedic Physiotherapy:** Orthopedic physiotherapists specialize in diagnosing and treating musculoskeletal conditions, including fractures, ligament injuries, and joint replacements. They design tailored exercise regimens and employ manual techniques to enhance joint mobility and alleviate pain. These therapists play a crucial role in postoperative rehabilitation, guiding patients through the recovery process.

2. **Cardiovascular and Pulmonary Physiotherapy:** Specializing in cardiac and pulmonary conditions, these physiotherapists aid patients recovering from heart surgeries or managing chronic lung diseases. Through aerobic conditioning, breathing exercises, and airway clearance techniques, they enhance cardiovascular fitness and respiratory function. Although this specialization was provided in hospitals, its usefulness was not widely acknowledged until the recent COVID-19 epidemic. Chest PT is often necessary for patients who are hospitalized for illnesses other than musculoskeletal or respiratory ones, such as gastrointestinal or renal. Following abdominal surgery, postoperative pulmonary complications (PPCs) are frequent and are to blame for higher morbidity and mortality, longer hospital stays, and higher healthcare expenses. Compared to lower abdominal surgical procedures, upper abdominal surgical operations often carry a higher risk of

complications. The reported risk of postoperative pulmonary issues following upper abdominal surgery ranged from 17% to 88% (Maity, 2023).

3. **Neurological Physiotherapy:** Neurological physiotherapists focus on patients with neurological disorders like stroke, spinal cord injuries, and Parkinson's disease. They address motor impairments, balance issues, and functional limitations through targeted interventions. Utilizing task-specific training and adaptive equipment, these therapists help individuals regain independence and improve their quality of life.

4. **Obstetrics and Gynecological Physiotherapy:** In present times, expecting mothers are participating in palliative care to control pregnancy issues in order to lower the risk and ensure a healthier and easier birth. Even after giving birth, women are urged to strengthen their core muscles and rehabilitate their pelvic floor muscles to help their bodies recover from pregnancy-related abnormalities. The innovative and advanced discipline of PT that is in high demand in maternity facilities is prenatal and postpartum care courses.

5. **Pediatric Physiotherapy:** Pediatric physiotherapists work with infants, children, and adolescents facing developmental delays, congenital disorders, or injuries. Their interventions stimulate motor skill acquisition, improve posture, and enhance mobility. Through play-based therapy, these professionals contribute to young patients' physical, cognitive, and emotional growth. Pediatric physiotherapists assist kids in developing physically to their full potential. They treat patients from one-day-old newborns to teenagers and have specialized understanding in the mobility, development, and conditions that are likely to harm the baby and developing child. Soft tissue massage, mobilization, stretching, certain therapeutic exercises, and posture instruction may all be used in the course of treatment. Because children are not miniature adults, these therapists encourage kids to move as best they can through play and developmentally appropriate games and activities.

6. **Sports Physiotherapy:** Sports physiotherapists collaborate with athletes to prevent injuries, optimize performance, and

expedite recovery. They conduct biomechanical assessments, design injury prevention programs, and provide immediate care during competitions. Rehabilitation plans are tailored to each athlete's sport-specific demands and goals. The possibility for this type of PT is expanding dramatically as a result of the flourishing sports scenario in India and the younger generation's involvement in various sports with a view to representing the nation globally.

3.2.1.2 EDUCATIONAL INSTITUTE

As the need for PT in the clinical setting grows, academic physiotherapists are needed to teach the next generation and prepare them to meet the high expectations of the outside world. This expands the job opportunities for physiotherapists in the academic setting. There is a significant need for academics in the institutions where one may study the latest developments and also aid fresh research to reinvent the current trending procedures for advanced rehabilitations due to the rising number of requests day by day in the clinical area.

3.2.1.3 RESEARCH AND ACADEMIA

Physiotherapists can engage in research to contribute to the advancement of the field. They can work in universities, research institutions, or hospitals to conduct studies that improve treatment methods, develop new techniques, or explore the effectiveness of interventions. This involves designing experiments, analyzing data, and publishing findings in scientific journals.

3.2.1.4 HEALTH AND WELLNESS CONSULTING

Physiotherapists with expertise in exercise, movement, and wellness can offer consulting services to individuals, corporations, or fitness centers. They can design customized wellness programs, provide ergonomic assessments for workplaces, and educate clients on injury prevention strategies.

3.2.1.5 MEDICAL DEVICE INDUSTRY

Physiotherapists can work with medical device manufacturers to develop and test new equipment or devices designed to aid in rehabilitation and mobility. This role involves providing insights based on clinical experience and collaborating with engineers and designers.

3.2.1.6 REHABILITATION ADMINISTRATION

In addition to direct patient care, physiotherapists can take on administrative roles within rehabilitation centers, hospitals, or healthcare organizations. They can manage teams, oversee treatment protocols, and ensure the quality of care provided.

3.2.1.7 TELEHEALTH AND DIGITAL HEALTH

The rise of telehealth has created opportunities for physiotherapists to provide virtual consultations and treatment sessions. They can develop online exercise programs, provide remote guidance, and contribute to digital health platforms.

3.2.1.8 GOVERNMENT AND POLICY ROLES

Physiotherapists can work in government agencies or healthcare policy organizations to contribute their expertise in shaping healthcare policies, regulations, and standards related to rehabilitation and mobility.

3.2.1.9 INTERNATIONAL AID AND DISASTER RELIEF

Physiotherapists can volunteer or work with organizations that provide rehabilitation services in disaster-stricken areas or regions with limited access to healthcare resources.

3.2.2 CAREER IN CARDIO VASCULAR TECHNOLOGY (CARDIOVASCULAR CREDENTIALING INTERNATIONAL, 2023)

A career in cardiovascular technology offers exciting opportunities to work at the intersection of healthcare and technology, specializing in the diagnosis and treatment of cardiovascular conditions. This field plays a crucial role in the diagnosis, monitoring, and treatment of heart and vascular diseases, contributing to patient care and improved cardiovascular health. Cardiovascular technologists, also known as cardiovascular technicians, are healthcare professionals who operate specialized equipment to perform diagnostic tests and procedures related to the cardiovascular system. They work alongside cardiologists, physicians, and nurses to provide crucial information for diagnosing and treating heart conditions. It is a comprehensive degree program that equips students with the knowledge and skills required for a successful career in this field. The curriculum typically covers anatomy, physiology, cardiovascular diseases (CVD), medical instrumentation, patient care techniques, and imaging technologies. Clinical internships and hands-on training are integral components of the program.

3.2.2.1 SPECIALIZATIONS WITHIN CARDIOVASCULAR TECHNOLOGY

Within the field of cardiovascular technology, there are several specializations you can pursue:

1. **Cardiac Sonography (Echocardiography):** Cardiac sonographers use ultrasound (USG) technology to create images of the heart's structures and functions, aiding in the diagnosis of heart conditions.
2. **Vascular Sonography:** Vascular technologists use USG to evaluate blood vessels, detecting blockages, clots, and other vascular abnormalities.
3. **Invasive Cardiology:** Invasive cardiovascular technologists assist during procedures such as cardiac catheterizations, angioplasties, and stent placements. They ensure the proper functioning of equipment and monitor patients' responses during procedures.

3.2.2.2 EDUCATIONAL PATHWAYS

A degree in cardiovascular technology is a comprehensive degree program that equips students with the knowledge and skills required for a successful career in this field. The curriculum typically covers anatomy, physiology, CVD, medical instrumentation, patient care techniques, and imaging technologies. Clinical internships and hands-on training are integral components of the program.

3.2.2.3 WORK SETTINGS

Graduates with a degree in cardiovascular technology can work in a variety of healthcare settings, including:

1. **Hospitals:** Cardiovascular technologists play a vital role in diagnostic imaging departments, cardiac catheterization labs, and surgical suites.
2. **Clinics and Private Practices:** Private cardiology clinics and physician practices hire cardiovascular technologists to perform diagnostic tests and assist in patient care.
3. **Diagnostic Imaging Centers:** These centers focus on non-invasive diagnostic imaging, and cardiovascular technologists contribute to the accurate diagnosis of heart and vascular conditions.
4. **Research and Education:** Some technologists choose to work in research institutions or educational settings, contributing to advancements in cardiovascular technology and training future professionals.

3.2.2.4 CAREER ADVANCEMENT AND GROWTH

As we gain experience and expertise, we can take on roles with more responsibilities, such as senior technologist, department supervisor, or educator. Continuing education and certifications from organizations like Cardiovascular Credentialing International (CCI) can enhance skills and open doors to leadership positions.

3.2.2.5 TECHNOLOGICAL ADVANCEMENTS

The field of cardiovascular technology is constantly evolving with advancements in medical technology. Staying updated on the latest equipment and techniques is essential for providing accurate and efficient patient care. A B.Sc. in Cardiovascular Technology opens doors to a rewarding career focused on cardiovascular health. The combination of medical knowledge and technical skills positions you as a vital member of the healthcare team, contributing to the diagnosis and treatment of heart and vascular conditions.

3.2.3 CAREER IN FORENSIC SCIENCES (AMERICAN ACADEMY OF FORENSIC SCIENCES, 2023)

A career in Forensic Science offers a captivating journey into the world of crime investigation, scientific analysis, and justice. Forensic science is the application of scientific principles and techniques to solve criminal cases, identify evidence, and support legal proceedings. Pursuing a degree in Forensic Science opens doors to a range of opportunities in law enforcement, laboratories, and legal settings. Forensic science combines various scientific disciplines, including biology, chemistry, physics, and more, to analyze physical evidence related to criminal investigations. Professionals in this field play a vital role in uncovering the truth, identifying perpetrators, and ensuring justice. It is a multidisciplinary program that provides a solid foundation in scientific principles and forensic techniques. The curriculum typically includes coursework in forensic chemistry, biology, crime scene investigation, forensic anthropology, forensic psychology, and legal aspects of forensic science. Hands-on laboratory experience and practical training are integral components of the program.

3.2.3.1 SPECIALIZATIONS WITHIN FORENSIC SCIENCE

Forensic Science encompasses several specializations that cater to different aspects of crime investigation:

1. **Forensic Chemistry:** Analyzing chemical substances like drugs, toxins, and explosives in evidence.
2. **Forensic Biology:** Examining biological evidence like Deoxyribonucleic acid (DNA), blood, and other bodily fluids.
3. **Crime Scene Investigation:** Collecting, preserving, and analyzing evidence at crime scenes.
4. **Forensic Anthropology:** Identifying human remains and analyzing skeletal evidence to determine identities and causes of death.
5. **Digital Forensics:** Recovering and analyzing digital evidence from computers, mobile devices, and electronic systems.

3.2.3.2 WORK SETTINGS

Graduates with a degree in Forensic Science can find employment in various sectors, including:

1. **Law Enforcement Agencies:** Police departments and federal agencies hire forensic scientists to analyze evidence and support criminal investigations.
2. **Forensic Laboratories:** Public and private laboratories offer roles in DNA analysis, toxicology, ballistics, and more.
3. **Medical Examiner's Office:** Forensic pathologists and scientists work in medical examiner's offices to determine causes of death and analyze remains.
4. **Legal and Law Firms:** Forensic experts can serve as consultants or expert witnesses in legal proceedings.
5. **Academia and Research:** Some forensic scientists teach, conduct research, and contribute to advancements in the field.

3.2.3.3 CAREER ADVANCEMENT AND GROWTH

As you gain experience, you can progress to senior roles, supervisory positions, or specialize further in specific areas of forensic science. Continuing education, certifications, and attending professional conferences can enhance your skills and credibility in the field.

3.2.3.4 ETHICAL CONSIDERATIONS

Forensic scientists must adhere to ethical guidelines, ensuring accurate analysis, unbiased reporting, and maintaining the integrity of evidence. A degree in Forensic Science equips you with the knowledge and skills to contribute to criminal investigations and justice systems. The role of a forensic scientist is instrumental in analyzing evidence, uncovering truths, and playing a crucial part in upholding the law and ensuring justice prevails.

3.2.4 CAREER IN RADIOLOGY IMAGING TECHNIQUES

A career in Radiology Imaging Techniques offers an exciting opportunity to work at the forefront of medical imaging technology, playing a critical role in diagnosing and treating various medical conditions. Radiology technologists use advanced equipment to create detailed images of the internal structures of the human body, aiding physicians in making accurate diagnoses and treatment plans. Pursuing a degree in Radiology Imaging Techniques opens doors to a range of roles in healthcare facilities, clinics, and imaging centers. Radiology imaging techniques involve using various imaging modalities, such as X-rays, computed tomography (CT), magnetic resonance imaging (MRI), and USG, to capture images of internal body structures. These images provide essential information to healthcare professionals for diagnosing and monitoring medical conditions. A degree in Radiology Imaging Techniques is a comprehensive program that provides students with a strong foundation in radiologic sciences. The curriculum typically includes courses in radiographic positioning, radiation protection, anatomy, and physiology, patient care, and the operation of imaging equipment. Practical clinical experience is a key component of the program, allowing students to apply their knowledge in real-world settings.

3.2.4.1 SPECIALIZATIONS WITHIN RADIOLOGY IMAGING TECHNIQUES

Radiology imaging encompasses several specializations, each focusing on a specific imaging modality:

1. **Diagnostic Radiography (X-ray):** Diagnostic radiographers use X-rays to create images of bones, organs, and tissues, aiding in the diagnosis of fractures, infections, and other conditions.
2. **Computed Tomography (CT):** CT technologists use advanced X-ray equipment to produce cross-sectional images of the body, allowing for detailed visualization of internal structures.
3. **Magnetic Resonance Imaging (MRI):** MRI technologists operate machines that use strong magnetic fields and radio waves to create detailed images of soft tissues, organs, and joints.

4. **Ultrasound:** Ultrasound technologists use sound waves to produce images of internal structures, making it valuable for assessing pregnancy, abdominal issues, and vascular conditions.

3.2.4.2 WORK SETTINGS

Graduates with a B.Sc. in Radiology Imaging Techniques can find employment in a variety of healthcare settings, including:

1. **Hospitals:** Radiology technologists are an integral part of hospital imaging departments, performing a wide range of imaging procedures.
2. **Diagnostic Imaging Centers:** These centers specialize in conducting various imaging exams, from X-rays to advanced modalities like MRI and CT scans.
3. **Outpatient Clinics:** Medical clinics offer imaging services, and radiology technologists play a crucial role in conducting diagnostic procedures.
4. **Physician Practices:** Some specialized medical practices have their imaging equipment, and technologists can work directly with physicians to perform imaging tests.

3.2.4.3 CAREER ADVANCEMENT AND GROWTH

As you gain experience and expertise, you can advance to supervisory roles, become a lead technologist, or specialize further in a specific imaging modality. Continuous education and certifications from organizations like the American Registry of Radiologic Technologists (ARRT) can enhance your career prospects.

3.2.4.4 SAFETY AND PATIENT CARE

Radiology technologists must adhere to strict safety protocols to minimize radiation exposure to patients and themselves. Ensuring patient comfort and providing clear instructions during procedures are essential aspects of the role. A degree in Radiology Imaging Techniques equips you with the skills to operate advanced medical imaging equipment, contribute to accurate diagnoses, and provide essential support to healthcare teams. Your role as a radiology technologist is vital in enabling medical professionals to visualize and understand complex medical conditions, ultimately leading to better patient care.

3.2.5 CAREER IN OPTOMETRY (AMERICAN OPTOMETRIC ASSOCIATION (AOA), 2023)

A career in optometry offers a fulfilling path focused on eye care and vision health. Optometrists are primary healthcare professionals who specialize in diagnosing and treating visual disorders, prescribing corrective lenses, and providing comprehensive eye care services. Pursuing a career in optometry opens up opportunities to work in various settings and contribute to the well-being of individuals' eyes and vision. Optometrists are essential members of the healthcare team, focusing on assessing and managing visual health. They examine patients' eyes for vision problems, refractive errors, and eye diseases. Optometrists also prescribe eyeglasses, contact lenses, and low vision aids to improve patients' visual acuity and comfort. To become an optometrist, you need to complete a degree from an accredited optometry school. The program typically spans four years and includes coursework in ocular anatomy, physiology, optics, pharmacology, and clinical techniques. Clinical rotations provide hands-on experience in diverse areas of optometry.

3.2.5.1 SPECIALIZATIONS WITHIN OPTOMETRY

Optometrists can specialize in various subfields, including:

1. **Pediatric Optometry:** Specializing in children's eye care, diagnosing, and managing visual conditions that affect young patients.
2. **Geriatric Optometry:** Focusing on age-related eye conditions and vision changes in older adults.
3. **Contact Lens Fitting:** Specializing in fitting and prescribing contact lenses for patients with refractive errors.

4. **Low Vision Rehabilitation:** Helping individuals with severe visual impairment make the most of their remaining vision.

3.2.5.2 WORK SETTINGS

Graduates with a degree in Optometry can work in diverse settings, including:

1. **Private Practice:** Many optometrists establish their private practices, providing comprehensive eye exams, vision correction, and eye health management.
2. **Retail Clinics:** Optometrists can work in retail settings, providing vision exams and prescribing eyewear.
3. **Hospitals and Medical Centers:** Some hospitals employ optometrists to provide eye care services to patients in various departments.
4. **Specialized Clinics:** Optometrists can work in clinics specializing in pediatric, geriatric, or medical eye care.

3.2.5.3 CAREER ADVANCEMENT AND GROWTH

Experienced optometrists can advance their careers by becoming clinic owners, specializing in a particular field, or engaging in research and academia. Continuing education and pursuing certifications in specialized areas can enhance career prospects.

3.2.5.4 TECHNOLOGICAL ADVANCEMENTS

The field of optometry benefits from technological advancements in diagnostic tools, treatment options, and corrective lenses. Staying updated on these advancements is crucial for providing optimal care. A career in optometry allows you to make a positive impact on people's lives by providing essential eye care services and improving vision. As an optometrist, one plays a crucial role in diagnosing eye conditions, prescribing corrective measures, and contributing to overall visual health.

3.2.6 CAREER IN NUTRITION AND DIETETICS (ACADEMY OF NUTRITION AND DIETETICS, 2023)

A career in Nutrition and Dietetics offers a rewarding pathway to becoming a registered dietitian or nutritionist, specializing in promoting healthy eating habits, preventing, and managing health conditions, and enhancing overall well-being through proper nutrition. Graduates of this program play a pivotal role in healthcare, education, research, and community settings. Nutrition and dietetics professionals focus on the science of food and its impact on health. They provide evidence-based guidance on diet, nutrition, and lifestyle to individuals, communities, and institutions. A degree in Nutrition and Dietetics is a comprehensive program that equips students with knowledge in nutritional science, physiology, food science, and dietary management. The curriculum typically includes courses in human nutrition, macronutrients, micronutrients, dietary assessment, therapeutic nutrition, and public health nutrition. Practical experiences, such as clinical rotations or internships, are essential for hands-on learning.

3.2.6.1 SPECIALIZATIONS WITHIN NUTRITION AND DIETETICS

Graduates of a Nutrition and Dietetics program can specialize in various areas, such as:

1. **Clinical Dietetics:** Working in healthcare settings, clinical dietitians assess patients' nutritional needs and create customized diet plans to manage medical conditions.
2. **Community Nutrition:** Community dietitians educate the public about healthy eating habits, develop nutrition programs, and work with community organizations.
3. **Sports Nutrition:** Sports dietitians provide nutritional guidance to athletes, helping them optimize performance, recovery, and overall health.
4. **Public Health Nutrition:** Public health dietitians focus on improving the nutritional health of populations through policy development, education, and interventions.

3.2.6.2 WORK SETTINGS

Graduates with a degree in Nutrition and Dietetics can find employment in various settings, including:

1. **Hospitals:** Clinical dietitians work as part of healthcare teams, assessing patients' nutritional needs and creating dietary plans.
2. **Clinics and Wellness Centers:** Nutritionists provide one-on-one counseling to clients seeking dietary guidance for weight management, disease prevention, or health improvement.
3. **Schools and Universities:** Nutrition educators teach students about healthy eating habits and promote nutrition awareness.
4. **Food Service Industry:** Dietitians work with food service establishments, ensuring menus meet nutritional standards and cater to specific dietary needs.
5. **Research and Industry:** Some professionals engage in research, product development, or nutritional consulting for food companies and research institutions.

3.2.6.3 CAREER ADVANCEMENT AND GROWTH

With experience and advanced degrees, professionals can pursue leadership roles, engage in research, or contribute to policy development. Obtaining Registered Dietitian Nutritionist (RDN) credentials and pursuing specialized certifications can enhance career prospects.

3.2.6.4 WELLNESS AND PREVENTIVE CARE

Nutrition and dietetics professionals focus on preventive care by promoting healthy eating habits and guiding individuals to make informed dietary choices. A career in Nutrition and Dietetics allows you to positively impact individuals' health and well-being through evidence-based nutritional guidance. As a nutritionist or dietitian, you'll have the opportunity to help individuals make healthier choices, manage medical conditions, and improve their quality of life through proper nutrition.

3.2.7 CAREER IN MEDICAL LABORATORY TECHNOLOGY (AMERICAN SOCIETY FOR CLINICAL PATHOLOGY, 2023)

A career in Medical Laboratory Technology (MLT) or Medical Laboratory Techniques offers an essential role in the healthcare system, involving the analysis of patient samples to diagnose diseases, monitor health conditions, and ensure accurate medical treatment. MLT professionals work behind the scenes to provide vital information that guides medical decisions. Pursuing a career in MLT involves specialized education, laboratory skills, and a commitment to precision and patient care. Medical Laboratory Technologists, also known as Medical Laboratory Scientists (MLS), play a critical role in conducting laboratory tests on patient samples, such as blood, urine, tissue, and other bodily fluids. These tests help physicians diagnose and treat diseases and monitor patients' health conditions. To pursue a career in MLT, you can typically complete an Associate's degree or a Bachelor's degree in Medical Laboratory Science or a related field. The curriculum includes courses in clinical laboratory procedures, clinical chemistry, hematology, microbiology, immunology, and laboratory safety. Hands-on training in laboratory settings is an integral part of the education.

3.2.7.1 SPECIALIZATIONS WITHIN MEDICAL LABORATORY TECHNOLOGY

Medical Laboratory Technologists can specialize in various areas of laboratory testing, including:

1. **Clinical Chemistry:** Analyzing blood and body fluids to assess chemical components and diagnose conditions like diabetes and kidney diseases.
2. **Hematology:** Examining blood samples to diagnose anemia, blood clotting disorders, and blood-related diseases.
3. **Microbiology:** Identifying and studying microorganisms to diagnose infections and recommend appropriate treatments.
4. **Immunology:** Analyzing the immune system's response to infections and autoimmune disorders.

5. **Blood Banking (Immunohematology):** Ensuring compatibility of blood for transfusions and organ transplants.
6. **Molecular Diagnostics:** Detecting genetic disorders and studying DNA and Ribonucleic acid (RNA) to diagnose diseases.

3.2.7.2 WORK SETTINGS

Graduates in Medical Laboratory Technology can find employment in various healthcare settings, including:

1. **Hospitals:** Clinical laboratories within hospitals employ the majority of Medical Laboratory Technologists.
2. **Diagnostic Laboratories:** Independent clinical laboratories offer specialized testing services to medical providers.
3. **Research and Academic Institutions:** Some technologists work in research settings or educational institutions.
4. **Public Health Departments:** Contributing to disease surveillance, outbreaks, and epidemiological research.

3.2.7.3 CAREER ADVANCEMENT AND GROWTH

With experience and specialized training, Medical Laboratory Technologists can take on supervisory roles, become laboratory managers, or engage in research and teaching. Obtaining certifications from organizations like the American Society for Clinical Pathology (ASCP) can enhance career prospects.

3.2.7.4 ACCURACY AND PRECISION

Medical Laboratory Technologists must perform tests with the utmost accuracy, as their results directly influence medical decisions and patient care. A career in MLT involves playing a vital role in patient care by providing accurate and reliable diagnostic information. As a Medical Laboratory Technologist, you contribute to the early detection and management of diseases, ensuring that patients receive appropriate and timely medical treatment.

3.2.8 CAREER IN OPERATION THEATER TECHNOLOGY (NATIONAL BOARD OF SURGICAL TECHNOLOGY AND SURGICAL ASSISTING (NBSTSA), 2023)

A career in Operation Theatre (OT) Technology offers a dynamic and crucial role in the healthcare sector, focusing on ensuring the smooth functioning of surgical procedures and maintaining a sterile and safe environment in the operating room. OT Technologists, also known as Surgical Technologists or Operating Room Technicians, play a vital part in assisting surgeons, preparing equipment, and maintaining sterile conditions during surgeries. Pursuing a career in OT Technology involves specialized training, technical skills, and a commitment to patient safety. OT Technologists are integral members of the surgical team. They prepare operating rooms, sterilize equipment, assist surgeons during procedures, and ensure that all necessary tools and supplies are available for surgeries. To pursue a career in OT Technology, you can complete a diploma, certificate program, or an Associate's degree in Surgical Technology or OT Technology. The curriculum covers anatomy, surgical procedures, sterilization techniques, patient positioning, infection control, and medical ethics. Practical hands-on training in simulated or real surgical environments is a vital component of the education.

3.2.8.1 RESPONSIBILITIES AND SKILLS

Operation Theatre Technologists perform various tasks, including:

1. **Preparing the Operating Room:** Setting up the operating room with surgical instruments, sterile drapes, and equipment.
2. **Assisting Surgeons:** Providing instruments and supplies to surgeons during procedures and anticipating their needs.
3. **Sterilization:** Ensuring that all instruments and equipment used in the operating room are properly sterilized and maintained.
4. **Patient Care:** Assisting with patient positioning, skin preparation, and monitoring during surgery.

5. **Emergency Situations:** Being prepared to handle unexpected situations and emergencies during surgeries.

3.2.8.2 WORK SETTINGS

Graduates in OT Technology can find employment in various healthcare settings, including:

1. **Hospitals:** Operating Theatre Technologists are an essential part of surgical teams in hospitals, where they assist in a wide range of surgical procedures.
2. **Outpatient Surgical Centers:** Ambulatory surgery centers offer a variety of outpatient surgeries, providing opportunities for Technologists to work in different specialties.
3. **Specialized Clinics:** Some clinics offer specialized surgical procedures, where Operating Theatre Technologists can contribute to patient care.
4. **Trauma Centers:** Trauma centers require skilled Technologists to assist in emergency surgeries.

3.2.8.3 CAREER ADVANCEMENT AND GROWTH

With experience and advanced certifications, OT technologists can become senior technologists, supervisors, or educators. Obtaining certifications from organizations like the National Board of Surgical Technology and Surgical Assisting (NBSTSA) can enhance career prospects.

3.2.8.4 ATTENTION TO DETAIL AND STERILITY

Operation theatre technologists must adhere to strict protocols for maintaining a sterile environment and ensuring patient safety during surgeries. A career in OT technology involves being an integral part of surgical teams, contributing to successful surgical outcomes, and ensuring patient safety. As an OT technologist, you'll play a crucial role in maintaining a sterile environment, assisting surgeons, and supporting the overall functioning of the operating room.

KEYWORDS

- **career and advancements**
- **operating room technicians**
- **operation theatre technology**
- **sterilizing equipment**
- **surgical procedures**
- **surgical technologists**
- **work settings**

REFERENCES

American Academy of Forensic Sciences. (2023). Retrieved from: https://www.aafs.org/forensic-sciences-foundation (accessed on 14 March 2025).

American Board of Physical Therapy Specialties. (2023). *Specialist certification.* Retrieved from: https://specialization.apta.org/ (accessed on 14 March 2025).

American Medical Technologists. (n.d.). Retrieved from: https://americanmedtech.org/ (accessed on 14 March 2025).

American Optometric Association. (2023). Retrieved from: https://www.aoa.org/?sso=y (accessed on 14 March 2025).

American Society for Clinical Pathology. (2023). Retrieved from: https://www.ascp.org/content/learning# (accessed on 14 March 2025).

Arcous, M., Putois, O., Dalle-Nazebi, S., et al. (2020). Psychosocial determinants associated with quality of life in people with Usher syndrome. *Disability and Rehabilitation, 42*(19), 2809–2820.

Association of Surgical Technologists. (n.d.). Retrieved from: https://www.ast.org/ (accessed on 14 March 2025).

Atwal, A., Sriram, V., & McKay, E. A. (2023). Mentoring for Black and minoritized allied health professionals in health and social care: A scoping review. *Journal of Multidisciplinary Healthcare, 16*, 2251–2259.

Ayton, L., Galvin, K., Johansen, L., O'Hare, F., & Shepard, E. (2023). Awareness of Usher syndrome and the need for multidisciplinary care: A cross-occupational survey of allied health clinicians. *Journal of Multidisciplinary Healthcare, 16*, 1927–1936.

Bennett, C. J., & Grant, M. J. (2004). Specialisation in physiotherapy: A mark of maturity. *Australian Journal of Physiotherapy, 50*(1), 3–5.

Bureau of Labor Statistics, U.S. Department of Labor. (2023). *Occupational Outlook Handbook: Optometrists.* Retrieved from: https://www.bls.gov/ooh/healthcare/optometrists.htm (accessed on 14 March 2025).

Bureau of Labor Statistics, U.S. Department of Labor. (2023). *Occupational Outlook Handbook: Clinical Laboratory Technologists and Technicians.* Retrieved from: https://www.bls.gov/ooh/healthcare/clinical-laboratory-technologists-and-technicians.htm (accessed on 14 March 2025).

Canadian Physiotherapy Association. (2023). *Specialization.* Retrieved from: https://physiotherapy.ca/education-events/clinical-specialist-program/ (accessed on 14 March 2025).

Cardiovascular Credentialing International. (2023). Retrieved from: https://cci-online.org/ (accessed on 14 March 2025).

Karthikeyan, G. (2021). Cardiovascular clinical examination: The need for an evidence-based approach. *European Heart Journal, 42*, 4101–4110.

Kumari, A. (2023). Admissibility and evidentiary value of forensic evidence in India. *Indian Journal of Law and Legal Research, 5*, 1–5.

National Board of Surgical Technology and Surgical Assisting. (2023). Retrieved from: https://www.nbstsa.org/careers (accessed on 14 March 2025).

Paynter, S., Iles, R., Hodgson, W. C., & Hay, M. (2023). Career intentions and satisfaction influences in early career Australian physiotherapists. *Physiotherapy Theory and Practice, 7*, 1–18.

Putter, T., van Staden, D., & Munsamy, A. (2023). Perceptions and experiences of employers and mentors of graduate optometrists' practice readiness in South Africa. *African Journal of Health Professions Education, 15*, 1–6.

Saxon, R., Gray, M., & Oprescu, F. (2014). Extended roles for allied health professionals: An updated systematic review of the evidence. *Journal of Multidisciplinary Healthcare, 7*, 479–488.

Schiro, S., Elwood, L. S., Streed, T., & Kivisto, A. J. (2023). Occupational exposure to traumatic evidence and posttraumatic stress symptoms in forensic science professionals: Prevalence and patterns. *Journal of Forensic Sciences, 68*(4), 1259–1267.

Sharma, K. (2012). Exploration of the history of physiotherapy. *Scientific Research Journal of India, 1*, 19–22.

Snell, R., Fyfe, S., Fyfe, G., Blackwood, D., & Itsiopoulos, C. (2020). Development of professional identity and professional socialization in allied health students: A scoping review. *Focus on Health Professional Education: A Multi-Professional Journal, 21*, 29–56.

The Chartered Society of Forensic Sciences. (2023). Retrieved from: https://www.csofs.org/ (accessed on 14 March 2025).

Toor, H., Kashyap, S., Yau, A., Simoni, M., Farr, S., Savla, P., Kounang, R., & Miulli, D. E. (2021). Efficacy of incentive spirometer in increasing maximum inspiratory volume in an outpatient setting. *Cureus, 13*(10), e18483.

U.S. Bureau of Labor Statistics. (2021). *Forensic Science Technicians.* Retrieved from: https://www.bls.gov/ooh/life-physical-and-social-science/forensic-science-technicians.htm (accessed on 14 March 2025).

CHAPTER 4

Educational Requirements and Career Advancements in Allied Health Professions

MEENAKSHI VERMA,[1*] RITIKA INDORIA,[2] and SUMEDHA RABRA[1]

[1]*Department of Physiotherapy, Sharda School of Allied Health Sciences, Sharda University, Greater Noida, Uttar Pradesh, India*

[2]*Consultant Physiotherapist, Shakti Physiotherapy Centre NOIDA, Uttar Pradesh, India*

*Corresponding author

ABSTRACT

Allied Health Professionals (AHPs) are described as "experts in a variety of therapeutic, diagnostic, and preventive interventions" by the U.S. Department of Health and Human Services. In terms of the level and fusion of clinical and technical skills, these specialists are leaders. Dental hygienists, diagnostic medical sonographers, dietitians, medical technologists, occupational therapists (OT), physical therapists, radiologists, respiratory therapists, and speech-language pathologists (SLP) would all be considered AHPs by this definition. India has a large and diversified pool of health human resources. They range from a variety of community- and household-based healers to highly educated biomedical professionals and super-specialists. The negative reputation of allied health sciences (AHS) is a result of the great diversity in how the idea of an AHP, more often known as a "paramedic," is understood, as well as the nomenclature and functions. The AHS area is extremely fragmented despite the enormous demand for services from this industry. AHPs and courses are now separated into smaller divisions and seem to be "regulated" by independent

Allied Healthcare in Practice: An Introduction to Integrated Patient Care. Sally Lukose, Karuna Singh (Eds.)

DOI: 10.1201/9781998511037-5

professional bodies at the national and state levels as a result of the lack of a centralized regulating body for AHPs and courses.

4.1 INTRODUCTION

The World Health Organization (WHO) defines health as a state of overall well-being rather than only the absence of disease. Overall well-being comprises physical, mental, and social well-being. That definition defines "health workers" as anybody who contributes to the enhancement, protection, or promotion of the general public's health. In the past 10 years, there has been a significant shift in how healthcare is delivered, mostly as a result of scientific and technical developments. More individuals than ever before are aware that other professionals besides physicians and nurses are now responsible for delivering health services. Now, it's a team effort with input from both clinical and non-clinical professionals. Historically, these people have been referred to as health technicians, paraprofessionals, or paramedical staff. The National Knowledge Commission was one of several organizations and experts that had previously stressed the significance of paramedics in the delivery of healthcare, prioritizing the creation of additional paramedical personnel above physicians despite the latter's acknowledged shortage. The opinions of 72 experts in the country during the last 40 years served as the basis for the study on the production and use of the health workforce toward the growth of health services in India (Dal et al., 2007).

They assert that there is an urgent requirement to focus on boosting the quantity and quality of human resources for nursing and paramedical/allied health services. They contend that improving the standard and focus of service delivery to better fulfill the demands of the public's health is more important than increasing the number of physicians. One of the biggest problems the Indian public health sector is now facing is the lack of qualified human resources. The Planning Commission's Working Group on Medical Education Training and Manpower Training prioritized the training of paraprofessional and auxiliary employees as follows (Report of Expert Committee 1987) in order to address the imbalance in human resources in 1984:

- Auxiliary staff development and training.
- Undergraduate medical education, postgraduate medical education.

- Basic and pre-service/induction training in public health and health management.
- Continuing education in those fields, training, and development of paraprofessional staff.

The Mudaliar Committee (Report of the Health Survey and Planning Committee, 1962) emphasized the necessity for restructuring healthcare delivery with greater roles for auxiliary and paramedical professionals, resulting in better use of doctors and nurses, in 1962, after acknowledging the scarcity of clinicians. Even after 50 years, the advice is still relevant for public health reforms in India since paramedics may save costs and improve service quality. The key to India's health sector reforms is a better understanding and usage of the full spectrum of abilities provided by these paraprofessionals, also known as Allied Health Professionals (AHPs), particularly in light of the nation's acute scarcity of physicians and nurses.

Over the last few decades, many new health vocations (physician assistants, nurse practitioners, certified nurses) have evolved to take over some of the work that doctors previously performed. In addition to becoming deskilled, the work is increasingly being done without the doctor's or physician's oversight as other professionals pursue their own identities and autonomy. AHPs can often do the same tasks just as successfully and efficiently for patients who must use them, according to controlled research, but managers who are continually looking for lower labor costs have backed these systems. Instead of "physician extender" or "physician assistant," the phrase "AHP" is used, which shows the development of this occupational division of labor.

Consumers of services are becoming more powerful as a result of health consumerism, which has enhanced information accessibility and user involvement in service design and delivery. The roles of the present professional groups may be affected by each of these factors, which makes the task of workforce planners more challenging. Many of the allied health programs that India's medical education system offers are not known to students. Their parents and classmates, who are not aware of the potential in this profession, frequently have an impact on the jobs they choose. By understanding that an entry-level profession is merely the first step, young people may realistically plan for their future and have a better understanding of what is necessary for long-term success. This tactic benefits employers who need a steady supply of labor as well.

All areas of social and public health care utilize AHPs. They typically provide the cross-border fusion necessary to provide patients and their caregivers with expedited care, creating a social solidarity paradigm. Thanks to some places where they offer open access to their services, AHPs are able to respond quickly to patient needs in therapeutic domains where locating a general practitioner (GP) or consultant always takes longer. Comparable services created using a consultant physician approach are significantly more costly than AHP-led services. They assist in providing tailored care while dealing with juvenile offenders, the elderly, cancer patients, and people with long-term illnesses like diabetes.

AHPs play a critical role in the treatment of persons with disabilities, such as amputees, those who have vision problems, and others. AHPs are essential to the treatment of individuals with mental and emotional health issues as well as their return to wellness. The assistance of AHPs significantly speeds up rehabilitation and returns to normal life for some patients, such as stroke survivors. The aforementioned table of AHP functions does not take into account the various patient populations and potential beneficiaries who gain from the tailored treatment delivered by AHPs. The role of the AHP has changed in terms of knowledge and expertise as medical care has evolved and become more specialized.

4.2 CLASSIFICATION OF ALLIED HEALTH PROFESSIONALS (AHP)

The two main groups of AHPs are technicians (assistants) and therapists/technologists. Technicians receive fewer than two years of schooling and are taught to carry out operations. Physical therapy assistants, medical laboratory technicians (MLT), radiographic technicians, occupational therapy assistants, recreation therapy assistants, and respiratory therapy technicians are some of the professionals who operate under the direction of technologists or therapists. On the other hand, therapists or technologists learn to evaluate patients, diagnose problems, devise suitable treatment plans by weighing probable side effects, ascertain therapy responses, and make suitable judgments.

1. **Para-Professional** – These are community volunteers who are not part of a formal organization. The community and the local self-government provide these volunteers with training and some type of recognition. This concept was used to attract traditional birth attendants and community health volunteers/guides. Such

programs are being started by many state governments, including Madhya Pradesh and Chhattisgarh, in numerous locations. A method is required to impartially assess their viability and effectiveness while maintaining community control.

2. **Paramedical** – They are linked to therapeutic, promotional, and preventative medical interventions. They consist of various types of nurses, social welfare/extension workers, pharmacists, computer professionals, and various types of technicians (such as laboratory X-ray technicians, ophthalmic assistants, and physiotherapists). Additionally, both male and female multifunctional employees Auxiliary Nurse and Midwife (ANM) exist.
3. **Peri-Medical** – They include group C employees (clerks, accountants, storekeepers, ward masters), general duty assistants, sweepers, and non-medical technical hands. They could be crucial in both curative and preventative treatments.

4.3 ROLE OF ALLIED HEALTH PROFESSIONALS (AHP)

A variety of tasks are performed by AHPs, including those in early intervention, health promotion, and assistance for people with chronic diseases, disabilities, and palliative care. Since the beginning of colonialism, mid-level practitioners (MLPs) have provided treatment to indigenous communities.

Currently, they work with experts or provide treatment on their own, especially in places where there aren't enough or no professionals like therapists, physicians, dentists, pharmacists, or nurses. AHPs offer services in health centers, primary, secondary, and tertiary care settings, as well as in urban and rural locations. An AHP must possess a variety of abilities in order to provide patients with specialized treatment. There is a need for specialized care provided by various members of the allied health team, including physiotherapists, OTs, SLPs, podiatrists, psychologists, and dieticians, to name a few. Non-communicable diseases like heart disease, stroke, cerebral palsy, and developmental disorders are on the rise. As a result, an AHP's function within the interdisciplinary team is flexible and is expected to grow with time.

The age range of human development from neonate to old age; working with people who have complex and difficult problems resulting from multisystem illnesses; working toward health promotion and injury prevention; and the assessment, management, and evaluation of interventions; working in a wide range of settings from the patient's home to acute, primary, and critical care settings; are all included in the breadth and scope of allied health practice, having knowledge of the medical problems caused by various cultures in society.

4.4 THE SITUATION IN INDIA

India has a large and diversified pool of health human resources. They range from a variety of community- and household-based healers to highly qualified biomedical professionals and super specialists. Qualified allopathic or contemporary biomedical physicians, a variety of paramedical professionals, policymakers, social workers, researchers, health educators, promoters, and technicians make up half of this workforce. The second part is rich in India's ancient medical practices.

The need for AHPs has skyrocketed as a result of these facts, as well as to keep up with the development of new diagnostic and treatment approaches and the advancement of medical knowledge. This led to the creation of several schools and centers that teach these professionals, many of which lack oversight and control over the educational standards and quality. Given the significant role AHPs play in the delivery of healthcare, maintaining suitable standards for their education and training is critical. On the other hand, since 1949, the private healthcare industry has risen rapidly in the nation, now accounting for 93% of hospitals and 85% of physicians in India. Therefore, it is vital to regulate these professions by establishing councils similar to those for nursing, pharmacy, and other professions. The Government of India suggested the creation of separate councils in 2007 for physiotherapists/OTs, radiology technicians, and MLTs. These councils would be in charge of registering competent individuals to practice their professions as well as maintaining standardized levels of education in the relevant disciplines.

The Ministry of Health and Family Welfare (MoHFW), India, informed the Parliamentary Standing Committee on Health and Family Welfare of the circumstances that necessitated the firming up of a Bill to establish the new council. The following issues were identified as needing legislation as soon as possible: The level of knowledge and skills is not uniform because training periods vary from place to place and are not consistent, course curricula are not consistent, fee structures are not regulated, facilities are not regulated in these institutions, and ethical standards are not consistent and are not enforced.

The government groups allied health services, ambulance services, and alternative health services (systems of medicine) together in its many policy documents on AHPs. Although a paramedic is not specifically defined in the Indian Public Health Standards (IPHS), the contents suggest that two categories of functionaries are included: those who directly contribute to the delivery of healthcare to patients and those who maintain the medical facilities. The Himachal Pradesh Paramedical Council Act and the Madhya Pradesh Paramedical Council Act, both approved in 2003, apply to medical practitioners who practice traditional systems of medicine (Ayurveda, Unani, or Homeopathy), each of which is governed by a different council at the national level.

Practitioners in these states must register with both councils since both federal and state laws apply to these professions. "An ECG technician, Electroencephalographic (EEG) technician, EMG technician, X-ray technician, MLT, or ophthalmic assistant, and includes such other technicians as may be specified and notified by the government as paramedical technicians from time to time," according to the Kerala Paramedical Council Bill.

The healthcare sector in India consists of hospitals, telemedicine, clinical trials, medical equipment and gadgets, health insurance, and medical tourism. As the middle class expands and an older population increasingly chooses preventative healthcare, these market sectors are projected to diversify. Furthermore, there is a growing need for specialist care services in metropolitan areas due to the prevalence of lifestyle disorders such as high cholesterol, high blood pressure, obesity, poor diet, and alcohol usage.

Along with these demographic and epidemiological trends, COVID-19 is likely to spark long-lasting changes in how people think about their own personal cleanliness, health insurance, fitness, and diet, as well as health monitoring and regular doctor visits. The spread of the epidemic has also increased the uptake of telemedicine and other digital technologies.

In India's healthcare industry, there is also an increasing focus on and introduction of Public-Private Partnership models. Medical Value Tourism is becoming more and more popular due to the nation's relative cost competitiveness and availability of trained workers.

4.5 PROFESSIONAL DEVELOPMENT AND ADVANCEMENT

In the field of allied health sciences (AHS) are crucial for staying competitive, improving patient care, and advancing your career. Whether you're a student, a recent graduate, or an experienced AHP, here are some strategies to help you achieve professional growth and advancement:

4.5.1 EDUCATION AND CERTIFICATION

Continue your education: Pursue advanced degrees, certifications, or specialized training in your area of interest within AHSs. This can open up new career opportunities and increase your expertise. Stay up-to-date: Allied health fields often evolve with new research and technologies. Attend workshops, seminars, conferences, and online courses to stay current in your field.

4.5.2 NETWORKING

Join professional organizations: Becoming a member of organizations like the American Association of Medical Assistants (AAMA) or the American Society of Radiologic Technologists (ASRT) can provide networking opportunities and access to resources. Attend conferences and workshops: These events offer opportunities to connect with peers, mentors, and potential employers. Networking can lead to job openings and career advice.

4.5.3 CLINICAL EXPERIENCE

Gain diverse experience: Seek out opportunities to work in different clinical settings or with various patient populations. This can make you more versatile and attractive to employers. Seek mentorship: Find experienced professionals who can guide you in your career. Mentors can provide valuable insights and help you navigate challenges.

4.5.4 SPECIALIZATION

Consider specialization: Many allied health professions have specialized areas, such as pediatric nursing or sports medicine. Specialization can make you more marketable and potentially lead to higher-paying roles.

Obtain specialized certifications: Earning certifications in your chosen specialization can demonstrate your expertise to employers and patients.

4.5.5 RESEARCH AND PUBLICATIONS

Engage in research: Contributing to research in your field can enhance your credibility and open up opportunities in academia or leadership roles. Publish articles or present findings: Sharing your research through publications or presentations at conferences can establish you as an expert in your area.

4.5.6 LEADERSHIP AND MANAGEMENT

Develop leadership skills: Pursue leadership training and roles within your organization. Leadership skills are often highly valued in allied health professions. Consider management roles: Advancing to supervisory or managerial positions can offer increased responsibilities and higher salaries.

4.5.7 CONTINUING EDUCATION CREDITS

Keep up with CE requirements: Many allied health professions require ongoing continuing education to maintain certification. Ensure you meet these requirements to remain employable.

4.5.8 SOFT SKILLS

Improve communication skills: Effective communication with patients and colleagues is vital. Enhancing your interpersonal skills can help you stand out in your profession. Develop problem-solving skills: The ability to think critically and solve complex problems is essential in healthcare.

4.5.9 JOB SEARCH AND CAREER PLANNING

Set clear career goals: Define your long-term career objectives and create a plan to achieve them. Utilize job search resources: Leverage job boards, professional networks, and career services to find job openings and career opportunities.

4.5.10 WORK-LIFE BALANCE

Maintain a healthy work-life balance: Burnout is common in healthcare. Prioritize self-care and maintain a balance between your personal and professional life. Remember that professional development is an ongoing process, and staying adaptable and willing to learn is key to advancing in the AHSs. Continuously assess your goals and make adjustments to your professional development plan as needed to achieve them.

Professional development and career advancement in physiotherapy (PT), also known as physical therapy in some regions, require a commitment to ongoing learning, skill development, and professional networking. Here are some key strategies for achieving growth and advancement in the field of PT:

1. **Specialized Certifications:** Seek out certifications in areas of interest or specialization, such as sports therapy, pediatric care, geriatric care, or orthopedics.
2. **Continuing Education:** Stay current with the latest research, techniques, and technologies by attending workshops, seminars, and conferences. Complete continuing education requirements to maintain your licensure or certification.
3. **Networking:** Join professional organizations like the American Physical Therapy Association (APTA) or regional PT associations. These organizations offer networking opportunities, resources, and access to the latest industry developments. Attend local and national PT conferences to connect with colleagues and potential mentors.
4. **Clinical Experience:** Seek opportunities to work in different clinical settings, such as hospitals, rehabilitation centers, sports clinics, or private practices, to gain a broad range of experience. Consider volunteering for mission trips or humanitarian work to diversify your experience.
5. **Specialization:** Choose a specific area of interest within PT and become an expert in that field. Specialization can lead to more specialized and higher-paying roles. Pursue advanced certifications related to your chosen specialization.

6. **Research and Publications:** Engage in research projects related to PT and aim to publish your findings in journals or present them at conferences. This can enhance your reputation and career opportunities. Collaborate with academic institutions or research centers on research initiatives.
7. **Leadership and Management:** Develop leadership skills by taking on roles like lead therapist, clinic manager, or supervisor. Consider pursuing a career path in management, which can lead to higher-paying administrative positions.
8. **Mentorship:** Find experienced physiotherapists who can mentor you in your career. A mentor can provide guidance, advice, and support as you work toward your professional goals.
9. **Teaching and Education:** Consider becoming a clinical instructor or adjunct professor at a physical therapy program to share your expertise with future physiotherapists. Pursue teaching opportunities through workshops, seminars, or online courses.
10. **Job Search and Career Planning:** Set clear career goals and regularly reassess them. Create a plan to achieve these goals, including the steps you need to take and the timeline for achieving them. Utilize job search resources like online job boards, professional networks, and career services to explore job openings and career opportunities.
11. **Soft Skills:** Improve communication skills, as effective communication with patients and colleagues is vital in PT. Develop strong problem-solving abilities and critical thinking skills to provide optimal patient care.
12. **Work-Life Balance:** Maintain a healthy work-life balance to prevent burnout. Balancing your personal life with your professional commitments is essential for long-term success.

Remember that the field of PT is dynamic, and staying adaptable and up-to-date with the latest developments is crucial for your professional growth and advancement. Continuously seek opportunities for learning and improvement to excel in your career.

4.6 LABORATORY TECHNOLOGY

4.6.1 EDUCATION AND CERTIFICATION

Pursue a bachelor's degree in medical laboratory science or a related field. Some roles may require a master's degree for advanced positions. Obtain relevant certifications, such as MLS or MLT, which may be required or preferred by employers.

4.6.2 CONTINUING EDUCATION

Stay up-to-date with advancements in laboratory technology by attending workshops, seminars, and conferences. Complete continuing education requirements to maintain your certification.

4.6.3 NETWORKING

Join professional organizations like the American Society for Clinical Laboratory Science (ASCLS) to access resources, network with peers, and stay informed about industry developments.

4.6.4 SPECIALIZATION

Consider specializing in a specific area of laboratory science, such as clinical chemistry, hematology, microbiology, or genetics. Specialization can lead to higher-paying roles. Pursue advanced certifications or specialized training related to your chosen specialization.

4.6.5 RESEARCH AND PUBLICATIONS

Engage in research projects within your laboratory or collaborate with researchers in your institution. Aim to publish your findings in scientific journals or present them at conferences to enhance your professional reputation.

4.6.6 LEADERSHIP AND MANAGEMENT

Develop leadership skills by taking on supervisory or management roles within your laboratory or department. Consider pursuing a career path in laboratory management, which can lead to higher-level administrative positions.

4.6.7 MENTORSHIP

Seek out experienced laboratory professionals who can mentor you in your career. A mentor can provide valuable guidance and support.

4.6.8 SOFT SKILLS

Effective communication, problem-solving, and teamwork are crucial in laboratory technology. Work on improving these skills to excel in your role.

4.7 FORENSIC SCIENCES

4.7.1 EDUCATION AND TRAINING

Obtain at least a bachelor's degree in forensic science, biology, chemistry, or a related field. Pursue advanced degrees or specialized training for career advancement.

4.7.2 CERTIFICATIONS AND LICENSURE

Depending on your role in forensic science, certifications may be required or advantageous. Examples include certifications in forensic photography, latent print examination, or digital forensics. Some forensic scientists may require licensure in certain jurisdictions.

4.7.3 NETWORKING AND PROFESSIONAL ORGANIZATIONS

Join organizations like the American Academy of Forensic Sciences (AAFS) for networking opportunities and access to the latest research. Attend forensic science conferences and seminars to meet professionals in the field and stay updated on developments.

4.7.4 INTERNSHIPS AND FELLOWSHIPS

Seek out internships or fellowships with forensic laboratories, law enforcement agencies, or government organizations to gain practical experience.

4.7.5 CONTINUING EDUCATION

Stay current with advancements in forensic science through ongoing training and workshops.

4.7.6 SPECIALIZATION

Consider specializing in a specific area of forensic science, such as forensic biology, forensic chemistry, digital forensics, or forensic anthropology.

4.8 NUTRITION AND DIETETICS

4.8.1 EDUCATION AND CERTIFICATION

Complete a bachelor's degree in nutrition and dietetics or a related field. Pursue dietetic internship programs accredited by the Accreditation Council for Education in Nutrition and Dietetics (ACEND). Obtain the Registered Dietitian Nutritionist (RDN) credential by passing the Registration Examination for Dietitians.

4.8.2 CONTINUING EDUCATION

Stay informed about the latest research, dietary guidelines, and nutritional therapies by completing continuing education requirements. Pursue advanced degrees, such as a Master's in Nutrition, to specialize in specific areas.

4.8.3 PROFESSIONAL ORGANIZATIONS

Join associations like the Academy of Nutrition and Dietetics (AND) to access resources, networking opportunities, and career support.

4.8.4 SPECIALIZATION

Consider specializing in areas like clinical nutrition, sports nutrition, pediatric nutrition, or gerontology. Obtain additional certifications, such as Certified Diabetes Educator (CDE) or Certified Specialist in Sports Dietetics (CSSD), to enhance your expertise.

4.8.5 RESEARCH AND PUBLICATIONS

Engage in research projects related to nutrition and dietetics and consider publishing your findings in professional journals.

4.8.6 CLINICAL EXPERIENCE

Gain diverse clinical experience in healthcare settings, including hospitals, private practices, and community health programs.

4.8.7 LEADERSHIP AND MANAGEMENT

Develop leadership skills for roles like clinical nutrition manager or director of nutrition services in healthcare organizations.

Remember that professional development is an ongoing process in all three fields. Continuously seek opportunities for learning and improvement to excel in your career and advance to higher-level positions.

KEYWORDS

- **AHP**
- **cerebral palsy**
- **developmental disorders**
- **multisystem illnesses**
- **non-communicable diseases**
- **physiotherapists**
- **podiatrists**
- **professional development**
- **psychologists**
- **speech-language pathologists**

REFERENCES

American Board of Physical Therapy Specialties. (2023). *Specialist Certification.*

Canadian Physiotherapy Association. (2023). *Specialization.* Retrieved from: https://physiotherapy.ca/ (accessed on 14 March 2025).

Dal Poz, M. R., Kinfu, Y., Dräger, S., & Kunjumen, T. (2007). *Counting Health Workers: Definitions, Data, Methods, and Global Results.* Geneva: Department for Human Resource for Health, World Health Organization.

Expert Committee on Health Manpower. (1987). *Health Manpower: Planning, Production, and Management.* Retrieved from: http://nrhm-mis.nic.in/ui/who/PDF/ (accessed on 14 March 2025).

Himachal Pradesh Paramedical Council Act, 2003. (2003). *24.*

Investment Opportunities in India's Healthcare Sector. (2021).

Kerala Paramedical Council Bill. (2002). Retrieved from: http://www.keralalawsect.org/law_cms/index.php/law-reforms-committee/132 (accessed on 14 March 2025).

Madhya Pradesh Paramedical Council Bill. (2004). Retrieved from: http://www.prsindia.org/uploads/ (accessed on 14 March 2025).

Mudaliar Committee. (1962). *Report of the Health Survey and Planning Committee* (Vol. I). Retrieved from: http://nihfw.org/NDC/Documentation Services/Reports/Mudalier Vol.pdf (accessed on 14 March 2025).

National Initiative for Allied Health Sciences. (2012). *A Study to Augment the Capacity and Quality of Allied Health Professionals in India.* Report commissioned by the Ministry of Health and Family Welfare, Government of India. Retrieved from: https://main.mohfw.gov.in/sites/default/files/NIAHS%20Report.pdf (accessed on 14 March 2025).

Sahni, A. (n.d.). Production and utilization of health manpower towards improvement of health services in India. *Health Administrator, XVII*(1), 1–4.

Saxon, R. L., Gray, M. A., & Oprescu, F. I. (2014). Extended roles for allied health professionals: An updated systematic review of the evidence. *Journal of Multidisciplinary Healthcare, 7*, 479–488.

Sequeira, R., & Nayar, U. (n.d.). *Faculty Development in Medical Education: International Perspectives.* Retrieved from: http://www.ncme.in/ppt-pdf-doc/ (accessed on 14 March 2025).

Snell, R., Fyfe, S., Fyfe, G., Blackwood, D., & Itsiopoulos, C. (2020). Development of professional identity and professional socialization in allied health students: A scoping review. *Focus on Health Professional Education: A Multi-Professional Journal, 21*, 29–56.

Summary report for medical records and health information technicians. (n.d.). Retrieved from: http://www.onetonline.org/ (accessed on 14 March 2025).

Thirty-first report on paramedical and physiotherapy central councils bill. (2007). Retrieved from: http://www.physiotherapyindia.org (accessed on 14 March 2025).

PART II

Basic Knowledge and Skills for Allied Health Professionals

CHAPTER 5

Overview of Human Anatomy and Physiology

HIBA AHMAD,* RAJESH YADAV,* and RAHAMATUN NISHA

Sharda School of Allied Health Sciences, Sharda University, Greater Noida, Uttar Pradesh, India

*Corresponding author

ABSTRACT

In the dynamic landscape of healthcare, Allied Health Professionals (AHPs) play a pivotal role in providing comprehensive and patient-centered care. At the core of their expertise lies a profound understanding of human anatomy and physiology, serving as the bedrock for informed decision-making, precise diagnostics, and effective treatment strategies. This chapter delves into the significance of a robust knowledge base in human anatomy and physiology for AHPs, exploring how this foundation contributes to the overall quality of healthcare services. The understanding of human physiology and anatomy plays a major role in the field of allied health science (AHS). Without the understanding of anatomy and physiology, it is very difficult to make radiodiagnoses. Anatomy is the basis of CT scans and MRIs, which play a crucial role in the diagnostic process for various neurological and other diseases. Physiology and anatomy provide information on how medicine performs its actions, how it binds with receptors, and how it achieves its goals inside the body. Physiology is the platform for various paramedical courses running in medical colleges. The chapter covers the requisite knowledge of each and every system and provides the significance of human physiology and anatomy in everyday life.

Allied Healthcare in Practice: An Introduction to Integrated Patient Care. Sally Lukose, Karuna Singh (Eds.)

DOI: 10.1201/9781998511037-7

5.1 INTRODUCTION OF ANATOMY AND PHYSIOLOGY

Human anatomy and physiology are two separate branches of medical sciences. Human anatomy is the study of the internal structure of various tissues, including blood supply, anatomical structure, and different compositions of tissues, while physiology covers the external structure of different physiological systems and their mechanisms (Aguilar and Ludwig, 2022). Human physiology includes various systems such as the digestive system, endocrine system, respiratory system, nervous system, musculoskeletal system, sensory system, circulatory system, excretory system, and reproductive system, which coordinate with each other to regulate homeostasis. The kidney is the main excretory organ in the human body, which participates in removing various kinds of acids from the body and maintaining the pH of tissues. The hypothalamus is one of the crucial areas of the brain that controls temperature, thirst, and hunger, and maintaining a constant temperature of the human body is an important part of homeostasis.

The study of neurons in different areas of the brain and spinal cord is included in the nervous system. The study of digestion in different areas of the alimentary canal falls under the digestive system. The special nervous system that connects the digestive system to the central nervous system (CNS) of the brain is called the enteric nervous system. In this way, every system of the body is connected to the nervous system via either the CNS or the peripheral nervous system. Knowledge of physiology and anatomy helps to solve the various mysteries associated with physiological disorders in the human body and provides assistance in understanding the pathology of diseases. Physiology and anatomy are the backbone of medical science, which supports the understanding of the mechanisms of physiological phenomena. It also reports how anomalies and physiological disturbances relate to biological and physical illness symptoms (Van et al., 1990). Anatomy is broadly classified into macroscopic (gross) anatomy, developmental anatomy, and microscopic anatomy, which is further subdivided and shown in Figure 5.1.

Before understanding physiology, we should understand the functional and structural organization of the human body. We start at the most fundamental level—the chemical level—and work our way up to cells, tissues, organs, and organ systems.

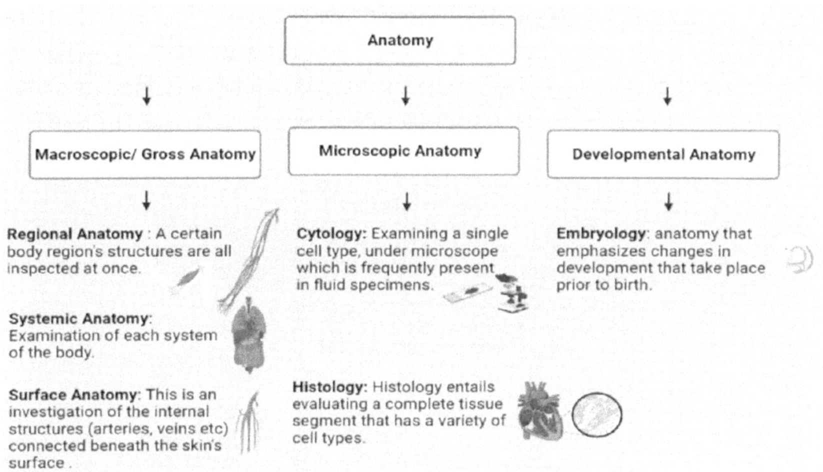

FIGURE 5.1 Classification of anatomy: Gross anatomy, microscopic anatomy, and developmental anatomy.

Source: Created with BioRender.com.

5.2 STRUCTURAL AND FUNCTIONAL ORGANIZATION OF HUMAN BODY

The human body constituents are divided into organic and inorganic ions at the chemical level. Inorganic ions include calcium, magnesium, sodium, potassium, and hydrogen, which are the most important constituents of extracellular fluid (ECF) and cerebrospinal fluid (CSF). Water is also the most copious and crucial component of cells, as it is a major part of cytoplasm and other body fluids. Sodium and potassium ions maintain osmotic balance between the nerve and cell cytoplasm. Sodium ions maintain blood pressure in the human body and are also responsible for the nerve conduction mechanism along with potassium ions. Organic constituents are made up of carbon, hydrogen, and oxygen, along with nitrogen, which form proteins, carbohydrates, lipids, and nucleic acids (DNA and RNA).

At the cellular level, a cell is the smallest structural as well as functional element of living things. The chief component of a cell is the nucleus, which contains Deoxyribonucleic acid (DNA) and other nuclear proteins that command the whole cell, along with the transportation of proteins in and out of the nucleus. The other constituents of a cell are mitochondria, the Golgi body, the endoplasmic reticulum, the plasma membrane, ribosomes, cytoplasm, microfilaments, microtubules, and others. These cell organelles are the functional components of the cell that perform various functions. Cells collectively form tissues at different locations in the body, so on the basis of similar structures and functions, tissues can be classified as epithelial tissue, connective tissue, muscular tissue, and nerve tissue (Figure 5.2).

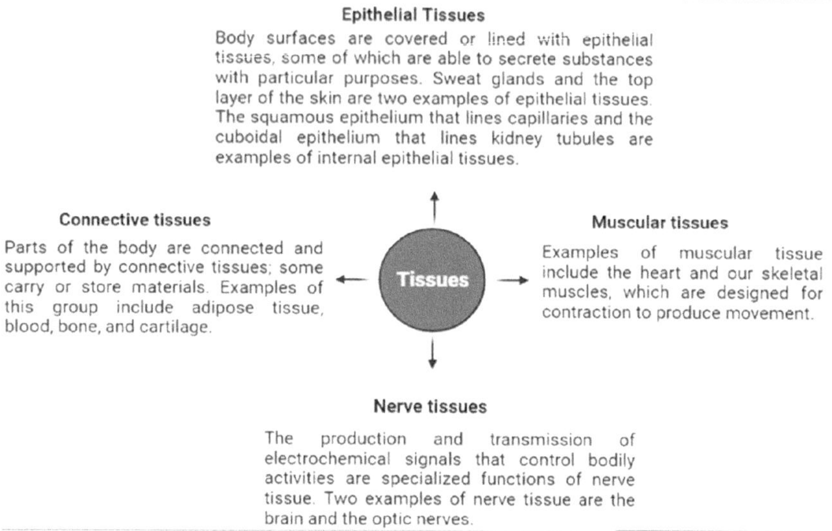

FIGURE 5.2 Classification of tissues: Epithelial tissues, connective tissues, muscular tissues and nerve tissues.

Source: Created with BioRender.com.

A collection of tissues that are carefully organized to perform particular responsibilities is called an organ. The liver, heart, lungs, stomach, individual bones, and kidneys are a few such organs. Collection of organs that participate together to provide a single function is called organ system. The respiratory system, circulatory system, gastrointestinal system, nervous system, musculoskeletal system, reproductive system and urinary systems and sensory system are example of organ system. Various system that works together inside body are described:

5.3 DIGESTIVE SYSTEM

The human digestive system comprises the gastrointestinal tract (GIT) along with the accessory organs that help in digestion. The accessory organs include the tongue, salivary glands, liver, gallbladder, and pancreas. Digestion is the breakdown of large insoluble food molecules into small water-soluble food molecules so that they can be absorbed into the watery blood plasma.

Three pairs of salivary glands are found in humans, which secrete saliva in the buccal cavity. Saliva contains the ptyalin enzyme (salivary amylase), which is responsible for the partial digestion of carbohydrates present in food. Saliva contains lysozyme enzyme and mucin (MUC) along with potassium bicarbonate. The lysozyme enzyme kills bacteria present in food by creating holes in the cell wall (peptidoglycan) of bacteria. Bicarbonates produce a slight alkaline medium in the buccal cavity. The food mixed with saliva is called bolus, and the bolus moves through the esophagus and comes to the stomach, where HCl acid is secreted from oxyntic cells/parietal cells of the oxyntic gland. HCl produces an acidic medium in the stomach, which is crucial for the digestion of protein and also kills microorganisms remaining in food.

The human stomach can be divided into various regions: the cardia, fundus, body, and pyloric region. The corpus or body of the stomach comprises D cells, which secrete somatostatin; enterochromaffin-like cells (ECL), which secrete histamine; EC cells, which secrete serotonin; X cells, which secrete ghrelin; chief cells; and parietal cells. The antral region contains G cells (gastrin), D cells, ECL cells, EC cells, and deep mucous cells (MUC6, TFF2). In the stomach, there are two types of glands present: one is the oxyntic gland, and the other is the pyloric gland. The oxyntic gland comprises chief cells, oxyntic cells, and mucous neck cells. Chief cells secrete the pepsinogen enzyme, which converts into pepsin with the help of HCl and is responsible for protein digestion (Guyton and Hall, 2015). Oxyntic cells produce intrinsic factor along with hydrochloric acid (HCL); intrinsic factor helps with vitamin B12 absorption. Mucous neck cells secrete MUC, which is glycoprotein in nature and acts as a lubricant in the GIT. The pyloric gland secretes mucus and the gastrin hormone, which regulates HCL secretion. Gastrin stimulates ECL cells, which secrete histamine, which further stimulates oxyntic cells to secrete HCl.

The vagal neuron of the enteric nervous system stimulates G cells by gastrin-releasing peptide (GRP) and acetylcholine and stimulates ECL for histamine secretion. The acetylcholine neurotransmitter inhibits somatostatin release from D cells of the stomach and promotes more acid secretion. Somatostatin acts as a negative regulator of gastrin and inhibits gastrin release from the antral region. Oxyntic cells also produce apelin, which employs regulatory effects on ECL cells. Histamine acts as a negative feedback mechanism and reduces ECL cell activity (Engevik et al., 2020).

After protein digestion in the stomach, food enters the small intestine. The small intestine encompasses three parts: the duodenum, jejunum, and ileum. The wall of the small intestine acts as an endocrine gland and secretes cholecystokinin, secretin, and pancreozymin. Cholecystokinin (CCK) was discovered by Ivy and Oldberg in 1928 in dogs (Rodger, 2003). CCK (33 amino acids) hormone secreted from I cells of the duodenum stimulates the pancreas and liver for pancreatic juice and bile juice, while secretin (27 amino acids) secreted from S cells of the duodenum stimulates the secretion of copious quantities of bicarbonate ions for the neutralization of acidic stomach chyme. CCK-8 and CCK-58 both stimulate the pancreas to secrete digestive enzymes, but only CCK-58 stimulates pancreatic juice (Travis et al., 2013). Pancreatic juice reaches the small intestine through the pancreatic duct, while bile juice secreted by the liver first concentrates in the gallbladder and then comes into the small intestine via the common bile duct. Bile juice comprises bile pigments and bile salts, which help with the emulsification of fat.

Pancreatic juice comprises trypsinogen, chymotrypsinogen, and procarboxypeptidase for protein digestion, as well as amylase and lipase for carbohydrate and fat digestion. The pancreas also secretes a large quantity of bicarbonate ions, which produce an alkaline medium in the small intestine where the precursors of enzymes are converted into their active forms, facilitating digestion. Trypsinogen is converted into trypsin with the help of the enterokinase enzyme, while chymotrypsinogen is converted into chymotrypsin by the trypsin enzyme. The Brunner's gland also secretes a large amount of bicarbonate solution in the small intestine. In the small intestine, a large number of microvilli are present, which aid in the absorption of food and water. In this way, the complete digestion of carbohydrates, lipids, and proteins occurs in the small intestine. After complete digestion, food enters the large intestine, which comprises the cecum, colon, and rectum. In the cecum, a huge number of symbiotic bacteria are available for the digestion of cellulose. The colon has three parts: the ascending colon, transverse colon, and descending colon, which are responsible for water absorption through haustra, and undigested material exits the body through the rectum. The GIT and its accessory glands are our initial line of defense against foreign substances and infections of all kinds since xenobiotics typically enter the body through food (Gelberg et al., 2014).

AHPs employ their comprehensive knowledge of the digestive system to play pivotal roles in diverse aspects of patient care. Dietitians and nutritionists draw upon their understanding of digestive processes to offer personalized dietary guidance, tailoring recommendations for optimal nutrient absorption while addressing conditions like celiac disease or inflammatory bowel disorders. In diagnostic roles, radiographers, and sonographers utilize their expertise to perform and interpret imaging studies, aiding in the identification of gastrointestinal issues such as obstructions or tumors. Physiotherapists, recognizing the interconnectedness of bodily systems, design rehabilitation programs that consider the impact of digestive conditions on patients' overall health, incorporating exercises to enhance core strength and mobility. Medical laboratory technicians analyze diagnostic tests related to the digestive system, providing valuable insights into conditions affecting organs like the liver and pancreas. Pharmacists, integral to patient education, impart knowledge on medications affecting the digestive tract, addressing potential side effects and advising on lifestyle modifications. This interdisciplinary approach underscores the integral role AHPs play in enhancing digestive health, contributing to accurate diagnostics, patient education, rehabilitation, and surgical interventions. Through their multifaceted contributions, AHPs significantly impact the quality of care for individuals with digestive system disorders, embodying the importance of their anatomical and physiological expertise in comprehensive healthcare delivery.

5.4 NERVOUS SYSTEM

The nervous system in humans is divided into the central and peripheral nervous systems. The CNS contains the brain and spinal cord, while the remaining body systems come under the peripheral nervous system. The brain is a crucial part of the nervous system, which contains billions of neurons. It comprises the forebrain or prosencephalon, midbrain or mesencephalon, and hindbrain or rhombencephalon. The forebrain has very crucial areas like the hypothalamus, basal ganglia, hippocampus, thalamus, and cerebral cortex. The midbrain comprises the auditory and balancing areas, while the hindbrain contains the pons, cerebellum, and medulla. The cerebral cortex is a highly important area of the forebrain, responsible for learning and reasoning. The brain's weight differs between men and women; the male brain weighs around 1300 grams, while the female brain weighs about 1200 grams. There are four lobes in the cortex: the frontal lobe, parietal lobe, temporal lobe, and occipital lobe (Jawabri et al., 2023). The cortex forms a major part of the brain, and the gyri and sulci found in the cortical region are responsible for intelligence. Different areas of the cerebral cortex have different functions. The cerebral cortex has four regions: the frontal lobe, temporal lobe, occipital lobe, and parietal lobe. The left and right cerebral cortices are connected by the corpus callosum. The left region of the cortex controls the right part of the body, while the right region controls the left part of the body.

Frontal lobe: In the frontal lobe, Broca's area is present; it is also called the speech area. Temporal lobe: Auditory area (ear) and smell area. Parietal lobe: Somatosensory area, pain, touch, and pressure. Occipital lobe: Visual area. The cerebral cortex comprises a large number of neurons (10^{10}), which are responsible for high-order cognitive processing in humans (David et al., 2002). The hippocampus is responsible for memory, while the hypothalamus contains areas for appetite, thirst, sexual reproduction, and sleep regulation. The preoptic area of the hypothalamus is a well-known area responsible for sleep and thermoregulation (Adamantidis et al., 2023; Boulant et al., 2000; Yadav et al., 2017). The ventromedial nucleus of the hypothalamus is the satiety center, which controls hunger along with the feeding center (Yadav et al., 2009). The basal ganglia maintain movements, and the thalamus is the relay center for information from the upper brain to the brainstem. The pons and medulla are regulatory centers for various physiological activities. The cerebellum, often called the mini-brain, contains more than 50% of the neurons in the brain and is responsible for locomotion.

The cerebellar cortex comprises various types of neurons: Purkinje, stellate, basket, Golgi, and granule cells. Except for granule cells, all are inhibitory neurons in nature. Afferent fibers to the cerebellar cortex are mossy and climbing fibers. They carry information from the cerebral cortex, brainstem, and other somatosensory, vestibular, acoustic, and visual origins. Purkinje neurons are the major neurons of the cerebellar cortex, which synapse with axons inside the deep nuclei of the brain. The axons of the cerebellar nuclei travel to the brainstem and thalamic relay nuclei (Delgado et al., 2001). Alcohol affects the cerebellum and causes toddler-like locomotion.

If any damage occurs in any part of the brain, it shows serious effects as very limited regeneration occurs in the brain. The hippocampus is the only area of the brain where axonal regeneration has been observed. People who have extensive damage on the medial undersides of both occipital lobes and along the medioventral surfaces of the temporal lobes are unable to recognize people, a condition called *prosopagnosia* (Barton et al., 2022). Some people are capable of understanding either the spoken word or the written word but are unable to interpret the thought that is expressed, which is called *Wernicke's Aphasia* (Levassort et al., 2022).

AHPs, like physiotherapists and occupational therapists (OT's), leverage their understanding of the nervous system to design rehabilitation programs tailored to individuals recovering from neurological injuries or conditions, promoting mobility and functional independence. Pharmacists and rehabilitation counselors educate patients on medications affecting the nervous system, addressing mechanisms of action and potential side effects. Meanwhile, radiographers and diagnostic medical sonographers use their expertise to interpret imaging studies like MRIs and CT scans, aiding in the visualization of brain and spinal structures for diagnoses ranging from tumors to traumatic injuries. Speech-language pathologists (SLP), specializing in neurological conditions affecting communication and swallowing, apply their knowledge to develop targeted interventions for individuals recovering from strokes or traumatic brain injuries.

5.5 MUSCULOSKELETAL SYSTEM

The musculoskeletal system includes the study of the muscle and skeletal systems. In the human body, three types of muscle are present: skeletal muscle, also called voluntary muscle, which is found all over the body; visceral muscle, which is involuntary and found in visceral organs like the lungs, liver, and kidneys; and cardiac muscle, which is specialized and found in the heart.

The skeletal and visceral muscles have actin and myosin fibers that slide past each other and are responsible for muscle contraction. Calcium is an important mineral for the muscle contraction process and Adenosine Triphosphate (ATP) formation. The actin filament is made up of F-actin, which has a double helical structure. G molecules, also called active sites, are covered by a spiral structure known as tropomyosin, along with troponin. One myosin filament is made up of 1000 molecules of myosin. Each myosin comprises two heavy chains and four light chains. The light chains form the head of the myosin, while the heavy chains form the body of the myosin. All light chains of myosin form cross-bridges, while all heavy chains form the body of myosin. The interaction of G molecules of actin and the cross-bridges of myosin filaments occurs during muscle contraction (Squire et al., 2019). The ATPase enzyme is utilized for the step called the power stroke. Cardiac muscle is unique as it contains gap junctions and well-developed T-tubules, which store mucopolysaccharides. The mucopolysaccharides have a negative charge that attracts calcium ions, resulting in more calcium being stored in the T-tubules. In cardiac muscle, the sarcoplasmic reticulum is less developed, which means it cannot store as much calcium, a limitation compensated for by the T-tubules during muscle contraction.

Depending on the axis and plane, there are various types of movements performed by the musculoskeletal system, such as (i) flexion and extension: bending and straightening the knee from a flexed position (Wilke et al., 2019); (ii) adduction and abduction: moving the arm away from the body and bringing it towards the body (Manzi et al., 2023); (iii) rotation: body parts rotate around the longitudinal axis in the transverse plane; and (iv) supination and pronation: supination is a lateral rotation of the forearm, while pronation is rolling the foot inwards (Soubeyrand et al., 2017).

This comprehensive understanding of the musculoskeletal system is utilized by physiotherapists to contribute significantly to patient care. They design rehabilitation programs tailored to musculoskeletal conditions, emphasizing exercises and therapies that enhance mobility, strength, and function. OT's collaborate with individuals recovering from injuries or surgeries, devising strategies to regain independence in daily activities by considering the impact of musculoskeletal health. Physiotherapists specializing in the orthopedic domain work alongside orthopedic surgeons, specializing in the application of casts, braces, and other orthopedic devices to support musculoskeletal healing.

Radiographers and diagnostic medical sonographers utilize their expertise in musculoskeletal anatomy to perform and interpret imaging studies such as X-rays, CT scans, and MRIs. This aids in the diagnosis of conditions affecting bones, joints, and soft tissues, informing treatment plans and surgical interventions. The integration of musculoskeletal knowledge across AHP specialties highlights its foundational role in promoting optimal musculoskeletal health and overall well-being.

5.6 CIRCULATORY SYSTEM

The circulatory system is a system of organs that comprises the heart, blood vessels, and blood, which is circulated throughout the entire body of a human or other vertebrate. The heart pumps oxygenated blood throughout the body via arteries and collects deoxygenated blood via veins. Blood contains cells including RBCs, WBCs, and platelets, along with plasma containing various proteins such as albumin and globulin (Hammond et al., 1982). RBCs carry oxygen via hemoglobin in circulation and deliver oxygen to every cell of the body, including the brain, while WBCs protect us against various pathogens, microorganisms, parasites, bacteria, viruses, and fungi, and maintain the immune system. Platelets are responsible for blood coagulation and protect us in trauma and injury through a blood clotting mechanism known as the intrinsic and extrinsic pathways to prevent excessive bleeding (Levi et al., 2010). Collectively, hematopoiesis is the phenomenon of blood formation from pluripotent hematopoietic stem cells (PHSCs). Erythropoiesis is the formation of RBCs from stem cells. HPSCs are found in the red bone marrow of long bones and produce RBCs. The erythropoietin hormone enhances the level of RBCs in hypoxic conditions, which is released from the kidney (90%) and liver (10%). Vitamin C, B12, B6, along with other growth hormones, interleukins, and minerals such as iron and calcium, are also required for the biosynthesis of RBCs. PHSCs are being used in the clinical implantation of stem cells in diseased individuals. Lajtha and McCulloch defined PHSCs as having extensive proliferative potential to differentiate into all types of blood cells. The properties of PHSCs, such as self-renewal and long-term repopulation, have been observed *in vitro* and *in vivo* studies, including in human recipients (Orlic, 1994). Proteins in blood maintain osmotic balance.

In humans, circulation is termed double circulation, as blood passes two times in one cardiac cycle through the heart. Through three large blood vessels called the superior vena cava, inferior vena cava, and coronary sinus, deoxygenated blood enters the right atrium of the heart. It then enters the right ventricle (RV) through the tricuspid valve.

When the pressure in the RV increases, blood enters the pulmonary aorta and reaches the lungs, where blood purification occurs after gaseous exchange, resulting in oxygenated blood. This oxygenated blood travels into the left atrium through the pulmonary vein. Blood again enters the left ventricle via the bicuspid valve or mitral valve, and finally, blood goes into the whole body via the systemic aorta. In this way, blood flows two times in one circulation. Once the blood has been oxygenated in the lungs, the systemic circulation ensures that blood containing oxygen and nutrients reaches the rest of the body. The heart's function can be measured by ejection fraction (EF). EF is a measurement, expressed as a percentage, of how much blood the left ventricle pumps out with each contraction. It is calculated from the end-diastolic and end-systolic volumes of the left ventricle (Bamira et al., 2018): EF = (EDV – ESV) / EDV. For a healthy person, the EF is around 60%, while below 50% is an alarming situation, and below 40% is indicative of heart failure. However, it does not always indicate heart failure; it may indicate damage to heart function and cardiomyopathy. EF can be divided into two types. The first is preserved EF, which is also referred to as diastolic heart failure. In this situation, the heart muscle contracts normally, but the ventricles do not relax properly. The second is reduced EF, also called systolic heart failure. In this case, the heart muscle does not contract effectively, and therefore less oxygen-rich blood is pumped out to the body.

This circulatory system knowledge is utilized by the Radio imaging technologists and cardiovascular technologists to perform and interpret imaging studies such as echocardiograms and vascular USGs, providing critical information on the structure and function of the heart and blood vessels. This aids in the diagnosis of conditions like heart disease, blood clots, and vascular disorders.

Cardiac rehabilitation specialists, including physiotherapists and exercise physiologists, design programs to enhance cardiovascular health. They incorporate exercise regimens that target the circulatory system, improving heart function, and promoting overall cardiovascular fitness.

In surgical settings, the cardiovascular technologists also assist during cardiovascular surgeries, ensuring the operating room is well-prepared for procedures such as coronary artery bypass grafting or valve replacements hence ensuring a comprehensive care for individuals with circulatory system disorders, emphasizing diagnostics, rehabilitation, and patient education to promote cardiovascular health and overall well-being.

5.7 RESPIRATORY SYSTEM

The respiratory system is essential to survival because it enables an exchange of gases between a living being and its surroundings. The respiratory zone, which corresponds to the lung parenchyma, is composed of the pulmonary bronchioles, alveolar ducts, and alveoli. The two functional and structural divisions of the lower respiratory system, which is an organizational structure, comprise the conducting tract (airways) and the zone of respiration. The conducting tract, which includes the airways that move gases into and out of the lungs, is made up of the trachea, bronchi, and bronchioles. For the lungs to operate properly, the airways that carry air must be open to the respiratory zone, where the exchange of gases occurs (Carlos et al., 2012). The heart and lungs work together to transport this oxygen and get rid of waste products of metabolism. The respiratory system also maintains homeostasis by regulating the amount of oxygen and carbon dioxide in the blood. In the lungs, type II alveolar cells are found, which secrete surfactant that reduces surface tension at the site of gaseous exchange. The mechanism of respiration can be studied as inhalation and exhalation. During the inhalation process, the first contraction occurs in the diaphragm and internal intercostal muscles; as a result, the diaphragm moves downward and the rib cage moves upward. Consequently, the volume of the thoracic cavity increases. According to Boyle's law, at a fixed temperature, volume is reciprocal to pressure; therefore, the pressure in the lung alveoli decreases compared to atmospheric pressure, so air goes inside the lungs to fulfill the pressure. This procedure is called inspiration or inhalation. Again, after inhalation, diaphragm relaxation occurs and contraction occurs in the external intercostal muscles; as a result, the rib cage moves back down, and the diaphragm returns to its original position upward. Consequently, the volume of the thoracic cavity decreases, and the pressure inside the alveoli in the lungs increases, so air goes outside of the lungs. This process is termed exhalation.

Speech and the production of sound are also part of the respiratory system, which depends on three factors. The pitch of the sound depends on the length as well as the tightness of the vocal cords. As the vocal cords grow, the pitch of the voice becomes lower; for example, in males, the pitch of the voice is lower in adulthood. The second factor is volume, which depends on the force with which the vocal cords vibrate. If the force of the expired air is greater, vocal cord vibration enhances, and the loudness of the sound increases. The third factor is tone, which depends on the shape of the mouth, the position of the lips and tongue, facial muscles, and air in the paranasal sinuses.

The molecular mechanisms of lung development are still an enigma; very little knowledge is available regarding lung development. Stem cells and transit-amplifying (TA) cells are two different types of regenerative cells known in the lungs (Mason et al., 1997). Clara/secretory cells, pulmonary neuroendocrine cells, and basal cells have been identified in conducting airways and have characteristics of Transit-Amplifying Cell (TA cell). Clara cells are the chief TA cells of the rodent conducting airway epithelium. Clara cells are non-ciliated columnar to cuboidal secretory cells in the respiratory epithelium, which secrete a 10 kDa secretory protein. Clara cells in the lungs are the site of xenobiotic metabolism, which is P450 cytochrome-dependent (Evans et al., 1978; Reynolds et al., 2000). In Clara cells, 40% of the volume is occupied by smooth endoplasmic reticulum in humans, while in dogs and cats, cytoplasmic glycogen is a major component. Neuroepithelial bodies (NEBs) in the lungs contain regenerative cells that are responsible for bronchiolar regeneration after the depletion of selective Clara cells (Reynolds et al., 2000, 2009).

The Physiotherapists especially those specializing in Cardio-pulmonary physiotherapy (PT) utilize their in-depth knowledge of the respiratory system to provide optimal patient care. These professionals play a crucial role in the assessment, treatment, and management of respiratory conditions such as asthma, chronic obstructive pulmonary disease (COPD), or pneumonia. Based on different levels of assessments, these therapists develop and implement individualized treatment plans, which may include breathing exercises, inhalation therapy, and mechanical ventilation support.

In critical care settings, the therapists collaborate with multidisciplinary teams to manage patients on ventilators, ensuring proper oxygenation and ventilation. They also provide education to patients and their families on respiratory care techniques and disease management.

Additionally, these therapists are involved in pulmonary rehabilitation programs, helping individuals with chronic respiratory conditions improve their lung function, exercise tolerance, and improve overall quality of life.

5.8 EXCRETORY SYSTEM

The excretory system, an essential biological function, removes waste and surplus material from the body in order to maintain homeostasis. The bulk of these substances is used and broken down to remove metabolic wastes from the body through sweat, urine, or feces. The term "excretory system" refers to those structures that are utilized entirely for the removal and elimination of these broken-down components, even though many organs are indirectly engaged in the process of getting rid of metabolic waste. The description of the system that eliminates waste will therefore mostly focus on the renal system, which is composed of two kidneys, ureters, a bladder, and a urethra (Peters, 2017).

In the kidney, various types of aquaporins are expressed, which are *AQP1, AQP2, AQP3, AQP4, AQP6, AQP7*, and *AQP11* (Su et al., 2020). Aquaporin is made up of a single peptide chain of 270 amino acids. *AQP2* is responsible for inherited central diabetes insipidus. The structure of the aquaporin channel was explained by the hourglass model. Aquaporin channel-forming integral protein (CHIP), also called *AQP1*, is highly permeable to water and is found at the proximal convoluted tubule (PCT) of the kidney. Antidiuretic hormone (ADH), also called vasopressin, acts at V2 receptors in the basolateral membrane of the distal convoluted tubule (DCT) and helps in water absorption. Although ADH is synthesized in hypothalamic neurons and transported into the pituitary gland, which secretes ADH in necessary conditions and acts on the kidney, it enhances the level of cyclic Adenosine monophosphate (AMP) by activating adenyl cyclase, which converts ATP to cyclic AMP. Cyclic AMP binds to protein kinase A and causes phosphorylation of AQP2, which forms a water channel by clustering aquaporin channels (Agarwal et al., 2000). Aquaporin 3 (*AQP3*) is localized along the basolateral membrane of the principal cells of the collecting ducts. Aquaporin 4 (*AQP4*), together with AQP3, is localized at the basolateral membrane of the principal cells of the late DCT (Ma et al., 2000).

Dialysis technicians are the primary AHPs who excel in utilizing their extensive knowledge of the excretory system for optimal patient care. Specializing in kidney health, these dialysis technicians work closely with nephrologists to provide comprehensive care for patients with kidney issues. They administer medications, monitor vital signs, and educate patients on managing their condition, including adhering to dietary restrictions and fluid intake recommendations.

Nutritionists and dietitians also contribute significantly to patient care related to the excretory system. For individuals with kidney disease, dietitians design nutrition plans that help manage electrolyte balance, control blood pressure, and reduce the workload on the kidneys. Their expertise ensures that dietary recommendations align with the specific needs of patients with impaired excretory function, ultimately enhancing the overall well-being of individuals with excretory system-related health challenges.

5.9 ENDOCRINE SYSTEM

The study of the complex network of glands and their hormones is reviewed under the endocrine system. There are mainly two types of glands: endocrine and exocrine glands. Endocrine glands are called ductless glands as their secretion is directly mixed into the blood, and their hormones are transported through the blood directly. The pituitary gland and adrenal gland are examples of endocrine glands; the wall of the small intestine also acts as an endocrine gland, as it secretes secretin and CCK hormones, which travel through the blood and reach the pancreas and liver, where they induce the secretion of pancreatic juice and bile juice consequently. While a duct is present in exocrine glands, exocrine gland secretions are transported through ducts. Sweat glands and sebaceous glands are examples of exocrine glands. The pancreas is referred to as a mixed gland, as it secretes insulin hormone from B cells and glucagon hormone from alpha cells of the islet of Langerhans of the pancreas, which are released into the blood; thus, the islet of Langerhans acts as the endocrine part of the pancreas. The cells of acini present in the pancreas secrete pancreatic juice, which is released inside the duct and transports pancreatic juice to the small intestine; therefore, the cells of acini act as exocrine glands. The pituitary gland is called the master gland as it secretes various types of hormones that perform many physiological functions. The hypothalamus is called the master of the master gland, as it regulates the secretion of the master gland by secreting hypothalamic releasing and inhibitory hormones that act on the pituitary gland (Pituitary gland) (Paul Gard, 1998). The hormones secreted by glands act on the target tissue through hormone-receptor interaction (Hackney et al., 2015). The anterior part of the pituitary gland secretes growth hormone, adrenocorticotropic hormone (ACTH) (Tomaschitz et al., 2014), thyroid-stimulating hormone (TSH), follicle-stimulating hormone (FSH), and luteinizing hormone (LH). Growth hormone acts on bone with IGF and somatomedin and promotes the growth of the body; it also promotes the growth and development of the female reproductive system (Chang et al., 2020). ACTH stimulates the adrenal gland cortex region for the secretion of adrenal gland hormones. TSH stimulates the thyroid gland for the secretion of T3 and T4 hormones. FSH and LH are male and female gonadal hormones responsible for the development of reproductive organ growth and maturation. Melanocyte-stimulating hormone is secreted by the middle part of the pituitary gland and is responsible for melanin formation, such as eumelanin (EM) and pheomelanin (PM), and trichomes, which produce the black and grey appearance of skin and eyes (Lee et al., 2011; Wakamatsu et al., 2020). The variation of colors in humans and animals depends upon the quantity and quality of the melanin pigments as well as the ratios of EM versus PM. The posterior part of the pituitary gland secretes oxytocin and vasopressin hormones. The oxytocin hormone is responsible for the contraction of vaginal muscles during pregnancy and for lactation. Vasopressin, also called antidiuretic hormone, helps with water absorption from the DCT and collecting tubule via interaction with V2 receptors (V2R) from the basal surface and via clustering of aquaporin channels (Ikeda et al., 2015). Other glands are the adrenal glands, which primarily produce mineralo-corticoid hormones like aldosterone, maintaining mineral absorption and metabolism, and glucocorticoid hormones like cortisol, which suppress the immune response by inhibiting histamine from mast cells and eosino-phils, suppress T cell activation, and release cytokines from macrophages. Ovaries and testes also act as glands that produce sex hormones testos-terone, estrogen, and progesterone. The thyroid gland produces thyroid hormones T3 and T4, which are responsible for growth and basal metabolic rate (BMR); the parathyroid produces parathyroid hormone, responsible for vitamin D and calcium absorption and regulation; and the pancreas produces insulin and glucagon, which regulate glucose metabolism by glycogenesis and glycogenolysis.

5.10 REPRODUCTIVE SYSTEM

1. **Female Reproductive System:** The major organs involved in the female reproductive system are the ovaries, fallopian tubes, uterus, and vagina. In females, two almond-shaped ovaries located inside the body produce ova through oogenesis, which travel through the fallopian tubes where sperm fuse with the ova

to form a zygote that moves into the uterus for further development. The lining of the uterus is called the endometrium, which breaks down and sheds during the menstrual cycle. The vagina is a muscular organ that contains the genital organs or vulva, which participate in intercourse during sexual reproduction. The labia majora and labia minora are the outer and inner lips of the vagina (Hofmeister et al., 1982). The clitoris is analogous to the penis in males and is responsible for providing stimulatory signals for reproduction. It comprises a supply of branches from the pudendal nerve and elicits an orgasmic response (Pauls et al., 2015). Endometriosis, polycystic ovarian syndrome (PCOS), fibroids (non-malignant tumors), infertility, and premenstrual tension are some complications related to the female reproductive system in humans. Estrogen and progesterone are the two major hormones involved in the development of the female reproductive system and the maturation of ova.

2. **Male Reproductive System:** The testes, vas deferens, epididymis, and penis are the major parts of the male reproductive system, while the prostate gland, seminal vesicles, and bulbourethral glands are accessory organs involved in the male reproductive system. During reproduction, the testes produce sperm through spermatogenesis, which travels through the vas deferens and epididymis, reaching near the seminal vesicle where prostate gland secretions mix, and finally, seminal fluid is released from the penis into the vagina, neutralizing the partially acidic medium of the vagina. Fructose present in seminal fluid provides energy to sperm for movement, and prostaglandins enhance sperm motility and viability, allowing sperm to move from the vagina to the uterus and fallopian tubes where fertilization occurs (Talluri et al., 2017). The major hormones are important androgens produced by the testes for the development of male reproductive organs. Testosterone is an example of an androgen secreted by Leydig cells of the testes, responsible for the maturity and development of sexual reproductive organs (Zirkin et al., 2018). Low total fertility rates (TFR), testicular dysgenesis syndrome (TDS), testicular germ cell cancer (TGCC), cryptorchidism, and hypospadias are some major reproductive organ disorders (Skakkebaek et al., 2016).

Sexual health is crucial for maintaining a healthy lifestyle and well-being, which can be affected by various disorders related to reproductive organs. Physiotherapists play a crucial role in maintaining good sexual health. Pelvic health issues and back pain are very common challenges in females. Such issues can be effectively managed by expert physiotherapists who promote exercise-based therapy to increase stamina, reduce back pain, and maintain the health of reproductive organs, as well as help achieve orgasm (Areskoug et al., 2015).

5.11 SENSORY SYSTEM

Sensory systems include the study of sensory organs such as the eye, ear, nose, and the receptors associated with pain, touch, and pressure (Hendry et al., 2012). The eye and ear are extensively discussed in this chapter. The eye is a very crucial part of the sensory system, which contains three layers: sclera, choroid, and retina. The sclera is the fibrous layer; the choroid is the vascular layer, while image formation occurs on the retina. The retina is differentiated into three layers: the first is the pigmented layer, which contains pigmented granules; the second is the layer of rods and cones; the third is the bipolar nerve layer, and the fourth is the ganglionic layer. Rods and cones have different kinds of pigments, such as outer rod cells that contain rhodopsin for night vision, while cone lamellae contain three types of pigments: iodopsin (red), porphyropsin (green), and cyanopsin (blue). Rhodopsin was first discovered in the animal retina in 1876, but to this day, various types of rhodopsin, including bacteriorhodopsin, have been described in the cell membrane of an extreme *Halophilic archaeon* and *Halobacterium salinarum* (Nagata et al., 2021). Retinol is required for the synthesis of pigments in rods and cones, and a deficiency of retinol causes night blindness or nyctalopia. The choroid layer has pigments for night vision. *Tapetum fibrosum* is found in hoofed mammals like cows and buffalo, *Tapetum lucidum* is found in elasmobranch fish, and tapetum cellulosum is found in carnivorous mammals. The *Tapetum lucidum* and fibrosum of the choroid layer are composed of densely packed long collagen fibers forming lamellae with a large number of blood vessels intertwined. The peripheral zone of this choroidal *Tapetum lucidum* and *fibrosum* is covered by a lightly pigmented retinal epithelial layer; the capillary vessel lamina is composed of fenestrated vessels and lacks melanocytes (Paszta et al., 2022). Myopia, hypermetropia, astigmatism, presbyopia, and glaucoma are common disorders of eye malfunctioning.

Another sensory organ is the ear, which comprises three parts: the external ear, middle ear, and inner ear. The external ear is responsible for the collection of different frequency sounds, so it has an irregular round curvature. It is closed at the eardrum, while the middle ear contains the ear ossicles, which are the malleus (hammer), incus (anvil), and stapes (stirrup). The inner ear contains the vestibular system, which includes the semicircular canals, utricle, and saccule for balance, while the cochlea is for hearing. Hair cells are found in the cochlea; the hair cells on the outer side are called outer hair cells (OHC), while the inner hair cells (IHC) are located inside. IHCs are connected to the spiral ganglion, which is further connected to the vestibulocochlear duct that moves to the temporal region of the cerebral cortex, where the understanding of hearing sensation occurs. Hair cells can be damaged by many factors, including age, noise, and genetics.

The high load noise and prolonged exposure to noise can lead to the loss of *ribbon synapses*. This loss reduces hearing ability in noisy environments, known as "hidden hearing loss" (Wagner et al., 2019). Other sensory receptors include pain, temperature, and pressure detectors. The transient receptor potential vanilloid type 1 (TRPV1) receptor is present on free nerve endings responsible for pain sensation. TRPV1 and TRPV4 type receptors are found in the preoptic area of the brain and are also responsible for temperature detection and regulation (Yadav et al., 2017). Baroreceptors are pressure receptors located on blood vessels. Two types of baroreceptors are present on blood vessels: first, high-pressure arterial baroreceptors, and second, low-pressure volume receptors. Both receptors are stimulated by the stretching of the blood vessel wall. Arterial baroreceptors are located within the aortic arch and carotid sinuses of the heart. Low-pressure volume receptors are located within the atria and ventricles. The low-pressure volume receptor is also called cardiopulmonary receptors (Al-Khazraji et al., 2018).

Taste receptors also play a crucial role in the sensory organ system. Taste receptors are present on taste buds. Taste buds are collections of columnar sensory cells that are rooted in the tongue and palate. Taste cells are of three types: type I, type II, and type III cells. Type I cells encompass around half the total number of cells in a taste bud. Type I cells have irregularly shaped nuclei and act as glial cells. They express enzymes, transporters, and ion channels on their surface. Transporters are needed to eliminate extracellular neurotransmitters, while ion channels are associated with the redistribution and buffering of potassium ions (K+) (Bartel et al., 2006; Lawton et al., 2000; Vandenbeuch et al., 2013). They are moderately heterogeneous in terms of their gene expression patterns and their functions.

KEYWORDS

- **bipolar nerve**
- **endocrine glands**
- **exocrine glands**
- **hoofed mammals**
- **nyctalopia**
- **pancreatic juice**
- **sebaceous glands**
- **sensory system**
- **sweat glands**

REFERENCES

Adamantidis, A. R., & de Lecea, L. (2023). Sleep and the hypothalamus. *Science, 382*(6669), 405–412.

Agarwal, S. K., & Gupta, A. (2008). Aquaporins: The renal water channels. *Indian Journal of Nephrology, 18*(3), 95–100.

Aguilar, L. E. (2022). *Biomaterial Science: Anatomy and Physiology Aspects*. De Gruyter.

Al-Khazraji, B. K., & Shoemaker, J. K. (2018). The human cortical autonomic network and volitional exercise in health and disease. *Applied Physiology, Nutrition, and Metabolism, 43*(11), 1122–1130.

Areskoug-Josefsson, K., & Gard, G. (2015). Physiotherapy as a promoter of sexual health. *Physiotherapy Theory and Practice, 31*(6), 390–395.

Bamira, M. H. (2018). Picard. In *Encyclopedia of Cardiovascular Research and Medicine*.

Bartel, D. L., Sullivan, S. L., Lavoie, E. G., Sevigny, J., & Finger, T. E. (2006). Nucleoside triphosphate diphosphohydrolase-2 is the ecto-ATPase of type I cells in taste buds. *Journal of Comparative Neurology, 497*, 1–12.

Barton, J. J. S., Davies-Thompson, J., & Corrow, S. L. (2021). Prosopagnosia and disorders of face processing. In *Handbook of Clinical Neurology, 178*, 175–193.

Bortolami, R., Callegari, E., & Lucchi, M. L. (1979). Ultrastructural observations on the tapetum lucidum fibrosum. *Anatomia, Histologia, Embryologia, 8*(1), 72–78.

Boulant, J. A. (2000). Role of the preoptic-anterior hypothalamus in thermoregulation and fever. *Clinical Infectious Diseases, 31*(Suppl. 5), S157–S161.

Cámara-Vázquez, M. Á., Hernández-Romero, I., Morgado-Reyes, E., Guillem, M. S., Climent, A. M., & Barquero-Pérez, O. (2021). Non-invasive estimation of atrial fibrillation driver position with convolutional neural networks and body surface potentials. *Frontiers in Physiology, 12*, 733449.

Cechetto, D. F., & Topolovec, J. C. (2002). Cerebral cortex. In V. S. Ramachandran (Ed.), *Encyclopedia of the Human Brain* (pp. 663–679). Academic Press.

Chang, C. W., Sung, Y. W., Hsueh, Y. W., Chen, Y. Y., Ho, M., Hsu, H. C., Yang, T. C., Lin, W. C., & Chang, H. M. (2022). Growth hormone in fertility and infertility: Mechanisms of action and clinical applications. *Frontiers in Endocrinology, 13*, 1040503.

Delgado-García, J. M. (2001). Estructura y función del cerebelo [Structure and function of the cerebellum]. *Revista de Neurología, 33*(7), 635–642.

Engevik, A. C., Kaji, I., & Goldenring, J. R. (2020). The physiology of the gastric parietal cell. *Physiological Reviews, 100*(2), 573–602.

Evans, M. J., Cabral-Anderson, L. J., & Freeman, G. (1978). Role of the Clara cell in renewal of the bronchiolar epithelium. *Laboratory Investigation, 38*, 648–655.

Gard, P. R. (1998). *Human Endocrinology*.

Gelberg, H. B. (2014). Comparative anatomy, physiology, and mechanisms of disease production of the esophagus, stomach, and small intestine. *Toxicologic Pathology, 42*(1), 54–66.

Hackney, A. C., & Lane, A. R. (2015). Exercise and the regulation of endocrine hormones. *Progress in Molecular Biology and Translational Science, 135*, 293–311.

Hall, J. E. (2015). *Guyton and Hall Textbook of Medical Physiology* (13th ed.).

Hammond, G. L., Lähteenmäki, P. L., Lähteenmäki, P., & Luukkainen, T. (1982). Distribution and percentages of non-protein bound contraceptive steroids in human serum. *Journal of Steroid Biochemistry, 17*(4), 375–380.

Hendry, C., Farley, A., & McLafferty, E. (2012). Anatomy and physiology of the senses. *Nursing Standard, 27*(5), 35–42.

Heusser, K., Tank, J., Engeli, S., Diedrich, A., Menne, J., Eckert, S., Peters, T., Sweep, F. C., Haller, H., Pichlmaier, A. M., Luft, F. C., & Jordan, J. (2010). Carotid baroreceptor stimulation, sympathetic activity, baroreflex function, and blood pressure in hypertensive patients. *Hypertension, 55*, 619–626.

Hofmeister, F. J. (1982). Pelvic anatomy of the ureter in relation to surgery performed through the vagina. *Clinical Obstetrics and Gynecology, 25*(4), 821–830.

Ikeda, M., & Matsuzaki, T. (2015). Regulation of aquaporins by vasopressin in the kidney. *Vitamins and Hormones, 98*, 307–337.

Jawabri, K. H., & Sharma, S. (2023). Physiology, cerebral cortex functions.

Lawton, D. M., Furness, D. N., Lindemann, B., & Hackney, C. M. (2000). Localization of the glutamate–aspartate transporter, GLAST, in rat taste buds. *European Journal of Neuroscience, 12*, 3163–3171.

Lee, D. Y., Kim, C. R., & Lee, J. H. (2011). Trichrome vitiligo in segmental type. *Photodermatology, Photoimmunology & Photomedicine, 27*(2), 111–112.

Levassort, H., Cluchet, M., Cudennec, T., & Levassort, M. (2022). Troubles phasiques et aphasie en gériatrie [Phasic disorders and aphasia in geriatrics]. *Soins Gérontologie, 27*(155), 38–42.

Levi, M., & van der Poll, T. (2010). Inflammation and coagulation. *Critical Care Medicine, 38*(2 Suppl), S26–S34.

Liddle, R. A. (2003). *Encyclopedia of Gastroenterology*.

Ma, T., Song, Y., Yang, B., Gillespie, A., Carlson, E. J., Epstein, C. J., et al. (2000). Nephrogenic diabetes insipidus in mice lacking aquaporin-3 water channels. *Proceedings of the National Academy of Sciences of the United States of America, 97*, 4386–4391.

Manzi, J. E., Dowling, B., Trauger, N., Hansen, B. R., Quan, T., Dennis, E., Fu, M. C., & Dines, J. S. (2023). The relationship between maximum shoulder horizontal abduction and adduction on peak shoulder kinetics in professional pitchers. *Sports Health, 15*(4), 592–598.

Mason, R. J., Williams, M. C., Moses, H. L., Mohla, S., & Berberich, M. A. (1997). Stem cells in lung development, disease, and therapy. *American Journal of Respiratory Cell and Molecular Biology, 16*, 355–363.

Nagata, T., & Inoue, K. (2021). Rhodopsins at a glance. *Journal of Cell Science, 134*(22), jcs258989.

Nagpal, M., Singh, S., Singh, P., Chauhan, P., & Zaidi, M. A. (2016). Tumor markers: A diagnostic tool. *National Journal of Maxillofacial Surgery, 7*(1), 17–20.

Orlic, D., & Bodine, D. M. (1994). What defines a pluripotent hematopoietic stem cell (PHSC): Will the real PHSC please stand up! *Blood, 84*(12), 3991–3994.

Paszta, W., Klećkowska-Nawrot, J. E., & Goździewska-Harłajczuk, K. (2022). Morphological evaluation of the orbit, eye tunics, eyelids, and orbital glands in young and adult aardvarks *Orycteropus afer*, Pallas, 1766 (Tubulidentata: Orycteropodidae): Similarities and differences with representatives of the Afrotheria clade. *The Anatomical Record, 305*(11), 3317–3340.

Pauls, R. N. (2015). Anatomy of the clitoris and the female sexual response. *Clinical Anatomy, 28*(3), 376–384.

Peters, S. (2017). Excretory system. In J. Vonk & T. Shackelford (Eds.), *Encyclopedia of Animal Cognition and Behavior*. Springer.

Reynolds, S. D., & Malkinson, A. M. (2010). Clara cell: progenitor for the bronchiolar epithelium. *International Journal of Biochemistry & Cell Biology, 42*(1), 1–4.

Reynolds, S. D., Giangreco, A., Power, J. H. T., & Stripp, B. R. (2000). Neuroepithelial bodies of pulmonary airways serve as a reservoir of progenitor cells capable of epithelial regeneration. *American Journal of Pathology, 156*, 269–278.

Reynolds, S. D., Hong, K. U., Giangreco, A., Mango, G. W., Guron, C., Morimoto, Y., & Stripp, B. R. (2000). Conditional ablation of Clara cells in transgenic mice reveals a self-renewing progenitor function of pulmonary neuroendocrine cells. *American Journal of Physiology, 278*, L1256–L1263.

Sembulingam, K., & Sembulingam, P. (2010). *Essentials of Medical Physiology* (5th ed.). Jaypee Brothers Medical Limited.

Skakkebaek, N. E., Rajpert-De Meyts, E., Buck Louis, G. M., Toppari, J., Andersson, A. M., Eisenberg, M. L., Jensen, T. K., Jørgensen, N., Swan, S. H., Sapra, K. J., Ziebe, S., Priskorn, L., & Juul, A. (2016). Male reproductive disorders and fertility trends:

Influences of environment and genetic susceptibility. *Physiological Reviews, 96*(1), 55–97.

Sokoloff, L. (1983). Measurement of local glucose utilization and its use in localization of functional activity in the central nervous system of animals and man. In R. O. Greep (Ed.), *Recent Progress in Hormone Research, 39*, 75–126. Academic Press.

Solomon, T. E., & Reeve, J. R. Jr. (2013). In *Handbook of Biologically Active Peptides* (2nd ed.).

Soubeyrand, M., Assabah, B., Bégin, M., Laemmel, E., Dos Santos, A., & Crézé, M. (2017). Pronation and supination of the hand: Anatomy and biomechanics. *Hand Surgery & Rehabilitation, 36*(1), 2–11.

Su, W., Cao, R., Zhang, X. Y., & Guan, Y. (2020). Aquaporins in the kidney: Physiology and pathophysiology. *American Journal of Physiology–Renal Physiology, 318*(1), F193–F203.

Suarez, C. J., Dintzis, S. M., & Frevert, C. W. (2012). *Comparative Anatomy and Histology* (pp. 121–134). Academic Press.

Talluri, T. R., Mal, G., & Ravi, S. K. (2017). Biochemical components of seminal plasma and their correlation to the fresh seminal characteristics in Marwari stallions and Poitou jacks. *Veterinary World, 10*(2), 214–220.

Thakkar, M., & Mallick, B. N. (1993). Rapid eye movement sleep-deprivation-induced changes in glucose metabolic enzymes in rat brain. *Sleep, 16*(8), 691–694.

Tomaschitz, A., Ritz, E., Pieske, B., Rus-Machan, J., Kienreich, K., Verheyen, N., Gaksch, M., Grübler, M., Fahrleitner-Pammer, A., Mrak, P., Toplak, H., Kraigher-Krainer, E., März, W., & Pilz, S. (2014). Aldosterone and parathyroid hormone interactions as mediators of metabolic and cardiovascular disease. *Metabolism, 63*(1), 20–31.

Van Ravenswaaij-Arts, C. M. A., Hopman, J. C. W., Kollée, L. A. A., & Stoelinga, G. B. A. (1990). The influence of physiological parameters on long-term heart rate variability in healthy preterm infants. *Journal of Perinatal Medicine, 18*(2), 131–138.

Vandenbeuch, A., et al. (2013). Role of the ectonucleotidase NTPDase2 in taste bud function. *Proceedings of the National Academy of Sciences of the United States of America, 110*, 14789–14794.

Wagner, E. L., & Shin, J. B. (2019). Mechanisms of hair cell damage and repair. *Trends in Neurosciences, 42*(6), 414–424.

Wakamatsu, K., & Ito, S. (2023). Recent advances in characterization of melanin pigments in biological samples. *International Journal of Molecular Sciences, 24*(9), 8305.

Wilke, J., Macchi, V., De Caro, R., & Stecco, C. (2019). Fascia thickness, aging, and flexibility: Is there an association? *Journal of Anatomy, 234*(1), 43–49.

Wolf, S. (1985). William Beaumont: The man, his time, and his legacy. *Federation Proceedings, 44*, 2887–2888.

Yadav, R., Jaryal, A. K., & Mallick, H. N. (2017). Participation of preoptic area TRPV4 ion channel in regulation of body temperature. *Journal of Thermal Biology, 66*, 81–86.

Yadav, R., Suri, M., Mathur, R., & Jain, S. (2009). Effect of procainization of ventromedial nucleus of hypothalamus on the feeding behavior of rats. *Journal of Clinical Biochemistry and Nutrition, 44*(3), 247–252.

Zirkin, B. R., & Papadopoulos, V. (2018). Leydig cells: Formation, function, and regulation. *Biology of Reproduction, 99*(1), 101–111.

CHAPTER 6

Interrelationship Between Physiological Systems and Organs

RAJESH YADAV

Sharda School of Allied Health Sciences, Sharda University, Greater Noida, Uttar Pradesh, India

ABSTRACT

Physiology and anatomy serve as the bridge between the foundational sciences and the field of medicine. The class of physiology lies in its ability to seamlessly integrate the diverse functions of cells, tissues, and organs into the functional unity of the human body. This chapter delves into the interconnectedness between organs and physiological systems, shedding light on how the harmonious functioning of various systems contributes to human well-being. Disruptions in these systems can lead to various diseases, underscoring the importance of their proper functioning. The discussion extends to the positive impact of mild exercise on osteogenesis, heart health, mental wellbeing, emotional balance, and overall physical development. Exploring the interplay between the nervous system and other physiological systems, such as the digestive, respiratory, and reproductive systems reveals the intricate connections that foster a healthy mind and body. A comprehensive overview of prevalent diseases associated with physiological systems is provided, drawing insights from recent research in allied health sciences (AHS). The chapter emphasizes the critical role of anatomy and physiology in cultivating a healthy lifestyle. Additionally, the chapter addresses how factors like stress, aging, and other variables influence memory and cognitive skills.

Allied Healthcare in Practice: An Introduction to Integrated Patient Care. Sally Lukose, Karuna Singh (Eds.)

DOI: 10.1201/9781998511037-8

6.1 INTERRELATIONSHIP BETWEEN EXERCISE PHYSIOLOGY AND DIFFERENT ORGANS

6.1.1 MECHANISM OF EXERCISE AND HEALTH IMPROVEMENT

Exercise physiology is a specific branch of physiology closely linked to the development of various physiological systems and organs. Its significance lies in promoting the proper functioning of crucial organs such as the heart, lungs, kidneys, liver, muscles, bones, and the brain. Additionally, exercise contributes to the maintenance of healthy skin, intestines, and reproductive organs. The positive impact of exercise on health is profound, as it enhances blood circulation throughout the body and improves tissue oxygenation. Furthermore, exercise plays a key role in enhancing glucose tolerance, increasing insulin sensitivity, maximizing oxygen uptake, and influencing the expression of uncoupling protein (Ucp1) mRNA. Notably, exercise contributes to elevated plasma levels of fibroblast growth factor 21 (FGF21), which, in turn, mediates the browning of white adipose tissue (WAT) to increase energy consumption (Reilly et al., 2021).

6.1.2 EXERCISE AND ITS IMPACT ON VARIOUS PHYSIOLOGICAL SYSTEMS

Aerobic exercise is a form of physical activity that utilizes oxygen to generate energy, contributing to the development of a healthy cardiovascular system. This type of exercise enables individuals to engage in prolonged physical activity without experiencing fatigue, as oxygen plays a vital role in various metabolic processes. Regular physical activity is particularly beneficial for patients with osteoporosis and other bone-related issues, promoting osteogenesis and increasing bone thickness (Benedetti et al., 2018). Moderate-intensity exercises have proven helpful for conditions like cholelithiasis and constipation (de Oliveira et al., 2009). With depression affecting around 12 million people globally and often linked to sedentary lifestyles (Moussavi et al., 2007), physical activity emerges as a powerful tool. Exercise raises endorphin levels, decreases cortisol levels, and improves Brain-Derived Neurotrophic Factor (BDNF), a hormone crucial for nerve growth regulation (Cotman et al., 2002; Ernst et al., 2006). Consequently, physical activity plays a crucial role in maintaining a healthy nervous system and addressing psychological concerns. However, for individuals with asthma, strenuous exercise may exacerbate respiratory issues. Andréanne Côté's 2018 study indicated that exercise-induced bronchoconstriction (EIB) could be a result of intense exercise for asthmatic individuals (Côté et al., 2018). It is essential to tailor exercise regimens to the type and intensity that best suits the needs of asthmatic patients.

Hence, physical activity and exercise contribute significantly to the well-being of the mind, body, and soul. Figure 6.1 illustrates various types of exercises that are important for human health.

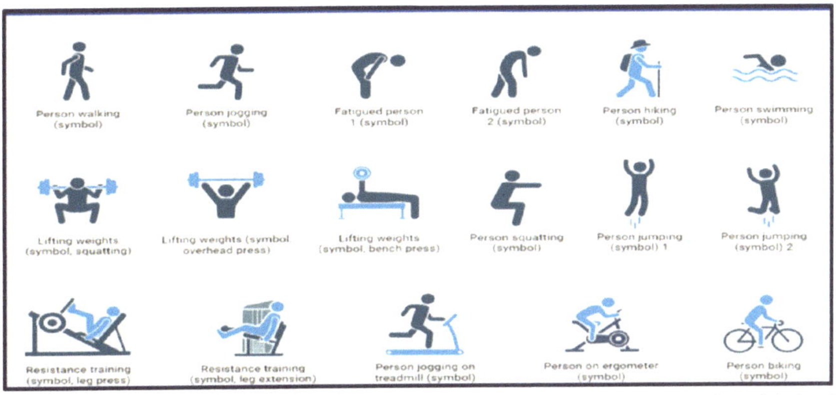

FIGURE 6.1 Schematic diagram created by Biorender.com showing various kind of exercise including aerobic and anaerobic exercise for being healthy.

6.1.3 OBESITY AND EXERCISE

Obesity poses a significant health risk, serving as the precursor to various diseases. Its association with conditions such as cancer, diabetes, infertility, kidney failure, and gallbladder complications is illustrated in Figure 6.2. Maintaining a healthy lifestyle, particularly for the digestive system, is crucial. One major cause of obesity is the imbalance between high energy intake and low energy expenditure. Diets rich in unhealthy fats contribute to the deposition of LDL cholesterol in the body. Adipose tissue plays a vital role in obesity, with three main types identified in the human body: WAT, BAT, and beige adipose tissue. WAT primarily stores triglycerides, with its differentiation into visceral and subcutaneous types based on the location of triglyceride storage. Visceral WAT breaks down triglycerides into fatty acids, mobilizing energy (Morigny et al., 2021). Brown adipose tissue functions in thermogenesis due to its abundant mitochondria, containing uncoupling proteins that generate heat through respiratory uncoupling (Fedorenko et al., 2012). In response to cold and exercise, WAT differentiates into beige adipose tissue, also contributing to heat generation or thermogenesis. Exercise induces the production of myokines, with Irisin being a crucial myokine produced after physical activity. *In vivo* studies on mice suggest that Irisin, released from skeletal tissue, enhances insulin sensitivity, promotes carbohydrate metabolism in adipose tissue, and induces browning of WAT (Boström et al., 2012). Regular exercise, especially over extended periods, results in an increased number of mitochondria. This increase allows for enhanced utilization of fat as fuel, leading to increased fatty acid oxidation. After a period of endurance training, the body exhibits a "carbohydrate-sparing effect," where the utilization of fat surpasses that of carbohydrates. This phenomenon emphasizes that fat becomes the preferred fuel for muscles during prolonged exercise (Talanian et al., 2010; Villiot et al., 2011).

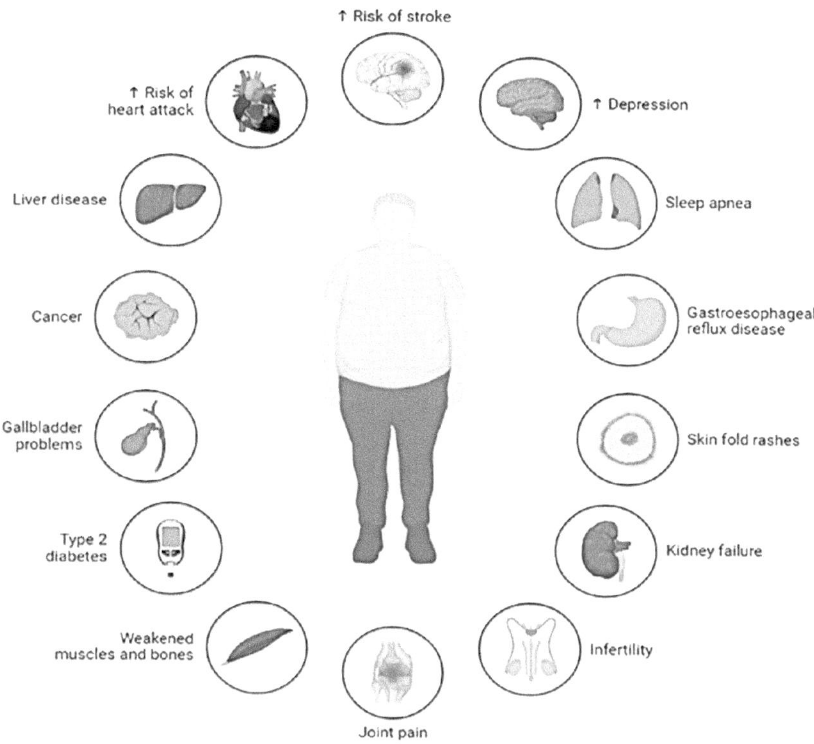

FIGURE 6.2 Schematic diagram showing the possible risk of obesity.

Source: Created by Biorender.com.

6.1.4 EXERCISE AND STRENGTHENING OF THE MUSCULOSKELETAL SYSTEM

Exercise induces an increase in the size of muscle cells without generating new cells. When exercise is coupled with higher protein intake, the diameter of muscle cells increases, leading to muscle growth known as hypertrophy. Consistent exercise promotes the development of blood capillaries around muscles, a process referred to as angiogenesis. Additionally, exercise recruits muscle fibers within the muscle.

The human body possesses three crucial types of muscle fibers, and the quantity of these fibers increases with different types of exercise. Lifting heavy weights recruits Type 2x fibers, responsible for tolerating heavy forces, leading to their increased numbers in activities such as weightlifting, jumping, and fast running. Moderate activities, such as swimming and dancing, engage Type 1 fibers, which are responsible for endurance work. Type 2a fibers, a combination of Type 1 and Type 2x fibers, see an increase in their numbers during light-intensity activities.

6.2 DISEASE ASSOCIATION WITH PHYSIOLOGICAL SYSTEMS AND ORGANS

6.2.1 CIRCULATORY SYSTEM AND CARDIOVASCULAR DISEASE

Cardiovascular disease stands as a major contributor to mortality in developed nations, posing a risk to 50% of the population in these regions today (North et al., 2012). Coronary heart disease (CHD), a chronic ailment, is characterized by the continuous deposition of LDL cholesterol in the blood. Risk factors for CHD include high blood pressure, smoking, physical inactivity, and diabetes, all exacerbating the condition of the disease (Jokinen et al., 2014). Obesity independently serves as a risk factor for CHD, and among individuals above 65 years old, CHD emerges as the leading cause of death. Dysfunction and hypertrophy in the sinoatrial (SA) node impair the electrical conduction of nerve impulses across all chambers of the heart. Other cardiovascular diseases (CVD) encompass atherosclerosis, hypertension, stroke, and myocardial infarction.

With advancing age, left ventricular (LV) contractility and ejection fraction diminish, accompanied by a reduced response to β-adrenergic receptor activation. Vascular tone, regulated by nitric oxide released from the endothelium of blood vessels, also declines with age (Lakatta et al., 2003). Recent observations in 2018 highlight the association between vitamin D and atherosclerosis, suggesting that plasma 25-hydroxyvitamin D levels might serve as a biomarker (Nista et al., 2018).

A study published in the Protein Cell journal in 2018 emphasizes the intricate relationship between the human gut and cardiovascular health. The gut harbors approximately 100 trillion microbes, including bacteria, fungi, and archaea, with 10 million microbiota genes yet to be sequenced. Gut microbiota play a crucial role in maintaining intestinal homeostasis. Disruptions in this equilibrium increase the likelihood of CVD, obesity, and cancer (Wang et al., 2018).

6.2.2 NERVOUS SYSTEM AND NEUROLOGICAL DISEASES

Neurons serve as channels for transmitting information between the body and the brain, establishing a bidirectional communication channel. They establish connections between the brain and the spinal cord and coordinate with the endocrine system. The digestive system boasts its own nervous system known as the enteric nervous system, intricately connected with the central nervous system (CNS). The CNS encompasses the study of the brain and spinal cord, while the peripheral nervous system involves the study of other nerves. Malfunctions in nerve cells give rise to various neurological problems, impacting both the brain and other bodily functions. Neurological disorders affect hundreds of millions of people worldwide, with staggering statistics from the World Health Organization (WHO) reporting six million deaths annually due to strokes and 50 million people being affected by epilepsy. Alzheimer's and dementia, prevalent neurological disorders, impact 7.7 million individuals globally. Furthermore, various bacteria, viruses, and certain fungi can also induce neurological problems in humans.

6.2.2.1 ALZHEIMER'S DISEASE

Amyloid precursor protein (APP) is a membrane protein that extends outward from the cell membrane, playing a crucial role in neuronal growth, repair, and survival. The B-Secretase enzyme cleaves APP into small fragments known as Beta amyloid (or AB). Beta amyloid tends to be sticky, causing fragments to cling together with other materials outside the cell, forming plaques (Figure 6.3). Neurons rely on an internal support structure composed of microtubules that contain the tau protein, contributing to the stabilization of microtubules. These microtubules act like tracks, guiding nutrients and molecules from the cell body to the ends of the axon and back. In Alzheimer's disease, changes in tau (hyperphosphorylation) lead to the collapse of microtubules, and tau proteins clump together, forming neurofibrillary tangles (Stein et al., 2014) as depicted in Figure 6.4.

The accumulation of Beta amyloid and neurofibrillary tangles in the brain is highly toxic, disrupting calcium homeostasis, and may result in apoptosis. Early symptoms include memory loss, impairment of semantic memory, mild cognitive impairment, and apathy. As the disease progresses, individuals may experience difficulty in language comprehension, agnosia, and apraxia, leading to challenges in motor planning and task execution. In the middle stage, individuals may struggle to recognize close relatives, while in the late stage, complete loss of speech and extreme apathy may occur (Lyketsos et al., 2011).

Recent research by Chunmei Jiang in 2017 has explored the association between gut microbiota and Alzheimer's disease. Bacteria in the gut microbiota secrete amyloids and lipopolysaccharides, which have the capacity to alter signaling pathways and produce cytokines associated with Alzheimer's disease (Jiang et al., 2017). Additionally, several proteins, including α-synuclein, presenilin-1, FUS, and TIA1, are associated with neurodegenerative disorders. Tau and α-synuclein mutually contribute to their fibrillization, and their interaction results in the formation of insoluble tau and α-synuclein aggregates, observed in Lewy bodies deposits found in Parkinson's disease (PD) (Giasson et al., 2003; Ishizawa et al., 2003).

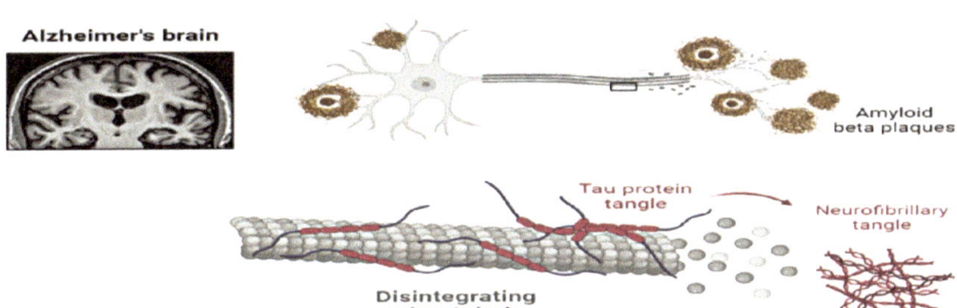

FIGURE 6.3 Schematic diagram created by Biorender.com illustrating nerve cell in Alzheimer's patient, showing deposition of tau protein and B amyloid plaque and formation of neurofibrillary tangle around nerve cell.

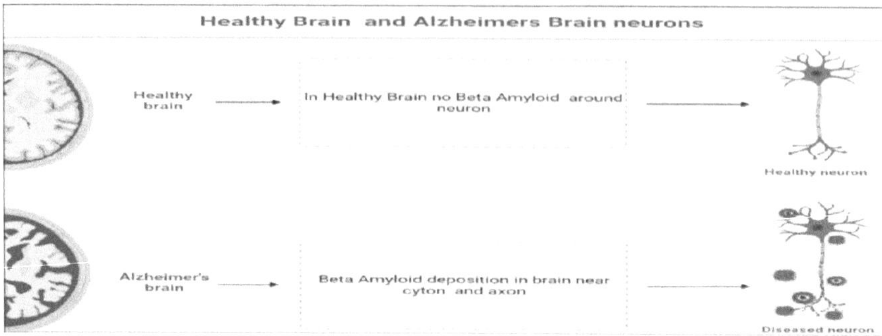

FIGURE 6.4 Schematic diagram created by Biorender.com shows nerve cell in healthy brain and Alzheimer's brain depicting formation of B amyloid plaque around nerve cell in Alzheimer's brain.

6.2.2.2 PARKINSON DISEASE

Another critical neurological disorder after Alzheimer's disease is Parkinson's disease, in which degeneration of dopaminergic neurons in the substantia nigra pars compacta occurs, resulting in a deficiency of the dopamine neurotransmitter in the substantia nigra and striatum. It is progressive with age and characterized by tremor, bradykinesia, and muscle rigidity. Gait and balance are also disturbed in Parkinson's disease. The exact mechanism of Parkinson's is not known, but protein misfolding and a major misfolded protein called amyloid protein are observed in the intercellular space of substantia nigra neurons. Numerous misfolded proteins observed in Parkinson's include alpha-synuclein, amyloid beta protein, and phosphorylated tau (Chouhan et al., 2015; Kim et al., 2014). These are termed Lewy bodies in Parkinson's disease. Motor symptoms are very common in Parkinson's, but as aging occurs, non-motor symptoms also appear, such as decreased cognition, loss of memory, increased stress, and serum cortisol. BDNF may act as a biomarker for non-motor symptoms. After 18 weeks of disease progression, serotonin (5-hydroxytryptamine) levels decrease in the prefrontal cortex, and the 5-HT transporter (SERT) is also reduced. Mitochondrial damage, oxidative stress, and prion infection can increase the possibility of the onset of the disease (Huot et al., 2017; Kim et al., 2014).

6.2.2.3 WERNICKE APHASIA AND GLOBAL APHASIA

Individuals afflicted with Wernicke's aphasia possess the ability to comprehend either spoken or written words but face difficulty expressing their thoughts. This condition arises when damage occurs in Wernicke's area and the posterior superior temporal gyrus in the dominant hemisphere. On the other hand, global aphasia involves the destruction or damage in Wernicke's area extending to the angular gyrus, temporal lobe, and Sylvian fissure. In this condition, individuals experience profound impairment in language comprehension, rendering them completely unable to grasp linguistic information.

6.2.3 DIGESTIVE SYSTEM AND GASTROLOGICAL DISEASES

The primary organs involved in digestion are the mouth, stomach, small intestine, and large intestine. The digestive system orchestrates the breakdown of various components of food across different organs, employing digestive enzymes and hormones. Digestion is the process of converting large, complex food into smaller chemical components that can be absorbed into the bloodstream, reaching every cell of the body. This intricate process involves the digestive tract, as well as accessory organs such as the liver, pancreas, teeth, tongue, salivary glands, and gallbladder, all under the control of the enteric nervous system and hormones (Bender et al., 2005; Saladin, 2017).

Protein digestion primarily occurs in the stomach and intestine, while carbohydrate and fat digestion take place in the intestine. Accessory organs like the liver and pancreas play crucial roles in ensuring the complete digestion of carbohydrates, proteins, and fats. Genetic digestive issues and autoimmune attacks on the digestive system can lead to various disorders such as irritable bowel syndrome, gallstones, celiac disease, diarrhea, constipation, and peptic ulcers. Maintaining a healthy lifestyle and good nutrition supports a robust digestive system. Practices like consuming balanced meals, engaging in regular exercise and yoga, and incorporating probiotics into the diet contribute to digestive well-being. Avoiding deep-fried and fast foods while opting for juices and health drinks over sugary beverages is recommended for digestive health.

The large intestine houses a myriad of microorganisms collectively known as gut microbiota, which possess 10 times more genes than the human genome. These microbiomes play a pivotal role in shaping health, behavior, brain health, and the immune system. Gut microbiota release metabolites that impact insulin sensitivity and are associated with type

2 diabetes (Cani et al., 2007; Pedersen et al., 2016; Vadder et al., 2014). Gram-negative bacteria, containing lipopolysaccharide, can translocate into the blood from the gut, binding to lipopolysaccharide binding protein (LBP) and altering interleukin-6 (IL-6) levels. Higher plasma LBP levels and IL-6 have been observed in type 2 diabetes (Tamaki et al., 2019). Lipopolysaccharide acts as an endotoxin in the blood, causing inflammation and affecting IL-7 levels. Probiotics play a crucial role in reducing lipopolysaccharide translocation, offering assistance in managing metabolic syndrome. Popular probiotic drinks like Yakult, containing 6.5 billion healthy bacteria, *Lactobacillus casei* strain Shirota (LcS) and *Bifidobacterium breve* strain, contribute to intestinal health.

The inclusion of millets in the diet is gaining global recognition due to their rich nutrient and phenolic compound content. Finger and pearl millets, exemplifying this category, contain significant amounts of flavonoids, tannins, and phenolic acids with potent antioxidant activity. Millets, known for their cholesterol-lowering properties, are particularly noteworthy. Pearl millet, the sixth-highest producing crop globally, offers essential vitamins (B1, B2, B3) and minerals such as calcium, phosphorus, and iron. Notably, finger millets exhibit lower carbohydrate content, constituting less than 10% compared to pearl millets (Hassan et al., 2021; Wankhede et al., 1979).

6.2.4 ENDOCRINE SYSTEM AND ASSOCIATED DISEASES

The endocrine system involves the study of various types of endocrine glands and their hormone functions. The pituitary gland, a chief endocrine gland, oversees numerous bodily functions, including body growth and development, kidney water absorption, milk formation and secretion in women, regulation of thyroid hormones, and other essential functions. The liver, the body's largest gland, and the pancreas, a mixed gland, play crucial roles in fat digestion through bile salt formation. Deficiencies in growth hormone and thyroid hormone can lead to conditions such as dwarfism and impaired brain development. Other endocrine disorders include Cushing's syndrome, goiter, acromegaly, hypopituitarism, and diabetes insipidus.

Numerous hereditary endocrine disorders, with around 300 genes responsible for causal mutations, are prevalent in humans (Ye et al., 2015). The antidiuretic hormone (ADH) secreted from the posterior pituitary gland facilitates water reabsorption in the distal convoluted tubule

(DCT) of the nephron. Seven types of aquaporins (AQP) expressed in the kidneys, particularly AQP-2, play a vital role in water reabsorption in the DCT. Mutations in the AQP2 channel can lead to inherited central diabetes insipidus (Agarwal et al., 2008). Glucocorticoids, hormones from the adrenal gland, are now utilized in treating various immune-related disorders (Cain et al., 2017). In 1948, at the Mayo Clinic in Minnesota, United States, glucocorticoid hormones were first used to treat arthritis, earning Philip S. Hench, Edward Kendall, and Tadeus Reichstein the Nobel Prize in 1950. Insulin, released from B cells of the pancreas, regulates glucose homeostasis. The GLUT4 transporter is responsible for insulin-responsive glucose absorption in adipose tissue and skeletal muscle via the insulin receptor signaling pathway. In the liver, kidney, and intestine, the GLUT2 transporter aids in the absorption of glucose from the proximal convoluted tubule of the nephron into the bloodstream (Marks et al., 2003; Yonamine et al., 2017). In the brain and testis, GLUT3 is found for glucose uptake in nerve cells. Mutations in glucose transporters decrease insulin response and increase the risk of type 2 diabetes (Naval et al., 2016).

6.3 SLEEP MEMORY AND TEMPERATURE

6.3.1 SLEEP CLASSIFICATION

Sleep can be categorized into two main types: Rapid Eye Movement (REM) sleep and non-Rapid Eye Movement (NREM) sleep. During REM sleep, dreams occur, accompanied by REMs. In non-rapid eye movement sleep (NREM), memory consolidation takes place, transforming short-term memory into long-term memory through a phenomenon known as long-term potentiation. NREM is commonly referred to as deep sleep. Throughout the sleep cycle, NREM and REM sleep alternate. The actual mechanism of dreaming is still unknown. The pineal body gland regulates the circadian rhythm and secretes the melatonin hormone. Melatonin production and secretion are more pronounced during dark periods and decrease in well-lit environments. Acting as an internal clock, melatonin regulates the sleep and wake cycle in response to changes in light intensity (Arendt et al., 2005). During the daytime, serotonin levels are high in the pineal gland, while at night, melatonin levels rise. Serotonin, also known as 5-hydroxytryptamine, is synthesized from the amino acid tryptophan through a four-step chemical reaction facilitated by different enzymes

(Borjigin et al., 1999). In melatonin synthesis, tryptophan hydroxylase 1 (TPH1) serves as the rate-limiting enzyme.

6.3.2 SIGNIFICANCE OF SLEEP IN HEALTH IMPROVEMENT

Sleep plays a crucial role in the overall development of both the body and the mind. Deficiencies in sleep can lead to irritability and challenging behavior. A sufficient amount of sleep is essential for optimal cognitive performance, especially in activities such as surgery, military operations, nuclear reactor maintenance, aviation, and traffic control (Smithies et al., 2021).

The recommended total sleep duration for humans is 8–10 hours, with 8 hours being necessary for young individuals. A reduction of two hours in nocturnal sleep adversely affects cognitive performance. However, compensating with 6.5 hours of nighttime sleep and an additional two hours during the day can boost cognitive abilities. Research indicates that a split sleep schedule, consisting of 6.5 hours of nocturnal sleep and a 1.5-hour nap, achieves comparable performance in basic cognitive tasks, subjective alertness, and mood compared to a nocturnal sleep-only schedule (Lo et al., 2020).

Irregular sleep patterns disrupt the circadian rhythm, leading to conditions like Shift Work Disorder and Jet Lag. People with irregular sleep times experience circadian rhythm sleep-wake disorders (CRSWD) (Duffy et al., 2021). The suprachiasmatic nucleus (SCN) was identified as the central circadian pacemaker in mammals in 1970. The retinal ganglion in our eyes sends light-dark information to the SCN, regulating 24-hour rhythms in most cells of the body (Moore et al., 1972).

Adequate quantity and quality of sleep are vital for daytime alertness, optimal work performance, and a high quality of life. Sleep deficiency can disrupt blood circulation, alter glucose metabolism, increase blood pressure, elevate the risk of obesity and cardiovascular disease, and impact mood, memory, and cognition. A 2011 WHO report highlighted that individuals in Europe and the United States were suffering from noise-induced sleep disturbances, particularly from aircraft, rail, and road traffic. In 2018, WHO issued advisories recommending minimum noise levels of 45 dBL and 44 dBL at night for road and rail traffic, and 40 dBL at night for air traffic to prevent noise-induced sleep disturbances (Basner et al., 2018).

6.3.3 MEMORY AND HEALTH

Memory encompasses the acquisition, storage, and retrieval of sensory information, allowing the recall of past events at both conscious and unconscious levels. It can be categorized into two main types: declarative and nondeclarative memory. Declarative memory involves the conscious storage and recollection of data (Graf et al., 1985) and can be further divided into semantic and episodic memory. Semantic memory includes information such as phone numbers, codes, and face recognition, while episodic memory involves recalling past events. Declarative memory is also known as explicit memory. On the other hand, nondeclarative memory, also referred to as procedural memory, requires motor skills for tasks like cycling, car driving, and performing procedural steps such as DNA isolation from onions (Figure 6.5A).

The hippocampus, located in the anterior part of the brain, is a major area associated with memory. Although neuron regeneration is generally limited in the brain, the hippocampus is one of the few areas where limited neurodegeneration occurs. Other brain areas, including the basal ganglia, striatum, amygdala, and mammillary body, are also considered in memory processes (Figure 6.5B). The basal ganglia are responsible for procedural memory, while the amygdala is linked to emotional memory. The exact roles of other areas in memory are not precisely defined (Šimić et al., 2021; Simonyan et al., 2019).

Lesions in the hippocampus can result in anterograde amnesia, where the individual is unable to establish new long-term memories, as the hippocampus plays a crucial role in long-term potentiation, converting short-term memory into long-term memory. Damage to the temporal lobe of the cerebral cortex can lead to retrograde amnesia, where recalling past memories becomes challenging. Memory-related problems are prevalent in Alzheimer's disease, and there is a specific condition called prosopagnosia, where individuals struggle to recognize faces. This condition is observed in people with extensive damage to the medial undersides of both occipital lobes and along the medioventral surfaces of the temporal lobes of the cerebral cortex.

Certain foods are considered beneficial for brain health and memory. Blueberries, fatty fish, caffeine, curcumin, broccoli, pumpkin seeds, dark chocolate, nuts, oranges, and green tea are known to support good memory.

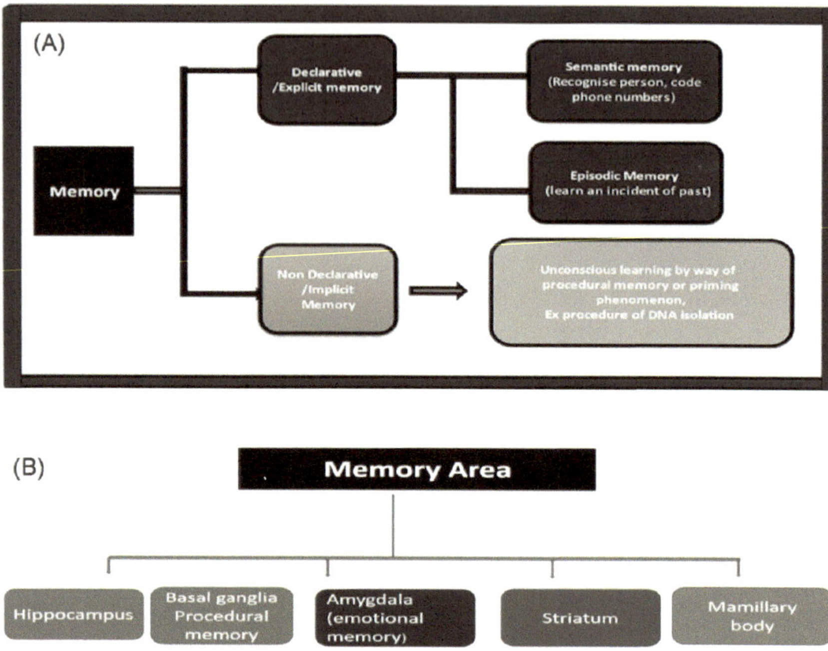

FIGURE 6.5 (A) Schematic diagram shows the memory classification including declarative and nondeclarative memory, declarative memory further classified into semantic and episodic memory. (B) shows the different area of brain responsible for memory.

6.3.4 TEMPERATURE AND HEALTH ASSOCIATION

The preoptic area of the hypothalamus plays a pivotal role in the regulation of body temperature. Within the preoptic area, both warm-sensitive neurons (WSN) and cold-sensitive neurons (CSN) contribute to the intricate process of temperature control. When exposed to warm environments, WSN activation leads to a downregulation of body temperature through mechanisms such as vasodilation and sweating. Conversely, in cold environments, CSN activation increases body temperature by promoting vasoconstriction, shivering, and inhibiting WSN function. Together, these warm and CSN work in tandem to maintain body temperature homeostasis.

A 2017 study highlighted the presence of transient receptor potential vanilloid type 4 (TRPV4) channels in the preoptic area. Immunohistochemistry revealed the location of TRPV4 in this crucial brain region (Yadav et al., 2017). Activation of TRPV4 by its agonist was found to decrease body temperature, emphasizing the significant role of TRPV4 in the preoptic area of the hypothalamus in the regulation of body temperature. TRPV4 is a cation channel activated at warm temperatures (>30°C) and is distributed in various areas of the body, including the brain.

Fever, a medical term indicating an elevation in body temperature, can occur under various conditions. In the presence of microbial infections, the release of pyrogens induces fever as part of the body's defense mechanism. It's important to note that fever itself is not a disease but rather a physiological response indicating the presence of a foreign invader or an abnormality within the cells. Understanding the intricate mechanisms of temperature regulation, including the role of TRPV4 in the preoptic area, contributes to our knowledge of how the body responds to environmental changes and potential threats.

KEYWORDS

- **cognitive performance**
- **cold-sensitive neurons**
- **exercise impact**
- **hypothalamus**
- **immunohistochemistry**
- **irregular sleep pattern**
- **memory association**
- **nervous system**
- **nocturnal sleep**
- **physiology**
- **warm-sensitive neurons**

REFERENCES

Agarwal, S. K., & Gupta, A. (2008). Aquaporins: The renal water channels. *Indian Journal of Nephrology, 18*(3), 95–100. https://doi.org/10.4103/0971-4065.43687.

Ansah, T. A., Ferguson, M. C., Nayyar, T., & Deutch, A. Y. (2011). Age- and duration-dependent effects of MPTP on cortical serotonin systems. *Neuroscience Letters, 504*(2), 160–164.

Arendt, J. (2005). *Melatonin and the Mammalian Pineal Gland.* Chapman & Hall.

Basner, M., & McGuire, S. (2018). WHO environmental noise guidelines for the European region: A systematic review on environmental noise and effects on sleep. *International Journal of Environmental Research and Public Health, 15*(3), 519. https://doi.org/10.3390/ijerph15030519.

Bender, L., Harding, D., Kennedy, D., Lee, G., & Stokes & Taylor, J. B. (2005). *The Facts on File Illustrated Guide to The Human Body: Digestive System.* Facts on File, Inc.

Benedetti, M. G., Furlini, G., Zati, A., & Mauro, G. L. (2018). The effectiveness of physical exercise on bone density in osteoporotic patients. *Biomedical Research International, 2018*, 4840531. https://doi.org/10.1155/2018/4840531.

Borjigin, J., Li, X., & Snyder, S. H. (1999). The pineal gland and melatonin: Molecular and pharmacologic regulation. *Annual Review of Pharmacology and Toxicology, 39*, 53–65.

Boström, P., Wu, J., Jedrychowski, M. P., Korde, A., Ye, L., Lo, J. C., Rasbach, K. A., Boström, E. A., Choi, J. H., Long, J. Z., et al. (2012). A PGC1-α-dependent myokine that drives brown-fat-like development of white fat and thermogenesis. *Nature, 481*, 463–468.

Cain, D. W., & Cidlowski, J. A. (2017). Immune regulation by glucocorticoids. *Nature Reviews Immunology, 17*(4), 233–247. https://doi.org/10.1038/nri.2017.1.

Cani, P. D., Amar, J., Iglesias, M. A., Poggi, M., Knauf, C., Bastelica, D., Neyrinck, A. M., Fava, F., Tuohy, K. M., Chabo, C., et al. (2007). Metabolic endotoxemia initiates obesity and insulin resistance. *Diabetes, 56*, 1761–1772. https://doi.org/10.2337/db06-1491.

Chauhan, A., & Jeans, A. F. (2015). Is Parkinson's disease truly a prion-like disorder? An appraisal of current evidence. *Neurology Research International, 2015*, 345285.

Cotman, C. W., & Berchtold, N. C. (2002). Exercise: A behavioural intervention to enhance brain health and plasticity. *Trends in Neurosciences, 25*, 295–301. https://doi.org/10.1016/S0166-2236(02)02143-4.

De Oliveira, E. P., & Burini, R. C. (2009). The impact of physical exercise on the gastrointestinal tract. *Current Opinion in Clinical Nutrition and Metabolic Care, 12*(5), 533–538. https://doi.org/10.1097/MCO.0b013e32832e6776.

De Vadder, F., Kovatcheva-Datchary, P., Goncalves, D., Vinera, J., Zitoun, C., Duchampt, A., Bäckhed, F., & Mithieux, G. (2014). Microbiota-generated metabolites promote metabolic benefits via gut-brain neural circuits. *Cell, 156*, 84–96. https://doi.org/10.1016/j.cell.2013.12.016.

Duffy, J. F., Abbott, S. M., Burgess, H. J., Crowley, S. J., Emens, J. S., Epstein, L. J., Gamble, K. L., Hasler, B. P., Kristo, D. A., Malkani, R. G., Rahman, S. A., Thomas, S. J., Wyatt, J. K., Zee, P. C., & Klerman, E. B. (2021). Workshop report. Circadian rhythm sleep-wake disorders: Gaps and opportunities. *Sleep, 44*(5), zsaa281. https://doi.org/10.1093/sleep/zsaa281.

Ernst, C., Olson, A. K., Pinel, J. P. J., Lam, R. W., & Christie, B. R. (2006). Antidepressant effects of exercise: Evidence for an adult neurogenesis hypothesis? *Journal of Psychiatry and Neuroscience, 31*, 84–92.

Fedorenko, A., Lishko, P. V., & Kirichok, Y. (2012). Mechanism of fatty-acid-dependent UCP1 uncoupling in brown fat mitochondria. *Cell, 151*, 400–417.

Giasson, B. I., et al. (2003). Initiation and synergistic fibrillization of tau and alpha-synuclein. *Science, 300*(5619), 636–640.

Graf, P., & Schacter, D. L. (1985). Implicit and explicit memory for new associations in normal and amnesic subjects. *Journal of Experimental Psychology: Learning, Memory, and Cognition, 11*(3), 501–518. https://doi.org/10.1037/0278-7393.11.3.501.

Hassan, Z. M., Sebola, N. A., & Mabelebele, M. (2021). The nutritional use of millet grain for food and feed: A review. *Agriculture & Food Security, 10*(1), 16. https://doi.org/10.1186/s40066-020-00282-6.

Huot, P., Sgambato-Faure, V., Fox, S. H., & McCreary, A. C. (2017). Serotonergic approaches in Parkinson's disease: Translational perspectives, an update. *ACS Chemical Neuroscience, 8*(5), 973–986.

Ishizawa, T., Mattila, P., Davies, P., Wang, D., & Dickson, D. W. (2003). Colocalization of tau and alpha-synuclein epitopes in Lewy bodies. *Journal of Neuropathology & Experimental Neurology, 62*(4), 389–397.

Jiang, C., Li, G., Huang, P., Liu, Z., & Zhao, B. (2017). The gut microbiota and Alzheimer's disease. *Journal of Alzheimer's Disease, 58*(1), 1–15.

Jokinen, E. (2015). Obesity and cardiovascular disease. *Minerva Pediatrica, 67*(1), 25–32.

Kim, W. S., Kagedal, K., & Halliday, G. M. (2014). Alpha-synuclein biology in Lewy body diseases. *Alzheimer's Research & Therapy, 6*(5), 73.

Lakatta, E. G., & Levy, D. (2003). Arterial and cardiac aging: Major shareholders in cardiovascular disease enterprises, part II: The aging heart in health: Links to heart disease. *Circulation, 107*, 346–354.

Lo, J. C., Leong, R. L. F., Ng, A. S. C., Jamaluddin, S. A., Ong, J. L., Ghorbani, S., Lau, T., Chee, N. I. Y. N., Gooley, J. J., & Chee, M. W. L. (2020). Cognitive effects of split and continuous sleep schedules in adolescents differ according to total sleep opportunity. *Sleep, 43*(12), zsaa129.

Lyketsos, C. G., Carrillo, M. C., Ryan, J. M., Khachaturian, A. S., Trzepacz, P., Amatniek, J., Cedarbaum, J., Brashear, R., & Miller, D. S. (2011). Neuropsychiatric symptoms in Alzheimer's disease. *Alzheimer's & Dementia, 7*(5), 532–539.

Marks, J., Carvou, N., Debnam, E., Srai, S., & Unwin, R. (2003). Diabetes increases facilitative glucose uptake and GLUT2 expression at the rat proximal tubule brush border membrane. *Journal of Physiology, 553*, 137–145.

McKee, A. C., Stein, T. D., Kiernan, P. T., & Alvarez, V. E. (2015). The neuropathology of chronic traumatic encephalopathy. *Brain Pathology, 25*, 350–364.

Moore, R. Y., et al. (1972). A retinohypothalamic projection in the rat. *Journal of Comparative Neurology, 146*(1), 1–14.

Morigny, P., Boucher, J., Arner, P., & Langin, D. (2021). Lipid and glucose metabolism in white adipocytes: Pathways, dysfunction and therapeutics. *Nature Reviews Endocrinology, 17*, 276–295.

Moussavi, S., Chatterji, S., Verdes, E., Tandon, A., Patel, V., & Ustun, B. (2007). Depression, chronic diseases, and decrements in health: Results from the World Health Surveys. *The Lancet, 370*, 808–809.

Navale, A. M., & Paranjape, A. N. (2016). Glucose transporters: Physiological and pathological roles. *Biophysical Reviews, 8*, 5–9.

Nitsa, A., Toutouza, M., Machairas, N., Mariolis, A., Philippou, A., & Koutsilieris, M. (2018). Vitamin D in cardiovascular disease. *In Vivo, 32*(5), 977–981.

North, B. J., & Sinclair, D. A. (2012). The intersection between aging and cardiovascular disease. *Circulation Research, 110*(8), 1097–1108.

Pedersen, H. K., Gudmundsdottir, V., Nielsen, H. B., Hyotylainen, T., Nielsen, T., Jensen, B. A. H., Forslund, K., Hildebrand, F., Prifti, E., Falony, G., et al. (2016). Human gut microbes impact host serum metabolome and insulin sensitivity. *Nature, 535*, 376–381.

Reilly, S. M., Abu-Odeh, M., Ameka, M., DeLuca, J. H., Naber, M. C., Dadpey, B., Ebadat, N., Gomez, A. V., Peng, X., Poirier, B., et al. (2021). FGF21 is required for the metabolic benefits of IKKε/TBK1 inhibition. *Journal of Clinical Investigation, 131*, 158.

Saladin, K. S. (2017). *Human Anatomy* (5th ed.). McGraw-Hill Education.

Šimić, G., Tkalčić, M., Vukić, V., Mulc, D., Španić, E., Šagud, M., Olucha-Bordonau, F. E., Vukšić, M., & Hof, P. R. (2021). Understanding emotions: Origins and roles of the amygdala. *Biomolecules, 11*(6), 827.

Simonyan, K. (2019). Recent advances in understanding the role of the basal ganglia. *F1000Research, 8*, F1000 Faculty Rev-122.

Smithies, T. D., Toth, A. J., Dunican, I. C., Caldwell, J. A., Kowal, M., & Campbell, M. J. (2021). The effect of sleep restriction on cognitive performance in elite cognitive performers: A systematic review. *Sleep, 44*(7), zsab008.

Stein, T. D., Alvarez, V. E., & McKee, A. C. (2014). Chronic traumatic encephalopathy: A spectrum of neuropathological changes following repetitive brain trauma in athletes and military personnel. *Alzheimer's Research & Therapy, 6*, 4.

Tamaki, S., Kanazawa, A., Sato, J., Tamura, Y., Asahara, T., Takahashi, T., Matsumoto, S., Yamashiro, Y., & Watada, H. (2019). Clinical factors associated with bacterial translocation in Japanese patients with type 2 diabetes: A retrospective study. *PLOS ONE, 14*, e0222598.

Wang, Z., & Zhao, Y. (2018). Gut microbiota derived metabolites in cardiovascular health and disease. *Protein & Cell, 9*(5), 416–431.

Wankhede, D. B., Shehnaj, A., & Rao, M. R. (1979). Carbohydrate composition of finger millet (*Eleusine coracana*) and foxtail millet (*Setaria italica*). *Plant Foods for Human Nutrition, 28*, 293–307.

World Health Organization (WHO) Regional Office for Europe. (2011). *Burden of Disease from Environmental Noise: Quantification of Healthy Life Years Lost in Europe*. WHO Regional Office for Europe.

Ye, L., & Ning, G. (2015). The molecular classification of hereditary endocrine diseases. *Endocrine, 50*(3), 575–579.

CHAPTER 7

Principles of Health Assessment and Diagnosis

RAHUL SAXENA,[1*] SUYASH SAXENA,[1] and AJIT PAL SINGH[2]

[1]*Department of Biochemistry, School of Allied Health Sciences, Sharda University, Greater Noida, Uttar Pradesh, India*

[2]*Medical Lab Technology, Sharda School of Allied Health Sciences, Sharda University, Greater Noida (UP)*

*Corresponding author

ABSTRACT

People have always been concerned with their health and well-being, and numerous scientific attempts have been made to help people live thriving and healthy lives. Though the enigma of immortality remains unsolved, it is now commonly accepted that physical and mental well-being will progressively decline with age, giving way to a myriad of health issues and, eventually, death. In this regard, it has been found that clinical health evaluation, a dynamic and multifaceted phenomenon, is associated with the identification of multiple pathophysiological diseases that impact different body systems, such as the respiratory, cardiovascular, musculoskeletal, and nervous systems. There is a dire need to recognize the steps involved in health assessment, sources of evidence, and levels of health assessment (HA) screening dimensions. Interestingly, guidelines pertaining to HA screening, along with coverage of HA practices, have been emphasized as an important step to create awareness among the general population. This chapter gives an introductory overview of the current HA principles and screening tactics connected to the many types of clinical conditions. It places an emphasis on the function of diagnostics in the prompt detection and effective treatment of pathophysiological incidents.

Allied Healthcare in Practice: An Introduction to Integrated Patient Care. Sally Lukose, Karuna Singh (Eds.)

DOI: 10.1201/9781998511037-9

7.1 INTRODUCTION OF HEALTH ASSESSMENT (HA)

In this mortal world, nothing is possible as a solitary effort and decision of any individual. It needs a lot of collective effort, both directly and indirectly, from all the contributors. Similarly, the diagnosis of any disease can be based on several factors, which include a well-defined assessment strategy of health. It's crucial to note that part of the process of evaluating a patient's health involves applying the clinician's knowledge and skills to distinguish between normal and abnormal data. Often, a health evaluation moves from a general assessment of a body system to more in-depth observations or functional testing. This clinical assessment and decision-making process is based on deductive reasoning. For instance, a doctor would perform a physical examination on a patient with known hypertension to check their blood pressure. The doctor would conclude that high blood pressure is most likely the source of these observations after measuring both the systolic and diastolic blood pressure, considering dietary habits and family history (Finkelstein, 2002). This would significantly limit the options available for medical decisions and diagnostic treatments. Advanced health evaluation is based on basic assessment and expands upon it. Through an inductive or inferential process—more frequently employed in advanced assessment—a broader diagnosis, or set of diagnoses, is usually determined based on the patient's history, physical findings, and the outcomes of laboratory and diagnostic tests. The professional gathers more data and analyzes it in order to formulate a hypothesis that narrows the field of possibilities even more. We call this method of thinking diagnostic.

7.2 STEPS OF HEALTH ASSESSMENT (HA) SCREENING

Start with a clinical issue first. It is necessary to determine a topic's value for public health before deciding whether it is appropriate to investigate it and create screening criteria. The burden of suffering from a disorder placed on a population and the efficiency of a preventive service or intervention in easing that burden are among the criteria. Next, pose a clinical question focused on the problem the patient is experiencing and any possible prophylactic measures (Finkelstein, 2002). The PICO structure, which comprises problem, intervention or exposure, comparison, and outcome (PICO), is beneficial as it integrates crucial components of a well-crafted investigation. An analytical framework can be used to show the chain of evidence that needs to be evaluated in order to get from screening or preemptive therapy to health outcomes, such as improved overall quantity and quality of life. After the main query, a series of inquiries are made in an effort to build the clinical case for the implementation of a preventive program in a primary care setting:

Does screening for X reduce morbidity and/or mortality?

i. Is it possible to identify a group with X high risk based on clinical evidence?
ii. Are accurate screening tests—that is, sensitive and specific—available?
iii. When the disease is discovered early or found by screening, are there treatments that affect intermediate outcomes?
iv. Are there any therapies that lower morbidity or mortality rates in cases where the illness is identified early on or via screening?
v. To what extent are the patient health outcomes and intermediate outcomes correlated?
vi. What are the screening test's drawbacks?
vii. What are the treatment's drawbacks?

To address the various potential for bias, the certainty and strength of evidence for each important question are evaluated while reviewing the chain of facts. Third, choose the appropriate sources and conduct a literature search on every main topic that contrasts different treatment approaches and techniques for examining relevant outcomes.

Think about the evidence's validity and applicability. To begin a search, major databases such as the Cochrane Library or PubMed will access original sources. A number of secondary sources, such as Clinical Evidence, Vital Evidence Plus, and the Journal Club of the American College of Physicians, review the original work. Examine the following terms when interpreting the findings:

i. The risk in the control group divided by the risk in the experimental group yields the relative risk (RR).
ii. The decision between statistical and clinical significance can be subjective and frequently hinges on the magnitude of the effect under investigation. Is there a significant enough difference between the groups to justify improvement? The likelihood of past exposure in a case divided by the probability of exposure in a

control patient is known as the odds ratio, or OR. For instance, an OR of 3.0 indicates that the risk of exposure in control cases was three times higher than in treated patients.

iii. Confidence intervals (CI) are a tool used to evaluate the accuracy of study results. Reduced precision is indicated by wider CI. For instance, "36 (CI 27 to 51)" means that, if the trial were to be repeated 100 times, the values would, in 95% of cases, fall between 27 and 51.

Subsequently, use your understanding of patients' preferences. It is critical to determine whether the population from which the evidence is collected is representative of the patient population. For example, population-based mammography screening guidelines would not apply to a woman who has previously had breast cancer (Kleinman and Benson, 2006).

7.3 EVIDENCES OF HEALTH ASSESSMENT (HA)

A study design that allows for less bias or systematic mistakes and may result in an incorrect conclusion is referred to as having a hierarchy of evidence. RCTs, or randomized controlled clinical trials, can eliminate bias and offer reliable proof of cause and effect. Threats to the research population's representativeness and inconsistent intervention implementation are other drawbacks of RCTs. In a meta-analysis, multiple credible studies on a subject are examined, and the data are computationally combined to present them as if they were from a single, sizable study. Clinical competence, group experience, and knowledge from professional groups such as the American College of Obstetrics and Gynecology or the American Heart Association serve as the foundation for expert opinion. Compared to higher levels of evidence, case reports, longitudinal studies, and qualitative investigations offer less reliable and valid evidence of cause and effect (Connelly, 1988).

7.4 LEVELS OF PREVENTION

The three categories are primary, secondary, and tertiary preventative levels. Primary prevention comprises focused disease defense measures combined with efforts to improve general health. Interventions include things like screening, counseling, and preventative medicine like vaccinations and dental sealants. Counseling on risky activities, such as riding a bicycle without a seatbelt or helmet, can reduce the number of accidents and fatalities. The 5 As approach is a popular one for behavioral counseling: Ask about the behavior, provide information on the health hazards and advantages of changing, set a goal-setting agreement; help in recognizing and removing obstacles; decide on follow-up. Finding and detecting disease early on, before symptoms appear, is known as secondary prevention. A test of hemoglobin A1C during screening interventions can reveal high blood pressure or diabetes risk. It may be possible to treat an illness, delay its progression, avoid or reduce consequences, and restrict disability with early detection and diagnosis. Through the provision of rehabilitative services, the reduction of disease intensity and progression, and the mitigation of complications and disabilities, tertiary preventive programs seek to improve the quality of life for those afflicted with a variety of illnesses (rehabilitation therapy to regain independence and functionality). Extended periods of time, such as those after the optimal management of chronic conditions like diabetes and hypertension, can be used for tertiary prevention. Unlike primary and secondary prevention, tertiary prevention involves treating the ailment.

7.5 GUIDELINES OF SCREENING

Not every disease or condition has to be checked for. The screening process must have ethically sound objectives, make appropriate use of information, employ high-quality tests, inform participants of the procedure and their results, provide counseling to assist participants in interpreting the results, and maintain participant confidentiality. Furthermore, a new urgency in recognizing and applying screening recommendations to evaluate the efficacy of population screening for genetic vulnerability to diseases and conditions has been brought about by genomic medicine (Barton et al., 2007). The following criteria can be used to decide if a disease or condition needs to be screened for:

i. The condition must be measured by quality of life, utilizing statistics on morbidity and mortality, and it must have a significant influence on either the quantity or quality of life. The incidence of the condition, or the number of new or undiagnosed instances, must be high enough to warrant the expense of the screening.
ii. Affordable tests that can detect the illness when it is asymptomatic must be made available to patients. Test acceptance is

evaluated using a variety of metrics, including validity (does the test measure what you think it measures?), reliability (reproducibility), and sensitivity (capacity to deliver a true positive) and specificity (capacity to deliver a true negative). Potential screening negatives include labeling and stigma, screening test-related morbidity, and patient preference are other factors to consider. Does the condition need to be screened? Acceptable treatments must be accessible prior to the recommendation of screening. Contextual factors like geographic location, social level, and cultural beliefs and traditions must be taken into account. For an illness to be eligible for screening, it must have both an asymptomatic phase and a period during which treatment and detection substantially enhance health outcomes above a diagnosis made only on the basis of symptoms.

7.6 PREVENTIVE SERVICE TASK FORCE

Because of how swiftly the healthcare industry is changing in India and globally, many individuals characterize the environment as dynamic, complex, and extremely uncertain. This is accurate for a number of reasons. In this regard, the CEOs Forum hosted by the (AAPI) brought together leaders in the healthcare industry, opinion leaders, and community organizers to discuss the significance of advancing preventive healthcare in India. In order to support India's 1.4 billion residents, the CEO Forum unanimously supported an appeal made by AAPI to the government of India to start the process of establishing an Indian Preventive Task Force (IPTF) and carrying out yearly preventive healthcare screenings across the country (Barton et al., 2007).

In addition, the United States Preventive Services Task Force was established in the year 1984 as a free-standing organization of professionals with a focus on evidence-based medicine and prevention. The task force's responsibility is to offer advice on clinical preventive services such as tests, counseling, and medication (Rockville, 1996). The USPSTF collaborates with Evidence-Based Practice Centers (EPCs), which carry out comprehensive systematic reviews of the current evidence and create an analytical framework or research plan with a list of important questions and outcomes that the study must address. For clinical preventive treatments, the USPSTF recommendations are regarded as the benchmark. Practitioners can electronically obtain USPSTF recommendations via the Electronic Preventive Services Selector (ePSS) site.

The Affordable Care Act (ACA) addresses the development of a customized preventive plan, an individual health risk assessment that considers medical and family history, an evaluation of current healthcare providers and medications, a physical and mental evaluation, and a review of a screening schedule. Wellness visits per year are also provided. The ACA mandates that evidence-based techniques for preventive treatments, including weight loss, smoking cessation, and the promotion of healthy lifestyles, be covered (Faulkner and Schauffler, 1997).

7.7 DIAGNOSTIC IMPORTANCE OF HEALTH ASSESSMENT (HA)

Before beginning any type of treatment, a doctor must make a medical diagnosis of the patient. For that, the patient is questioned and frequently has physical measurements taken. The doctor conducts an analysis of the data after receiving all the responses and medical reports before beginning the patient's corrective therapy. The treatment continues until the patient achieves the targeted level of physical wellness. For example, before a nephrologist can initiate the treatment of a patient, it is essential to know the health status of the patient's kidneys. A diagnostic assessment of renal function tests provides diagnostic information to the nephrologist about the patient's current health status and functioning of the kidneys. The nephrologist can determine the patient's present health status and the preconditions that need to be controlled as the diagnostic data is analyzed. A nephrologist can accurately and efficiently develop a treatment plan with the use of this crucial information, allowing the patient to recover from their illness.

7.8 CONCLUSION

In the context of an assisted living facility, the introduction to knowledge should be comprehensive, general, and focused on the most common or prevalent conditions within that particular population group. It is necessary for the expert professional to develop inductive thinking skills in order to arrive at a conclusion and design a treatment plan that is worthy of the patient in this introduction. A long-term relationship with the patient greatly enhances the database, which the expert uses to make the best treatment decisions. In primary care settings, treatment strategies prioritize low-tech stress reduction, open and effective patient-provider communication, and self-care.

Additionally, experts need to be able to locate and assess the best available evidence in order to recommend appraisal, treatment, and assessment of indicative adequacy on well-being outcomes. By asking the right questions, searching for pertinent and high-quality information from readily available logical proof, and applying clinical reasoning to apply the best proof to clinical settings, a specialist can progress from amateur to master and become more proficient in determining clinical judgment.

7.9 SUMMARY

Thus, HA has a positive impact on the provision of various clinical preventative services and may have a positive impact on patient worry, offering evidence in support of its continued use in clinical practice. Additional data from studies is required to determine the long-term advantages, disadvantages, and costs of HA, as well as to assess the benefits of getting therapeutic preventative care and anxiety reduction in the absence of evidence indicating such long-term clinical advantages. Despite this, current research supports HA's obvious advantages for the general population. Additionally, while using their own discretion on the best manner to administer the HA, clinicians could be confident that HA may confer comparable advantages in their own practices according to evidence-based literature. It is clear from this that experience and intuition cannot be replaced by evidence alone. In clinical decision-making, human issues must constantly be taken into consideration. However, the provision of both preventative and acute care services will increasingly fall under the purview of primary care physicians. Practitioners must be aware of this and base their judgments on both clinical judgment and high-quality scientific data when treating specific patients.

KEYWORDS

- **clinical assessment**
- **decision-making process**
- **diastolic blood pressure**
- **hypertension**
- **low-tech stress reduction**
- **patient database**
- **population group**
- **systolic blood pressure**
- **treatment strategies**

REFERENCES

Barton, M. B., Miller, T., & Wolff, T. (2007). How to read the new recommendation statement: Methods update from the U.S. Preventive Services Task Force. *Annals of Internal Medicine, 147*, 123–125.

Bernacki, E. J., Tsai, S. P., & Malone, R. D. (1988). Participation in a periodic physical examination program and group health care utilization and costs. *Journal of Occupational Medicine, 30*, 949–952.

Connelly, J. E. (1988). Periodic health examination. In D. M. Becker & L. B. Gardner (Eds.), *Prevention in Clinical Practice* (Vol. 1, pp. 419–434). Springer.

Faulkner, L. A., & Schauffler, H. H. (1997). The effect of health insurance coverage on the appropriate use of recommended clinical preventive services. *American Journal of Preventive Medicine, 13*, 453–458.

Finkelstein, M. M. (2002). Preventive screening: What factors influence testing? *Canadian Family Physician, 48*, 1494–1501.

Kleinman, A., & Benson, P. (2006). Anthropology in the clinic: The problem of cultural competency and how to fix it. *PLoS Medicine, 3*, e294.

U.S. Preventive Services Task Force. (1996). *Guides to Clinical Preventive Services*. Agency for Healthcare Research and Quality.

CHAPTER 8

Physical Examination Techniques

SUYASH SAXENA,[1,*] RAHUL SAXENA,[1] and AJIT PAL SINGH[2]

[1]*Department of Biochemistry, Sharda School of Allied Health Sciences, Sharda University, Greater Noida, Uttar Pradesh, India*

[2]*Department of Medical Laboratory Technology, Sharda School of Allied Health Sciences, Sharda University, Greater Noida, Uttar Pradesh, India*

*Corresponding author

ABSTRACT

Diagnosis of a disease has important repercussions for patient care and recovery. Clinical decision making will be based on an accurate understanding of the patient's health problem, when a diagnosis is accurate and made promptly, a patient has the highest chance for a favorable health outcome. Correct diagnosis of the disease is the most important part of treatment. There are three pillars for making a correct diagnosis, which involve detailed history taking, physical examination, and lastly, diagnostic testing. Physical examination can help to confirm a lot of diseases along with careful history taking, even without the extra burden of expenditure on diagnostics, or if required, it can help the health worker to choose wisely for the correct investigations. Physical examination also helps in judging the severity of the disease and can assist in deciding the prognosis. Physical examination can be divided into three stages: anthropometric measures, vital signs, and the hands-on observational examination. In this chapter, we are going to discuss all the measures of physical examination, the techniques to perform the physical examination, and their clinical importance.

Allied Healthcare in Practice: An Introduction to Integrated Patient Care. Sally Lukose, Karuna Singh (Eds.)

DOI: 10.1201/9781998511037-10

8.1 INTRODUCTION

The physical examination is a crucial component of the diagnostic evaluation. It provides a way to verify a history-based suspicion of a diagnosis without spending further money. Additionally, a physical examination can help choose the right laboratory investigations by revealing information about the nature and severity of the condition. The physical examination still plays a crucial part in the diagnosis process, even though the etiology of a disease is hypothesized based on history and validated through laboratory tests (Jain and Jain, 2021). Lack of a thorough physical examination might raise the possibility of diagnostic mistakes and oversights, endangering patient safety.

A thorough physical examination can assist a doctor in fine-tuning the next steps in the diagnostic procedure, avoiding needless diagnostic tests, and building patients' trust through tactile engagement. Although physical examination traditionally involves four techniques: inspection, palpation, percussion, and auscultation, it is equally important to measure anthropometric values and vital signs, which provide crucial information about general health and help identify and monitor medical problems.

8.2 ANTHROPOEMETRIC MEASURES

According to the Centre for Disease Control and Prevention, anthropometric measurements are quantitative, non-invasive measurements of the body used to evaluate nutritional status in both children and adults (Fryar et al., 2021). According to the Academy of Nutrition and Dietetics (the Academy) and the American Society for Parenteral and Enteral Nutrition (A.S.P.E.N.), accurate and serial tracking of anthropometric measurements can aid in identifying underlying medical, nutritional, or social issues in children (Corkins et al., 2015).

Anthropometry can be performed on humans to assess diet and health, identify obesity, forecast illness risk in the future, and estimate body composition. The major components of anthropometry include height, weight, head circumference, body mass index (BMI), body circumferences (waist, hip, and limbs to evaluate adiposity), and skinfold thickness. However, isolated measurements need to be compared to relative norms for the relevant group in order to yield useful insights. Pediatricians must regularly plot anthropometric data on suitable growth charts up until the age of 18 since anthropometry is a key tool for tracking a child's growth. Through doing this, you can avoid the need for pricey investigations through early identification of the root causes of failure to thrive. While WHO simple growth charts are advocated for newborns and young children under the age of five, the Indian Academy of Pediatrics (IAP) has recommended using the IAP 2015 Growth charts to track the growth of Indian children between the ages of 5 and 18 (Khadilkar et al., 2015). The IAP 2015 BMI charts also define overweight and obesity as 23 and 27 kg/ m^2 adult equivalents, respectively.

Analyzing body composition in athletes and nutritional status in children and adults using anthropometric measurements can improve performance and identify underlying medical issues like eating disorders. Strength and cardio-respiratory fitness can be increased in athletes using anthropometry-based training programs. Additionally, anthropometric measurements can be used to evaluate individuals with obesity and pregnant women's nutritional health.

Specific methods are advised in order to obtain accurate anthropometric measurements. These techniques include using a stadiometer to measure height, a calibrated scale to measure weight, a non-stretchable tape to measure head circumference, a caliper to measure skinfold thickness, and a BMI calculator to determine weight in relation to height squared. All measurements must be carried out in accordance with defined processes to ensure accuracy and consistency.

In conclusion, anthropometric measurements are an invaluable tool for evaluating a person's health since they provide vital details about nutritional status, growth, and body composition. Healthcare providers can gather precise and helpful data to assist in uncovering underlying medical, nutritional, or social concerns and provide relevant interventions by adhering to standardized methods and comparing measures to suitable population norms.

8.2.1 HEAD CIRCUMFERENCE

When measuring the head circumference of infants and toddlers younger than two years of age, it is crucial to use a non-stretchable measuring tape and take the measurement surrounding the largest circumference of the head, which is typically around the most prominent part of the head to the middle of the forehead. The measuring tape should be stretched tightly around the skull, squeezing the hair and delicate tissue underneath. To ensure precision, the measurement should be performed twice with readings that are within 0.2 cm or 0.25 inches of one another. The final head circumference measurement should be the average of the two closest readings. This measurement is important in monitoring the growth and development of infants and toddlers, as abnormal head growth may indicate underlying medical issues that require intervention.

8.2.2 HEIGHT

A stadiometer needs to be used to measure the height of an individual precisely. The subject should be erect, with their heels, buttocks, and shoulder blades touching the stadiometer's back. If the patient has knock-knees, their feet should be separated to prevent overlapping the knees while preserving contact between them. The toes are supposed to face outward at a 60° angle. The palms of the arms must be facing the thighs and should dangle lightly at the sides. To compress the hair to the crown of the head, the horizontal bar of the stadiometer should be lowered. Remove any items from the hair or from the head that might prevent the bar from squeezing the hair to the crown of the head. It is recommended to read the measurement to the nearest 0.1 cm (1/8 inch). The measurement should be done twice for precision, with the two readings being within 0.2 cm or 0.25 inches of one another. The mean of the two closest values should be used as the final height measurement. This measurement is essential for figuring out an adult's height for medical reasons as well as monitoring a child's or adolescent's growth and development.

8.2.3 WEIGHT

Children older than 2 years of age can have their weight measured using a balanced floor scale or an electronic floor scale. The child should stand in the middle of the scale with their arms at their sides and bare feet. To the nearest 0.1 kg or 0.5 pounds, the weight should be calculated. The weight of the wheelchair or stroller should be deducted from the overall weight if the child is unable to stand and must instead be weighed while seated in one. To get precise measurements, it's crucial to make sure the scale is correctly calibrated before use.

8.2.4 BODY MASS INDEX (BMI)

For determining a person's body weight in both adults and children, the BMI is a typical measurement. The BMI is not a perfect indicator of body fatness or health, although it is useful for assessing weight status and any health problems related to it. As you noted, there are restrictions on its application, particularly in certain demographics like athletes and the elderly. Waist circumference, skinfold thickness, and bioelectrical impedance analysis are a few other measurements that could offer more details on body composition and potential health hazards.

8.2.5 WAIST CIRCUMFERENCE

In addition to height and weight, waist circumference can be used to evaluate a person's risk for cardiovascular disease (CVD). Men are considered to have a high waist circumference if it measures more than 102 cm (40 inches), while women are considered to have a high waist circumference if it measures more than 88 cm (35 inches). These cut-off numbers, however, can differ by ethnicity because some groups may have a higher risk of CVD at lower levels of waist circumference. In order to determine overall CVD risk, waist circumference should be used in conjunction with other measurements like BMI and blood pressure rather than as a sole indicator of health risk.

8.2.6 WAIST TO HIP RATIO (WHR)

Another body composition metric used to evaluate how body fat is distributed is the Waist to Hip Ratio (WHR). It is a measurement of central obesity, which is linked to a higher risk of cardiovascular and metabolic disorders. A high WHR suggests more abdominal fat being stored, which is thought to be more metabolically active and consequently more hazardous to health. The WHR is determined by dividing the waist circumference by the hip circumference.

8.3 VITAL SIGNS

Vital signs are measurements of the body's most basic functions. The four main vital signs routinely checked by healthcare providers include:

- Body temperature.
- Pulse rate.
- Breathing rate (respiration).
- Blood pressure.

8.3.1 BODY TEMPERATURE

Body temperature can change depending on a number of variables, including gender, activity level, time of day, and dietary consumption. Body temperature for an adult should range from 97.8°F (36.5°C) to 99°F (37.2°C). An elevated body temperature can be a sign of fever (a high body temperature) or hypothermia (low temperature). Hypothermia occurs when the body temperature drops below 95°F, while a fever occurs when it rises by 1° or more above 98.6°F. There are numerous ways to take someone's body temperature, depending on the circumstance and the individual, including orally, rectally, under the armpit (axillary), by the ear, by the skin, or internally. Each method is used for different things and has differing levels of accuracy.

8.3.2 PULSE RATE

The pulse rate, which also serves as a gauge for heart rate, heart rhythm, and pulse force, is the number of times the heart beats per minute. The expansion and contraction of the arteries as the heart pumps blood through them allows one to feel the pulse. The average pulse rate in healthy persons is 60 to 100 beats per minute; however, it might differ based on factors like exercise, disease, injury, and emotions. Heart rates in women over the age of 12 are typically higher than in men, and athletes undergoing cardio-vascular conditioning may experience heart rates as low as 40 beats per minute. The neck, elbow, wrist, or groin are just a few places on the body where the pulse can be taken. The wrist is usually the most convenient place to check the pulse, but it's important to be careful not to press too firmly when examining the pulse at the lower neck because doing so can result in a blockage of the blood supply to the brain.

8.3.3 BREATHING RATE

The number of breaths an individual takes per minute while at rest is referred to as their respiration rate. One only needs to count how many times their chest rises during a minute to establish their breathing rate. Exercise, a fever, an illness, or other medical problems are just a few of the factors that might cause the respiration rate to rise. While monitoring the respiration rate, it's crucial to take notice of any breathing problems. Adults typically breathe between 12 and 20 times per minute while at rest.

8.3.4 BLOOD PRESSURE

The force of the blood pressing against the artery walls during a heartbeat is measured as blood pressure. When the heart beats and forces blood into the arteries, the pressure is at its maximum. Its technical name is systolic pressure. Diastolic pressure is the term used to describe the pressure that forms as the heart contracts and fills with blood. Millimeters of mercury are used to measure blood pressure (mm Hg). Because high blood pressure makes it harder for the heart to circulate blood throughout the body, it can raise the risk of myocardial infarction, congestive heart failure, and stroke. Stage 1 and 2 of high blood pressure can be distinguished from values of normal and raised blood pressure.

Less than 120/80 mm Hg is considered normal blood pressure. Elevated blood pressure is systolic pressure of 120 to 129 mm Hg and diastolic pressure less than 80 mm Hg. Stage 1 high blood pressure is systolic pressure 130 to 139 mm Hg or diastolic pressure of 80 to 89 mm Hg. Stage 2 high blood pressure is when systolic pressure is 140 mm Hg or higher or diastolic pressure is 90 mm Hg or higher.

8.4 HANDS-ON OBSERVATION

Inspection, palpation, percussion, and auscultation are the four procedures typically used in a physical examination. By observing, touching, hearing, and interpreting the data, these techniques aid in learning about the patient's condition. In order to spot any anomalies, it's critical to grasp what is regarded as typical. Additionally, understanding typical presentation or manifestation patterns linked to various illnesses is crucial for the physical examination procedure. The data collection from these techniques can help medical professionals diagnose a patient's functional health problems or make a clinical diagnosis.

8.4.1 INSPECTION

Healthcare personnel examine the patient as a whole throughout the inspection process, taking into account many aspects such as their attire, facial expressions, body form, and stride. Inspection may concentrate on certain body parts connected to a system if it is deemed to be problematic. The patient's general appearance, posture, symmetry, and nutritional state should all be evaluated before anything else. Poor grooming or signs of wasting could be a sign of depression or a chronic illness. The doctor should also perform a thorough examination of the skin, looking for any changes that might point to early cancer, moles, or other pigmented spots, infections, or other symptoms. In addition, areas like the scalp, back, and buttocks that are difficult for the patient to see should be inspected.

The skin and nails play a significant role in diagnosis. For instance, a nail examination can reveal important details regarding systemic disorders. The condition known as clubbing of the nails, which is characterized by widened nail beds and curled, polished nails, may be a sign of bronchogenic cancer, chronic obstructive pulmonary disease, or congenital cardiac disease. On the other hand, onycholysis of the nails is a common symptom in psoriasis sufferers. It is imperative to screen for cancer when inspecting the skin, even if it can be difficult to tell a dangerous lesion from a benign mole (nevus).

Procedure: Each physiological system is examined visually, olfactorily, and auditorily to determine both healthy and unhealthy conditions. Each system's color, size, location, movement, texture, symmetry, scents, and sounds should be assessed throughout this assessment.

8.4.2 PALPATION

Palpation is the process of learning about the organs beneath the skin of the body by feeling the surface with the hands. It can be done with one or both hands, and it can be shallow or deep. An abdomen's stiffness, muscle spasms, or discomfort can all be felt with light probing. When stomach discomfort is present, gently palpating in the opposite direction of the pain will reveal the area that is the most painful. Localized discomfort and muscle rigidity are signs of acute abdominal inflammation, such as acute appendicitis. Deep abdominal palpation is used to feel the size of internal organs such as the liver, spleen, or kidneys, as well as to feel for abnormal masses like an abdominal aortic aneurysm. An inflamed gallbladder is most likely the source of an acutely sore lump in the right upper abdomen that is more uncomfortable on inspiration. A non-tender abdominal mass could be dangerous like a tumor or benign like a firm stool. Additionally, suspicious lesions in the breast, prostate, lymph nodes, or testes can be found and assessed using palpation. Regular monthly self-examinations and an annual medical evaluation are required for proper breast examination.

Procedure: It's crucial to utilize various regions of your hands and exert different amounts of pressure when palpating. As your main tools, it's also crucial to keep your hands warm and your fingernails short. Gloves should be worn when touching mucous membranes or places that have come into contact with bodily fluids. Additionally, to reduce pain for the patient, painful areas should be palpated last. Methods of palpation:

8.4.2.1 LIGHT PALPATION

Use the following method to check for surface abnormalities:

- Use your finger pads to gently push the skin, about 1/2 to 3/4 inch down (about 1 to 2 cm).
- Evaluate the mass's presence, texture, tenderness, temperature, wetness, flexibility, and pulsations.

8.4.2.2 DEEP PALPATION

Using the deep palpation technique, one can assess the size, shape, tenderness, symmetry, and motion of internal organs and masses. It entails using deep, firm pressure to depress the skin by 1.5 to 2 inches (approximately 4 to 5 cm). In some circumstances, stacking one hand on top of the other can aid in applying more force as necessary. This method can be useful for measuring the size of various organs, including the liver, spleen, and kidneys, as well as for finding any abnormal masses or tumors. However, it's crucial to proceed with caution and keep your hands off the patient if you don't want to hurt them. To reduce the danger of infection, palpation should also be carried out methodically and with strict adherence to cleanliness standards.

8.4.2.3 PERCUSSION

Percussion is a diagnostic procedure that involves giving a bodily part a few brief, sharp taps to determine its density. This can help with the diagnosis of diseases such as liver enlargement, intestinal blockage, and ascites, which is an accumulation of fluid in the abdomen. Nevertheless, it is most frequently used to assess the chest because it can find lung tissue anomalies there. When tapped, a healthy lung emits a resonant note, but a dull sound may be caused by fluids, as in respiratory infections, or a solid mass, like the heart. On the other hand, a lung with emphysema will emit a hyper-resonant note because it has more air than typical. The amount of air in the stomach can also be determined by percussion; tympanic noises that are high-pitched and hollow are indicative of a bloated stomach.

8.4.2.4 DIRECT PERCUSSION

Direct percussion is a method that is used to cause tenderness in a particular location of the body. Adults frequently utilize it to evaluate their sinuses. The healthcare provider asks the patient to identify any areas of discomfort or pain while tapping directly on the area of concern with one or two fingers. The medical professional also looks for indications of discomfort in the patient's facial expressions. A good method for locating localized soreness that might be a sign of underlying pathology is direct percussion.

8.4.2.5 INDIRECT PERCUSSION

Indirect percussion is a clinical method that uses sound to assess the underlying tissue. The process entails firmly pressing the non-dominant hand's middle finger's distal end against the body part while flexing the wrist. The middle finger of the hand with control is then quickly tapped over the region where the other finger meets the patient's skin. When the noises are listened to, they can reveal information about the underlying tissue's makeup. This method is frequently employed to determine whether the lungs contain fluid or air and to measure the dimensions of internal organs like the liver or spleen. It is a crucial component of the physical examination and can assist the healthcare professional in the diagnosis of a variety of illnesses.

8.4.2.6 AUSCULTATION

Auscultation is a medical procedure in which a stethoscope is used to listen for sounds coming from the bowels, respiratory system, or cardiovascular system. By listening to these sounds, doctors can gain a better understanding of how these organs function as well as listen for any irregularities or disorders that might require further investigation. For instance, a paralyzed or non-functioning intestine could be indicated by the absence of bowel sounds, whereas a bowel obstruction might be indicated by high-pitched "tinkling" sounds. On the other hand, the "growling" of the digestive tract accentuates these noises when the bowel is acting hyperactively.

Another type of sound that can be heard by auscultation is bruit. It is a blowing vascular sound that is heard over partially clogged blood arteries and sounds like a heart murmur. A bruit heard over the carotid arteries may signal an elevated risk of stroke, whereas a bruit heard from the belly may signal aortic or other major artery partial obstruction, such as that of the renal, iliac, or femoral arteries.

In order to identify a blockage or inflammation, such as that caused by asthma, bronchitis, or pneumonia, it can also be helpful to listen to the sound of air moving into and out of the lungs. Crackles, wheezes, and rubs are examples of adventitious sounds, which are those heard in addition to regular breathing noises. Crackles, referred to as rales, are brought on by fluid in the tiny passages that stick to the walls during inhalation and imitate the sound created by stroking hair between the fingers adjacent to the ear. Rapid airflow across a partially blocked airway, as in asthma or bronchitis, results in wheezes, which are melodic noises heard predominantly during expiration. Pleural rubs, which occur in patients with pneumonia and pulmonary infarction, are characterized by the sound of cracking leather and are brought on by the movement of two pleural surfaces that have been roughened by inflammation.

Finally, cardiac auscultation entails listening for murmurs that could be caused by turbulence in the blood flow or vibrations from a heart valve abnormality in the noises made by the heart valves, including the aortic, pulmonary, tricuspid, and mitral valves. Heart murmurs can be pathogenic, which means they need to be treated, especially if they reflect restriction of normal blood flow, or physiological, which means they have no clinical significance. Heart murmurs differ depending on their location, duration, severity, pitch, and quality, as well as when they occur in the cardiac cycle.

Procedure: When performing auscultation, it is important to use the appropriate part of the stethoscope to pick up different types of sounds. Use the stethoscope's diaphragm to apply firm pressure to the patient's skin while listening for high-pitched sounds like the first and second heart sounds (S1 and S2). This will leave a faint ring on the skin. With the stethoscope's bell, low-pitched noises like the final two sounds of the heart (S3 and S4) can be more easily detected. However, pressing too firmly causes the skin to behave as a diaphragm, which may limit the identification of low-pitched noises; therefore, the bell should only be held softly against the skin to establish a seal.

It's crucial to recognize the unique qualities of each sound when you listen for them. To better identify it from other noises that could be present, try to concentrate on just one sound at a time.

8.5 STANFORD 25

The Stanford Medicine 25 is a program designed to teach and promote bedside medicine skills to healthcare professionals (Elder et al., 2020). The program is named after the famous William Osler quote, "Listen to your patient; he is telling you the diagnosis." The program's objective is to educate medical professionals in the proper use of physical examination methods for patient diagnosis and care. The Stanford Medicine 25 program was started by Dr. Abraham Verghese, a well-known physician and author who is committed to improving bedside medical skills. The program offers a range of resources, including workshops, podcasts, and videos, to help medical practitioners improve their physical examination methods.

The program places a strong emphasis on educating "traditional" physical examination techniques like palpation, auscultation, and percussion that are typically ignored in modern medicine. By mastering these techniques, medical professionals can accurately diagnose and treat their patients, which can eventually lead to improved outcomes and a higher standard of care. The Stanford Medicine 25 program is a terrific resource for medical professionals who want to improve their bedside medicine skills and provide the best care for their patients in general.

KEYWORDS

- **blood supply blockage**
- **bowel obstruction**
- **cardiovascular conditioning**
- **carotid arteries**
- **clogged arteries**
- **heart rate**
- **heart rhythm**
- **paralyzed intestine**
- **pulse rate**
- **respiratory system**

REFERENCES

Corkins, M. R., Jessica, & Monczka, R. D. (2015). Consensus statement of the Academy of Nutrition and Dietetics/American Society for Parenteral and Enteral Nutrition: Indicators recommended for the identification and documentation of pediatric malnutrition (undernutrition). *Nutrition in Clinical Practice, 30*(1), 147–161.

Elder, A., Chi, J., Ozdalga, E., Kugler, J., & Verghese, A. (2020). The road back to the bedside. *JAMA, 323*(17), 1672–1673.

Fryar, C. D., Carroll, M. D., Gu, Q., Afful, J., & Ogden, C. L. (2021). Anthropometric reference data for children and adults: United States, 2015–2018. *Vital and Health Statistics, 3*(36), 1–44. PMID: 33541517.

Jain, R., & Jain, Y. (2021). The importance of physical examination in primary health care provided by NPHW is being threatened in COVID-19 times. *Journal of Family Medicine and Primary Care, 10*(1), 19.

Khadilkar, V., Yadav, S., Agrawal, K. K., Tamboli, S., Banerjee, M., Cherian, A., Goyal, J. P., Khadilkar, A., Kumaravel, V., Mohan, V., & Narayanappa, D. (2015). Revised IAP growth charts for height, weight, and body mass index for 5-to 18-year-old Indian children. *Indian Pediatrics, 52*, 47–55.

CHAPTER 9

Diagnostic Tools and Techniques in Cardiovascular Technology

NAJMUS SAQUIB

Department of Allied Health Sciences, Sharda University, Greater Noida, Uttar Pradesh, India

ABSTRACT

Cardiovascular diagnostic techniques are a series of medical tests that record two main activities, such as the electrical conduction system and muscular movement or parts of the heart, on graph paper or a digital screen. These diagnostic tools and techniques help cardiologists obtain a range of static images and electrical indications to understand the condition of the cardiovascular system. Cardiovascular diagnostic techniques are one of the essential parts of human health diagnosis and treatment. Besides, they also indicate future critical medical issues in the early stage. Cardiovascular technology is divided into two categories: the first and most common category is known as non-invasive cardiovascular techniques (which involve ECG, echocardiography, stress tests, and CTA), and the second category is known as invasive cardiovascular techniques (which involve coronary angiography, cath study, and EPS).

9.1 INTRODUCTION

The cardiovascular system is the most important system of the human body, supplying oxygen, nutrients, hormones, and other vital substances to cells and organs (Braunwald et al., 2019). Parts of the cardiovascular system include the heart (a muscular organ having four chambers: right

Allied Healthcare in Practice: An Introduction to Integrated Patient Care. Sally Lukose, Karuna Singh (Eds.)

DOI: 10.1201/9781998511037-11

atrium, right ventricle (RV), left atrium, left ventricle) and four valves: the tricuspid valve located between the right atrium and the RV, the pulmonary valve located between the RV and the pulmonary artery, the mitral valve located between the left atrium and the left ventricle, and the aortic valve located between the left ventricle and the aorta (Braunwald et al., 2019). These valves work as doors; when open, they allow blood to move farther, and when closed, they help fill the chamber with blood and maintain chamber pressure. The superior and inferior vena cava (two central veins) collect deoxygenated blood from the body and deposit it into the right atrium. During atrial depolarization, blood moves from the right atrium to the RV. Then, during the ventricle depolarization phase, blood moves towards the pulmonary artery from the RV. The pulmonary artery is further divided into two branches: the right and left pulmonary arteries (through these two branches, blood moves towards the lungs and gets filtered). After filtration, blood moves towards the left atrium through the pulmonary veins, then blood moves from the left atrium to the left ventricle, and then towards the aorta (the main artery), which supplies oxygenated blood to the heart (the coronary arteries are the first branches of the aorta that supply blood to heart cells) and other organs of the body (Braunwald et al., 2019) (World Health Organization, 2022). (Figure 9.1).

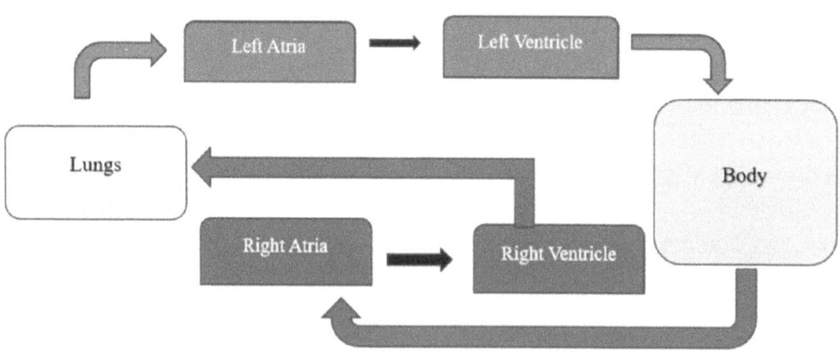

FIGURE 9.1 Cardiovascular system.

9.2 CARDIOVASCULAR DISEASE

A disease of the heart (structural problems) or blood vessels (deposition of cholesterol, calcium, blood clots) is generally known as cardiovascular disease (American Heart Association, 2023) (World Health Organization, 2022).

i. **Some of the common heart diseases are as follows:** (American Heart Association, 2023) (European Society of Cardiology, 2022)

- Unstable angina (undiagnosed chest pain or a sudden worsening of existing angina).
- Heart attack.
- Heart failure.
- Arrhythmia.
- Valve disease.
- High blood pressure.
- Inherited heart conditions.
- Congenital heart conditions.

ii. **Common Causes that lead to these problems are:** (American Heart Association, 2023) (Benjamin et al., 2019).

- High blood pressure.
- Diabetes.
- Smoking.
- High low-density lipoprotein cholesterol.
- Poor diet.
- Obesity.
- Physical inactivity.

The pathophysiology of heart failure includes maladaptive remodeling and neurohormonal activation, whereas atherosclerosis causes coronary artery constriction and ischemia (Braunwald et al., 2019) (Kannel, 2000) (McMurray et al., 2014). Arrhythmias frequently result from ischemic tissue, atrial remodeling, or anomalies in electrical conduction (January et al., 2019). Both congenital and acquired valve dysfunction can lead to regurgitation or stenosis with chronic chamber overload (Otto & Prendergast, 2014).

9.3 DIAGNOSTIC TOOLS AND TECHNIQUES

Various techniques used to the assessment of these ailments are divided into two categories:

1. **Non-Invasive cardiovascular techniques** are those techniques or tests, we perform without inserting fluids or medical devices in the body.

2. **Invasive cardiovascular techniques** are those techniques or procedures, we perform with the insertion of fluids, medical equipment, and so forth.

9.3.1 NON-INVASIVE CARDIOVASCULAR TECHNIQUES

9.3.1.1 CHEST X-RAY

It is an imaging procedure that focuses on the organs and structures in the chest using X-rays. Because certain disorders might alter the structure of the heart or lungs, it can be useful to assess how well the lungs and heart function (Fihn et al., 2012) (Figure 9.2).

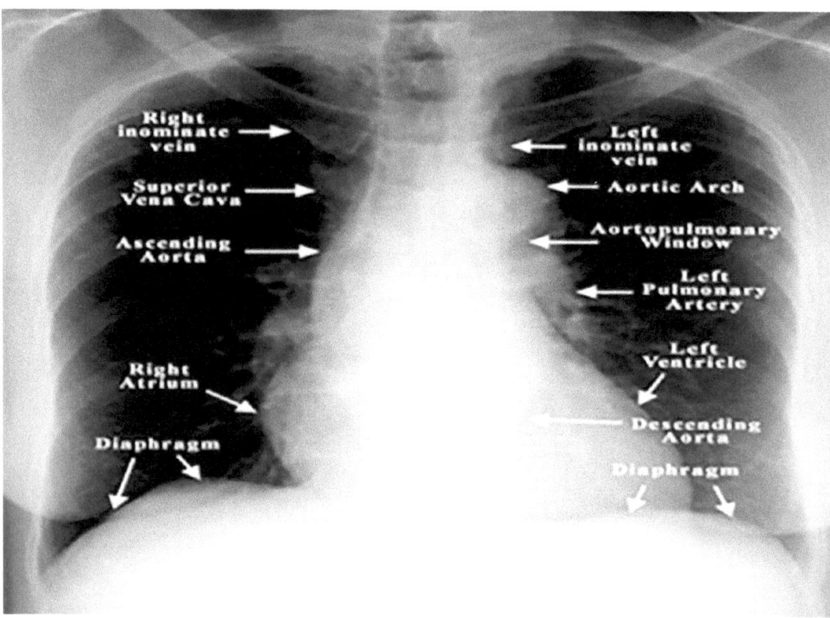

FIGURE 9.2 Normal chest x-ray.

9.3.1.2 ELECTROCARDIOGRAM (ECG)

An ECG machine monitors the electrical activity of the heart through repeated cardiac cycles with the use of 10 electrodes applied to the skin. It is an electrogram, or graph, showing the electrical activity of the heart as a function of time and voltage. The heart is a pumping muscular organ that pumps through its own conducting system.

- SA node – Starting point or natural pacemaker – generates electrical impulses.
- Inter-nodal pathways and Bachmann's Bundle – carry electrical impulses inside the right and left atria for atrial depolarization.
- AV node – receives the signal coming from the right and left atria, then slows down the speed of the signal (to give time to fill blood into the ventricles) and transfers it to the bundle of His (HIS) or ventricles.

In the ventricles, through the HIS, right and left bundle branches.

- Purkinje fibers – receive the signals from the AV node at actual speed and perform ventricular depolarization.

If any area or pathway becomes damaged, diseased, or unable to transfer/conduct the electrical signals properly, the heart is not able to pump effectively.

With the help of an ECG, we can easily identify which area of the conduction system is diseased, and it also provides information about the condition of heart muscles, valve disease, and any other abnormalities related to the heart (Figures 9.3–9.6).

In ECG graph, there are five main waves and important three segment.

- Five main waves – P, Q, R, S, T.
- Three segment – PQ/PR Segment, ST Segment and QT Segment.

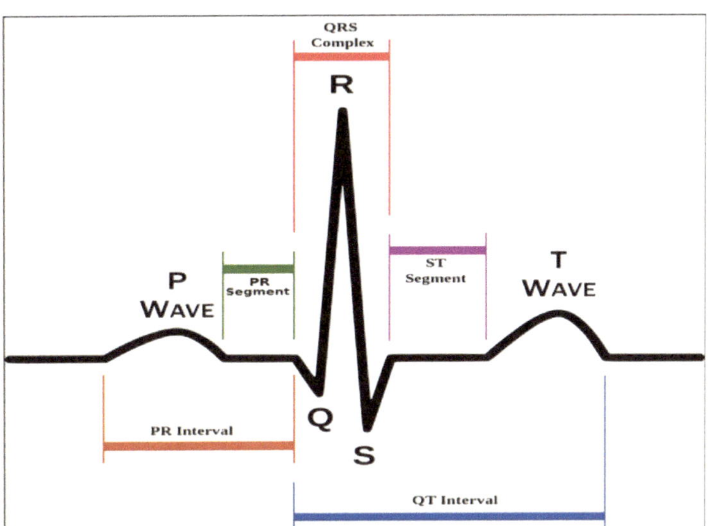

FIGURE 9.3 ECG important waves and segments.

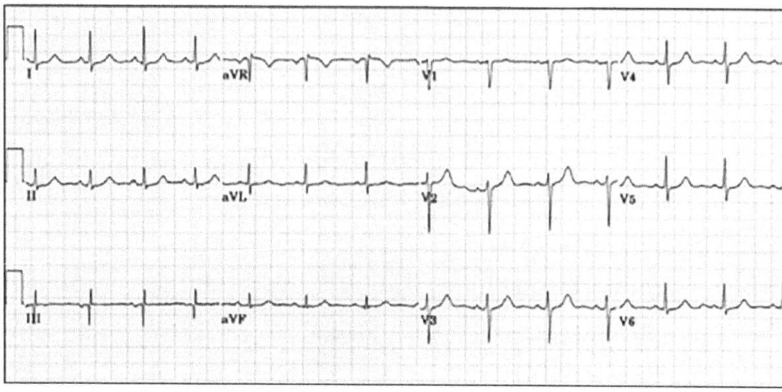

FIGURE 9.4 Normal ECG.

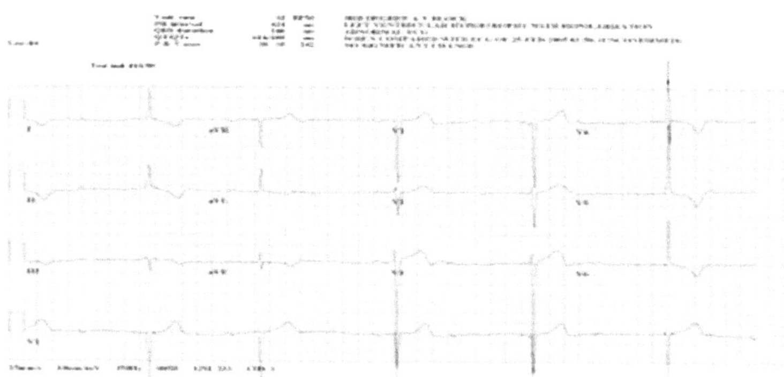

FIGURE 9.5 Third degree heart block.

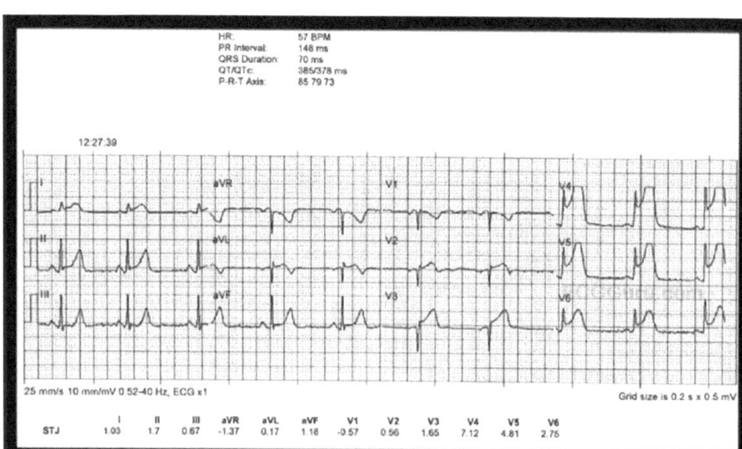

FIGURE 9.6 Lateral wall myocardial infarction.

9.3.1.3 CARDIAC STRESS TEST

During a controlled clinical setting, a cardiac stress test assesses the heart's capacity to respond to external stress. Exercise, intravenous pharmaceutical stimulation, or occasionally a combination of the two can trigger the stress response. In other words, this test is recommended for those patients who complain that they feel normal at rest, but when they engage in physical activity, the symptoms begin.

- **Treadmill Test (TMT):** On a treadmill, cardiovascular stress testing combines physical activity with electrocardiography (ECG) and blood pressure monitoring. Usually, this kind of stress testing is done on a treadmill or bicycle while exercising according to a regimen. Furthermore, for those who are unable to exercise, an injection of a pharmacologic medication that mimics the effects of exercise and raises heart activity may be helpful. Healthcare providers can assess a patient's functional ability, risk and severity of coronary artery disease (CAD), prognosis, and treatment outcomes using treadmill stress testing (Garner et al., 2017) (Beller and Zaret, 2000).

  Results from the Henry Ford exercise testing (FIT) study appear to indicate a graded and inverse relationship between the incidence of atrial fibrillation and cardiorespiratory fitness, particularly for obese patients.
  In TMT, there are three main phases:

  1. **Rest Phase** – This is the first phase of the test in which we record at least two ECGs in different positions of the body (mostly supine and standing position). These ECGs are also considered as a baseline of the patient's conduction system.
  2. **Exercise Phase** – The second phase starts after taking two baseline ECGs, in which the patient has to walk on the treadmill (speed and elevation change according to some protocols, mostly Bruce Protocols). During the exercise phase, all the ECG changes are recorded by the TMT machine. The exercise phase is over when the patient achieves a target heart rate, is unable to continue, or if any symptoms are shown by the patient.

3. **Recovery Phase** – After the end of the exercise phase, the recovery phase immediately starts. In the recovery phase, the TMT machine again records ECG changes and how much time the heart takes to become normal or reach baseline.

The final diagnosis depends on the basis of ECG changes during these three phases. If a patient is unable to walk on a treadmill or is physically challenged, pharmacological drugs are used in place of a treadmill, which also increases the stress in the patient's body, and the same three phases are recorded.

- **Contraindications (Absolute prohibitions)** (Garner et al., 2017)
    - Within two to three days, an acute myocardial infarction.
    - Unstable angina that has not yet been treated medically to stabilize it.
    - Hemodynamic compromise or uncontrolled cardiac arrhythmias that cause symptoms.
    - Severe aortic stenosis symptoms.
    - Uncontrolled symptomatic heart failure.
    - A pulmonary infarction or embolism.
    - Very high pulmonary blood pressure.
    - Acute pericarditis, endocarditis, myocarditis, or pericarditis.
    - Aortic acute dissection.
- **Contraindications Relative (May be Disregarded if Advantages of Treadmill Stress Testing Exceed Disadvantages)**
    - Superior AV blocks.
    - Hypertension that is severe (systolic above 200 mmHg, diastolic over 19 mmHg, or both)
    - Severe obesity or other physical or mental impairments prevent you from exercising.
    - Coronary stenosis in the left main.
    - Heart disease with moderately stenotic valves.
    - Abnormal electrolytes.
    - Both Brady-arrhythmias and tachy-arrhythmias.
    - Including any additional types of outflow tract blockage and hypertrophic cardiomyopathy.
    - Having a mental or physical disability that prevents you from exercising properly.

9.3.1.4 HOLTER MONITOR

One kind of portable electrocardiogram (ECG) is the Holter monitor. It continually captures the electrical activity of the heart for at least 24 hours. Holter monitors, which are among the simplest and fastest tests used to check the heart, are advised for patients whose standard or resting ECGs and stress tests occasionally do not reveal certain alterations, but the patient is still complaining of symptoms (Holter, 1961). Specific locations on the chest and belly are used for electrodes, which are tiny plastic patches that adhere to the skin. Wires are used to connect the electrodes to the ECG equipment. The electrical activity of the heart can then be monitored, noted, and printed (Figure 9.7).

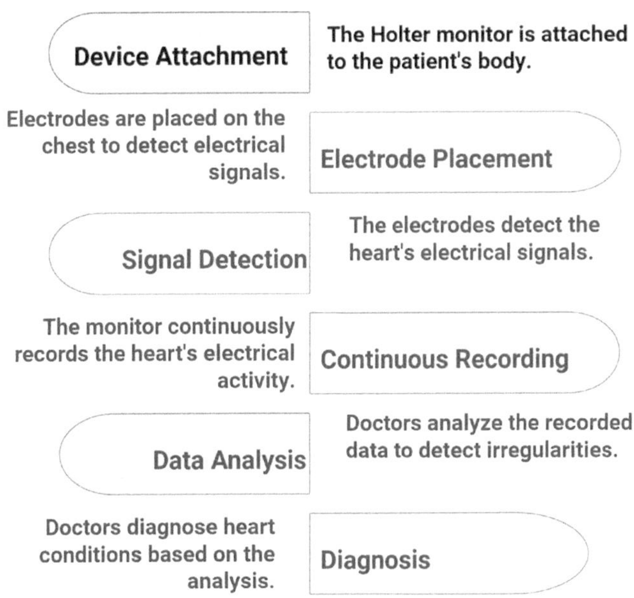

FIGURE 9.7 Holter monitor.

9.3.1.5 ECHOCARDIOGRAPHY

Using sound waves, an examination known as echocardiography produces real-time images of your heart. This test allows us to monitor the heart's overall health, muscle, and valves.

The pictures can be used to determine things like the heart's size, whether the chambers' proportions have changed due to enlargement or thickening, blood clots in the heart chambers, problems with the aorta, fluid in the sac surrounding the heart, problems with the major artery leading to the heart, problems with the heart's pumping or relaxing mechanisms, problems with the heart valves, and more.

- **Transthoracic Echocardiography:** (This is the most typical kind of echocardiography). A transducer will be positioned over your heart on your chest (Nagueh et al., 2016). Ultrasound (USG) waves are sent through your chest and toward your heart via the transducer. The sound waves are decoded by a computer as they return to the transducer. This results in the real-time visuals seen on a monitor (Figures 9.8–9.10).

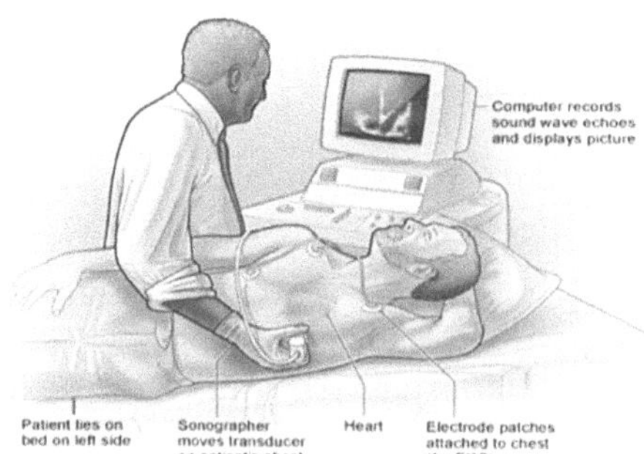

FIGURE 9.8 Transthoracic echocardiography.

Source: https://southerncrosscardiology.com.au/project/transthoracic-echocardiography/

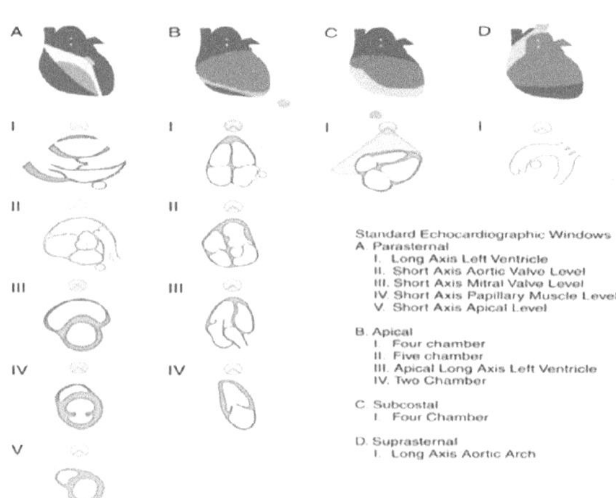

FIGURE 9.9 Echocardiography view.

Source: https://radiologykey.com/echocardiography-2/

- **Transesophageal Echocardiography:** A transesophageal echocardiography is advised for images that are more detailed (Nagueh et al., 2016). In this process, the throat is first numbed to make it easier and to stop the gag reflex before a smaller transducer is guided into the throat through the mouth. The esophagus, the tube that connects your throat to your stomach, is used to guide the transducer tube. The transducer behind your heart allows the doctor to see more of any issues and to observe several heart chambers that are not seen on a transthoracic echocardiogram.

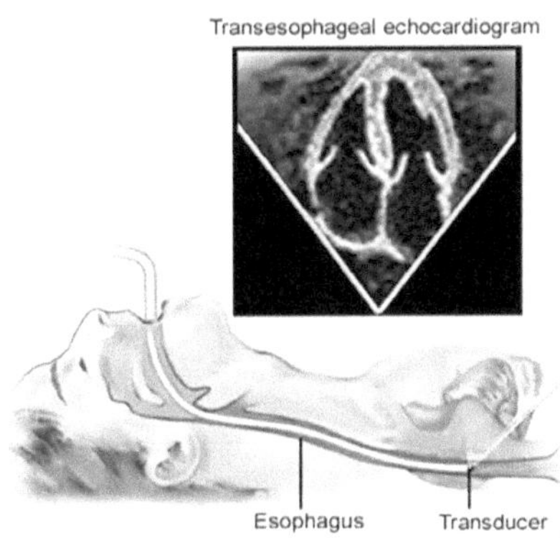

FIGURE 9.10 Transesophageal echocardiography.

Source: https://cardiovascularconsultantsofsouthgeorgia.com/our-services/transesophageal-echocardiography

- **Stress Echocardiography**

Transthoracic echocardiography is used in a stress echocardiogram, but the patient is given medicine to speed up the heartbeat, or the doctor takes pictures before and after they exercise. This enables the clinician to examine how the heart responds to stress (Beller and Zaret, 2000). It can also show any signs of high blood pressure, heart failure, or other problems. The procedure for stress echocardiography is almost similar to the TMT; the only change is that just after the exercise phase, we have to perform echocardiography.

9.3.1.6 COMPUTED TOMOGRAPHY ANGIOGRAPHY (CTA)

An injection of a specialized dye is combined with a CT scan in a medical technique known as CT angiography to create images of the blood vessels and tissues in a particular area of your body (Sun and Choo, 2010). The dye is administered via an intravenous (IV) line that was started in your hand or arm.

A computed tomography scan, or CT scan, is a kind of X-ray that uses technology to produce cross-sectional images of your body. Since the dye used in CT angiography "lights up" the tissues and blood vessels under examination, it is also known as a contrast substance (Figure 9.11).

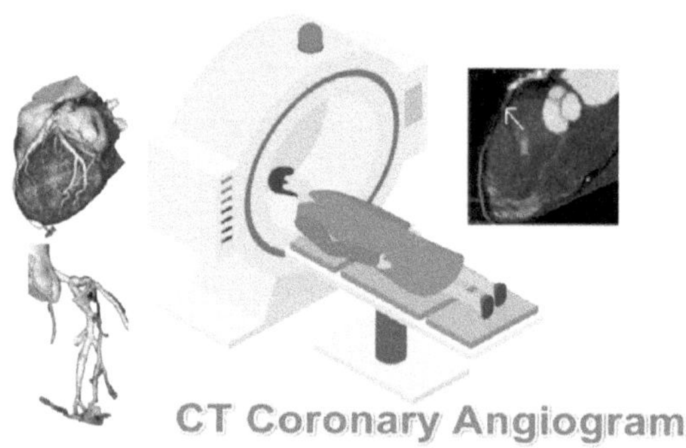

FIGURE 9.11 Computed tomography coronary angiogram.

9.4 INVASIVE CARDIOVASCULAR TECHNIQUES

9.4.1 CORONARY ANGIOGRAM

The most popular kind of cardiac catheterization technique is coronary angiography, in which the heart's blood arteries are visualized or diagnosed using X-ray imaging and specialized catheters, wires, and contrast medium (Anderson and Morrow, 2017). Usually, the purpose of the test is to determine whether the heart's blood flow is restricted. A coronary angiography involves the patient lying on their back while an IV line, ECG electrodes, and fluo- roscopy machine are attached to them. A tiny incision is made at the entry site, and a short plastic tube (sheath) is inserted into the artery after the groin or arm has been cleaned or sterilized. The catheter is gently threaded to the heart or coronary arteries after being placed into the blood vessel through the sheath. Through the catheter, dye (contrast material) is administered. Fluoroscopy makes the dye easy to see (multiple views are acquired from different angles). The physician can watch it pass through the coronary arteries and see any narrowed or blocked spots. Based on the observation, the doctor makes the final diagnosis and recommendation.

9.4.1.1 CONTRAINDICATIONS

- Severe uncontrolled hypertension
- Active bleeding
- Renal dysfunction.
- Unstable arrhythmias.
- Acute cerebrovascular accidents.
- Allergy to radiographic contrast.
- Acute pulmonary oedema (patient unable to lie flat).
- Untreated active infection/Sepsis.
- Severe coagulopathy.
- Significant peripheral vascular disease.
- Encephalopathy.

Depending on risk-benefit, the procedure can be considered in these Situations (Anderson & Morrow, 2017).

9.4.2 RIGHT AND LEFT HEART STUDY

A right and left heart study is a type of cardiac catheterization procedure in which special types of catheters, contrast media, and a cardiac monitor (to record pressure) are used under X-ray imaging to see or diagnose the heart's chambers or chamber pressures (Anderson and Morrow, 2017). The test is generally done to identify any abnormalities (increased size or disease in chamber size and oxygen level due to congenital heart defects or arrhythmias) in the heart.

The patient lies on the fluoroscopy table or X-ray table while the ECG electrodes, IV line, and patient are prepared for the heart investigation. A tiny incision is made at the entrance site after the groin or arm has been cleaned and sterilized. A short plastic tube, called a sheath, is then introduced into the vein (during the right heart study) and the artery (during the left heart study). The catheter is gently threaded to the heart (left or right) after being placed into the blood vessel through the sheath. Through the catheter, dye (contrast material) is administered. Fluoroscopy makes the dye easy to see (multiple views are acquired from different angles). As it moves inside the heart chamber, the doctor can observe its flow and identify areas of size, and with the help of the cardiac monitor and catheter (Swan-Ganz or Berman), the doctor can also record the chamber's internal pressure. Based on the observations, the doctor makes the final diagnosis and recommendations (Figure 9.12).

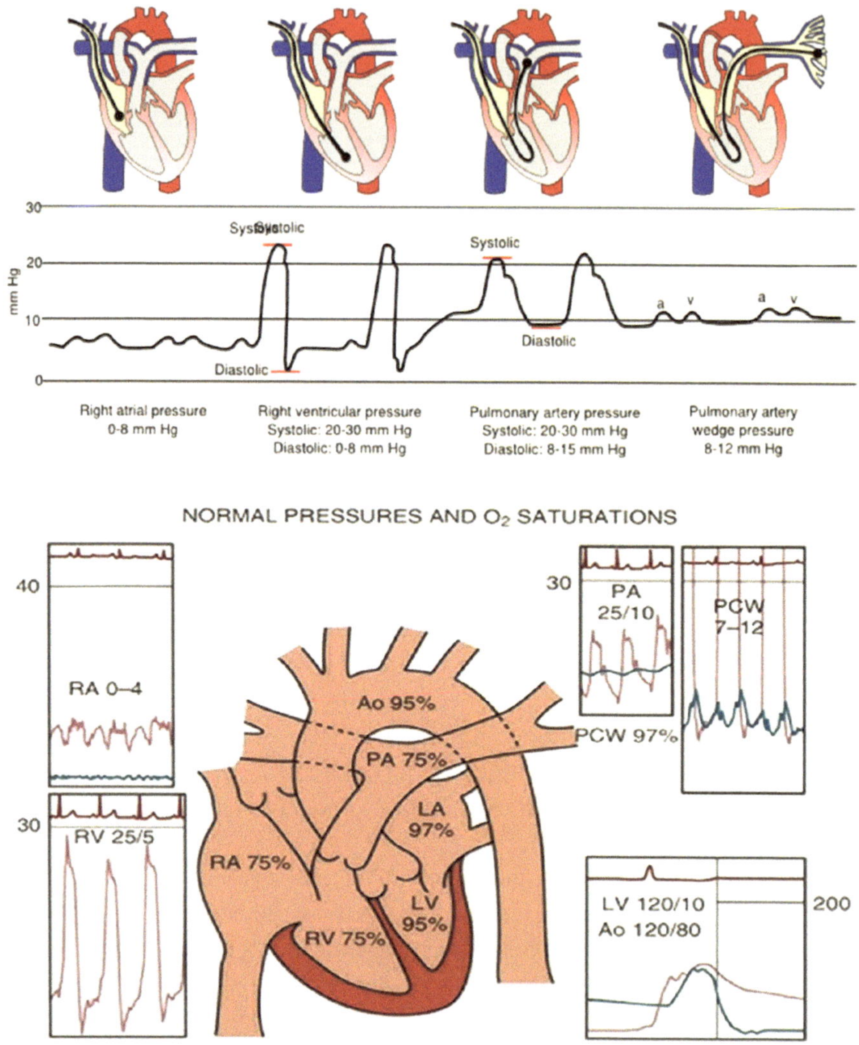

FIGURE 9.12 Right heart study and left heart study.

9.4.3 ELECTROPHYSIOLOGY STUDY (EPS)

An EPS (electrophysiology study) is a procedure in which special catheters (having electrodes on their tips) are used to examine how well your heart's "internal electrical circuit" works. It is the best procedure to identify irregular heartbeats (arrhythmias) because electrical activities are recorded directly from conduction pathways (Figure 9.13).

During EPS, multiple catheters are inserted through the femoral and jugular veins towards the heart. In the heart, these catheters are placed in individual and fixed positions to record the conduction signals and pathways (January et al., 2019). The catheter placement positions are:

- **HRA** – High Right Atria – near to SVC and right atria junction.
- **HIS** – Bundle of His – just below to tricuspid valve in contact with the septum.
- **RV** – Right Ventricle – near to the apex of right ventricle.
- **CS** – Coronary Sinus – through CS towards left ventricle.

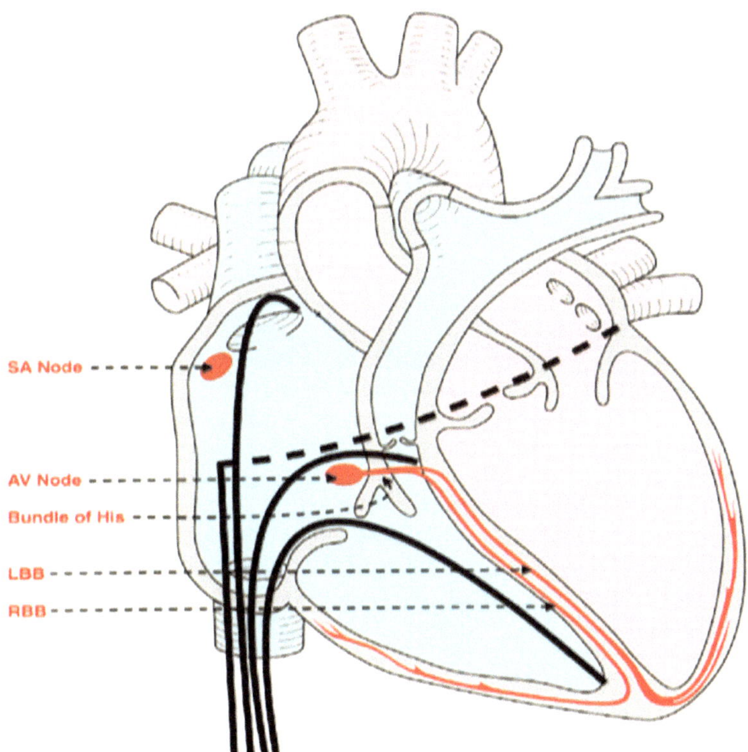

FIGURE 9.13 Electrophysiology study (heart and catheters placement).

Source: https://www.drhirenkevadiya.com/Svc_4h_2D_RF_ablation

KEYWORDS

- **cardiac catheterization**
- **cardiac monitor**
- **cardiovascular diagnostic techniques**
- **catheters**
- **conduction signals**
- **congenital heart defects**
- **electrophysiology study**
- **heart disease**
- **internal electrical circuit**
- **invasive cardiovascular techniques**
- **jugular veins**
- **non-invasive cardiovascular technique**

REFERENCES

American Heart Association. (2023). 2023 AHA/ACC Guideline on the Primary Prevention of Cardiovascular Disease. *Circulation, 148*(10), e804–e890. https://doi.org/10.1161/CIR.0000000000001140

Anderson, J. L., & Morrow, D. A. (2017). Acute myocardial infarction. New England Journal of Medicine, 376, 2053–2064. https://doi.org/10.1056/NEJMra1606915

Beller, G. A., & Zaret, B. L. (2000). Contributions of nuclear cardiology to diagnosis and prognosis of patients with coronary artery disease. *Circulation, 101*(12), 1465–1478. https://doi.org/10.1161/01.CIR.101.12.1465

Benjamin, E. J., Muntner, P., Alonso, A., Bittencourt, M. S., Callaway, C. W., Carson, A. P., ... & Virani, S. S. (2019). Heart disease and stroke statistics—2019 update. *Circulation, 139*(10), e56–e528. https://doi.org/10.1161/CIR.0000000000000659

Braunwald, E., Zipes, D. P., Libby, P., & Bonow, R. O. (2019). Braunwald's Heart Disease: A Textbook of Cardiovascular Medicine (12th ed.). Elsevier.

European Society of Cardiology. (2022). 2022 ESC Guidelines on Heart Failure. *European Heart Journal, 43*(36), 3599–3729. https://doi.org/10.1093/eurheartj/ehac937

Fihn, S. D., Gardin, J. M., Abrams, J., Berra, K., Blankenship, J. C., Dallas, A. P., ... & Smith, S. C. (2012). 2012 ACCF/AHA/ACP/AATS/PCNA/SCAI/STS guideline for the diagnosis and management of patients with stable ischemic heart disease. *Journal of the American College of Cardiology, 60*(24), e44–e164. https://doi.org/10.1016/j.jacc.2012.07.013

Garner, K. K., Pomeroy, W., & Arnold, J. J. (2017). Exercise stress testing: Indications and common questions. *American Family Physician, 96*(5), 293–299A.

Holter, N. J. (1961). New method for heart studies: Continuous electrocardiography of active subjects over long periods is now practical. *Science, 134*(3486), 1214–1220. https://doi.org/10.1126/science.134.3486.1214

January, C. T., Wann, L. S., Calkins, H., Chen, L. Y., Cigarroa, J. E., Cleveland, J. C., ... & Yancy, C. W. (2019). 2019 AHA/ACC/HRS Focused Update on Atrial Fibrillation. *Journal of the American College of Cardiology, 74*(1), 104–132. https://doi.org/10.1016/j.jacc.2019.01.011

Kannel, W. B. (2000). Risk stratification in hypertension: New insights from the Framingham Study. *American Journal of Hypertension, 13*(9 Pt 2), 3S–10S. https://doi.org/10.1016/S0895-7061(00)00271-4

McMurray, J. J. V., Packer, M., Desai, A. S., Gong, J., Lefkowitz, M. P., Rizkala, A. R., ... & Solomon, S. D. (2014). Angiotensin–neprilysin inhibition versus enalapril in heart failure. *New England Journal of Medicine, 371*(11), 993–1004. https://doi.org/10.1056/NEJMoa1409077

Nagueh, S. F., Smiseth, O. A., Appleton, C. P., Byrd, B. F., Dokainish, H., Edvardsen, T., ... & Waggoner, A. D. (2016). Recommendations for the evaluation of left ventricular diastolic function by echocardiography. *European Heart Journal–Cardiovascular Imaging, 17*(12), 1321–1360. https://doi.org/10.1093/ehjci/jew082

Otto, C. M., & Prendergast, B. (2014). Aortic-valve stenosis — from patients at risk to severe valve obstruction. *New England Journal of Medicine, 371*, 744–756. https://doi.org/10.1056/NEJMra1303500

Sun, Z., & Choo, G. H. (2010). Coronary CT angiography: Current status and continuing challenges. *British Journal of Radiology, 83*(985), 290–303. https://doi.org/10.1259/bjr/31401950

World Health Organization. (2022). Cardiovascular diseases (CVDs).

CHAPTER 10

Overview of Pharmacology

HAMID RAZA MOQADDASI

Department of Pharmacology, Sharda School of Allied Health Sciences, Sharda University, Greater Noida, Uttar Pradesh, India

ABSTRACT

Our understanding of the effects of drugs and therapeutic interventions has greatly benefited from the study of pharmacology, which is the science of how substances interact with organisms. This introduction delves deeply into the varied topic of pharmacology, exploring its origins, underlying ideas, and current uses. It begins with an investigation into the discovery and development of drugs, then examines the complex processes of drug absorption, distribution, metabolism, and excretion, shedding light on how these elements affect a drug's effectiveness and safety. The review provides more detail about pharmacodynamics, clarifying the ways that drugs behave at the molecular, cellular, and systemic levels. The importance of concepts like receptor theory, enzyme inhibition, and signal transduction pathways in rational drug design and personalized medicine methods is highlighted. The significance of optimizing drug administration regimens is further emphasized by discussions on dose-response relationships, pharmacokinetic-pharmacodynamic modeling, and therapeutic indices.

Allied Healthcare in Practice: An Introduction to Integrated Patient Care. Sally Lukose, Karuna Singh (Eds.)

DOI: 10.1201/9781998511037-12

10.1 INTRODUCTION

10.1.1 DEFINITIONS

1. **Pharmacology:** It is the branch of science that studies the pharmacokinetics and pharmacodynamics of drugs.
2. **Drug:** It is a chemical or compound that, when consumed, exerts physiological effects on the body. Drugs are frequently administered therapeutically to treat, prevent, or diagnose diseases or medical conditions. They can also be employed for research or diagnostic purposes. Drugs can come from a variety of sources, such as plants, animals, minerals, or chemical synthesis. They alter biochemical processes and physiological activities by interacting with specific molecules or receptors in the body. Drugs can have both positive effects (like treating illnesses) and potential hazards or side effects if they are not taken properly.
3. **Pharmacokinetics:** The study of a drug's absorption, distribution, metabolism, and elimination by the body is referred to as pharmacokinetics. In simple terms, pharmacokinetics is what the body does to the drugs.
4. **Pharmacodynamics:** It deals with the investigation of how medications act on the body as well as the relationship between drug concentration and pharmacological response. In simple terms, pharmacodynamics is what the drugs do to the body.
5. **Pharmacy:** It is a profession and scientific discipline that deals with manufacturing medications, distributing them, and ensuring that they are used properly. It includes all of the information and skills necessary to guarantee the secure and efficient use of medications.
6. **Therapeutic:** It encompasses all that has to do with managing a sickness, injury, or medical condition. It relates to activities or interventions that are meant to improve someone's health or well-being.
7. **Chemotherapy:** It is a form of treatment where medications, also referred to as cytotoxic drugs, are used to either kill or stop

the growth of rapidly proliferating cells, particularly cancer cells. Although it is mainly used to treat cancer, it can also be used to treat some autoimmune illnesses and other non-cancerous conditions. Chemotherapy medications function by targeting and disrupting the cell division and proliferation mechanisms.

8. **Toxicology:** It is a scientific study of poisons or toxins and how they affect organisms. It involves investigating the adverse effects of chemical, physical, or biological agents on biological systems and determining how toxicants work.
9. **Clinical Pharmacology:** It is the area of pharmacology that focuses on how pharmacological concepts are applied in clinical settings. It entails the investigation of how medications affect both individuals and populations, with a focus on patient-centered drug therapy optimization.
10. **Essential Medicines:** These drugs should always be made available and accessible in sufficient quantities and at reasonable costs because they are regarded as essential for the healthcare system. These medications are chosen based on their applicability to the demands of public health, evidence of their effectiveness and safety, and their capacity to treat important medical diseases.
11. **Orphan drugs:** A pharmacological or therapeutic agent known as an orphan drug is one that was manufactured to treat a rare medical disease, also known as an orphan disease. The term "orphan diseases" refers to conditions that typically affect fewer than 200,000 persons in the United States or fewer than 5 in 9000 people in the European Union (Product Development, Field and Boat, 209).
12. **Over-the-Counter drugs:** Over-the-Counter (OTC) drugs are those that can be bought by customers straight from a pharmacy without a doctor's prescription. When taken as prescribed, these medications are often regarded as secure and useful for self-medication.
13. **Prescription drugs:** These medicines are only available with a legitimate prescription from a qualified healthcare provider, like a doctor, nurse practitioner, or dentist. These medications are

frequently used to treat more severe or complex medical disorders that require expert diagnosis, observation, or management.

14. **Pharmacopeia:** A pharmacopoeia (or pharmacopoeia) is a comprehensive encyclopedia that provides details on the manufacturing, composition, and quality of medicines. Pharmacopoeias are reliable sources of drug information for regulatory bodies, chemists, medical practitioners, and researchers.
15. **Formulary:** A formulary is a list or collection of drugs and medications that have been authorized for use in a hospital, health insurance program, or pharmacy. It is used as a reference manual by medical practitioners when writing prescriptions and handing out drugs.

10.1.2 BRANCHES OF PHARMACOLOGY

1. **Clinical Pharmacology:** The study of pharmaceuticals in humans, including their therapeutic applications, efficacy, safety, and interactions, is known as clinical pharmacology.
2. **Pharmacokinetics:** The study of drug absorption, distribution, metabolism, and elimination by the body is the main subject of pharmacokinetics.
3. **Pharmacodynamics:** Pharmacodynamics is the study of how medications interact with the body and the resulting biochemical and physiological effects. It investigates how medications affect target receptors or molecules, stimulate or inhibit biological functions, and have either beneficial or harmful effects.
4. **Toxicology:** The study of how harmful compounds like drugs and other substances affect organisms is known as toxicology. It involves investigating the effects of prolonged drug exposure, as well as assessing the hazardous characteristics of medications, possible risks, and safe dosage levels.
5. **Pharmacogenomics:** Pharmacogenomics investigates how genetic variations affect patients' reactions to medication. It looks at how a person's genetic makeup affects drug metabolism,

effectiveness, and safety with the goal of individualized drug therapy.

6. **Ethnopharmacology:** The traditional uses of therapeutic plants and natural products are studied in ethnopharmacology. It looks into how these organic compounds can be used therapeutically and whether they can be used to create novel pharmaceuticals.
7. **Psychopharmacology:** Focused on the study of medications that have an impact on the brain and behavior, psychopharmacology investigates how drugs affect neurotransmitter systems, mental health issues, and the mechanisms that underlie drug addiction and substance abuse.
8. **Pharmaceutical Chemistry:** The development, synthesis, and optimization of new medicinal molecules are all part of pharmaceutical chemistry.

10.1.3 DRUG NOMENCLATURE

The system or set of guidelines used to give medications names is referred to as drug nomenclature. It ensures the promotion of accurate identification, communication, and understanding among healthcare professionals, researchers, regulatory authorities, and the general public. There are several aspects of drug nomenclature:

1. **Chemical Name:** This is the name that, in accordance with accepted chemical nomenclature guidelines, represents the chemical composition of a medicine. Although it provides details regarding the molecular makeup and composition of the substance, non-experts may find it difficult to comprehend or recognize.
2. **Generic Name:** The term "generic name" refers to a non-proprietary name given to a medication that is unrelated to its particular manufacturer. Regardless of the brand or manufacturer, it is often shorter and easier to remember than the chemical name. When referring to the same active ingredient, generic names facilitate medicine identification and communication.
3. **Brand Name (Trade Name):** The brand name is the name that a particular manufacturer chooses to advertise a drug under.

It is also referred to as the trade name or proprietary name. Brand names can be trademarked and are frequently distinctive. They act as a marketing technique and aid in setting one product apart from others on the market. Due to regional laws and trademarks, brand names can differ between nations.

4. **International Non-Proprietary Name (INN):** The World Health Organization (WHO) created the INN, a generic name that is widely used, to encourage the use of drug common names internationally. INNs reduce confusion brought on by various brand names and make it easier to identify and provide medications internationally (Guidance on the use of International Nonproprietary Names (INNs) for Pharmaceutical Substances, 2017)

Numerous institutions and organizations, including the WHO, national drug regulatory agencies, and pharmacopoeias, govern drug nomenclature. In order to improve patient safety, reduce medication errors, and foster clear communication within the healthcare system, these organizations set rules and standards to guarantee uniformity and correctness in drug nomenclature.

10.2 SOURCES OF DRUGS

Drugs can come from various sources, including:

1. **Synthetic or Chemical Synthesis:** In laboratories, chemical procedures are used for manufacturing a variety of medications. Molecules with desirable pharmacological characteristics are designed and made by organic chemists, who subsequently evaluate them for efficacy and safety (Lombardino and Lowe, 2004).

2. **Natural Sources:** Many medicines come from organisms like plants, animals, or microorganisms. Examples include medications derived from plants, such as aspirin from willow bark, antibiotics from fungi, such as penicillin, and anticoagulants from animal tissues, such as heparin.

3. **Biotechnology and Genetic Engineering:** Genetic engineering techniques have made it possible to produce medications thanks to

advancements in biotechnology. This entails altering the genetic material of organisms, such as bacteria, yeast, or mammalian cells, in order to manufacture particular therapeutic proteins or other physiologically active compounds (Khan et al., 2016).

4. **Semi-Synthetic Drugs:** Some medications come from natural sources, but they are chemically altered or partially synthesized to improve their medicinal effects or stability. For instance, semi-synthetic opioids like oxycodone are made from opium but are chemically altered to make them more potent (Pathan and Williams, 2012).
5. **Marine Organisms:** Unique species with potential medical use can be found in abundance in the oceans and marine settings. Marine organisms, including sponges, corals, and algae, have been used to make pharmaceuticals, including antibiotics and anti-cancer medications (Malve, 2016).
6. **Traditional Medicine:** Ayurveda and Traditional Chinese Medicine (TCM) are two traditional medical systems that employ the therapeutic use of natural products and herbal medicines. Some contemporary medications have their origins in conventional medical procedures and have undergone scientific research and development to enable wider use ("WHO Traditional Medicine Strategy," 2013) (Figure 10.1).

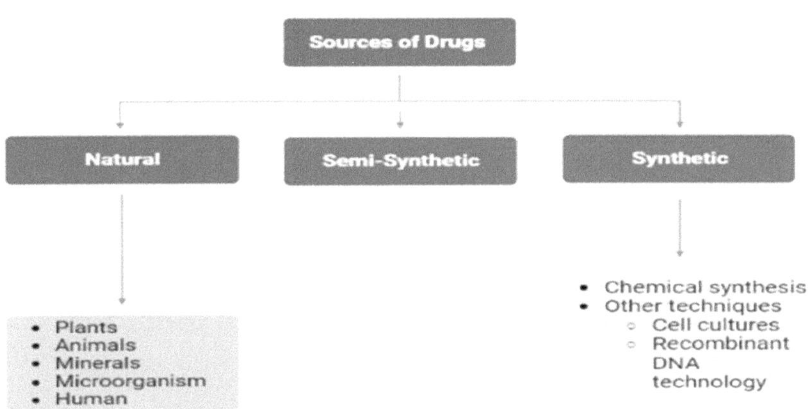

FIGURE 10.1 Sources of drugs.

10.3 ROUTE OF DRUG ADMINISTRATION

Depending on the desired therapeutic impact, the drug's properties, and patient considerations, there are a variety of ways that drugs can be administered into the body. Typical medication administration routes include:

1. **Oral:** Drugs are ingested after being taken orally. This is one of the most popular routes because it is quick and non-invasive. The medicine enters the bloodstream after being absorbed through the digestive system. Tablets, capsules, and liquids are a few examples.
2. **Sublingual/Buccal:** Drugs are administered buccally (between the cheek and gum) or sublingually (under the tongue). The medication dissolves or passes through the mucous membranes to the bloodstream. Examples include buccal film formulations and sublingual nitroglycerin.
3. **Inhalation:** Drugs are inhaled as a gas or aerosol into the lungs. This method utilizes the large surface area of the lung to enable quick absorption into the bloodstream. Inhalation is frequently used to administer drugs like asthma inhalers or to treat respiratory disorders (Figure 10.2).

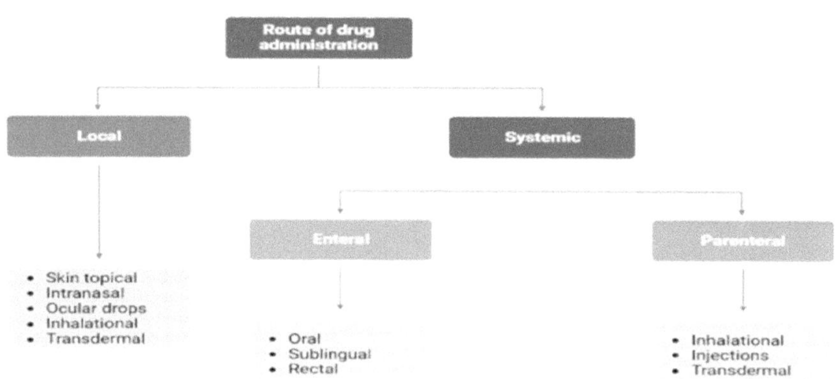

FIGURE 10.2 Route of drug administration.

4. **Topical:** For local effects, medications are applied to the skin or mucous membranes. They can be applied as creams, ointments,

patches, sprays, or lotions. Skin diseases, localized pain alleviation, or transdermal drug delivery are all treated using topical administration.

5. **Injection:** Using a needle and syringe, medications are directly injected into the body. Subcutaneous, intradermal, intramuscular, intravenous, and intramuscular injections are all possible ways to do this. Drug delivery is accelerated and dosing is exact with injection.
6. **Transdermal:** Drugs are administered via skin-attached patches or gels. The medication enters the bloodstream after being absorbed through the skin. For continuous medicine distribution, such as with hormone patches or nicotine patches, transdermal patches are frequently utilized.
7. **Rectal:** Suppositories or enemas are used to insert drugs into the rectum. The medication enters the bloodstream after being absorbed through the rectal mucosa. When oral administration is not an option or when localized effects are needed, this method is employed.

Intranasal (through the nose), intrathecal (into the spinal fluid), intraocular (into the eye), and intra-articular (into a joint) injection are other drug delivery methods. The qualities of the medicine, the patient's state, the desired time for action, and the precise therapeutic goal all play a role in the route selection.

10.4 PHARMACOKINETIC

In simple language, pharmacokinetics means what the body does to the drug and includes Absorption, Distribution, Metabolism, and Excretion.

10.4.1 ABSORPTION

When a medicine is administered, it must first enter the bloodstream in order to be disseminated throughout the body and have its desired pharmacological effects. This process is known as drug absorption. The many ways by which drugs are absorbed can change based on the physicochemical makeup of the drug and the route of delivery. Here are a few typical drug absorption mechanisms:

1. **Passive Diffusion:** The most typical method of absorbing drugs is this one. It happens when medications move from an area of higher concentration to an area of lower concentration across cell membranes. Drug lipophilicity (ability to dissolve in lipids), molecular size, degree of ionization, and the concentration gradient across the membrane are some parameters that affect passive diffusion.

2. **Facilitated Transport:** Some medications rely on transporters or carrier proteins to help them pass cell membranes. Drugs can move against concentration gradients or improve their uptake with the help of facilitated transport. The P-glycoprotein efflux pump and the solute carrier (SLC) family of transporters are two examples of drug transporters.

3. **Active Transport:** Energy is used in active transport to carry medicines across cell membranes. Drugs can be transported by this method against concentration gradients and normally need carrier proteins. Active transport is quite specialized and has the potential to saturate. Some antibiotics and antiviral treatments are examples of pharmaceuticals that move through active transport.

4. **Endocytosis and Exocytosis:** Some larger molecules, like peptides or macromolecular drugs, can be taken in by the body through a process called endocytosis, in which the cell engulfs the medication into a vesicle. On the other hand, exocytosis entails the release of medications from the cell via vesicles. These processes are important for targeted therapeutics and specialized drug delivery systems.

5. **Ion Trapping:** When a medication is ionized in one compartment and becomes trapped in that compartment as a result of pH variations, this is known as ion trapping. For instance, weak bases tend to accumulate in alkaline compartments (such as urine) while weak acids tend to build in acidic compartments (such as the stomach). Drug distribution and elimination are impacted by ion trapping (Figure 10.3).

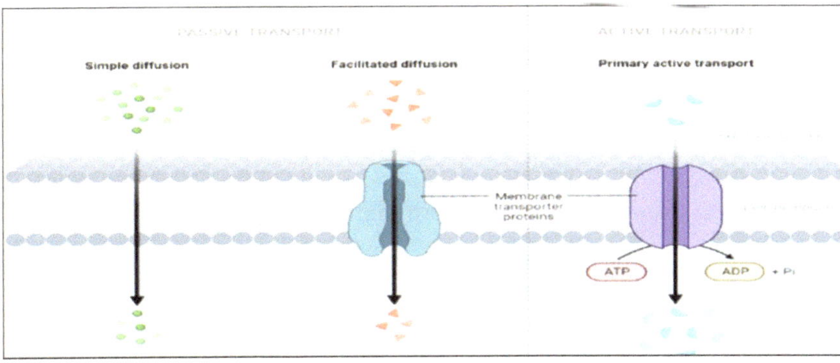

FIGURE10.3 Mechanism of drug absorption.

10.4.2 BIOAVAILABILITY

In order for a drug to have an impact on the body, it must reach the systemic circulation in an unaltered or active state. This is known as bioavailability. It shows the quantity and rate of medication absorption and availability at the site of action. Numerous variables, such as the method of administration, drug formulation, and physiological processes, have an impact on bioavailability. The following key ideas in bioavailability are important to understand:

1. **Routes of Administration:** The bioavailability of a medicine is influenced by the method of administration. For instance, oral delivery may result in decreased bioavailability due to possible degradation in the gastrointestinal tract and first-pass metabolism in the liver, whereas intravenous (IV) administration bypasses the absorption process and provides total bioavailability.
2. **Absorption:** Bioavailability is influenced by the rate and extent of medication absorption. Drug absorption and, thus, bioavailability can be impacted by factors such as drug solubility, formulation, gastrointestinal transit time, and the presence of food or other substances.
3. **First-Pass Metabolism:** When a medication is given orally, the liver may be the first place it is processed before it enters the bloodstream. First-pass metabolism is what causes this, and it can dramatically lower a drug's bioavailability. Drugs supplied

by alternative means, including intravenous injection, avoid first-pass metabolism and have better bioavailability as a result.

4. **Drug Formulation:** The bioavailability of a drug product can be impacted by its formulation. Drug absorption and subsequent bioavailability can be influenced by elements such as drug particle size, dissolving rate, and formulation excipients.

5. **Drug-Drug Interactions:** Drug interactions resulting from concurrent use can have an impact on bioavailability. Drug interactions can influence a drug's metabolism, elimination, or absorption, changing the drug's bioavailability.

By tracking the drug's levels in the blood or plasma over time, bioavailability is commonly evaluated. In relation to the drug's bioavailability when given intravenously, it is expressed as a percentage. Low bioavailability suggests inefficient absorption or considerable metabolism prior to systemic exposure, whereas high bioavailability indicates more effective absorption and higher systemic circulation.

10.4.3 DRUG DISTRIBUTION

The process by which a medicine is carried from the bloodstream to various tissues and compartments inside the body is referred to as drug distribution. Drugs are delivered to their target sites of action or other tissues by the circulatory system after absorption, where they may exert their pharmacological effects.

Factors that affect drug distribution are as follows:

1. **Plasma Protein Binding:** Numerous medications bind to plasma proteins, including albumin. Drugs that are bound are less easily distributed to tissues. The only part of a medication that can normally pass cell membranes and interact with its target is the unbound (free) fraction (Talevi and Bellera, 2022).

2. **Tissue Perfusion:** Blood flow to various tissues affects how medications are distributed. The liver, heart, kidneys, and brain are among the highly perfused organs that receive a substantial amount of the medication. Poorly perfused tissues, however, might only absorb low medication concentrations (Talevi and Bellera, 2022).

3. **Capillary Permeability:** For drugs to reach tissues, capillary barriers must be crossed. Depending on the tissue and the properties of the drug, such as its molecular size and lipophilicity, capillary permeability can change. Specific systems in some organs, such as the blood-brain barrier, limit medication penetration (Talevi and Bellera, 2022).
4. **Volume of Distribution (VD):** A pharmacokinetic metric known as the volume of distribution measures the apparent area in the body where a medicine seems to be spread. It illustrates the link between the plasma concentration and the overall amount of the drug in the body. A low VD denotes a restricted distribution, largely in the blood, while a high VD denotes a wide diffusion into tissues (Talevi and Bellera, 2022).
5. **Drug Accumulation:** Drugs may build up in particular tissues as a result of active transport mechanisms, tissue binding, or retention. Accumulation may result in hazardous effects or prolonged drug effects (Talevi and Bellera, 2022).
6. **Physiological Barriers:** Due to physiological limitations, the distribution of some medications is further complicated. For instance, the blood-brain barrier prevents many medications from entering the central nervous system (CNS). Drug delivery to the fetus during pregnancy may be impacted by placental barriers (Talevi and Bellera, 2022).

10.4.4 DRUG METABOLISM

The metabolic processes that take place in the body to convert medications or other foreign chemicals into metabolites are referred to as drug metabolism, also known as biotransformation. The process of metabolism is essential for the removal, inactivation, or activation of medications since these metabolites are frequently chemically altered versions of the parent substance. Although other organs and tissues, including the colon, lungs, and kidneys, can also participate, the liver is where drug processing largely takes place. Drug metabolism is divided into two distinctive phases:

1. **Phase I Metabolism:** Phase I reactions entail adding or exposing a functional group to the drug molecule (such as a hydroxyl, amino,

or carboxyl group) through procedures like oxidation, reduction, or hydrolysis. These processes could make the medication more polar, increasing its susceptibility to phase II metabolism or aiding in its excretion. A significant part of many phase I processes is played by the superfamily of enzymes known as cytochrome P450 (CYP) enzymes.

2. **Phase II Metabolism:** Phase II reactions involve glucuronic acid, sulfate, glutathione, or amino acids as conjugates of the drug or its phase I metabolites with endogenous molecules. Drugs become more water-soluble as a result of conjugation processes, which makes them easier to excrete. Glucuronidation, sulfation, acetylation, methylation, and conjugation with glutathione are typical phase II processes.

10.4.5 DRUG EXCRETION

Drug excretion is the process through which drugs or their metabolites are eliminated from the body. It is an essential procedure that gets rid of medications that have been metabolized or are no longer needed, stopping their build-up and potential toxicity. Drug excretion primarily happens through the kidneys via urine, but it can also happen through other elimination processes such as bile, feces, perspiration, saliva, breast milk, and exhaled air.

Routes of drug excretion are as follows:

1. **Renal Excretion:** Through the processes of renal filtration, reabsorption, and secretion, the kidneys play a crucial part in the excretion of drugs. The glomerulus filters medicines and their metabolites into the renal tubules as the blood flows through it. Some medications are then actively secreted into the urine, while others are reabsorbable by the tubules and returned to the bloodstream. The overall outcome determines how much of the medicine is eliminated in the urine.

2. **Biliary Excretion:** Bile, which the liver produces and releases into the small intestine, can be used to remove some medications and metabolites. Drugs that are expelled by the bile eventually pass through the feces. For medications that undergo significant

hepatic metabolism or are highly lipophilic and not suitable for renal clearance, biliary excretion is especially crucial.

3. **Other Routes of Excretion:** Drugs can be eliminated through various channels besides urine and feces. Some medicines and their metabolites can be excreted through sweat, saliva, and tears. Volatile or highly vaporized drugs may be expelled by exhaled air, especially through the lungs. Drug excretion in breast milk is a possibility in nursing individuals.
4. **Enterohepatic Circulation:** Drugs that are discharged into the bile, reabsorbed in the intestines, and subsequently re-enter the systemic circulation are known as enterohepatic circulators. This procedure can delay a drug's excretion or extend the time it takes for it to take effect (Figure 10.4).

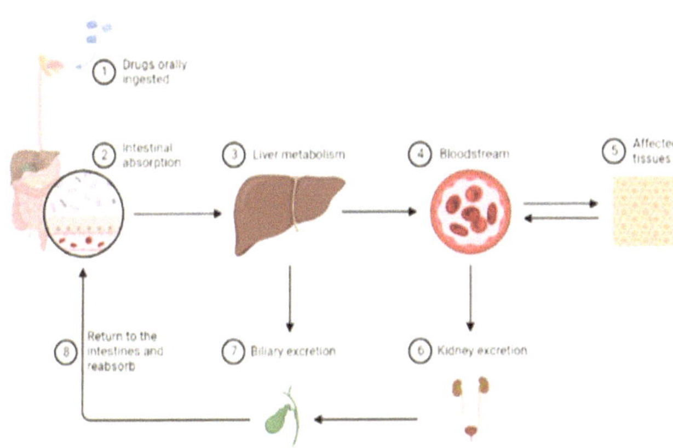

FIGURE 10.4 Fate of the drug in body.

10.5 DRUG DOSE

A drug dose is the precise amount of medication or other substance that is given to a person or patient. The dosage of a medication that has been prescribed is meant to have the desired therapeutic effect. Healthcare specialists, such as doctors or pharmacists, often determine drug doses depending on the patient's age, weight, medical condition, severity of the ailment, and the exact drug being used, among other variables. The dosage can change based on how it is administered (oral, intravenous, topically, etc.) and how frequently (once a day, twice daily, etc.).

Different pharmacological dosage kinds are frequently employed in clinical settings. Some of the most typical varieties are listed below:

1. **Single Dose:** This refers to a single drug administration. It is frequently utilized for treatments or procedures that call for the administration of drugs on an as-needed basis.
2. **Maintenance Dose:** This is a medication's recommended daily dosage in order to keep the desired therapeutic effect. For chronic illnesses that call for ongoing care, it is frequently employed.
3. **Loading Dose:** In order to quickly reach a therapeutic drug level in the body, a loading dose is a greater initial dose of a medication. It is frequently employed when swift or immediate action is sought.
4. **Maximum Dose:** This is the maximum amount of a medicine that can be safely taken within a certain time frame. It is based on elements like the drug's effectiveness, toxicity, and unique patient features.
5. **Minimum Effective Dose:** This is the lowest dosage of a drug needed to achieve the desired therapeutic result. To reduce the possibility of side effects or negative responses, the lowest effective dose should be used.
6. **Titration Dose:** Titration is the process of modifying a medication's dose to produce the desired therapeutic result. When a medicine requires individualized dosing based on the patient's response, titration doses are utilized.
7. **Cumulative Dose:** The entire dosage of a medicine given over a predetermined time period is referred to as the cumulative dose. To track and stop the accumulation of dangerous levels, it is frequently included in drugs with a limited therapeutic index.

The right medicine dosage for a specific person depends on a number of variables. When deciding the dosage for a certain medication, healthcare experts take these variables into consideration. Following are some typical variables that may impact medicine dosage:

1. **Age:** The dosage of a medicine is greatly influenced by age. Because everyone's metabolism, organ function, and body

composition are different, infants, children, adults, and the elderly may need to take varying amounts.

2. **Body Weight:** A person's weight is a significant consideration when prescribing medication, particularly for weight-based treatments. To guarantee that the body receives the right amount of the drug, the dosage can be adjusted.

3. **Gender:** Males and females may have different medication metabolisms in specific situations. Body composition and hormonal changes can affect how medications are metabolized and removed from the body.

4. **Renal Function:** In the process of eliminating drugs, the kidneys are crucial. To prevent drug accumulation and potential toxicity, the dosage of some drugs may need to be adjusted if a person has compromised renal function.

5. **Hepatic Function:** Numerous medicines are metabolized by the liver. Drug metabolism may be impacted by impaired liver function, necessitating possible dose modifications to avoid side effects.

6. **Genetic Factors:** The way a person reacts to drugs can vary genetically. Pharmacogenetics is a field that investigates how genetic variations can impact drug efficacy and metabolism. Genetic testing may occasionally be used to recommend a specific medicine dosage.

7. **Concurrent Medications:** Drug interactions can have an impact on the efficacy or safety of a given medication. When calculating the right dose of a medication, medical experts take possible drug interactions into account.

8. **Disease State:** The metabolism and clearance of medications might be affected by underlying medical problems. To guarantee the most effective therapy results and to reduce side effects, certain disorders may require dosage modifications.

9. **Therapeutic Goal:** The dosage of a medicine might be affected by its intended therapeutic effect and desired result. For instance,

compared to long-term maintenance therapy, a greater dose could be required for the alleviation of acute pain.

10. **Route of Administration:** It is possible for a drug's absorption, distribution, and bioavailability to be impacted by the route through which it is taken (oral, intravenous, topical, etc.). To obtain the intended effect, different delivery methods might need to use different doses.

10.6 DRUG DOSAGE CALCULATION

When calculating medicine dosages for both children and adults, a number of variables are taken into account, including body weight, age, and occasionally body surface area. Here are a few typical formulas for figuring out drug dosages:

1. **Body Weight-Based Dosing:** Based on a child's weight, Clark's Rule is a formula that determines the right pediatric dosage of a medication. Since children frequently require different dosages than adults due to their smaller stature, it is frequently utilized when figuring out the right dosage of medication for kids (Delgado et al., 2022).

(Weight* divided by 150 lbs.) x Adult Dose** = Pediatric Dosage

(Weight*** divided by 68 kg) x Adult Dose** = Pediatric Dosage

The adult dose here refers to the average dosage given to an adult, while the child's weight is typically expressed in pounds. Based on the child's weight in relation to the 150-pound typical adult weight, the outcome of this formula shows the recommended dosage for the youngster. In body weight-based dosing, the dose is adjusted in accordance with the patient's weight. Based on the particular drug and condition being treated, the healthcare practitioner determines the dose per kilogram (kg).

2. **Surface Area-Based Dosing:**

   i. **Pediatric Dose:** Pediatric dose (in mg) = Child's body surface area (BSA, in m^2) × Dose per m^2.

   ii. **Adult Dose:** Adult dose (in mg) = Adult body surface area (BSA, in m^2) × Dose per m^2.

Body surface area-based dosing accounts for the body surface area of the individual, which is determined using methods like the Mosteller formula or DuBois formula. When precise dosing is necessary or when a treatment has a limited therapeutic index, this method is frequently used (Pai, 2012).

3. **Age-Based Dosing:** Another formula used to determine a drug's pediatric dosage depending on a child's age is called Young's Rule. Although it is less frequently used than Clark's Rule, this rule might be used as a substitute to determine pediatric doses (Wade and Martinez, 2023).

[Age / (Age + 12)] x Recommended Adult Dose = Pediatric Dose

The adult dose here refers to the average dosage given to an adult, and the child's age is typically indicated in years. Based on the child's age in relation to the reference age of 12 years, the outcome of this formula shows the recommended dosage for the youngster.

10.7 DRUG TOXICITY

When a prescription or substance is used at levels that are higher than those advised, or when it builds up in the body due to a disordered metabolism or elimination process, it is referred to as drug toxicity. Drug interactions with other drugs, substances, or pre-existing medical disorders can potentially lead to drug toxicity. A drug's adverse effects can range from moderate and reversible to severe and life-threatening when it reaches toxic levels in the body. The precise signs and effects of drug toxicity depend on the medication being taken, as well as the patient's sensitivity, metabolism, and general health.

Some common signs and symptoms of drug toxicity may include:

- **Gastrointestinal disturbances:** Nausea, vomiting, diarrhea, or abdominal pain.
- **Central nervous system effects:** Drowsiness, confusion, dizziness, seizures, or coma.
- **Cardiovascular effects:** Irregular heart rhythms, changes in blood pressure, or chest pain.
- **Respiratory effects:** Difficulty breathing, shortness of breath, or respiratory depression.

- **Renal or hepatic impairment:** Impaired kidney or liver function, leading to changes in urine output or jaundice.
- **Dermatological reactions:** Skin rashes, hives, or severe allergic reactions.
- **Hematological abnormalities:** Blood disorders, such as decreased platelet counts or impaired clotting.

The severity of drug toxicity, the type of medication used, and the patient's clinical condition are all important considerations in managing drug toxicity. If drug poisoning is suspected, immediate medical assistance should be sought. The broad guidelines and potential treatments for managing medication toxicity are as follows:

- **Supportive Care:** In order to stabilize the patient and maintain crucial organ function, supportive care must be given. This can entail keeping an eye on vital signs, ensuring that oxygenation and ventilation are working properly, keeping hydrated, and addressing electrolyte imbalances.
- **Decontamination:** Techniques for decontaminating the medicine may be employed to lessen absorption if it was just consumed. In order to adsorb the drug and stop further absorption, these methods may include inducing vomiting, gastric lavage (stomach pumping), or giving activated charcoal.
- **Antidotes:** There are specific antidotes available for particular pharmaceuticals or drug classes. Antidotes function by either reducing the drug's hazardous effects or speeding up the body's ability to eliminate them. To manage medication toxicity, antidotes may need to be administered quickly. Naloxone for opioid overdoses, flumazenil for benzodiazepine overdoses, and N-acetylcysteine for paracetamol overdoses are a few examples of antidotes.
- **Enhanced Elimination:** Sometimes it may be advantageous to speed up the body's medication disposal. When the drug is dialyzable or rapidly binds to molecules that resemble charcoal,

methods like hemodialysis or hemoperfusion can be employed to remove it from the bloodstream.

- **Symptomatic Treatment:** Treatment for specific signs and symptoms of medication toxicity seeks to reduce them. For instance, drugs may be given to treat cardiac arrhythmias, control seizures, or maintain blood pressure.
- **Continuous Monitoring:** To evaluate the effectiveness of the treatment and identify any complications or changes in the clinical situation, it is crucial to closely monitor the patient's vital signs, cardiac function, renal function, electrolyte levels, and other pertinent measures.

10.8 CONCLUSION

It has become clear how diverse this field is as a result of the trip through drug discovery, pharmacokinetics, pharmacodynamics, and specialized fields of pharmacology. The ideas outlined in this overview continue to serve as the cornerstone upon which the improvements in healthcare that are about to bring in a new era of personalized medicine, precision medicines, and novel drug delivery technologies are created. Understanding pharmacokinetics and pharmacodynamics gives us knowledge of how medications are taken up, transported, metabolized, and eliminated, as well as how they interact with molecular targets to have beneficial or harmful effects. This information serves as the cornerstone on which logical drug development, dosing protocols, and therapeutic approaches are built. The study of general pharmacology also emphasizes the dynamic aspect of the subject as it develops in tandem with scientific and medical discoveries. The importance of having a solid understanding of general pharmacology increases as we approach personalized medicine, genetic insights, and novel drug delivery technologies. These developments have the potential to completely alter the healthcare industry by providing individualized treatments with increased efficacy and reduced adverse reactions.

KEYWORDS

- **drug delivery technologies**
- **drug discovery**
- **drug dosage**
- **general pharmacology**
- **pharmacodynamics**
- **pharmacokinetics**
- **pharmacology**
- **therapeutic approaches**

REFERENCES

Cascorbi, I. (2012). Drug interactions—Principles, examples, and clinical consequences. *Deutsches Ärzteblatt International, 99*(33, 34), 546.

Delcò, F., Tchambaz, L., Krähenbühl, S., Biollaz, J., & Rudin, D. (2005). Dose adjustment in patients with liver disease. *Drug Safety, 28*(6), 529–545.

Delgado, B. J., Safadi, A. O., & Bajaj, T. (2022). Clark's rule. *StatPearls* [Preprint]. Retrieved from: https://www.ncbi.nlm.nih.gov/books/NBK54194/ (accessed on 14 March 2025).

Fernandez, E., Perez, R., Hernandez, A., Tejada, P., Arteta, M., & Ramos, J. T. (2011). Factors and mechanisms for pharmacokinetic differences between pediatric population and adults. *Pharmaceutics, 3*(1), 53.

Heldin, C. H., Lu, B., Evans, R., & Gutkind, J. S. (2016). Signals and receptors. *Cold Spring Harbor Perspectives in Biology, 8*(4).

Heller, F. (2013). Genetics/genomics and drug effects. *Acta Clinica Belgica, 68*(2), 77–80.

Institute of Medicine (US) Committee on Accelerating Rare Diseases Research and Orphan Product Development, Field, M. J., & Boat, T. F. (2009). Introduction. Retrieved from: https://www.ncbi.nlm.nih.gov/books/NBK56194/ (accessed on 14 March 2025).

Khan, S., Ullah, M. W., Siddique, R., Nabi, G., Manan, S., Yousaf, M., Hou, H., & Zhang, X. (2016). Role of recombinant DNA technology to improve life. *International Journal of Genomics, 2016,* 2405954.

Kyriakopoulos, C., & Gupta, V. (2022). Renal failure drug dose adjustments. *StatPearls* [Preprint]. Retrieved from: https://www.ncbi.nlm.nih.gov/books/NBK560512/ (accessed on 14 March 2025).

Lombardino, J. G., & Lowe, J. A. (2004). The role of the medicinal chemist in drug discovery—Then and now. *Nature Reviews Drug Discovery, 3*(9), 853–862.

Malve, H. (2016). Exploring the ocean for new drug developments: Marine pharmacology. *Journal of Pharmacy & Bioallied Sciences, 8*(2), 83.

Mangoni, A. A., & Jackson, S. H. D. (2004). Age-related changes in pharmacokinetics and pharmacodynamics: Basic principles and practical applications. *British Journal of Clinical Pharmacology, 57*(1), 6.

Niederberger, E., & Parnham, M. J. (2021). The impact of diet and exercise on drug responses. *International Journal of Molecular Sciences, 22*(14).

Pai, M. P. (2012). Drug dosing based on weight and body surface area: Mathematical assumptions and limitations in obese adults. *Pharmacotherapy, 32*(9), 856–868.

Pathan, H., & Williams, J. (2012). Basic opioid pharmacology: An update. *British Journal of Pain, 6*(1), 11.

Pichai, E., & Lakshmanan, M. (2022). Drug elimination. In *Introduction to Basics of Pharmacology and Toxicology: Volume 1: General and Molecular Pharmacology: Principles of Drug Action* (pp. 117–129).

Talevi, A., & Bellera, C. L. (2022). Drug distribution. In *ADME Processes in Pharmaceutical Sciences: Dosage, Design, and Pharmacotherapy Success* (pp. 33–53).

Verhaegen, A. A., & Van Gaal, L. F. (2019). Drugs that affect body weight, body fat distribution, and metabolism. *Endotext* [Preprint]. Retrieved from: https://www.ncbi.nlm.nih.gov/books/NBK537590/ (accessed on 14 March 2025).

Wade, C. I., & Martinez, T. (2023). Young's rule (pp. 51–53).

World Health Organization. (2013). *WHO Traditional Medicine Strategy*. Retrieved from: www.who.int (accessed on 14 March 2025).

World Health Organization. (2017). *Guidance on the Use of International Nonproprietary Names (INNs) for Pharmaceutical Substances*. Retrieved from: http://apps.who.int/bookorders (accessed on 14 March 2025).

CHAPTER 11

Overview of Infection, Prevention, and Control

SUMEDHA RABRA,[1,*] MEENAKSHI VERMA,[1] RITIKA INDORIA,[2] and SUMEET BHARTI[3]

[1]*Department of Physiotherapy, Sharda School of Allied Health Sciences, Sharda University, Greater Noida, Uttar Pradesh, India*

[2]*Consultant Physiotherapist, Shakti Physiotherapy Centre NOIDA, Uttar Pradesh, India*

[3]*Kessler Rehabilitation Center, Weehawken, New Jersey, USA*

*Corresponding author

ABSTRACT

Infection prevention and control (IPC) is a crucial aspect of healthcare delivery that aims to minimize the spread of infectious diseases among patients, healthcare workers, and the community. IPC strategies involve a comprehensive set of measures that are designed to prevent the transmission of infections, including hand hygiene (HH), personal protective equipment, and environmental cleaning and disinfection. Effective IPC requires a multi-disciplinary approach and a commitment to continuous quality improvement, including ongoing education and training, as well as regular surveillance and monitoring of infection rates. In addition, IPC practices must be adapted and modified to reflect changes in the epidemiology of infectious diseases and the emergence of new pathogens. By implementing and maintaining effective IPC measures, healthcare facilities can reduce the risk of healthcare-associated infections (HCAIs), protect patients, and contribute to public health efforts to control the spread of infectious diseases.

Allied Healthcare in Practice: An Introduction to Integrated Patient Care. Sally Lukose, Karuna Singh (Eds.)

DOI: 10.1201/9781998511037-13

11.1 INTRODUCTION

Infection prevention and control (IPC) is a crucial aspect of healthcare delivery, aimed at minimizing the spread of infectious diseases among patients, healthcare workers, and the broader community. At least one in 10 patients who receive care in hospitals in low- and middle-income countries (LMICs) contract an infection, making healthcare-associated infections (HCAIs) the most common adverse outcome in healthcare delivery worldwide. While the rising use of antibiotics to treat HAIs contributes to the spread of antimicrobial resistance, HAIs also cause disability and cost to healthcare systems and individuals. HCAIs are infections that initially manifest 48 hours or more after being admitted to the hospital or within 30 days of receiving medical attention. Adverse medication events, HCAIs, and surgical complications are the most frequent categories of adverse events (AE) affecting hospitalized patients, according to several studies. Effective IPC is essential for delivering safe, efficient, and high-quality healthcare services and for putting an end to preventable HAIs. According to the World Health Organization (WHO), effective IPC interventions can lower HAI rates by 30%. The eight essential elements for the implementation of effective IPC are outlined in the 2016 WHO recommendations for IPC at the national and facility levels. By implementing and maintaining effective IPC measures, healthcare facilities can reduce the risk of healthcare- associated infections, protect patients and contribute to public health efforts to control the spread of infectious diseases (Williams et al., 2002).

11.2 SOURCES OF INFECTION

In the community and in the hospital, bacteria and viruses live in the environment naturally. Most of these organisms are not diseases and may even be helpful to human health. The organisms in the natural environment may act as a reservoir from which they might infect additional patients. Despite this, there are several reservoirs; the source is the one from which infections start. To stop the spread, accurate source identification is crucial. Similar to how infections are categorized, so are the sources of dissemination: Transmission of community-acquired illnesses to hospital patients can occur through blood contamination, respiratory diseases, Salmonella, Shigella, and Vibrio-infected feces. The skin's scales or the air, as in cases of chickenpox, herpes, or staphylococcal streptococci bacteria, and pus-like infections or discharges. Interventions tailored to the particular infected person are needed for the prevention of such spread (Haque et al., 2023).

Infections typically occur in patients receiving hospital care. Surgical or other invasive operations performed in operating rooms, wards, or other healthcare facilities can result in infections, which can come from a variety of sources. The resident microbial flora of medical personnel and other patients, the patient's mouth, gastrointestinal tract, vagina, or skin, inside the ward. Temporary germs that are spread from one healthcare worker to another, contaminated tools, bandages, needles, and other supplies used during invasive operations (Figure 11.1).

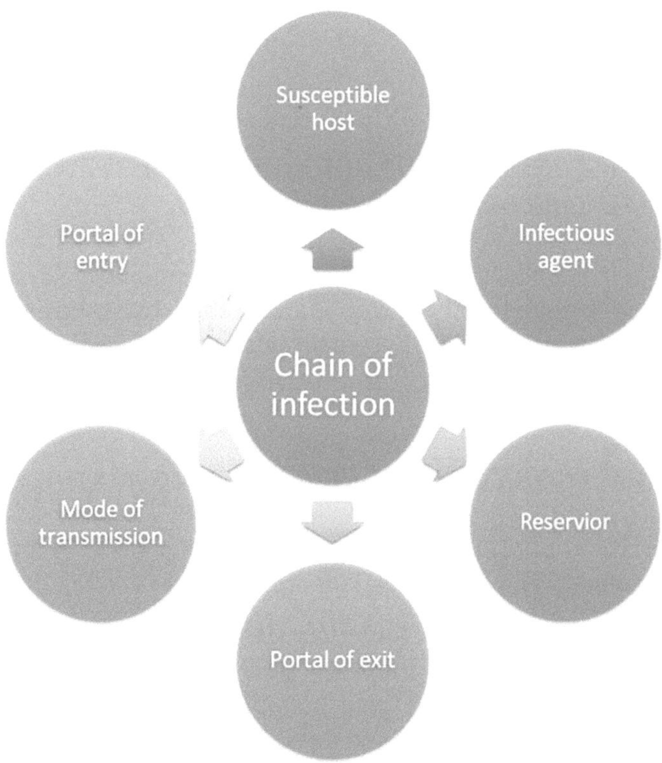

FIGURE 11.1 The sequence of events that must occur for an infection to be transmitted from one person to another. Breaking any link in the chain can prevent the spread of infection.

11.3 INFECTION CONTROL PROGRAM (ICP)

Hospitals must create policies to follow effective infection control practices and to protect the safety and well-being of both patients and workers.

11.3.1 OBJECTIVES OF THE INFECTION CONTROL PROGRAM (ICP)

Authorities should monitor outbreaks and put an end to the epidemic by addressing any technological errors. Staff health monitoring is essential to prevent staff-to-patient and patient-to-staff transmission of contamination. Guidance on isolation techniques and infection prevention methods should be provided. Audits for infection control, including examinations of handwashing, waste disposal, antibiotic safety checks, and recommendations, should be conducted.

11.3.2 RESPONSIBILITY OF HOSPITAL ADMINISTRATOR/ HEAD OF HEALTH CARE FACILITY

The head should allocate necessary funding and resources for controlling any disease. Ensure that the premises are clean and safe. Ensure that safe food and water are available. Ensure that materials are sterilized and establish a committee and team for infection control.

11.3.3 INFECTION CONTROL ORGANIZATIONS IN A HOSPITAL

Infection control organizations are essential components of an infection control program. These organizations are:

1. **Infection Control Committee (ICC):** Members are drawn from the departments of medicine, nursing, engineering, administration, pharmacy, CSSD, and microbiology. The group develops the policy for infection control and prevention. The chairperson of the committee, who has access to the top hospital administrators, is chosen from among its members. The member secretary serves as the infection control officer (ICO). The group convenes at least three times a year on a regular basis.

2. **Infection Control Team (ICT):** Members should identify the day-to-day measures for the control of infection.
3. **Infection Control Officer (ICO):** A medical microbiologist or another physician with expertise in hospital-associated illnesses typically serves as the ICO. The secretary of the Infection Control Committee is responsible for taking minutes and scheduling meetings. Pathogen identification and antibiotic sensitivity reporting should be conducted. Regular analysis and distribution of information on emerging diseases, antibiotic resistance, and unusual testing results should occur. Hospital infection surveillance and outbreak detection should be initiated. Investigations into outbreaks should be ongoing. Instruction and training in infection control practices should be conducted regularly.
4. **Infection Control Nurse (ICN):** A senior nursing staff member should be appointed for this role. Full- or part-time nursing personnel should be provided to support the course. The ICN should coordinate efforts between the clinical and microbiological divisions to identify and prevent HCAIs. They should work with the ICO on infection monitoring and outbreak detection. The ICNs should receive basic training in specimen collection and preliminary processing, as well as microbiological methods. Instruction and training should be conducted under the direction of the ICO to raise awareness of infection management among patients and visitors.
5. **Infection Control Manual (ICM):** It is advised that every institution create its own infection control handbook based on preexisting materials but customized for local hazards and situations (Williams, et al., 2002).

11.4 THE HOSPITAL ENVIRONMENT AND HOSPITAL-ASSOCIATED INFECTIONS

11.4.1 ENVIRONMENT

Hospital-acquired illnesses are often caused by factors related to the hospital environment. Several elements make up the hospital setting.

Air quality, water supply, diet, and the management of medical waste and laundry are just a few of the factors that directly affect HAIs.

11.4.2 PREMISES/BUILDINGS

Any new construction or remodeling project should engage a member of the infection control team. In this procedure, infection control's job is to reduce infections that are linked to hospitals. These include things like ensuring suitable facilities for hand washing, a reliable water source facility, adequate hospital isolation facilities, and sufficient ventilation in high-risk locations such as operating rooms, transplant centers, and critical care units. Advising traffic flow to reduce high-risk patients' exposure and facilitate easy patient transfer is also important. Additionally, avoiding fungal spore exposure for patients during repairs is crucial.

11.4.3 AIR

During coughing or sneezing, airborne droplet nuclei are a possible source of infection transmission, either directly through inhalation or indirectly through infected medical equipment. Droplets produced by infected respiratory tracts can spread diseases including TB, viral respiratory disorders, and antibiotic-resistant hospital germs over extended periods of time.

Cleaning tasks that involve sweeping or using dry mops or rags can release dust particles that may carry microorganisms into the air. Wet wiping is thus preferable. The number of particles in the air in a room will vary depending on how many people are present, how much activity is occurring, and how quickly the air is changing. Lint and skin squamae are significant causes of contamination.

11.4.4 VENTILATION

Since airborne microorganisms can cause certain HAIs, proper ventilation is required. Following significant building work in the facility, some laboratory observations may be required in high-risk areas such as operating rooms for heart surgery, neurosurgery, and transplant surgery. Fresh, filtered air is circulated, which reduces and eliminates airborne bacterial contamination as well as odors. All hospital spaces, especially the high-risk ones, should have as good ventilation as is practical. To reduce microbiological contamination, ventilation systems should be designed and maintained in good condition. In high-risk settings, fans that might transmit airborne diseases should be avoided, and the air conditioning filters should be cleaned regularly.

In high-risk situations, good housekeeping should prevent clutter and obstruction from empty boxes and other unnecessary items. Positive air pressure is advised for dangerous locations that need to be kept clean. For contaminated areas, negative air pressure vented to the atmosphere is recommended. It is also necessary to isolate people with illnesses transmitted through the air. In high-risk settings, filtration systems (air handling units) designed to produce clean air should incorporate HEPA filters. In the hospital's construction, unidirectional laminar airflow systems should be accessible when necessary. Some forms of heart surgery, neurosurgery, and implant surgery theaters benefit from ultraclean air unit transplants. Maintenance and verification of filters' effectiveness are two crucial aspects of air quality. Critical parameters for air quality include air changes each hour, with a minimum of 15 air changes. To prevent the growth of germs, the temperature and humidity should be kept between 20 and 22°C and 30 and 60%, respectively. Maintenance and validation of the efficacy of filters, as well as the pressure gradient across the filter bed and in the operating theater, are essential (Williams et al., 2002).

11.4.5 WATER

Hospitals utilize water for a variety of purposes. The standards for water quality are determined by the intended usage of the water. Most of the time, the requirements for drinking water are insufficient for the medicinal purposes of water. Water should be safe to consume orally.

11.4.5.1 STANDARDS FOR SAFE WATER TO CONSUME

The water supply system should ensure that clean water is available. Regular cleaning of storage tanks and sampling of the water's quality are also recommended. Periodically check for contamination from feces. Several hospitalized microorganisms have caused infections in wounds and lungs. In areas without access to potable water, water should be boiled for five minutes to make it safe. Alternatives include using water purifying devices. Water should be stored as hygienically as possible. The storage container shouldn't be touched with hands. Water should be released from the storage container through a tap or outlet that is equipped with a closing mechanism. Water coolers and storage containers need to be cleaned often.

11.4.6 KITCHENS AND FOOD HANDLING

Food safety is a crucial service provided by healthcare institutions since poor food handling techniques allow for bacterial contamination, survival, and development. The following mistakes are frequent causes of food poisoning outbreaks: consuming contaminated raw food, avoiding preparing food in advance for more than half a day, cross-contamination of prepared or stored cooked food with uncooked food, food handlers contaminating the food, improper refrigeration or storing food at room temperature, inadequate reheating, and preparing enteral or infant feeding in an unhygienic manner.

11.5 CLEANING THE HOSPITAL ENVIRONMENT

To maintain a clean and dust-free medical environment, periodic cleaning is essential. "Visible dirt" typically contains a large number of microorganisms, and regular cleaning helps to get rid of this filth. The cleaning method mostly relies on mechanical action because soap and detergents lack antibacterial activity. The amount of asepsis that is required and the possibility of contamination must be considered while choosing a method. The majority of patient care areas are cleaned by wet mopping. Administrative and office spaces without patient interaction require standard household cleaning. Using a dry broom is not recommended. Utilizing a detergent mixture enhances the quality of places that have been visibly contaminated by blood or other fluids. Areas with a high risk of infection, such as isolation rooms, require a detergent/disinfectant solution for clean-up. Daily cleaning of all horizontal surfaces and bathroom areas is recommended. Using hot water (80°C) to clean the environment is beneficial and effective.

11.6 HOSPITAL WASTE

Hospital garbage needs to be handled carefully since it might contain harmful microorganisms. Contaminated metallic wastes have been shown to be the most frequent method of recorded illness transmission from waste to healthcare professionals.

11.6.1 PRINCIPLES OF WASTE MANAGEMENT

Hospital waste must be managed at every stage, from generation to final disposal, including collection, transportation, storage, and treatment. Wastes must be separated into the designated categories at the point of generation, or the source. Internationally recognized color-coded bags must be placed in containers with the proper labels and logos, such as the biohazard sign for infectious waste. For the collection of metallic waste, it should be possible to find biohazard-marked, puncture-proof containers at the blood collection facilities, injection carts, nursing stations, and operating rooms. It is necessary to develop a cart-based collecting system for the transportation of separated garbage. Prior to treatment, a designated area must be set aside for waste storage (Figure 11.2).

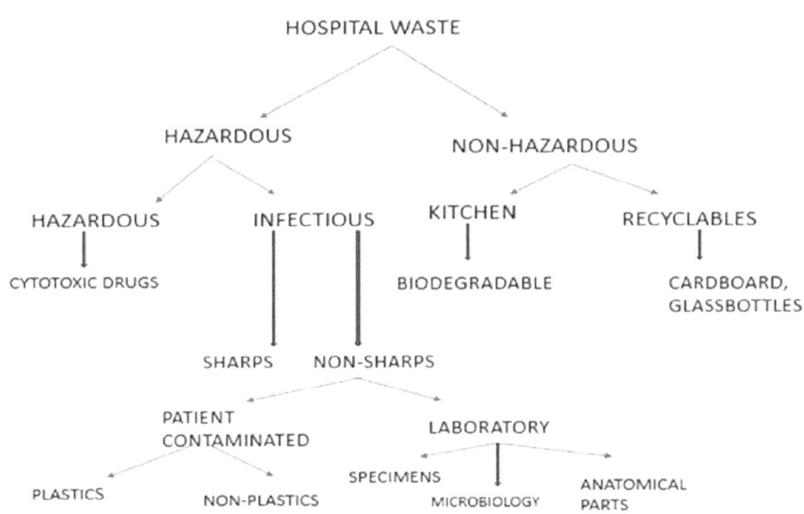

FIGURE 11.2 Classification of hospital waste.

Hospital waste is classified into hazardous and non-hazardous and further divided into different categories. It is crucial to prevent the spread of infections.

11.6.2 TREATMENT OF HAZARDOUS AND INFECTIOUS WASTES

1. **Sharps:** Alternatives available include: needle burners at the workstation, puncture-proof containers that can be microwaved, autoclaved, or treated with plasma pyrolysis before being shredded and placed in the ground; deep burial in a safe location, cutting of needles, a mechanical technique to prevent deformity. Recycling, however, is not a method of disinfection.
2. **Wastes Requiring Incineration:** Animal corpses, anatomical fragments, cytotoxic medications (outdated), and hazardous lab compounds other than mercury, non-plastics, and non-chlorinated plastics used by the patient that were contaminated.
3. **Laundry:** There are two recognized groups of used linen. It is referred to as "contaminated" when blood, excrement, or other biological fluids are clearly present. "Soiled" refers to several types of linen. These two groups ought to be separated and handled differently. To prevent the aerosolization of harmful microorganisms, all linen should be handled as little as possible. Contaminated linen should be transported in impermeable bags since it might be a source of infection for both patients and personnel. The use of hot water, bleach, heavy-duty gloves, eye protection, and splash-proof masks is necessary for disinfection. It is advised to use heavy-duty washers and dryers for hospital laundry.

11.7 HAND HYGIENE AND ITS IMPORTANCE

Several researchers, including Labarraque, Semmelweis, and Wendell Holmes, were striving to avoid hospital-acquired, nosocomial HCAIs in the middle of the 19th century in both Europe and the U.S. Even though they were conducting separate investigations, their findings led them to come up with a similar theory, namely that health care workers (HCWs) spread infectious agents to susceptible patients by carrying dangerous microbes on their hands from one patient to the next. Over the following century, a tone of evidence accumulated to show that HCWs often handled harmful germs. Semmelweis is credited as being the first medical professional to recognize the significance of HH in preventing communicable contagious illnesses (Haque et al., 2020).

1. **Hand Decontamination:** With the right hand cleanliness, the role of hands in the spread of hospital illnesses has been significantly reduced. However, handwashing compliance is typically not at its best. This is due to a number of factors, including the accessibility of equipment, a high patient-to-worker ratio, handwashing allergy products, and inadequate staff training on dangers and protocols. The single most crucial method of avoiding the transmission of germs is handwashing, especially between interactions with patients and following contact with blood, bodily fluids, secretions, excretions, and infected tools or objects.
2. **Facilities Requirements For Handwashing:** Large washbasins with running water, hands-free controls, low-maintenance construction, and splash guards. Depending on the operation, dry soap or liquid antiseptic may be used. Disposable towels, sterile single-use towels, or properly maintained roller towels are all suitable materials for drying hands.
3. **Hand Disinfection:** Specific hand sanitizers and antiseptics such as 2–4% chlorhexidine, 5–7.5% povidone iodine, 1% triclosan, or alcohol rubs are advised. Except for quick hand decontamination between patient interactions, alcohol-based hand massages are not a replacement for washing your hands. In order to prepare the hands for surgical procedures, the existing approach requires training. Three to five minutes of hand washing is adequate. The suggested antiseptics are either 7.5% povidone iodine or 4% chlorhexidine. Not all nations or medical facilities provide the same items and equipment. Compliance will increase if goods and processes are adaptable and sensitive to regional demands. In every situation, the optimal course of action should be implemented.

11.8 PERSONAL PROTECTIVE EQUIPMENT

Various additive manufacturing techniques have been shown to be efficient and practical in distant medical settings as well as in emergency or catastrophe scenarios. Our society has been greatly impacted by the coronavirus disease 2019 (COVID-19), which is brought on by the Severe Acute Respiratory Syndrome Coronavirus 2 (SARS-CoV-2) virus. This includes the ongoing availability of personal protective equipment (PPE) (Rendeki et al., 2020) (Figure 11.3).

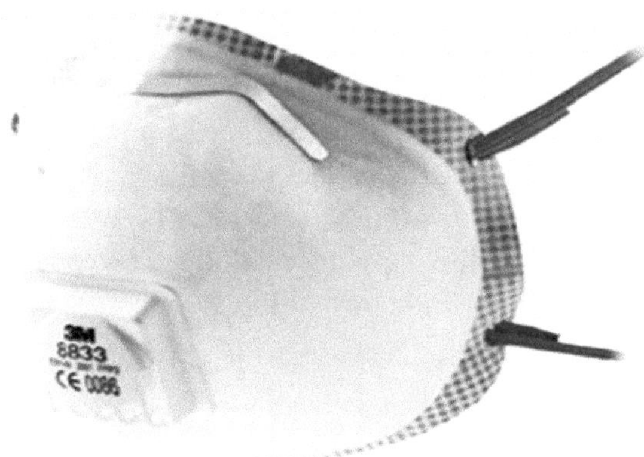

FIGURE 11.3 Face mask is a protective covering designed to be worn over the nose and mouth to reduce the spread of respiratory droplets that may contain virus.

Types of personal protective equipment: For healthcare professionals providing direct care (within 1 m) to patients with confirmed or suspected COVID-19, Public Health England (PHE) offers standard PPE recommendations. These recommendations include a disposable apron, gloves, a fluid-repellent surgical mask, and eye protection in the form of either goggles or a face shield. A respirator (N99 or FFP3 equivalent, which can be either valved or unvalved) is advised in place of a surgical mask when working in high-risk units (ICU, high-dependency unit, accident, and emergency, resuscitation, wards with non-invasive ventilation or continuous positive airway pressure ventilation, operating theatres, endoscopy units), or in the operating room where AGPs are being performed. According to the European Union (EU)-defined Filtering Face Piece (FFP) scale, respirator masks are categorized based on their capacity to filter tiny particles as small as 0.01–1 m in size, whereas SARS-CoV-2 measures

0.07–0.09 m in diameter on electron microscopy. FFP3 masks, which can filter over 99% (providing 90–9000-fold protection), are the gold standard in safety, as opposed to ordinary surgical masks, which can only filter 63% (6-fold). The National Health Service (NHS) is aware of its limitations; however, both FFP2 and N95 equivalent respirators, when properly worn, provide significant levels of protection with minimum efficiencies of 92–98% (providing 90-fold protection) (Jessop et al., 2020).

11.9 CONCLUSION

In conclusion, IPC are fundamental aspects of public health and healthcare delivery. By implementing comprehensive IPC measures at various levels, we can significantly reduce the transmission of infectious diseases, enhance patient safety, and contribute to healthier communities and a safer world. The lessons learned from previous infectious disease outbreaks, including COVID-19, underscore the need for ongoing investment in IPC to protect individuals and communities worldwide.

KEYWORDS

- **COVID-19**
- **healthcare delivery**
- **healthier communities**
- **infectious diseases**
- **intensive care unit**
- **non-invasive ventilation**
- **particle filtration**
- **personal protective equipment**
- **SARS-CoV-2**

REFERENCES

Association of Practitioners in Infection Control. (1996). *APIC Infection Control and Applied Epidemiology: Principles and Practice.* Mosby Inc.

Ayeliffe, G. A. J. (1992). *Control of Hospital Infection: A Practical Handbook* (3rd ed.). Chapman & Hall.

Ayeliffe, G. A., Hambraeus, A., & Mehtar, S. (1995). *Education Programme for Infection Control: Basic Concepts and Training.* International Federation of Infection Control.

Centers for Disease Control and Prevention. (1995). *Guidelines for Prevention of Intravascular Infections.* U.S. Department of Health and Human Services, National Center for Infectious Diseases, Hospital Infections Program.

Centers for Disease Control and Prevention. (1996). Guideline for isolation precautions in hospitals. *American Journal of Infection Control, 24*(4), 24–52.

Centers for Disease Control and Prevention. (n.d.). *Guidelines for Infection Control in Hospital Personnel.* U.S. Department of Health and Human Services.

Gardner, J. F., & Peel, M. M. (1991). *Introduction to Sterilization, Disinfection, and Infection Control.*

Haque, M., McKimm, J., Sartelli, M., Dhingra, S., Labricciosa, F. M., Islam, S., Jahan, D., Nusrat, T., Chowdhury, T. S., Coccolini, F., Iskandar, K., Catena, F., & Chara, J. (2020). Strategies to prevent healthcare-associated infections: A narrative overview. *Risk Management and Healthcare Policy, 13*, 1765–1780.

Haque, M., Sartelli, M., McKimm, J., & Abu Bakar, M. (2023). Healthcare-associated infections–An overview. *Infection and Drug Resistance, 11*, 2321–2333.

Jessop, Z. M., Dobbs, T. D., Ali, S. R., Combellack, E., Clancy, R., Ibrahim, N., Jovic, T. H., Kaur, A. J., Nijran, A., O'Neill, T. B., & Whitaker, I. S. (2020). Personal protective equipment for surgeons during COVID-19 pandemic: Systematic review of availability, usage, and rationing. *British Journal of Surgery, 97*(9), 1162–1180.

Lowe, H., Woodd, S., Lange, I. L., Janjanin, S., Barnet, J., & Graham, W. (2021). Challenges and opportunities for infection prevention and control in hospitals in conflict-affected settings: A qualitative study. *BMC, 15*(1), 1–9.

Medscape. (2001). *Preventing Infections in Healthcare Settings.* Retrieved from: http://www.medscape.com/govmt/CDC/EID/2001/v07.n02/e0702.14.nich/e0702.14.nich-01.html (accessed on 14 March 2025).

Nichols, R. L. (2001). Preventing surgical site infections: A surgeon's perspective. *Emerging Infectious Diseases, 7*(2).

Rendeki, S., Nagy, B., Bene, M., Pentek, A., Toth, L., Szanto, Z., Told, R., & Maroti, P. (2020). An overview on personal protective equipment (PPE) fabricated with additive manufacturing technologies in the era of the COVID-19 pandemic. *Polymers, 11*, 1–18.

Wenzel, R. P. (1997). *Prevention and Control of Nosocomial Infections.* Williams & Wilkins.

Williams, J. D., Sharma, K. B., Lolekha, S., Unahalekhaka, A., Atukorala, S. D., Kelkar, R., Sharma, A., Wattanasri, S., & Bhatia, R. (2002). *Guidelines on Prevention and Control of Hospital-Associated Infections.*, 1–13.

World Health Organization. (1993). *Guidelines for Drinking Water Quality* (Vol. 2, Issue 1). WHO.

World Health Organization. (1996). *Guidelines for Preventing HIV, HBV, and Other Infections in the Healthcare Setting.* WHO Regional Office for South-East Asia.

CHAPTER 12

Strategies for Prevention and Control of Infection for Health and Well-Being

VANDANA SINGH,[1,*] VAISHALI KUMAR,[2] HARSH SABLE,[2] ANKUSH VERMA,[3] and AMIT PRATAP SINGH CHOUHAN[3]

[1]*Department of Microbiology, Sharda School of Allied Health Sciences, Sharda University, Greater Noida, Uttar Pradesh, India*

[2]*Department of Forensic Science, Sharda School of Allied Health Sciences, Sharda University, Greater Noida, Uttar Pradesh, India*

[3]*Department of Radiology, School of Allied Health Sciences, Galgotias University, Greater Noida, Uttar Pradesh, India*

*Corresponding author

ABSTRACT

Infections arise as a result of the infiltration and rapid multiplication of microorganisms within a vulnerable host, including bacteria, fungi, viruses, and parasites. Infection prevention and control (IPC) encompass the protocols implemented to minimize the potential transmission of causative agents from one individual to another. These measures generally include hand hygiene (HH) practices, health education initiatives, utilization of personal protective equipment, implementation of cleaning and hygiene protocols, sterilization, and disinfection procedures, and adherence to vaccination protocols. Moreover, infection prevention and control (IPC) is a pivotal component of healthcare that seeks to impede the transmission or acquisition of communicable diseases in healthcare environments. This chapter mainly emphasizes a comprehensive examination of Infection Prevention and Control (IPC), encompassing its historical

Allied Healthcare in Practice: An Introduction to Integrated Patient Care. Sally Lukose, Karuna Singh (Eds.)

DOI: 10.1201/9781998511037-14

context, the significance of IPC, the transmission dynamics, the role of healthcare personnel in IPC, the components of precautionary programs, approaches for IPC, surveillance and management of outbreaks, implementation/assessment, and prospective advancements in the field of IPC. Furthermore, through the provision of a comprehensive elucidation of IPC, this chapter also furnishes healthcare professionals and policymakers with the requisite understanding and resources to execute efficacious IPC methodologies, thereby mitigating the prevalence of infectious diseases within healthcare environments.

12.1 INTRODUCTION

Throughout human history, infections have posed a serious threat to public health. A wide variety of infectious agents, including viruses, parasites, fungi, and bacterial strains, can cause them. It is possible for these pathogens to penetrate and multiply within the host, causing a range of symptoms as well as serious problems, or sometimes fatal outcomes. These pathogens use specific adhesion molecules to attach to the host cells in order to begin an infection, which facilitates their invasion and subsequent multiplication within the host cells. In order to successfully eliminate these invasive pathogens, the host's immune system responds to infections by enlisting the help of a variety of defensive mechanisms, such as phagocytes, the complement system, and antibody production, and so forth. However, some pathogens have developed resistance mechanisms to evade or compromise the host's immune system, which allows them to survive and multiply inside the host organism and also develop resistance to antibiotics. Fever, discomfort, swelling, rashes, and other similar manifestations are commonly observed symptoms of an inflammatory response, which represents the immune system's reaction in the host organism to an infection. Chronic infections have the potential to lead to sepsis, a potentially fatal condition characterized by significant organ and tissue injury (Fauci, 2001). Over the past few years, the emergence of infectious diseases like Ebola, Zika, and COVID-19 has brought attention to the persistent danger presented by infectious diseases and the necessity for efficient IPC strategies.

Infection Prevention and Control (IPC) is critical in reducing the spread of harmful microbiomes in healthcare settings with a high risk of transmission. By limiting the spread of infectious agents, IPC aims to effectively manage and attenuate diseases, along with the associated sickness and mortality. This is achieved by exploiting a thorough approach that concentrates on the infection's source, its mode of transmission, and its susceptible host. The sources of the infection could be endogenous (self-flora) or exogenous (animal, human, bird, or elements of the surrounding environment). Several strategies are available to prevent infections at their source level, which include vaccination, screening for infectious diseases, and treating infected patients. Additionally, vaccination is one of the most effective ways to stop the spread of infectious diseases because it makes the immune system work and produce protective antibodies that attack specific microbes to provide immunity. In contrast, the process of screening for infectious diseases, such as hepatitis, AIDS, tuberculosis (TB), and others, serves the purpose of detecting people who have acquired these diseases and necessitate prompt medical intervention (Kim et al., 2021). The simultaneous reduction of infection transmission can be accomplished by implementing efficacious measures among those who are afflicted. The processes through which pathogens are disseminated from one individual or location to another are commonly known as the mode of transmission. Direct contact, droplet transmission, airborne transmission, and vector-borne transmission are among the different types of transmission. In order to reduce the spread of infections through these channels, measures like wearing personal protective equipment (PPE), practicing strict hand hygiene (HH), and following extensive cleaning and disinfection procedures must be put into place. A "susceptible host" is a person who is exceptionally vulnerable to acquiring an infection. Several measures are used to reduce the risk of infections in people who are susceptible to them. These include vaccination, screening for underlying medical disorders, and the use of both standard and transmission-based precautions. Regardless of whether a patient has a confirmed infection or only a suspicion, standard precautions are a set of infection control practices that are applied consistently to all patients. Transmission-based precautions are extra procedures taken for patients who have confirmed or suspected infections that require extra control measures over and beyond standard precautions (Harun et al., 2022).

IPC techniques should be diversified, empirically supported, and informed by international and national standards and recommendations. The implementation of efficient IPC programs has been shown to have an additive impact on monitoring and reducing nosocomial disease, enhancing outcomes for patients, and also reducing healthcare delivery expenses. Therefore, it is imperative to consistently monitor and assess IPC measures in order to ascertain their effectiveness and mitigate the impact of healthcare-associated infections (HCAIs) and antibiotic resistance (Vandijck et al., 2012). This chapter mainly emphasizes the thorough analysis of the pivotal role played by IPC in reducing the transmission of infectious agents and the infections they may cause. This comprehensive guide encompasses the fundamental components, strategies, techniques for surveillance, and management of epidemics linked to IPC. Furthermore, it also explains the significance of ongoing monitoring and evaluation of IPC programs and explores potential future advancements in the same. Ultimately, the chapter highlights the significance of implementing efficient IPC strategies to diminish the occurrence of HCAIs, enhance patient outcomes, and optimize healthcare expenses.

12.2 TRANSMISSION OF INFECTIONS

The transmission of infections is a multifaceted phenomenon that encompasses various elements, including the infectious agent, the host, and the surrounding environment. A comprehensive understanding of the various modes of transmission is imperative for the formulation and implementation of effective IPC strategies (Daschner, 1985). Listed below are some additional elaborations concerning the transmission of infections:

12.2.1 DIRECT CONTACT TRANSMISSION

This mode of transmission entails the physical interaction between an infected host and a susceptible host. This phenomenon can manifest via direct dermal interaction or through the exchange of biological fluids, including but not limited to blood, saliva, or semen. Sexually transmitted infections (STIs), hepatitis B and C, and Methicillin-resistant *Staphylococcus aureus* (MRSA) infections are all examples of infections that can be spread through direct contact.

12.2.2 INDIRECT CONTACT TRANSMISSION

This mode of transmission is observed when a susceptible host encounters an infected object or surface that has been touched or handled by an infected individual. Frequently encountered instances of objects and surfaces that are susceptible to contamination include doorknobs, keyboards, and cell phones. Infections that can be transmitted via indirect contact encompass pathogens such as *Clostridium difficile* (*C. diff*), norovirus, and respiratory viruses, including influenza.

12.2.3 DROPLET TRANSMISSION

This mode of transmission is characterized by the release of respiratory droplets that contain infectious agents. These droplets subsequently come into contact with the mucous membranes of a susceptible individual, specifically targeting the eyes, nose, or mouth. This mode of transmission commonly occurs when an infected individual expels respiratory droplets through coughing, sneezing, or speaking. Instances of infectious diseases that can be transmitted via droplets include COVID-19, influenza, and pertussis.

12.2.4 AIRBORNE TRANSMISSION

This mode of transmission is observed when pathogenic microorganisms are found in minuscule droplets that persist as aerosols in the surrounding environment for an extended duration and are subsequently inhaled by a susceptible individual. This particular mode of transmission commonly takes place within enclosed environments characterized by inadequate air circulation. Instances include airborne pathogens such as *Mycobacterium tuberculosis*, influenza viruses, measles virus, H1N1 influenza virus (swine flu), and varicella-zoster virus (chickenpox).

12.2.5 VECTOR-BORNE TRANSMISSION

This refers to the process by which pathogens are transmitted from one organism to another through the intermediary of a vector. This mode of transmission is observed when a pathogenic organism is transmitted through a vector, such as mosquitoes, ticks, or fleas. The vector obtains the pathogenic organism from an infected host and subsequently transfers it to a host that is susceptible to infection. Examples of vector-borne infections include malaria, Lyme disease, and Zika virus.

In order to optimize IPC, it is crucial to customize strategies based on the distinct mode of transmission associated with each infection. These approaches involve implementing interventions such as strict adherence to protocols for HH, meticulous practices for sanitizing the surroundings, the adoption of respiratory etiquette, and the utilization of safety gear. It is imperative to consider that certain infections possess the capacity to be transmitted via diverse modalities, thereby necessitating the integration of preventive measures to effectively control the spread of infection (Devrim and Bayram, 2020; Khubrani et al., 2018).

12.3 HISTORICAL PERSPECTIVE OF IPC

The historical roots of IPC can be traced back to ancient civilizations, where the recognition of the importance of cleanliness and hygiene for reducing the spread or transmission of infectious diseases/pathogens was acknowledged. In the late 19th century, the area of germ theory of illnesses made significant strides that led to the formalization of IPC as a scientific subject. The widely regarded French chemist Louis Pasteur proposed the germ theory of disease in 1861. According to this novel viewpoint, microbes are responsible for infectious diseases. One of the most important developments in the history of IPC was the germ theory of illness, which stressed the critical need to control the spread of infectious diseases and offered a solid scientific basis for understanding their genesis. Preventive interventions were based more on empiricism and folk wisdom than on scientific reasoning prior to this paradigm-shifting development, as the agents responsible for infectious diseases were mostly unknown. With the development of his germ hypothesis, Louis Pasteur clarified that infectious diseases began and spread because of dangerous microorganisms like bacteria and viruses. Following a number of groundbreaking investigations and observations, Pasteur and his colleagues provided evidence for this theory. A modern understanding of infection control and transmission is largely owed to his work. Based on this, the germ theory of illness highlighted how important it is to have strict controls in place to stop the spread of microorganisms that might cause deadly infections. Because evidence-based tactics focused on preventing and controlling infections at their microbiological roots replaced anecdotal practices, this discovery radically changed the way that IPC was approached. Furthermore, it produced vaccinations, antimicrobial drugs, and infection control procedures that are still essential for preserving human health today. These advancements in the domains of microbiology, immunology, and public health were made possible by the foundation it laid. Similarly, in the year 1882, the bacterial strain responsible for causing TB was effectively isolated by German physician Robert Koch, who also presented evidence of its transmission from infected animals to humans. The scientific investigation carried out by Koch regarding TB and other contagious illnesses also established the fundamental groundwork for the progression of modern IPC strategies, which include the application of specific isolation protocols, sterilization procedures, and disinfection methodologies and prevention approaches (Birgand et al., 2022).

During the initial decades of the 20th century, there was a swift advancement in IPC methodologies, propelled by the advent of innovative tools such as sterilization, disinfection, vaccines, and so forth. The discovery of antibiotics in the 1940s led to a profound revolution in the treatment of infectious and most acute/chronic diseases, while simultaneously leading to the emergence and spread of antibiotic-resistant microbial strains. In the latter half of the 20th century, there was a notable transition within the domain of IPC. This shift involved a change in focus from the treatment of particular diseases/causative agents to placing greater emphasis on prevention, specifically from HCAIs. The successful execution of policies and evidence-based guidelines, encompassing protocols for the prevention of HAIs such as HH, proper disposal of waste, PPE kits, and so forth., has led to significant reductions in the incidence of these infections. Presently, the domain of IPC is experiencing many ongoing advancements to tackle emerging challenges, such as the emergence of novel infectious diseases, the escalating issue of antimicrobial resistance (AMR), and the potential peril of bioterrorism (Meng et al., 2019). The progression of innovative technologies, such as accelerated diagnostic tests and electronic surveillance systems, is enhancing the effectiveness of IPC measures. The ongoing progression of IPC strategies is crucial to ensure the safety and protection of individuals, patients, healthcare personnel, the environment, and the community (Birgand et al., 2022; Hillier, 2020).

12.4 THE IMPORTANCE OF IPC

Infection prevention and control (IPC) is critical in healthcare settings because it protects patients, healthcare personnel, and the general community from the spread of infectious illnesses. IPC techniques are conducted with the goal of preventing pathogen transmission or dissemination within healthcare settings, hence reducing the occurrence of HAIs. The impact of HAIs on patient outcomes and the financial burden on healthcare expenses demonstrates the need for IPC (IPC). Hospital-acquired infections (HAIs) are a significant cause of illness and mortality on a global scale, with roughly 1.7 million HAIs occurring in the United States alone each year (Septimus and Moody, 2016). These infections have been observed to exhibit a positive linear relationship with extended durations of hospitalization, elevated rates of re-hospitalization, and augmented healthcare expenditures, thereby imposing a substantial burden on healthcare systems. In the realm of emerging infectious diseases, such as the ongoing COVID-19 pandemic, the execution of IPC measures holds significant importance. IPC strategies, encompassing protocols such as meticulous HH, respiratory etiquette, and thorough environmental sanitation, have played a pivotal role in proficiently mitigating the transmission of COVID-19 within healthcare establishments and the broader populace (Alharbi et al., 2019). The importance of IPC is further exemplified by the emergence of antibiotic-resistant infections. AMR presents a worldwide health threat due to its ability to reduce the efficacy of various current antibiotics. The successful execution of effective IPC strategies holds promise in reducing the incidence of AMR infections, thereby preserving the efficacy of existing antimicrobial agents. Hence, it is crucial to incorporate effective IPC strategies within the context of emerging infectious diseases and AMR (Murhekar et al., 2009).

12.5 ELEMENTS OF INFECTION PREVENTION AND CONTROL

Infection prevention and control programs exhibit complexity and a multifaceted nature, necessitating the implementation of diverse components to accomplish their objectives (Popovich et al., 2019). The following are some supplementary particulars regarding each component of IPC programs.

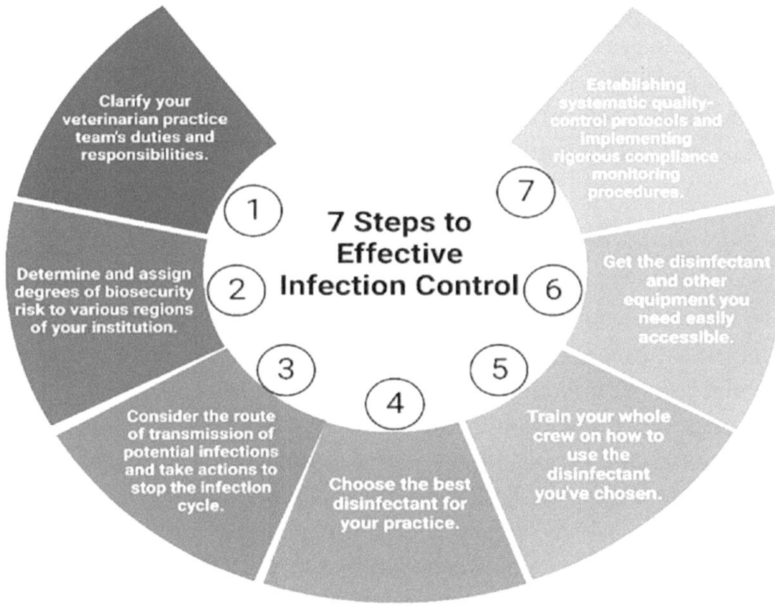

FIGURE 12.1 The key components of infection prevention and control (IPC), highlighting a systematic approach to safeguarding health and well-being by adhering seven effective steps.

12.5.1 EDUCATION AND TRAINING

Continuous education and training are imperative, and it is essential for all healthcare professionals to receive regular updates on optimal methodologies and novel investigations pertaining to IPC. Education should be customized based on the distinct roles and responsibilities of individual healthcare practitioners, and it should be delivered through a diverse range of formats, such as didactic lectures, interactive workshops, and online e-learning modules. Education should be facilitated by the implementation of monitoring and feedback mechanisms to ascertain the extent to which healthcare professionals are effectively applying the knowledge and skills acquired through their educational endeavors.

12.5.2 EPIDEMIOLOGICAL MONITORING

Epidemiological monitoring should encompass a comprehensive approach that incorporates all pertinent data sources, including laboratory findings, patient health records, and records of infection control measures. Regular analysis of surveillance data is essential for the identification of trends, patterns, and potential areas of enhancement. The design of surveillance systems should prioritize the prompt detection of outbreaks of infectious diseases and enable a timely response.

12.5.3 RISK ASSESSMENT AND MANAGEMENT

It is imperative to conduct regular and rigorous risk assessments and management procedures in order to systematically identify and mitigate potential risks of infection transmission. These protocols ought to include a thorough comprehension of the pathophysiology of infectious diseases as well as a careful examination of the various variables affecting the spread of those diseases. Risk assessment ought to investigate the complex mechanisms by which infectious organisms spread and take into account the dynamic interactions between variables that affect their transmission in the healthcare setting. Using empirical data and rigorous science is essential for developing risk mitigation plans. To provide the most efficient and specialized strategy to risk reduction and elimination, these tactics should be modified to account for the unique quirks and peculiarities present in healthcare settings.

12.5.4 STANDARD AND TRANSMISSION-BASED PRECAUTIONS

Standard precautions should be maintained and applied consistently throughout the procedure with all patients, regardless of their prognosis or anticipated health condition. These precautions usually include practices like HH, using PPE kits, following safe injection protocols, wearing masks for respiratory hygiene, and properly handling or disposing of sharps and other hazardous materials, such as needles and syringes. On the other hand, transmission-based precautions should be used when normal precautions alone are insufficient to prevent the spread of infectious pathogens. The exact mechanism by which infectious agents are transferred, such as contact, droplet, or airborne pathways, determines transmission-based measures. To reduce the risk of infection transmission, these precautions demand the use of additional PPE and the deployment of biological controls.

12.5.5 ENVIRONMENTAL DECONTAMINATION AND DISINFECTION

It is imperative to engage in routine environmental decontamination and disinfection protocols in order to effectively mitigate the potential transmission of pathogenic microorganisms. The process of cleaning should be executed utilizing suitable apparatus and cleaning substances while adhering to guidelines that are grounded in empirical evidence. Disinfection should be conducted utilizing suitable disinfectants that demonstrate efficacy against the particular pathogens under consideration.

12.5.6 ANTIMICROBIAL STEWARDSHIP

These programs need to be put in place to ensure that antibiotics and other antimicrobial agents are used correctly. The proposed programs ought to incorporate comprehensive protocols for the administration of antibiotics, systematic tracking of antibiotic utilization, and provision of informative assessments to healthcare providers. Antimicrobial stewardship programs have been shown to effectively decrease the occurrence of HAIs and mitigate the emergence of AMR (Haque et al., 2018).

12.5.7 IMPLEMENTATION OF OUTBREAK MANAGEMENT

It is imperative to establish outbreak management protocols to facilitate a prompt and efficient response to instances of infectious disease outbreaks. The management protocols for outbreaks should encompass systematic procedures for conducting investigations, implementing patient isolation measures, conducting contact tracing activities, and facilitating effective communication with public health authorities (Dexter et al., 2020).

12.6 STRATEGIES FOR PREVENTING AND CONTROLLING INFECTIONS

In healthcare settings, there are numerous ways for infection control and prevention. The subsequent strategies delineate the most efficacious methodologies through which healthcare facilities can proficiently avert and manage the dissemination of infectious diseases, thereby safeguarding the well-being of healthcare personnel and patients alike (Cheng et al., 2020; Goldmann et al., 1996).

12.6.1 HAND HYGIENE

Hand hygiene is an essential element of IPC protocols. It represents the most effective approach for reducing the transmission of infections and pathogenic microorganisms. HH should be performed before and after coming into contact with patients, after removing gloves, and after engaging in any activity that could lead to contamination. HH can be accomplished by employing different disinfecting agents, consisting of both soap-based products and alcohol-based hand rubs. Based on empirical evidence, the World Health Organization (WHO) has officially supported the use of alcohol-based hand rubs because of their higher effectiveness in comparison to soap, along with their decreased likelihood of causing harm to the skin. Furthermore, complying with established HH procedures has been scientifically proven to significantly reduce the occurrence of HAIs (Allegranzi and Pittet, 2009; Suetens et al., 2018).

12.6.2 PERSONAL PROTECTIVE EQUIPMENT (PPE)

Personal protective equipment (PPE) is primarily engineered to provide an additional layer of protection for healthcare professionals, effectively mitigating the risk of being exposed to pathogenic substances and subsequent infections. PPE comprises a range of articles, for example, gloves, clothing, masks, and eye protection. Healthcare professionals are recommended to employ appropriate PPE based on the specific circumstances related to patient care. In the realm of patient monitoring, it is advised to utilize gloves and an apron as a method for implementing contact precautions. Moreover, the utilization of masks functions as a preventive strategy to mitigate the spread of infectious agents present in droplets or suspended in the air. The proper utilization of PPE has the potential to effectively impede the transmission of infectious agents, both from patients to healthcare workers and vice versa.

12.6.3 SAFE INJECTION PRACTICE

Unsafe injection practices have the potential to facilitate the spread or transmission of pathogenic agents, such as hepatitis viruses, HIV, and so forth. Adherence to safe injection practices is imperative in order to mitigate the potential transmission of infectious agents via contaminated needles, syringes, and related apparatus. These practices encompass the utilization of aseptic technique, employing sterile equipment for every patient, and refraining from the reuse of syringes and needles. Healthcare professionals must adhere to protocols regarding the appropriate disposal and safe management of sharps and other injection waste that may be contaminated (Jones et al., 2020).

12.6.4 RESPIRATORY HYGIENE AND COUGH ETIQUETTE

Droplets produced by coughing or sneezing can spread respiratory illnesses including the flu, TB, pneumonia, and so forth. In order to mitigate the spread of respiratory infections, it is imperative for both patients and healthcare workers to adhere to respiratory hygiene and cough etiquette protocols. It is recommended that individuals cover their mouth and nose during episodes of coughing or sneezing, and that they dispose of used tissues in a suitable manner. It is recommended that healthcare workers utilize facial masks while monitoring and providing care to patients with respiratory infections (Lu et al., 2020).

12.6.5 THE PROPER MANAGEMENT AND DISPOSAL OF SHARPS AND OTHER INFECTIOUS WASTE

Sharps, including needles and scalpels, possess the potential to inflict harm upon healthcare personnel and facilitate the transmission of infectious pathogens. In order to mitigate the transmission of infectious agents, it is imperative to adopt appropriate handling and disposal procedures for infectious waste, including but not limited to utilized dressings and contaminated linens. Sharp objects should be appropriately discarded in containers that are resistant to punctures and disposed of in accordance with established protocols (Suetens et al., 2018).

12.6.6 ENVIRONMENTAL CLEANING AND DISINFECTION

Environmental cleaning and disinfection should be undertaken on a regular basis to limit the risk of illness and infectious agent transmission.

The process of cleaning should be executed utilizing suitable apparatus and cleaning agents while adhering to guidelines that are grounded in empirical evidence. Disinfection should be conducted utilizing suitable disinfectants that have demonstrated efficacy against the particular pathogens of interest (Doll et al., 2018).

12.6.7 ANTIMICROBIAL STEWARDSHIP

Antimicrobial stewardship programs are designed to promote the judicious utilization of antibiotics and other antimicrobial agents. The aforementioned programs ought to incorporate protocols pertaining to the administration of antibiotics, surveillance of antibiotic utilization, and provision of feedback to prescribers. Antimicrobial stewardship programs have been shown to effectively decrease the occurrence of HAIs and mitigate the emergence of AMR.

12.6.8 INFECTION SCREENING AND ISOLATION

It is recommended that patients undergo infection screening upon their admission to healthcare facilities, and appropriate measures should be taken to implement isolation precautions in order to mitigate the transmission of infectious agents. The selection of precautionary measures should be determined by the specific mode of transmission and the implementation of environmental controls (Organization, 2020).

12.6.9 IMMUNIZATION

Immunization is a highly efficacious approach for mitigating the spread and etiology of pathogens, particularly within healthcare environments. It is recommended that healthcare workers receive vaccinations against various infectious pathogens, including but not limited to influenza, hepatitis B, and measles, mumps, and rubella. The administration of vaccines has well-demonstrated efficacy in mitigating the transmission of pathogenic organisms or agents, particularly within populations that have elevated risk, such as individuals experiencing prolonged medication, highly sophisticated surgeries, immunosuppressant medication, malnutrition, or pre-existing immunocompromised states, and so forth (Dinleyici et al., 2021; Dooling et al., 2021).

12.6.10 EDUCATION AND TRAINING

It is a necessity for medical staff and associates to have intense, ongoing education and training in order to effectively stop the spread of infectious diseases in medical facilities. The pedagogical process holds significant importance and encompasses a diverse and multidimensional curriculum. The subject matter pertains to a thorough education on a range of protocols for preventing and controlling infections. This education begins with a detailed analysis of practices related to HH. It also includes precise guidance on correctly putting on and taking off PPE kits, which consist of gowns, gloves, masks, and eye protection. The importance of employing safe and aseptic methods for administering injections is highlighted, in addition to strictly adhering to the use of masks, practicing respiratory hygiene, and following proper cough/sneeze etiquette in order to minimize the transmission of respiratory pathogens. Moreover, healthcare professionals should undergo extensive training in the complexities of environmental sanitation protocols, personal hygiene upkeep, and effective disinfection methodologies. This comprehensive approach guarantees that healthcare professionals possess the necessary knowledge and abilities required for the efficient detection and control of infectious diseases in their medical settings (Kim et al., 2021).

12.6.11 EPIDEMIOLOGICAL SURVEILLANCE

Epidemiological surveillance is a crucial element in the systematic observation and scientific examination of the occurrence, frequency, and geographical distribution of infectious diseases. This aids in the prompt identification of outbreaks. The establishment of resilient surveillance systems is of utmost significance, especially when it comes to monitoring nosocomial or HAIs, tracking patterns of antibiotic resistance, and observing the emergence of new infectious diseases. The appropriate use of surveillance data acquires essential importance since it allows the identification of specific areas that require focused improvement initiatives within healthcare settings and supports evidence-based IPC policies. Data-driven insights are essential in reducing the transmission of infections and improving healthcare outcomes (Emmanuel et al., 2020).

12.6.12 COMMUNICATION

The implementation of efficient communication strategies plays a pivotal role in mitigating the transmission of pathogens or infectious diseases within healthcare settings. It is imperative to disseminate information regarding IPC practices to patients, healthcare workers, visitors, and all individuals associated with the healthcare sector. Furthermore, it is crucial to promote adherence to these practices among these individuals. Effective communication among healthcare workers is essential for maintaining consistent and efficient IPC practices (Ku et al., 2018) (Figure 12.1).

12.7 SURVEILLANCE AND OUTBREAK MANAGEMENT

Surveillance and outbreak management are integral facets of public health practice, particularly in the context of infectious disease outbreaks. Surveillance pertains to the ongoing gathering, examination, and interpretation of health data for the purpose of monitoring and identifying alterations in the occurrence, frequency, and spread of diseases. On the contrary, outbreak management encompasses the expeditious examination, regulation, and prophylaxis of disease outbreaks with the aim of mitigating their repercussions on the well-being of the general population (Van Seventer and Hochberg, 2017).

Surveillance systems can be categorized as either passive or active, based on the type of data being collected. Passive surveillance encompasses the systematic documentation of disease occurrences by healthcare providers, laboratories, or other relevant entities. On the other hand, active surveillance entails the deliberate and proactive identification of instances of a specific disease through focused surveys or investigations. Both forms of surveillance play a crucial role in the identification and response to outbreaks of infectious diseases (Ameli, 2015).

Surveillance systems can be categorized into two types: syndromic and specific. Syndromic surveillance entails the systematic observation of nonspecific clinical manifestations or ailments that could potentially signify the occurrence of an epidemic, whereas specific surveillance concentrates on the identification of particular pathogens or diseases. Syndromic surveillance has the capability to offer timely detection of an epidemic, while specific surveillance can validate the existence of a specific pathogen and direct focused control strategies (Choi et al., 2021; Karampatakis et al., 2018).

The outbreak's control strategy usually starts with the recognition of an impending crisis through the utilization of surveillance methods or medical suspicion. When there is a suspicion of an outbreak, it is recommended that the facility initiates an investigation to determine the cause and extent of the outbreak. Examining infection control procedures, conducting patient and staff interviews, and conducting laboratory experiments are all possible components of this investigation. Once the cause and scale of the epidemic have been determined, it is recommended that the governing body implement measures to hinder the further spread of the disease (Arun et al., 2019; Murhekar et al., 2009). These preventive measures can encompass enhanced sanitation and cleaning protocols, implementation of isolation precautions, meticulous contact tracing efforts, and the utilization of PPE kits. Outbreak management generally encompasses the subsequent stages:

1. **Scientific Investigation:** The outbreak is subjected to rigorous investigation in order to ascertain the etiology, infectious agent(s), transmission dynamics, and impacted population. This may entail conducting experiments in controlled laboratory settings, conducting large-scale studies/research to analyze patterns of disease and its transmission, and identifying and tracking individuals or patients who have come into contact with infected ones.

2. **Control Measures:** Once the origin of the outbreak has been identified, control measures are applied to stop the disease from spreading further. This may involve the implementation of strategies/measures such as the segregation of affected patients, the confinement of those who have been exposed, and the decontamination of specific areas that have been contaminated.

3. **Treatment:** Affected people are administered suitable treatment and receive proper care in response to the outbreak, which may necessitate the administration of pharmaceuticals, medical facilities, and the implementation of various medical protocols.
4. **Evaluation:** Once the outbreak has been tamed, an evaluation needs to be carried out to determine the success and also to recommend areas for improvement.

Efficient monitoring and outbreak control are imperative for the prevention and management of infectious disease outbreaks. The utilization of surveillance data enables the identification of patterns and shifts in the occurrence and prevalence of diseases, thereby informing the decision-making process and allocation of resources in the field of public health. The implementation of outbreak management strategies can effectively restrict the spread of outbreaks prior to their extensive dissemination, thereby mitigating their adverse consequences on the well-being of the general population (Madigan et al., 2018).

12.8 IMPLEMENTATION AND EVALUATION OF IPC PROGRAMS

The implementation and evaluation of IPC programs play an essential role in the surveillance and management of HAIs. These programs utilize a synergistic integration of engineering controls, administrative controls, and educational measures to guarantee adherence to optimal procedures and uphold the preservation of patient safety. The numerical value provided by the user is 20. The successful execution of IPC programs necessitates a methodical methodology that encompasses the subsequent stages:

1. **Assess the Current IPC Practices:** The first phase of executing effective IPC programs is to evaluate the existing IPC protocols within the medical setups. This may entail a comprehensive examination of established protocols, SOPs, and methodologies, meticulous monitoring of medical personnel conduct, and discernment of specific domains necessitating enhancement.
2. **Develop Policies and Procedures:** Policies and Standard Operating Procedures (SOPs) ought to be formulated in accordance with evidence-based principles in order to guarantee adherence to

optimal procedures. The policies and procedures should encompass all facets of IPC, such as HH, quarantine precautions, sanitization, and disinfection, and utilization of personal protective kits.

3. **Educate Healthcare Professionals:** Healthcare professionals should be educated and trained well on all policies and procedures developed for the effective IPCs of the healthcare setting. Continuous education is imperative to ensure that healthcare professionals remain cognizant of evolving policies, procedures, SOPs, and advancements related to IPC.
4. **Deploy Engineering Controls:** It is always recommended to deploy engineering controls, such as air-filtration systems and negative pressure rooms, in order to mitigate the potential spread or transmission of aerosols (airborne infections). These controls may also include the application of UV-based germicidal irradiation and other advanced sterilization technologies to mitigate potential contaminants.
5. **Execute Administrative Controls:** The implementation of administrative controls, such as the screening of infected patients, their attendants, and visitors, and the enforcement of isolation precautions, is recommended to effectively mitigate the risk of infection transmission. These controls may also encompass standard operating procedures for the management of outbreaks and the prompt response to emerging infectious agents along with diseases.
6. **Conduct Surveillance and Assessment of the Program:** In order to ascertain the efficacy of IPC programs in managing infections from spreading, it is imperative to consistently monitor and evaluate their performance. This may entail the implementation of regular surveillance programs to monitor the incidence rates of HAIs and adherence to the policies/procedures. Additionally, regular audits and surveys may be conducted to evaluate the level of current knowledge and attitudes of medical staff/workers towards effective IPC.

Evaluation of IPC programs is necessary to determine the program's effectiveness in limiting the transmission or spread of diseases and infectious agents in hospitals (Magill et al., 2018; Murhekar et al., 2009; Organization, 2020). The following procedures can be undertaken to assess the effectiveness of IPC programs:

1. **Determine Evaluation Metrics:** It is imperative to identify appropriate evaluation metrics in order to determine the efficacy of the IPC program developed or implemented in the hospital or healthcare settings. These metrics may encompass the frequency of nosocomial infections, adherence to precautionary and isolation protocols, and also include the level of healthcare personnel's understanding of the current protocols of IPC procedures.
2. **Data Acquisition:** It is imperative to collect data pertaining to the designated evaluation metrics. This data can be acquired from the systematic and regular surveillance of programs, rigorous audits, and comprehensive surveys. Consistent data collection and its statistical analysis over time is crucial for monitoring pattern and evaluation of the effective interventions.
3. **Conduct Data Analysis:** The collected data should be subjected to rigorous statistical analysis in order to ascertain the effectiveness of the followed IPC program in mitigating the transmission of infection and infectious agents in hospital or healthcare settings. Statistical analysis serves as a valuable tool for detecting and characterizing trends and patterns of infection control while also enabling the evaluation of the effects of targeted interventions.
4. **Implementation of Changes:** Based on the findings of the statistical data analysis, it is advisable to make modifications to the followed IPC program in order to improve its effectiveness in reducing the transmission of infectious agents along with infections. This may require alterations in the policies and protocols, the provision of additional or current education and training to healthcare personnel, or the implementation of innovative engineering or administrative strategies, among other things.
5. **Monitor and Evaluate the Program:** The IPC program necessitates ongoing monitoring and analysis to ascertain its sustained efficacy in combating the transmission of pathogenic microbes and the infections they cause, which may include continuing monitoring programs, timely audits, and surveys to assess compliance and identify areas for improvement.

12.9 PRECAUTIONS

12.9.1 STANDARD PRECAUTIONS

1. **Hand Hygiene:** Hand hygiene is one of the most essential components of standard precautions, which aims to prevent the spread of pathogenic agents and the infections they may cause. It involves the thorough removal of microbes from the hands to reduce the likelihood of transmitting infections. The recommended protocol entails the utilization of disinfectant (soap) and running water to cleanse the hands for a minimum duration of 20 seconds. This should be followed by a comprehensive rinsing process and subsequent drying using either a hygienic, disposable towel or an air dryer. Alcohol-based hand sanitizers containing a minimum of 60% alcohol are viable substitutes in situations where hands do not exhibit visible dirt or grime. Consistent adherence to HH protocols is essential, encompassing the practice of cleansing hands both before and after every interaction with patients, after the removal of gloves, and following any instances of contact with surfaces or equipment that may be contaminated. Strict adherence to established HH protocols is crucial in mitigating the occurrence of HCAIs (Zivich et al., 2018).
2. **Personal Protective Equipment** (PPE): PPE is a fundamental component of Standard Precautions, encompassing a range of protective barriers. Gloves, commonly composed of latex, nitrile, or alternative substances, are utilized as a protective barrier against direct exposure to blood, bodily fluids, mucous membranes, and compromised skin. Gowns, typically composed of impermeable fabric, function as a barrier to safeguard the attire and dermal layers of healthcare professionals against potential contamination. Masks and ocular protection, such as goggles or face shields, are employed in situations where there exists a possibility of encountering splashes, sprays, or aerosolized particles containing infectious agents. The precise methodology for donning and doffing PPE is of utmost importance in order to minimize the potential for self-contamination. It is imperative to strictly adhere to established guidelines in this regard (Khubrani et al., 2018).

3. **Respiratory Hygiene/Cough Etiquette:** Respiratory hygiene and cough etiquette are essential elements of Standard Precautions aimed at reducing the transmission of respiratory infections. It is imperative for both patients and healthcare workers to adhere to respiratory hygiene protocols, which involve the act of covering the mouth and nose during episodes of coughing or sneezing. Ideally, the recommended practice entails utilizing a tissue for the purpose of capturing respiratory droplets. In the event that a tissue is not readily available, an alternative approach involves directing coughing or sneezing towards the inner region of the elbow. To mitigate the potential transmission of infectious respiratory secretions, it is imperative to promptly dispose of used tissues in specifically designated waste receptacles (Huijghebaert et al., 2021).
4. **Safe Injection Practices:** Ensuring the implementation of proper injection protocols is of utmost importance in mitigating the spread of infections within healthcare environments. The strict observance of aseptic techniques is imperative in the process of preparing and administering injections. It is recommended to utilize single-use needles and syringes for every patient and properly dispose of them in puncture-resistant containers after use. It is advisable to refrain from reusing needles in order to minimize the potential for inadvertent needle stick injuries, which may result in exposure to blood-borne pathogens (Dooling et al., 2021).
5. **Environmental Cleaning:** Regular and thorough environmental cleaning and disinfection are essential components of Standard Precautions. This involves the regular cleaning and disinfection of areas where patient care is provided, surfaces that are frequently touched, and medical equipment. A suitable antimicrobial agent, capable of effectively targeting the specific pathogens of interest, should be employed in accordance with the instructions provided by the manufacturer to efficiently neutralize potentially infectious microorganisms (Doll et al., 2018).
6. **Waste Disposal:** The appropriate management of infectious waste, which encompasses sharps like needles and syringes, is a crucial element of Standard Precautions. Healthcare facilities are required to furnish specialized receptacles that possess the qualities of

being impervious to leakage and resistant to puncturing, in order to ensure the secure disposal of infectious waste. Strict adherence to appropriate waste disposal protocols is of utmost importance in order to mitigate the occurrence of injuries and effectively restrict the transmission of infections (Ahmed et al., 2020).

7. **Occupational Health:** Occupational health measures are essential components of Standard Precautions, which aim to prioritize the safeguarding and welfare of healthcare personnel. This entails providing immunizations for vaccine-preventable illnesses, such as hepatitis B, to personnel. In the occurrence of unintentional contact with blood-borne pathogens or infectious substances, it may be necessary to consider post-exposure prophylaxis (PEP). PEP, or Post-Exposure Prophylaxis, entails the prompt administration of suitable medications to minimize the likelihood of infection transmission. Healthcare facilities ought to implement comprehensive occupational health programs to guarantee the continual well-being and safety of their workforce (Mhango et al., 2020).

12.9.2 TRANSMISSION-BASED PRECAUTIONS

Transmission-Based Precautions encompass a collection of supplementary infection control strategies employed in healthcare environments when patients are identified or suspected to be infected or harboring particular pathogens that necessitate additional precautions beyond the baseline Standard Precautions. Transmission-Based Precautions have been developed with the purpose of inhibiting the dissemination of pathogens. These precautions can be classified into three primary types: Contact precautions, droplet precautions, and airborne precautions, as outlined in Table 12.1. Following is a comprehensive elucidation of a few components:

1. **Contact Precautions:** Contact precautions are implemented in cases where patients are identified or suspected to be infected or colonized with contagious pathogens that have the potential to be transmitted through direct or indirect contact with the patient or their surroundings. These pathogens frequently comprise multidrug-resistant organisms (MDROs) such as MRSA VRE

(Vancomycin-Resistant *Enterococcus)*, and *C. difficile*. The primary metrics for implementing Contact Precautions encompass the utilization of hand coverings and protective garments by healthcare personnel upon entering the patient's designated area. Ideally, it is recommended to allocate patients to individual rooms in order to mitigate the transmission of the pathogen. The utilization of specialized patient care equipment is recommended in order to minimize the occurrence of cross-contamination. Rigorous adherence to HH protocols prior to and following patient interaction is imperative in order to mitigate the risk of transmission. Thorough and frequent environmental cleaning and disinfection are essential elements of Contact Precautions, as these pathogens have the ability to endure on various surfaces (Table 12.1) (Turkistani, 2020).

2. **Droplet Precautions:** Droplet precautions are recommended in cases where patients are confirmed or suspected to be harboring pathogens that are transmitted via respiratory droplets, which are produced during activities such as coughing, sneezing, talking, or performing procedures like suctioning. The respiratory droplets in question are known to harbor various pathogens, including influenza viruses, *Streptococcus pneumoniae*, and *Neisseria meningitidis*. In order to mitigate the risk of respiratory droplet exposure, it is recommended that healthcare personnel who come into close proximity (within 6 feet) of the patient utilize appropriate personal protective equipment, including masks and eye protection such as face shields or goggles. Ideally, it is recommended that patients be accommodated in individualized isolation chambers, and they should utilize facial coverings when traversing beyond their designated spaces and during instances where direct proximity with others cannot be avoided. Maintaining proper HH is of utmost importance in mitigating the risk of transmission, and it is imperative for healthcare professionals to also adhere to respiratory hygiene and cough etiquette. Regular environmental cleaning is essential in order to mitigate the risk of surface contamination (Table 12.1) (Hassan, 2018).

3. **Airborne Precautions:** Airborne precautions are enacted when patients are identified or suspected to be harboring pathogens that

have the potential to be transmitted via small respiratory droplets, characterized by their size being less than 5 microns. These minuscule droplets have the ability to stay afloat in the atmosphere and can be inhaled by individuals, resulting in the heightened transmissibility of pathogens such as *Mycobacterium tuberculosis* (TB), varicella-zoster virus (chickenpox), and respiratory viruses like measles. Healthcare professionals are advised to utilize respiratory protection, such as an N95 respirator or respiratory protection of a higher level, upon entering the patient's room. Ideally, it is recommended that patients be accommodated in an airborne infection isolation room (AIIR) that maintains negative air pressure. This precautionary measure aims to effectively contain and prevent the dispersion of infectious particles into the surrounding environment. It is recommended to maintain the closed state of the door to the patient's room, and patients are advised to wear masks during necessary instances of transportation outside their rooms. HH, respiratory hygiene, and thorough environmental cleaning are fundamental elements of Airborne Precautions aimed at minimizing the potential for transmission (Wong et al., 2021).

Furthermore, it is imperative for healthcare facilities to establish precise protocols for the assessment of when and how to implement Transmission-Based Precautions, taking into account the particular pathogen, its method of transmission, and the patient's clinical state. Strict adherence to these precautions is of utmost importance in the prevention of HCAIs and the maintenance of safety for both patients and healthcare personnel.

12.10 FUTURE DIRECTIONS

The discipline of IPC is subject to continuous development as a result of the introduction of new infectious diseases and the dissemination of antibiotic-resistant microbiomes. Hence, future developments in IPC revolve around the investigation and use of innovative approaches and technology designed to reduce the spread and transmission of infectious agents and the diseases they cause inside healthcare settings. The further instructions are as follows:

TABLE 12.1 Precautions for the Prevention of Transmission of Infections

Purpose	Precaution based on		Room preference		Precaution		Measures to be taken	References
	Organism	Syndromic	Private	Negative pressure	Visitor	Staff		
Contact	*Clostridium difficile*, scabies, MRSA	Diarrhea, Infestation, Draining wound	Private	No	Gloves and PPE	Gloves and PPE	Hand should be sanitized Disinfecting contactable surfaces Enforcing PPE	Turkistani (2020)
Droplet	Streptococcus, Influenza invasive Group A, mumps, norovirus, *N. meningitidis*	Toxic shock	Private	No	Gloves, PPE, and surgical grade fluid resistant mask	Gloves, PPE, and surgical grade fluid resistant mask	The distance between one or more subjects to where the droplets can reach; distance between the beds, curtains, and so forth.	Hassan (2018)
Airborne	Measles, pulmonary tuberculosis, disseminated zoster, chicken pox	High tuberculosis risk, weight loss, fever, cough	Private	Yes	Surgical grade fluid resistant mask	Gloves, PPE, and N95 mask	The private rooms with private bathroom. Use of PAPR or N95 masks, gloves, and aprons.	Wong et al. (2021)

1. **The Utilization of Novel Technologies:** Tcchnologies such as ultraviolet-based germicidal irradiation, antimicrobial coatings, nanomaterials, and robotic devices for sterilization and disinfection are currently being explored in order to mitigate the potential transmission of infections within hospitals. These technological advancements are specifically engineered to complement current IPC strategies and also hold significant potential in mitigating the transmission of antibiotic-resistant pathogenic organisms.
2. **Emphasizing Antimicrobial Stewardship:** Antimicrobial stewardship initiatives are generally being formulated to promote the judicious utilization of antibiotics within healthcare settings or hospitals. The primary objective of these programs is to mitigate the emergence and proliferation of antibiotic-resistant microbial strains while simultaneously enhancing patient outcomes. This is achieved by implementing specific strategies that promote the judicious and appropriate utilization of antibiotics, ensuring that they are prescribed only when necessary and in the appropriate dosage.
3. **Enhancing Global Health Security:** The COVID-19 pandemic has underscored the significance of global health security and the imperative for robust IPC initiatives to mitigate the transmission of communicable diseases. Future directions in the field of infectious disease control may prioritize the enhancement of global health security by means of enhanced surveillance, preparedness, and response mechanisms to address the emergence of transmissible infectious diseases.
4. **Collaboration and Interdisciplinary Approaches:** IPC programs necessitate the establishment of collaborative efforts among healthcare professionals, public health authorities, and researchers representing diverse fields of research. Future directions in the field of IPC may prioritize the advancement of interdisciplinary methodologies and collaborative efforts aimed at formulating novel strategies to effectively hinder the transmission of pathogenic agents and infections.

5. **Emphasis on Education and Training:** Education and training play a crucial role in ensuring effective implementation and adherence to best practices in IPC. Future directions in IPC may prioritize the enhancement of education and training programs to ensure that healthcare professionals possess the necessary knowledge and skills to effectively mitigate the spread of diseases and infections.

12.11 CONCLUSION

In hospitals or healthcare settings, the implementation of effective IPC measures is crucial for the prevention and control of infectious diseases caused by pathogenic agents, such as fungi, bacteria, parasites, and viruses. The historical development of IPC, and past experiences is always significant in guiding current practices. This chapter has underlined the vital importance of IPC in protecting both healthcare professionals and patients by highlighting the many components and SOPs of IPC programs, such as infection control measures, surveillance and response frameworks, and assessment strategies, which will be essential in reducing the risk of infectious disease transmission, especially in the context of emerging infectious diseases such as COVID, Ebola, and TB, and so forth. In order to improve the timely identification and swift reaction to outbreaks of infectious diseases, it will be imperative to broaden the scope of surveillance and response frameworks. Furthermore, it is imperative to foster the advancement of a proficient healthcare workforce in order to guarantee the ability of healthcare personnel to efficiently address infectious disease outbreaks. Therefore, the implementation of effective IPC programs is of utmost importance in order to enhance patient outcomes, mitigate healthcare expenses, and bolster public health. This chapter is mainly emphasized on the information that can aid policymakers and healthcare workers in the process of designing and executing successful IPC programs that can prevent and control the spread of infectious diseases. Continued efforts in the development and implementation of novel IPC measures, the expansion of surveillance and response systems, and the support of a professional healthcare workforce will be required to ensure the long-term viability of IPC programs.

KEYWORDS

- **COVID-19**
- **disease transmission**
- **emerging infectious diseases**
- **infection prevention and control**
- **pathogenic agents**
- **standard operating procedures**
- **tuberculosis**

REFERENCES

Ahmed, M. A., Jouhar, R., Adnan, S., Ahmed, N., Ghazal, T., & Adanir, N. (2020). Evaluation of patient's knowledge, attitude, and practice of cross-infection control in dentistry during COVID-19 pandemic. *European Journal of Dentistry, 14*, S1–S6.

Alharbi, G., Shono, N., Alballaa, L., & Aloufi, A. (2019). Knowledge, attitude and compliance of infection control guidelines among dental faculty members and students in KSU. *BMC Oral Health, 19*, 1–8.

Allegranzi, B., & Pittet, D. (2009). Role of hand hygiene in healthcare-associated infection prevention. *Journal of Hospital Infection, 73*(4), 305–315. https://doi.org/9.916/j.jhin.2009.04.019.

Ameli, J. (2015). Communicable diseases and outbreak control. *Turkish Journal of Emergency Medicine, 15*(Suppl 1), 20–26. https://doi.org/9.5505/1304.7361.2015.19970.

Arunkumar, G., Chandni, R., Mourya, D. T., Singh, S. K., Sadanandan, R., Sudan, P., & Bhargava, B. (2019). Outbreak investigation of Nipah virus disease in Kerala, India, 2018. *The Journal of Infectious Diseases, 219*(11), 1867–1878.

Birgand, G., Ahmad, R., Bulabula, A. N. H., Singh, S., Bearman, G., Sánchez, E. C., & Holmes, A. (2022). Innovation for infection prevention and control—Revisiting Pasteur's vision. *The Lancet, 400*(9369), 2250–2260. https://doi.org/9.916/S0140-6736(22)02459-X.

Cheng, V. C., Wong, S. C., To, K. K., Ho, P. L., & Yuen, K. Y. (2020). Preparedness and proactive infection control measures against the emerging novel coronavirus in China. *Journal of Hospital Infection, 94*(3), 254–255.

Choi, U. Y., Kwon, Y. M., Kang, H. J., Song, J. H., Lee, H. Y., Kim, M. S., Kahm, S. H., Kwon, J. Y., Kim, S. H., Lee, S. H., Choi, J. H., & Lee, J. (2021). Surveillance of the infection prevention and control practices of healthcare workers by an infection control surveillance-working group and a team of infection control coordinators during the COVID-19 pandemic. *Journal of Infection and Public Health*, 454–460.

Daschner, F. D. (1985). The transmission of infections in hospitals by staff carriers, methods of prevention and control. *Infection Control: IC, 6*(3), 97–99. https://doi.org/9.917/s0195941700062755.

Devrim, I., & Bayram, N. (2020). Infection control practices in children during COVID-19 pandemic: Differences from adults. *American Journal of Infection Control, 48*(8), 933–939.

Dexter, F., Parra, M. C., Brown, J. R., & Loftus, R. W. (2020). Perioperative COVID-19 defense: An evidence-based approach for optimization of infection control and operating room management. *Anesthesia and Analgesia.*

Dinleyici, E. C., Borrow, R., Safadi, M. A. P., van Damme, P., & Munoz, F. M. (2021). Vaccines and routine immunization strategies during the COVID-19 pandemic. *Human Vaccines & Immunotherapeutics, 17*(2), 400–407.

Doll, M., Stevens, M., & Bearman, G. (2018). Environmental cleaning and disinfection of patient areas. *International Journal of Infectious Diseases, 67*, 52–57.

Dooling, K., Marin, M., Wallace, M., McClung, N., Chamberland, M., Lee, G. M., Talbot, H. K., Romero, J. R., Bell, B. P., & Oliver, S. E. (2021). The Advisory Committee on Immunization Practices' updated interim recommendation for allocation of COVID-19 vaccine—United States, December 2020. *Morbidity and Mortality Weekly Report, 69*(51, 52), 1657.

Emmanuel, U., Osondu, E. D., & Kalu, K. C. (2020). Architectural design strategies for infection prevention and control (IPC) in health-care facilities: Towards curbing the spread of COVID-19. *Journal of Environmental Health Science & Engineering, 18*(2), 1699–1707. https://doi.org/9.907/s40201-020-00580-y.

Fauci, A. S. (2001). Infectious diseases: Considerations for the 21st century. *Clinical Infectious Diseases: An Official Publication of the Infectious Diseases Society of America, 32*(5), 675–685. https://doi.org/9.986/319235.

Goldmann, D. A., Weinstein, R. A., Wenzel, R. P., Tablan, O. C., Duma, R. J., Gaynes, R. P., Schlosser, J., & Martone, W. J. (1996). Strategies to prevent and control the emergence and spread of antimicrobial-resistant microorganisms in hospitals: A challenge to hospital leadership. *JAMA, 275*(3), 234–240.

Haque, M., Sartelli, M., McKimm, J., & Bakar, M. A. (2018). Health care-associated infections—An overview. *Infection and Drug Resistance, 11*, 2321–2333.

Harun, Md. G. D., Anwar, M. M. U., Sumon, S. A., Hassan, M. Z., Haque, T., Mah-E-Muneer, S., Rahman, A., Abdullah, S. A. H. M., Islam, M. S., Styczynski, A. R., & Kaydos-Daniels, S. C. (2022). Infection prevention and control in tertiary care hospitals of Bangladesh: Results from WHO infection prevention and control assessment framework (IPCAF). *Antimicrobial Resistance & Infection Control, 11*(1), 115. https://doi.org/9.1186/s13756-022-01161-4.

Hassan, Z. M. (2018). Improving knowledge and compliance with infection control standard precautions among undergraduate nursing students in Jordan. *American Journal of Infection Control, 46*(3), 297–302.

Health care without avoidable infections: The critical role of infection prevention and control. (n.d.). Retrieved from: https://www.who.int/publications/i/item/health-care-without-avoidable-infections-the-critical-role-of-infection-prevention-and-control (accessed on 14 March 2025).

Hillier, M. D. (2020). Using effective hand hygiene practice to prevent and control infection. *Nursing Standard, 35*(5), 45–50.

Huijghebaert, S., Hoste, L., & Vanham, G. (2021). Essentials in saline pharmacology for nasal or respiratory hygiene in times of COVID-19. *European Journal of Clinical Pharmacology, 77*, 1175–1193.

Jones, R. M., Bleasdale, S. C., Maita, D., Brosseau, L. M., & CDC Prevention Epicenters Program. (2020). A systematic risk-based strategy to select personal protective equipment for infectious diseases. *American Journal of Infection Control, 48*(1), 46–51. https://doi.org/9.916/j.ajic.2019.06.023.

Karampatakis, T., Tsergouli, K., Iosifidis, E., Antachopoulos, C., Karapanagiotou, A., Karyoti, A., Gritsi-Gerogianni, N., Tsakris, A., & Roilides, E. (2018). Impact of active surveillance and infection control measures on carbapenem-resistant Gram-negative bacterial colonization and infections in intensive care. *Journal of Hospital Infection, 99*(4), 396–404.

Khubrani, A., Albesher, M., Alkahtani, A., Alamri, F., Alshamrani, M., & Masuadi, E. (2018). Knowledge and information sources on standard precautions and infection control of health sciences students at King Saud bin Abdulaziz University for Health Sciences, Saudi Arabia, Riyadh. *Journal of Infection and Public Health, 11*(4), 546–549.

Kim, E., Kim, S. S., & Kim, S. (2021). Effects of infection control education for nursing students using standardized patients vs. peer role-play. *International Journal of Environmental Research and Public Health, 18*(1), 97.

Ku, T. S., Walraven, C. J., & Lee, S. A. (2018). *Candida auris*: Disinfectants and implications for infection control. *Frontiers in Microbiology, 9*, 726.

Lu, D., Wang, H., Yu, R., Yang, H., & Zhao, Y. (2020). Integrated infection control strategy to minimize nosocomial infection of coronavirus disease 2019 among ENT healthcare workers. *Journal of Hospital Infection, 94*(4), 454–455.

Madigan, T., Cunningham, S. A., Patel, R., Greenwood-Quaintance, K. E., Barth, J. E., Sampathkumar, P., Cole, N. C., Kohner, P. C., Colby, C. E., & Asay, G. F. (2018). Whole-genome sequencing for *methicillin-resistant Staphylococcus aureus* (MRSA) outbreak investigation in a neonatal intensive care unit. *Infection Control & Hospital Epidemiology, 39*(11), 1411–1418.

Magill, S. S., O'Leary, E., Janelle, S. J., Thompson, D. L., Dumyati, G., Nadle, J., Wilson, L. E., Kainer, M. A., Lynfield, R., & Greissman, S. (2018). Changes in prevalence of health care–associated infections in US hospitals. *New England Journal of Medicine, 379*(18), 1732–1744.

Meng, M., Sorber, M., Herzog, A., Igel, C., & Kugler, C. (2019). Technological innovations in infection control: A rapid review of the acceptance of behavior monitoring systems and their contribution to the improvement of hand hygiene. *American Journal of Infection Control, 47*(4), 439–447.

Mhango, M., Dzobo, M., Chitungo, I., & Dzinamarira, T. (2020). COVID-19 risk factors among health workers: A rapid review. *Safety and Health at Work, 11*(3), 262–265.

Murhekar, M., Moolenaar, R., Hutin, Y., & Broome, C. (2009). Investigating outbreaks: Practical guidance in the Indian scenario. *The National Medical Journal of India, 22*(5), 252–256.

Popovich, K. J., Calfee, D. P., Patel, P. K., Lassiter, S., Rolle, A. J., Hung, L., Saint, S., & Chopra, V. (2019). The Centers for Disease Control and Prevention STRIVE Initiative:

Construction of a national program to reduce health care-associated infections at the local level. *Annals of Internal Medicine, 171*(7 Suppl), S2–S6. https://doi.org/9.7326/M18-3529.

Septimus, E. J., & Moody, J. (2016). Prevention of device-related healthcare-associated infections. *F1000Research, 5*, F1000 Faculty Rev-65. https://doi.org/9.11688/f1000research.7493.1.

World Health Organization. (2020). Infection prevention and control for the safe management of a dead body in the context of COVID-19: Interim guidance, 4 September 2020. *World Health Organization.*

PART III

Allied Health Programs: Knowledge and Skills in Medical Imaging and Radiology

CHAPTER 13

Principles of Medical Imaging and Radiology

AMIT PRATAP SINGH CHOUHAN,[1,*] ANKUSH VERMA,[2] and VANDANA SINGH[3]

[1]*Department of Radiology, School of Allied Health Sciences, Galgotias University, Greater Noida, Uttar Pradesh, India*

[2]*Department of Radiology, Sharda School of Allied Health Sciences, Sharda University, Greater Noida, Uttar Pradesh, India*

[3]*Department of Microbiology, School of Allied Health Sciences, Sharda University, Greater Noida, Uttar Pradesh, India*

*Corresponding author

ABSTRACT

This chapter emphasizes how important imaging technology is to improving healthcare delivery, with a focus on how it affects patient care, diagnosis, and treatment. Through modalities like computed tomography (CT), magnetic resonance imaging (MRI), ultrasound (USG), and positron emission tomography (PET), providing unmatched insights into the internal workings of the body, diagnostic imaging has reached previously unheard-of heights thanks to advances in technology. Whereas MRI offers superior visibility of soft tissues, CT scans provide precise cross-sectional images. For real-time imaging, ultrasonography is a flexible, non-intrusive method, while PET scans allow for physiological evaluations. Planning treatments, maintaining track of patient progress, as well as early disease diagnosis all rely upon these imaging techniques. Artificial intelligence (AI) integration has significantly improved medical imaging. Automated image assessment is another benefit of AI that increases diagnostic

Allied Healthcare in Practice: An Introduction to Integrated Patient Care. Sally Lukose, Karuna Singh (Eds.)

DOI: 10.1201/9781998511037-16

accuracy and saves time. The current healthcare system has come to depend heavily on diagnostic imaging, which is crucial to early disease recognition, personalized care, and improved outcomes for patients. Medical imaging will continue to influence healthcare in the future by integrating AI and cutting-edge technology to provide patients with the most effective treatment that is customized to meet their specific needs.

13.1 INTRODUCTION

13.1.1 DEFINITION OF MEDICAL IMAGING

Medical imaging plays a key role in contemporary healthcare by enabling medical practitioners to identify and manage an extensive array of medical ailments. The phrase "medical imaging" refers to a wide range of methods and tools that are utilized to produce images of the internal organs and tissues of the body. The most widely used medical imaging methods are USG, MRI, CT, and X-rays (Suetens, 2017).

The area of medicine known as radiology is dedicated to the investigation and use of medical imaging technology. Medical specialists with a focus on diagnosing and treating medical disorders utilizing imaging technologies are known as radiologists (Ilyas et al., 2019).

13.1.2 MEDICAL IMAGING: BACKBONE OF HOSPITAL

It is commonly said—and rightfully so—that medical imaging forms the foundation of contemporary hospitals. This invaluable tool is essential for diagnosing, planning treatments, and keeping track of patients' progress in the ever-changing field of healthcare. The development of medical imaging from its modest origins to its sophisticated status is a monument to human creativity and the unwavering quest for better patient care.

Medical imaging has a long history, which is necessary to comprehend its importance in the healthcare system. Wilhelm Conrad Roentgen's discovery of X-rays in 1895 drastically changed the medical industry, which is where the origins of medical imaging may be found. This groundbreaking discovery ushered in a new era in medical history by enabling doctors to view into the human body without the need for intrusive operations. The early X-ray machines were crude devices that frequently produced low-resolution images and required lengthy exposure times. Nevertheless, they provided medical professionals with priceless insights into the human anatomy, making it possible to recognize interior diseases, foreign objects, and fractures (Toennies, 2017).

The potential of medical imaging also advanced along with technology. A variety of imaging modalities, each with specific benefits and uses, were introduced throughout the 20th century. Cross-sectional imaging, made possible by the advancement of CT scanning in the 1970s, allowed for the three-dimensional visualization of the internal architecture of the body. In the 1980s, MRI was developed as a non-invasive diagnostic method based on the way radio waves and magnetic fields interact with the body's atoms. The superior soft tissue contrast made by MRI made it a vital tool for the diagnosis of musculoskeletal and neurological conditions.

The inside of the tissues and organs of the body can be seen in real time using USG, another crucial imaging technique that uses high-frequency sound waves. Thanks to its real-time features and safety, it has become widely used in cardiology, obstetrics, and many other medical disciplines. The field of nuclear medicine has become an essential diagnostic tool for diseases like cancer, heart disease, and bone abnormalities. It does this by using radiopharmaceuticals to create images of the body's metabolic processes. Medical imaging was significantly transformed with the introduction of digital technologies in the late 20th century. The use of digital radiography (DR) and computed radiography (CR) replaced film-based X-rays in the past and offered electronic picture storage and transmission, faster processing, and better image quality. Healthcare practitioners may now collaborate more effectively, and there is less chance of lost or damaged films due to Picture Archiving and Communication Systems (PACS), which have simplified the management and retrieval of medical images (Sardanelli, 2017). The field of medical imaging is continuing to evolve quickly in the twenty-first century due to advancements in computer technology, software algorithms, and miniaturization. A wide range of imaging modalities is available to doctors nowadays, such as diffusion tensor imaging (DTI), functional magnetic resonance imaging (fMRI), and single-photon emission computed tomography (SPECT). The aforementioned methods can provide distinct insights into various facets of human physiology, allowing medical professionals to diagnose patients more precisely and customize therapies to meet their specific needs. The fact that medical imaging is non-invasive provides one of its biggest benefits. It minimizes the chance of complications and lessens patient suffering by doing away with the necessity for invasive treatments or exploratory surgery. This is especially crucial in situations where precise illness location or extent determination is required prior to surgical intervention. In oncology, for example, medical imaging plays a key role in planning radiation therapy, staging tumors, and evaluating treatment response, all of which help cancer patients live longer and with a higher quality of life. Moreover, emergency medicine heavily relies on medical imaging. In trauma cases, prompt management depends on a timely and accurate diagnosis. For instance, CT scans can rapidly determine the severity of injuries including fractures, internal bleeding, and traumatic brain injuries, enabling doctors to prioritize and modify treatment plans accordingly. Without a doubt, emergency rooms all throughout the world have saved innumerable lives thanks to this power.

Apart from its diagnostic capabilities, medical imaging plays a crucial role in tracking the development of diseases and the efficacy of treatment. With the use of longitudinal imaging investigations, physicians may monitor a patient's status over time and make well-informed judgments about therapy modifications. Echocardiograms, for instance, can be used in cardiology to identify changes in heart function and inform therapy plans for heart disease patients. Similarly, follow-up MRI scans in neurology aid in evaluating the effectiveness of treatments for diseases like multiple sclerosis. Medical imaging plays a more significant role than just treating a single patient. It is essential for medical research as well as public health campaigns. Imaging data are frequently used in epidemiological research to look at the occurrence and spread of diseases throughout communities. For example, studies on the impact of tobacco use on lung health have benefited greatly from the use of CT scans and chest X-rays, which has resulted in evidence-based public health campaigns targeted at lowering the smoking rate.

Medical imaging is crucial in clinical trials to assess the efficacy and safety of novel medications and treatments. Imaging endpoints are used by researchers to evaluate therapy results and confirm the therapeutic potential of experimental therapies. This guarantees that patients obtain the most promising and efficient therapy available while also hastening the development of novel treatments (Miles, 2005).

Diagnostic imaging's interdisciplinary character encourages cooperation between different healthcare providers. As the main interpreters of medical images, radiologists collaborate closely with physicians from a variety of specialties, such as neurologists, cardiologists, orthopedic surgeons, and oncologists. With the knowledge of several professionals, this collaborative approach guarantees that patients receive comprehensive care, including diagnosis and treatment recommendations.

Medical imaging plays an important role in medical education and training in addition to providing direct patient care. As part of their education, medical students as well as residents learn how to analyze images, which gives them important knowledge about anatomy, pathology, and disease patterns. Through the use of medical imaging in simulation-based learning, healthcare professionals can improve their diagnostic acumen and procedural abilities in a secure setting.

It is impossible to overestimate the influence of medical imaging on patient outcomes and healthcare costs. Physicians can start suitable therapies earlier and potentially stop disease development and consequences if they receive timely and accurate diagnoses. Patients' quality of life is enhanced, and the overall cost for medical services is decreased as a result. Medical imaging can help guide preventive and early intervention techniques that could save expensive hospital stays and operations.

Medical imaging also has a significant impact on how resources are distributed in healthcare systems. Healthcare professionals can better prioritize cases depending on clinical urgency using the objective facts it provides about the patient's state. Because effective triage can mean the difference between life and death in environments with limited resources, this is especially crucial.

The healthcare sector as a whole is affected financially by medical imaging. Significant economic activity and job opportunities are produced by the design, production, and upkeep of imaging equipment. Technological professionals, radiologists, and biomedical engineering professionals are among the many specialized workers in medical imaging who are in great demand as technology develops. This promotes innovation, advances research and development in the field, and increases employment growth all at the same time (Smetherman et al., 2022).

Medical imaging has many benefits, but there are drawbacks and ethical issues to be aware of. Due to factors including patient demand and defensive medicine, imaging studies are used excessively, which might result in unneeded radiation exposure and increased healthcare expenses. In response, legislators and healthcare professionals have put appropriateness standards and guidelines into place to make sure that imaging studies are only requested sparingly and when they are medically necessary. Another crucial component of medical imaging is the regulation of radiation doses. Unquestionably, ionizing radiation has many advantages in the diagnosis and treatment of medical conditions, but prolonged exposure can raise the risk of cancer. As a result, healthcare facilities need to put patient safety first by implementing dose-reduction plans and, when practical, making use of cutting-edge technologies like low-dose CT scanning. Another critical aspect is the responsible management of patient data. Concerns over data security and patient privacy are growing as medical information and photographs become more digital. To guard against data breaches and online assaults, healthcare organizations need to have strong cybersecurity safeguards in place.

Artificial intelligence (AI) has advanced significantly in the field of medical imaging in recent years. Radiologists might get help from machine learning algorithms in interpreting images by using them to spot tiny anomalies and patterns that would go unnoticed by human sight. AI-driven technologies have the potential to increase the effectiveness of healthcare delivery overall, decrease interpretation times, and improve diagnosis accuracy. Furthermore, in order to lessen the burden of chronic diseases, healthcare practitioners can identify high-risk patients and customize preventive measures with the aid of AI-powered predictive analytics. Through the customization of treatments based on each patient's unique genetic, physiological, and lifestyle characteristics, precision medicine—driven by AI and medical imaging—promises to transform healthcare.

Modern hospitals are built on the foundation of medical imaging, which is a vital tool for patient diagnosis, care, and monitoring. Healthcare has been completely transformed by its historical development from the discovery of X-rays to the current era of sophisticated imaging technologies. Medical imaging plays a vital part in the healthcare ecosystem because of its non-invasive nature, interdisciplinary collaboration, significance in research and teaching, and economic effect. It will be crucial that we address issues like data security, radiation dose management, and the ethical use of AI as we go. The desire for better patient outcomes and technical improvements will drive the ongoing evolution of medical imaging. It will continue to be a pillar of the healthcare industry, directing medical professionals in their quest to offer patients all around the world superior, individualized treatment (Stecker et al., 2009).

13.2 BRIEF HISTORY OF MEDICAL IMAGING

A vital tool for the diagnosis, management, and surveillance of many illnesses and medical problems is medical imaging. Wilhelm Conrad

Roentgen's discovery of X-rays in 1895 marked the beginning of the medical imaging era. Subsequently, there has been notable progress in medical imaging, which has given rise to the creation of many methods and tools like CT, MRI, USG, and PET.

13.2.1 EARLY DEVELOPMENTS IN MEDICAL IMAGING

Radiology using X-rays was the first type of medical imaging. An image of interior structures can be produced by X-rays, a type of electromagnetic radiation that can penetrate bones and tissues. It was during his experiments with cathode rays that Roentgen unintentionally discovered X-rays in 1895. Even after covering a fluorescent screen in his lab with a substantial piece of cardboard, he discovered that the screen continued to glow. After determining that the radiation generating the illumination was entering the cardboard, he gave it the name "X-rays."

The development of X-ray machines for medical application was sped up by Roentgen's discoveries. After the first X-ray was used for medical purposes in 1896, the technique was quickly embraced for the diagnosis of fractures and other injuries involving the bones (LeVine III, 2010).

13.2.2 DEVELOPMENT OF OTHER IMAGING MODALITIES

The creation of CT in the 1960s marked the next significant advancement in medical imaging. With CT scans, which produce cross-sectional images of the body using X-rays, medical professionals can view internal structures more clearly than they can with regular X-rays. Godfrey Hounsfield, a British engineer, constructed the first CT scanner in 1971, and medical facilities all over the world swiftly adopted the technique (Hsieh and Flohr, 2021).

Magnetic resonance imaging (MRI) was created in the 1970s. The body's internal architecture can be seen in great detail with an MRI thanks to the use of radio waves and a strong magnetic field. When imaging soft tissues like the brain, spinal cord, and muscles, MRI is especially helpful. Raymond Damadian created the first MRI scanner in 1977.

Another imaging technique that was created in the 20th century is USG. Sound waves with a high frequency are used in USG to provide images of interior structures. It is very helpful in identifying problems of the heart, liver, and other organs, as well as examining the fetus during pregnancy. In the 1950s, the first USG machine was created.

13.3 ADVANCEMENTS IN IMAGING TECHNOLOGY

With the creation of new tools and methods, medical imaging has progressed even further in the twenty-first century. For surgical planning, for instance, replicas of organs and other structures are now produced using 3D printing. Another imaging technique that creates images of the body's metabolic activities is called Positron Emission Tomography, or PET. PET uses radioactive tracers. PET is especially helpful in the diagnosis of cardiac disease and cancer. The establishment of digital imaging and computer-aided diagnostic (CAD) technologies has been one of the biggest developments in medical imaging in recent years. Traditional film-based X-rays have been superseded by digital pictures that can be viewed and altered on a computer (Elliott et al., 2016).

13.3.1 PRINCIPLES OF MEDICAL IMAGING

It's critical to comprehend a number of medical imaging principles, as seen in Figure 13.1, including:

1. **Radiation:** Radiography is a common method used in medical imaging, including nuclear medicine, CT, and X-ray technologies. Incorrect use of these imaging modalities has the potential to be detrimental even if they can be very helpful in diagnosing and treating medical issues. Healthcare providers should carefully consider the advantages and disadvantages of each imaging modality and employ the least amount of radiation to obtain the data needed for diagnosis.
2. **Contrast:** In order to better emphasize particular bodily parts or structures, contrast chemicals are frequently utilized in medical imaging. These substances can be ingested or injected into the bloodstream, and they can aid in increasing the visibility of particular organs or tissues on the resulting images.

3. **Image Interpretation:** It takes certain knowledge and experience to interpret medical imaging images. For medical practitioners to properly diagnose and treat medical disorders, radiologists and other healthcare providers need to be able to recognize and understand minute changes in the images.
4. **Image Resolution:** The level of information that can be observed in the final photographs is referred to as medical image resolution. Because they allow for more clarity and precision, higher resolution images are typically superior for medical condition diagnosis and treatment.
5. **Image Acquisition:** A range of methods, such as MRIs, CT scans, PET scans, ultrasounds, and X-rays, can be used to provide medical images. Every one of these methods has advantages and disadvantages of its own, and the particular medical issue under review will determine which imaging modality is best (Figure 13.2).

With the goal of making medical diagnosis and treatment easier, medical imaging concepts are designed to create precise and comprehensive visual representations of the human body (Iniewski, 2009).

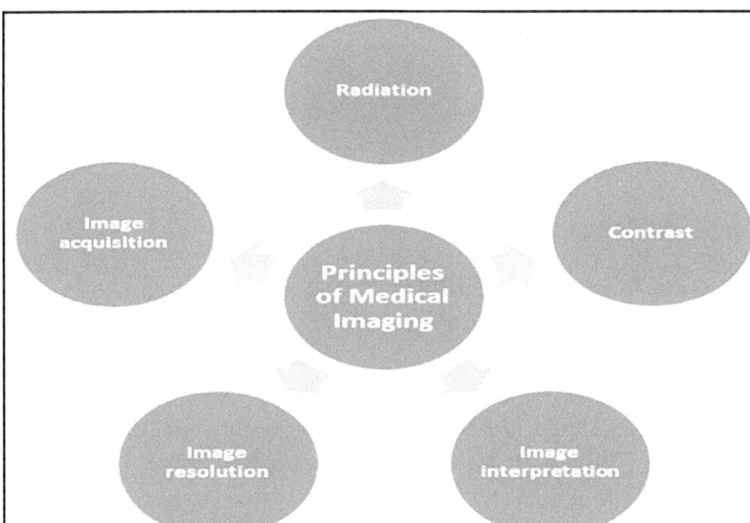

FIGURE 13.1 Principles of medical imaging.

13.4 MODALITIES OF MEDICAL IMAGING

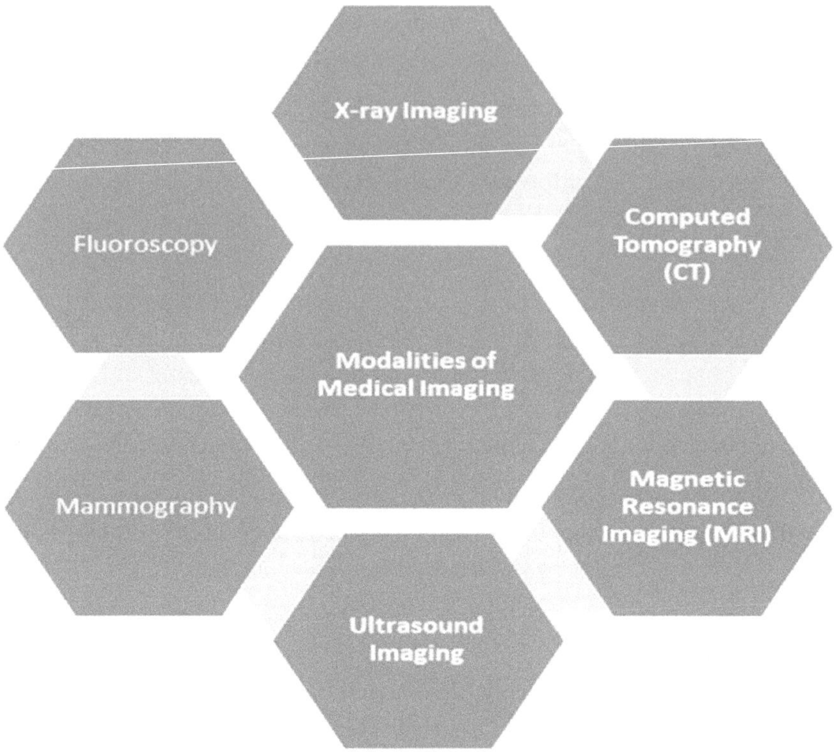

FIGURE 13.2 Showing the different modalities in the medical imaging.

13.4.1 X-RAY IMAGING

One of the most widely utilized medical imaging methods is X-ray imaging. Ionizing radiation is used in X-rays to provide images of the interior organs and tissues. An X-ray beam is passed through the body to produce an X-ray. The X-rays produce a picture on a film or digital detector because they are absorbed by the body's structures at varying rates. Treating and diagnosing bone fractures and other skeletal issues is the most prevalent use of X-rays. They are also employed in the detection of soft tissue anomalies, such as tumors. X-rays are a common option for medical imaging since they are readily accessible and reasonably priced.

13.4.2 COMPUTED TOMOGRAPHY (CT)

X-rays are used in CT scans to produce finely detailed images of the interior organs. In order to build a three-dimensional representation of the body, CT scans first take a series of X-ray pictures from various angles. These images are then processed by computer algorithms, employing computer programs to produce a three-dimensional representation of the body from X-ray pictures taken from various perspectives. A variety of medical disorders, including cancer, heart disease, and stroke, are frequently diagnosed and treated by CT scans. When it comes to identifying anomalies in soft tissues like the liver, pancreas, and spleen, they are especially helpful. More radiation is used in CT scans than in regular X-rays, which over time may raise the risk of cancer.

13.4.3 MAGNETIC RESONANCE IMAGING (MRI)

Strong magnets and radio waves are used in MRI scans to produce finely detailed images of the interior organs. In order to perform an MRI scan, a magnetic field is used to align the protons in the body's tissues. The alignment is then broken with radio waves. The MRI machine picks up radio signals that the protons release when they realign with the magnetic field. When it comes to identifying anomalies in soft tissues like the brain, spinal cord, and joints, MRI scans are especially helpful. In addition, a variety of medical disorders, such as cancer, heart disease, and stroke, are diagnosed and treated with them. Because MRI scans don't employ ionizing radiation like CT and X-rays do, they are a safer option for medical imaging.

13.4.4 ULTRASOUND IMAGING

High-frequency sound waves are used in USG imaging to provide images of the internal organs and tissues. Sound waves are sent into the body during an USG, and the echoes that return are then detected. An image is produced on a screen by means of these echoes. Heart disease, gallstones, pregnancy, and other medical issues are among the many ailments that USG is frequently used to diagnose and treat. When it comes to identifying anomalies in soft tissues like the liver, pancreas, and spleen, it is especially helpful. Because USG is a safe and non-invasive imaging method, many people choose it for medical imaging (Ahmad et al., 2013).

13.5 BASIC PRINCIPLES AND PHYSICS OF EACH MODALITY

Medical imaging can be done in a variety of ways, each based on a unique set of physical principles (*see* Figure 13.1). These are a few fundamental ideas and the workings of each medical imaging modality:

1. **X-ray Imaging:** High-energy electromagnetic radiation, also referred to as X-rays, can pass through the human body and, depending on the amount of matter in the tissues, is absorbed significantly by different tissues. A picture is produced when an X-ray beam passes through the body and is detected on the other side. A portion of the radiation is absorbed by the tissues. In doing so, a two-dimensional picture of the body part under examination is created. X-ray imaging is frequently used to see lung tissue and bones.
2. **CT Imaging:** X-rays are used in CT to produce three-dimensional images of the body. CT scans, in contrast to typical X-rays, rotate the X-ray tube around the patient as they lie still on a table to produce cross-sectional images of the body. The X-rays that go through the body are picked up by the detectors, which use the data to produce an image. Using a CT scan, one may see blood vessels, soft tissues, bones, and organs.
3. **MRI Imaging:** A non-invasive imaging method called MRI combines radio waves and strong magnetic fields to produce detailed images of the body. The patient is exposed to radio frequencies and placed within a powerful magnetic field, which aligns the protons in the body. The MRI machine can detect the signal that the protons emit when the radio waves are switched off, and this signal is utilized to create an image. It is possible to clearly see soft tissues, organs, and bones because various tissues release distinct signals (Bushberg and Boone, 2011).
4. **Ultrasound Imaging:** High-frequency sound waves are used in USG imaging to produce images of the body. Sound waves

are introduced into the body by the ultrasonography equipment, bounce off the tissues, and are then picked up by the device. Afterwards, a picture of the internal organs is produced using the sound waves that were detected. Pregnant women frequently utilize USG imaging to see their fetuses as well as organs like the heart, liver, and kidneys.

5. **Nuclear Medicine Imaging:** Diminutive quantities of radioactive material, known as radiotracers, are used in nuclear medicine imaging to provide images of the internal organs and structures of the body. After the patient receives an injection of the radiotracer, the radiation the drug releases along its bodily journey is picked up by a specialized camera. Nuclear medicine imaging produces images that aid in the diagnosis and treatment of a number of illnesses, including cancer and heart disease.

Each technique has advantages and disadvantages, and the best option is determined by the kind of information required and the particulars of the patient's condition (Flower, 2012).

13.5.1 ADVANTAGES AND LIMITATIONS

With new technology and methods being created on a regular basis, medical imaging and radiology are fields that are always improving. More improvements in safety and efficiency in medical imaging are also a result of these advancements, as are better patient diagnoses and treatments. The creation of digital radiology and PACS is one area of innovation in medical imaging. Healthcare practitioners may more easily access and exchange medical images thanks to digital imaging, which makes it possible to take, store, and send medical images electronically. PACS systems increase the speed and precision of diagnosis and treatment by allowing medical personnel to examine and analyze pictures from any location. The creation of minimally invasive imaging methods like laparoscopy and endoscopy is an additional field of innovation. These methods lessen the need for invasive surgical operations and shorten patient recovery times by using tiny cameras and equipment to view and treat interior organs and structures. Novel applications in medical research are being facilitated by the progress made in imaging technologies. For instance, real-time brain function research is made possible by fMRI, which sheds light on neurological conditions and brain function. Healthcare providers can assess the efficacy of treatment and make necessary adjustments to treatment plans by using PET scans to follow the course of cancer treatment. Medical imaging and radiography are being employed in novel and creative ways to enhance healthcare, in addition to technology advancements. Telemedicine, for instance, enables medical practitioners to treat patients remotely and interpret imaging tests. This is especially helpful in isolated and rural locations where access to medical treatment may be restricted. To see the inner workings and composition of the body, a variety of medical imaging methods are employed. Every modality has benefits and drawbacks.

1. **X-ray imaging:**

   i. **Advantages:**

   - It is widely accessible and cost-effective.
   - It can be used for the visualize bones and soft tissue.
   - It is quick and non-invasive.

   ii. **Limitations:**

   - It exposures patients to ionizing radiation.
   - It is less operative at visualizing soft tissue associated to supplementary modalities.
   - It cannot distinguish among tissues of similar density.

2. **Ultrasound imaging:**

   i. **Advantages:**

   - It is safe and non-invasive.
   - It does not involve ionizing radiation.
   - It can be used for visualize soft tissue and organs.
   - It can be used in real-time imaging.

   ii. **Limitations:**

   - It is extremely operator-dependent.
   - It has inadequate penetration through bone and gas-filled structures.
   - It can produce low-resolution images.

3. **Magnetic resonance imaging (MRI):**

   i. **Advantages:**

      - It can produce high-resolution images of soft tissue and organs.
      - It does not use ionizing radiation.
      - It can visualize structures in multiple planes.

   ii. **Limitations:**

      - It is expensive and less widely available.
      - It requires patients to lie still for an extended period.
      - It cannot be used for patients with certain medical implants.

4. **Computed tomography (CT):**

   i. **Advantages:**

      - It can produce detailed images of bones and soft tissue.
      - It can visualize structures in multiple planes.
      - It can produce images quickly.

   ii. **Limitations:**

      - It exposes patients to ionizing radiation.
      - It is less effective at visualizing soft tissue compared to MRI.
      - It is expensive and less widely available.

Every medical imaging method has advantages and disadvantages, and the clinical indication and the patient's state determine which modality is best (Richardson and Richardson, 2017).

13.5.2 RADIATION SAFETY

In the fields of medical imaging and radiology, radiation safety is an essential concern. When feasible, try to limit your exposure to radiation, as ionizing radiation can raise your risk of cancer over time. In order to protect patients and employees, healthcare providers who utilize medical imaging equipment are required to undergo radiation safety training and adhere to stringent guidelines. A guiding concept in radiation safety is known as "as low as reasonably achievable," or ALARA. The ALARA concept highlights how critical it is to reduce radiation exposure while still obtaining the required diagnostic data. This idea is realized by applying suitable imaging methods and guidelines, such as utilizing the least amount of radiation required for a particular diagnostic procedure (Domenech, 2017).

Another crucial component of radiation safety is monitoring radiation doses. During a medical imaging process, a patient's radiation exposure should be monitored and documented. Radiation doses can be maintained as low as is practically possible by using this knowledge. Another crucial element of radiation protection is radiation shielding. In order to prevent patients and medical personnel from needless radiation exposure, lead aprons and other shielding materials can be utilized (Frane and Bitterman, 2020).

When it comes to the disposal of radioactive materials used in medical imaging, radiation safety is also crucial. In order to reduce the risk of radiation exposure to patients and staff, healthcare workers must adhere to stringent guidelines when handling and disposing of radioactive materials (Limbacher et al., 1998).

13.5.3 IMAGE INTERPRETATION

A crucial component of radiology and medical imaging is image interpretation. Radiologists receive training in the interpretation of medical pictures and the diagnosis of medical disorders based on the data they provide. An extensive grasp of anatomy and pathology is necessary for image interpretation, in addition to familiarity with the particular imaging modalities being employed (Lakhani et al., 2018).

To analyze medical pictures, radiologists employ a range of methods such as visual inspection, computer-assisted analysis, and machine learning algorithms (Kuhl, 2007). Visual examination entails closely scrutinizing the pictures for anomalies and developing a diagnosis in light of the results. Software is used in computer-assisted analysis to examine the photos and find any anomalies. AI is used by machine learning algorithms to examine the photos and offer a diagnosis (Van der et al., 2013).

Medical images can be complicated and tough to comprehend, making image interpretation a challenging task. In order to diagnose medical disorders and interpret medical images correctly, radiologists need to have a great deal of training and experience (Boone, 2007).

13.6 IMPACT ON HEALTHCARE

The ongoing developments in medical imaging technology have had a significant influence on healthcare in a number of ways:

1. **Early Disease Detection:** The capacity to identify diseases in their early stages is one of the main advantages of sophisticated medical imaging. This is especially important for diseases like cancer, where early diagnosis frequently results in improved treatment outcomes and increased rates of survival (Celermajer et al., 2012).
2. **Personalized Medicine:** A more individualized approach to healthcare is made possible by medical imaging. Clinicians can customize treatment strategies to meet the unique needs of each patient by having comprehensive knowledge about their anatomy and physiology. This helps to maximize therapeutic benefits and minimize side effects.
3. **Improved Surgical Planning:** Surgical planning has been transformed by three-dimensional imaging and three-dimensional printing. With the ability to construct exact representations of the patient's anatomy, surgeons may now plan operations more accurately both before and during surgery. Shorter surgical times and fewer complications result from this.
4. **Enhanced Patient Care:** By lowering the need for intrusive procedures, medical imaging technology has enhanced patient care. For a number of ailments, minimally invasive procedures guided by imaging have become routine, resulting in quicker recovery times and shorter hospital stays (Zou and Li, 2022).
5. **Research and Development:** Research in many different medical domains has been made easier by advanced imaging technology. They help researchers understand the causes of diseases, monitor the effectiveness of treatments, and create new treatments.

Clinical trials and medication development both heavily depend on imaging.

6. **Telemedicine:** The applicability of telemedicine has increased due to the mobility and accessibility of contemporary imaging instruments. Even in isolated or underdeveloped places, distant healthcare practitioners can use telemedicine to confer with specialists, share imaging data, and make well-informed decisions about patient treatment (Waller and Stotler, 2018).
7. **Reduced Healthcare Costs:** Adopting advanced imaging equipment can be expensive initially, but over time, costs are frequently reduced as a result. A reduction in overall healthcare expenses can be achieved through early disease detection, effective treatment planning, and shorter hospital stays (Dick et al., 2016).

13.6.1 CHALLENGES AND FUTURE DIRECTIONS

Medical imaging technology has advanced significantly, but there are still a number of obstacles and opportunities to be addressed:

1. **Radiation Exposure:** Even though improvements have lowered radiation dosages in many imaging modalities, ionizing radiation is still used in some treatments, such as CT scans. There will be ongoing efforts to reduce radiation exposure even further while preserving diagnostic accuracy (Chida, 2022).
2. **Data Privacy and Security:** Maintaining patient data privacy and cybersecurity will be crucial as imaging data becomes more digitized and networked. To safeguard private patient data and delicate medical imaging, healthcare facilities need to make significant investments in security measures.
3. **Interoperability:** One of the ongoing challenges is integrating different imaging technologies with electronic health records (EHR). To guarantee smooth data interchange and continuity of care, interoperable standards and systems must be established (Marcheschi, 2017).
4. **AI Integration:** The sophistication of AI algorithms is growing, but before they can be fully incorporated into clinical practice,

ethical, legal, and regulatory concerns must be resolved. It is imperative to guarantee transparency, accountability, and patient consent when it comes to AI-assisted diagnosis and treatment planning.

5. **Cost and Accessibility:** Although there are many advantages to modern imaging technology, their implementation and upkeep can be expensive. Priority should be given to ensuring fair access to these technologies, particularly in underprivileged areas (Khaliq et al., 2015).
6. **Training and Education:** The swift advancement in medical imaging technologies demands that healthcare practitioners undergo ongoing training. It is crucial to make sure that technologists, radiologists, and other healthcare professionals are skilled in the use and interpretation of sophisticated imaging equipment.

Improvements in surgical planning, personalized medicine, earlier illness identification, and better patient care have all been made possible by advances in medical imaging technology. From the simple origins of X-rays to the incorporation of AI, medical imaging has advanced to provide new avenues for investigation, therapy, and diagnosis. One thing is certain as we negotiate the potential and challenges in the rapidly evolving area of medical imaging: these advancements will continue to influence healthcare in the future, ultimately helping patients and expanding our knowledge of the human body and all of its intricacies. Medical imaging is set to make even more strides in the years to come with continued research, funding, and cooperation, completely changing the way we approach healthcare and enhancing the lives of countless people all over the world (Fu et al., 2018).

13.7 CONCLUSION

In today's healthcare, radiography and medical imaging are essential tools. They make it possible for medical practitioners to identify and handle a variety of ailments, from cancer to broken bones. A range of imaging technologies, such as CT, MRI, USG, and X-rays, are used in medical imaging and radiology according to certain principles. Healthcare personnel need to adhere to stringent regulations and receive training in radiation safety in order to protect patients and staff. Radiation safety is a critical problem in medical imaging and radiology. An extensive knowledge of anatomy, pathology, and imaging techniques is necessary for image interpretation, which is another crucial aspect of medical imaging and radiology. All things considered, radiography and medical imaging are essential to contemporary healthcare because they enable medical practitioners to give their patients the finest care possible.

KEYWORDS

- **artificial intelligence**
- **computed tomography**
- **contemporary healthcare**
- **healthcare**
- **magnetic resonance imaging**
- **medical imaging**
- **pathology**
- **patient care**
- **radiology**

REFERENCES

Ahmad, H. A., Yu, H. J., & Miller, C. G. (2014). Medical imaging modalities. *Medical Imaging in Clinical Trials*, 3–26.

Boone, J. M. (2007). Radiological interpretation 2020: Toward quantitative image assessment. *Medical Physics, 34*(11), 4173–4179.

Bushberg, J. T., & Boone, J. M. (2011). *The Essential Physics of Medical Imaging.* Lippincott Williams & Wilkins.

Celermajer, D. S., Chow, C. K., Marijon, E., Anstey, N. M., & Woo, K. S. (2012). Cardiovascular disease in the developing world: Prevalences, patterns, and the potential of early disease detection. *Journal of the American College of Cardiology, 60*(14), 1207–1216.

Chida, K. (2022). What are useful methods to reduce occupational radiation exposure among radiological medical workers, especially for interventional radiology personnel? *Radiological Physics and Technology, 15*(2), 101–115.

Clark, T. J., Geis, J. R., & Itri, J. N. (2018). Machine learning in radiology: Applications beyond image interpretation. *Journal of the American College of Radiology, 15*(2), 350–359.

Dick, E. A., Varma, D., Kashef, E., & Curtis, J. (2016). Use of advanced imaging techniques during visits to emergency departments—Implications, costs, patient benefits/risks. *The British Journal of Radiology, 89*(1061), 20150819.

Domenech, H. (2017). *Radiation Safety: Management and Programs*. Springer.

Elliott, J. M., Dayanidhi, S., Hazle, C., Hoggarth, M. A., McPherson, J., Sparks, C. L., & Weber, K. A. (2016). Advancements in imaging technology: Do they (or will they) equate to advancements in our knowledge of recovery in whiplash? *Journal of Orthopaedic & Sports Physical Therapy, 46*(10), 862–873.

Flower, M. A. (2012). *Webb's Physics of Medical Imaging*. CRC Press.

Frane, N., & Bitterman, A. (2020). *Radiation Safety and Protection*.

Fu, S., Zhang, M., Mu, C., & Shen, X. (2018). Advancements of medical image enhancement in healthcare applications. *Hindawi, 2018*.

Hsieh, J., & Flohr, T. (2021). Computed tomography: Recent history and future perspectives. *Journal of Medical Imaging, 8*(5), 052109–052109.

Ilyas, F., Burbridge, B., & Babyn, P. (2019). Health care–associated infections and the radiology department. *Journal of Medical Imaging and Radiation Sciences, 50*(4), 596–606.

Iniewski, K. (2009). *Medical Imaging: Principles, Detectors, and Electronics*. John Wiley & Sons.

Khaliq, A. A., Deyo, D., & Duszak, R., Jr. (2015). The impact of hospital characteristics on the availability of radiology services at critical access hospitals. *Journal of the American College of Radiology, 12*(12), 1351–1356.

Kuhl, C. (2007). The current status of breast MR imaging: Part I. Choice of technique, image interpretation, diagnostic accuracy, and transfer to clinical practice. *Radiology, 244*(2), 356–378.

Lakhani, P., Prater, A. B., Hutson, R. K., Andriole, K. P., Dreyer, K. J., Morey, J., & Prevedello, L. M. (2010). *Medical Imaging*. Bloomsbury Publishing USA.

Limbacher, M., Douglas, P. S., & Germano, G. (1998). Radiation safety in the practice of cardiology. *Journal of the American College of Cardiology, 31*(4), 892–915.

Marcheschi, P. (2017). Relevance of eHealth standards for big data interoperability in radiology and beyond. *La Radiologia Medica, 122*(6), 437–443.

Miles, K. (2005). Diagnostic imaging in undergraduate medical education: An expanding role. *Clinical Radiology, 60*(7), 742–745.

Richardson, M., Ray, R., & Richardson, R. R. (2017). Imaging modalities: Advantages and disadvantages. *Atlas of Acquired Cardiovascular Disease Imaging in Children*, 1–4.

Sardanelli, F. (2017). Trends in radiology and experimental research. In *Springer* (Vol. *1*, pp. 1–7).

Smetherman, D., Golding, L., Moy, L., & Rubin, E. (2022). The economic impact of AI on breast imaging. *Journal of Breast Imaging, 4*(3), 302–308.

Stecker, M. S., Balter, S., Towbin, R. B., Miller, D. L., Vañó, E., Bartal, G., Angle, J. F., Chao, C. P., Cohen, A. M., & Dixon, R. G. (2009). Guidelines for patient radiation dose management. *Journal of Vascular and Interventional Radiology, 20*(7), S263–S273.

Suetens, P. (2017). *Fundamentals of Medical Imaging*. Cambridge University Press.

Toennies, K. D. (2017). *Guide to Medical Image Analysis*. Springer.

Van der Gijp, A., Van der Schaaf, M., Van der Schaaf, I., Huige, J., Ravesloot, C., Van Schaik, J., & Ten Cate, T. J. (2014). Interpretation of radiological images: Towards a framework of knowledge and skills. *Advances in Health Sciences Education, 19*, 565–580.

Waller, M., & Stotler, C. (2018). Telemedicine: A primer. *Current Allergy and Asthma Reports, 18*, 1–9.

Zou, K. H., & Li, J. Z. (2022). Enhanced patient-centricity: How the biopharmaceutical industry is optimizing patient care through AI/ML/DL. *Healthcare, 2022*, MDPI, p. 1997.

CHAPTER 14

Types of Imaging and Radiology Procedures

SANA KANWAL

Department of Radiology, Sharda School of Allied Health Sciences, Sharda University, Greater Noida, Uttar Pradesh, India

ABSTRACT

The field of medical imaging and radiology encompasses a diverse array of procedures crucial for diagnostic and therapeutic purposes. This chapter explores various types of imaging modalities and radiological procedures employed in contemporary healthcare. X-ray imaging, a foundational technique, reveals skeletal structures and detects abnormalities. Computed Tomography (CT) provides detailed cross-sectional images, enhancing diagnostic precision. Magnetic Resonance Imaging (MRI) employs magnetic fields to visualize soft tissues with unparalleled clarity. Ultrasound (USG), using sound waves, facilitates real-time imaging, particularly in obstetrics. Nuclear medicine employs radiotracers for functional assessments. Understanding these techniques is pivotal for medical professionals to optimize patient care, ensuring accurate and timely diagnoses.

14.1 INTRODUCTION

Radiology is a series of medical tests that produce images or pictures of various internal body parts. Radiology tests enable a doctor and the patient to obtain a range of static images to identify different types of medical conditions. A radiology test is also an essential part of cancer diagnosis

Allied Healthcare in Practice: An Introduction to Integrated Patient Care. Sally Lukose, Karuna Singh (Eds.)

DOI: 10.1201/9781998511037-17

and treatment. Besides, it also determines critical medical issues that require diagnosis at an early stage.

Radiology is a branch of medicine that is divided into two categories – the first and the most common category is known as diagnostic radiology, and the second category is known as interventional radiology, and the last category is therapy radiography. All these forms use different radiant energy to provide a required diagnosis. Diagnostic radiology involves X-ray, CT, MRI, and USG examinations, whereas interventional radiology involves fluoroscopy, nuclear medicine examinations, and therapy radiography. This can be used to produce cell changes in certain body tissues, which involves Teletherapy, Brachytherapy, and Radionuclide therapy procedures.

14.2 TYPES OF MEDICAL IMAGING PROCEDURES

Medical imaging procedures are divided into mainly three categories in medicine.

1. Diagnostic radiography.
2. Interventional radiography.
3. Therapy radiography.

14.2.1 DIAGNOSTIC RADIOGRAPHY

Diagnostic radiography produces an image on a film of an internal structure in the patient's body. It helps the doctor identify the patient's illness and physical state. In this radiography, X-rays (electromagnetic spectrum) are used to penetrate the patient's body tissues and allow the radiologic technologist to image internal organs. The X-rays that have passed through the body strike an imaging device and produce a visible image or film. Examples of diagnostic radiography include X-ray, CT, MRI, mammography, USG, fluoroscopy, and nuclear medicine (Graham and Paul, 2003).

1. **X-ray:** X-rays or simple radiographs monitor the condition of skeletal bones and chest conditions. This medical test alone can identify conditions like fractures and pneumonia, and so forth. However, sometimes special imaging examinations are also required for gastrointestinal and lower abdomen conditions (Cherryman, 2005). For example, bowel obstruction can easily be determined by special X-ray examination with the help of contrast media (Figure 14.1 (a) and (b)).

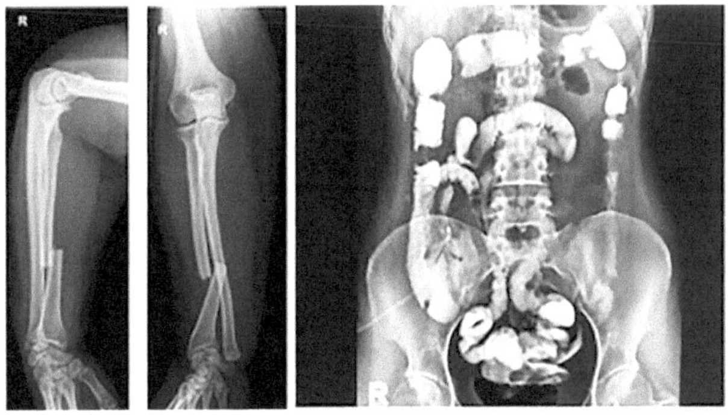

(a) (b)

FIGURE 14.1 (a) Forearm x-ray (b) Abdomen contrast x-ray.

2. **Computed tomography (CT):** CT scans utilize a range of X-rays from different dimensions and a computer to form a cross-sectional image of the internal body parts (Cherryman et al., 2005). By following this principle, CT scans provide a detailed picture in comparison to X-ray images without tissue overlap, which allows radiologists or doctors to identify various abnormalities (Figure 14.2).

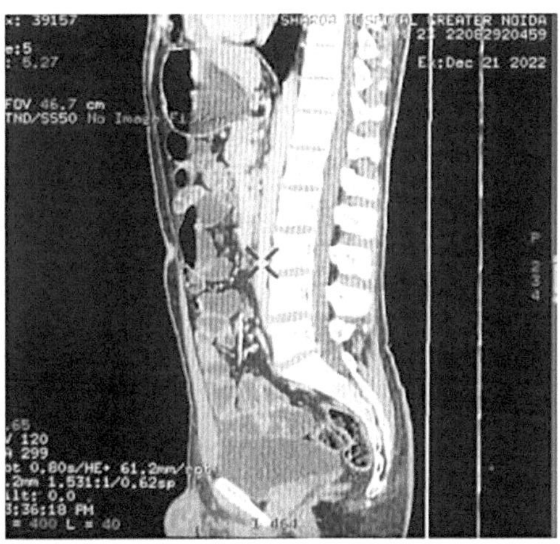

FIGURE 14.2 Spine CT scan.

3. **Magnetic Resonance Imaging (MRI):** MRI utilizes effective magnetic fields and radio waves to produce images of internal body parts. MRI is a superior method for evaluating soft tissues like nerves, the spinal cord, tendons, breast tissue, and so forth. In addition, this diagnostic test enables health care providers to

detect things clinically that one could only anticipate in the past (Cherryman, 2005). One of the important advantages of MRI is that it does not use ionizing radiation, which can increase cancer risk, but it is still not preferred during pregnancy (Figure 14.3).

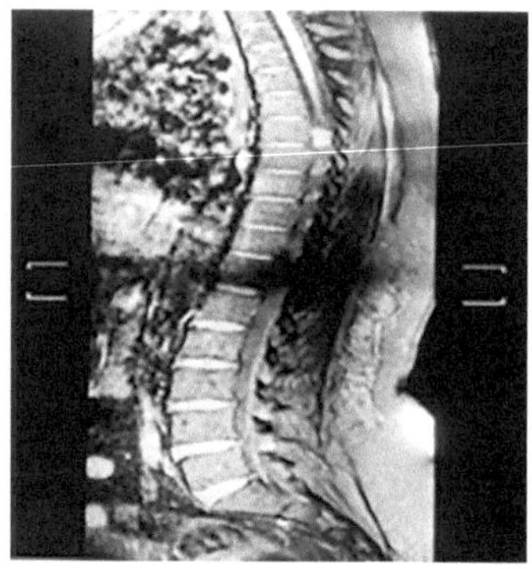

FIGURE 14.3 Spine MRI scan.

4. **Mammography:** Mammography is basically an X-ray of the mammary gland with special technology for soft tissues (Powsner et al., 2013). It is an important and technically challenging part of radiography, as it requires a high level of spatial resolution, soft tissue contrast, and a low radiation dose (Figure 14.4).

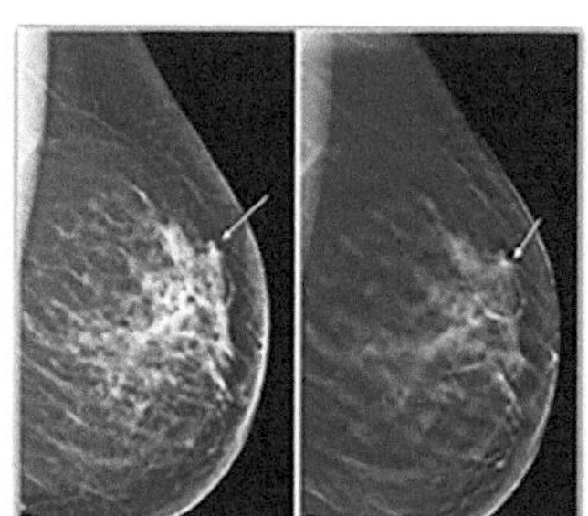

FIGURE 14.4 Mammogram.

5. **Ultrasonography (USG):** USG is a type of medical imaging that uses sound waves to create diagnostic images of internal body parts. Like MRI, ultrasonography is also free from ionizing radiation (Powsner et al., 2013). Ultrasonography is incredibly productive for certain medical conditions, such as echocardiograms, thyroid USGs, breast USGs, pelvic USGs, and abdominal USGs. USG is considered the safest medical imaging examination; therefore,

it is widely known as a method for inspecting fetal health and development during pregnancy (Figure 14.5(a) and (b)).

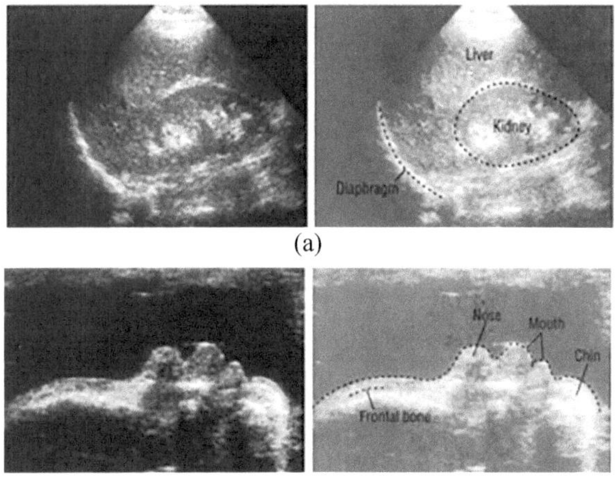

(b)

FIGURE 14.5 (a) Abdominal USG. (b) Fetal USG.

6. **Fluoroscopy:** It is a type of diagnostic radiography that uses X-rays to produce moving images or a live video of the internal body parts. In some cases, these authentic images are necessary (Powsner et al., 2013). For example, fluoroscopy monitors the changes in the flow of contrast in the digestive tract, while a barium enema study supervises progress during the insertion of a pacemaker. Due to continuous images, radiation exposure in this examination is higher than in X-ray examinations (Figure 14.6).

7. **Nuclear Medicine Scans:** Also commonly known as nuclear imaging, radionuclide imaging, or nuclear scans, this examination includes a radioactive material that is swallowed by the patient, making the patient's body a radiation source. A device known as a gamma camera detects the emitted radiation from the patient's body and creates images of the internal body parts. It helps doctors find tumors and determine how much the cancer has spread in the patient's body, which describes the cancer's stage (Gupta et al., 2013). These nuclear scans may also be used to assess the effectiveness of treatment. Some of the nuclear medicine scans include PET scan, thyroid scan, arthrogram, thallium, and cardio Lyte test, virtual colonoscopy, and bone scan (Figure 14.7).

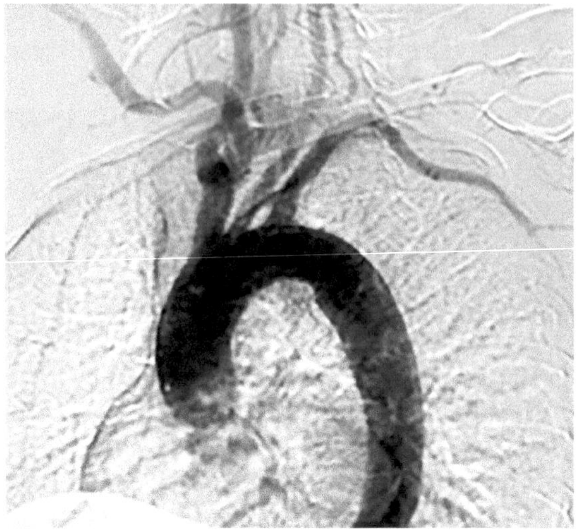

FIGURE 14.6 Aorta fluoroscopy scan.

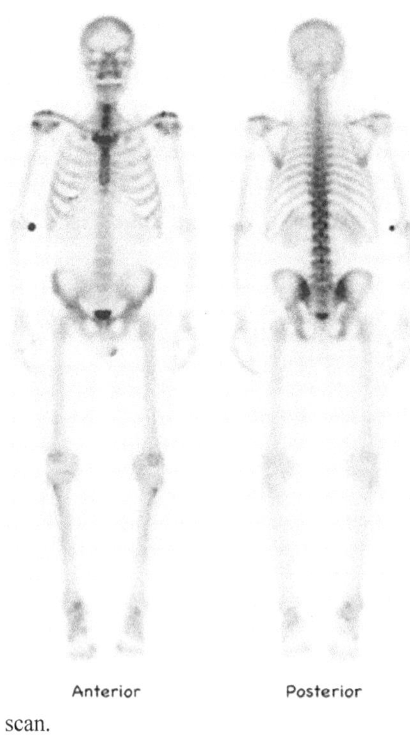

FIGURE 14.7 Bone scan.

14.2.2 INTERVENTIONAL RADIOGRAPHY

Interventional radiography uses imaging techniques like CT, MRI, USG, and fluoroscopy to help and guide procedures. This radiography is also helpful for physicians to insert wires, catheters, and other required instruments and tools into the patient's body. This basically involves small cuts (incisions) (Powsner et al., 2013).

Interventional technology can identify or cure conditions in almost any part of the human body by looking inside the patient's body directly through a camera (scope) or by open surgery. An interventional radiologist is also involved in curing cancers or tumors, blockages in veins and arteries, uterine fibroids, and pain in the back, as well as kidney and liver problems. Interventional procedures include angioplasty, embolization, tube ablation, vertebroplasty, kyphoplasty, breast biopsy, placement of feeding tubes, and catheter placement such as ports and Peripherally Inserted Central Catheter (PICC) (Powsner et al., 2013).

1. **Angioplasty:** It is a procedure for widening a narrowed or obstructed blood vessel mechanically due to atherosclerosis. In an angioplasty procedure, under fluoroscopic guidance, a balloon-tipped catheter is passed into an artery and positioned at the area of the narrowed vessel. The balloon part of the catheter is then inflated, which opens the vessel. Once the obstruction is removed, the balloon is deflated and removed. During the angioplasty procedure, a small wire or a mesh tube called a stent may also be placed in the newly opened artery permanently to help it remain open and work properly (Powsner et al., 2013). Therefore, it is also known as a stent placement procedure (Figure 14.8).

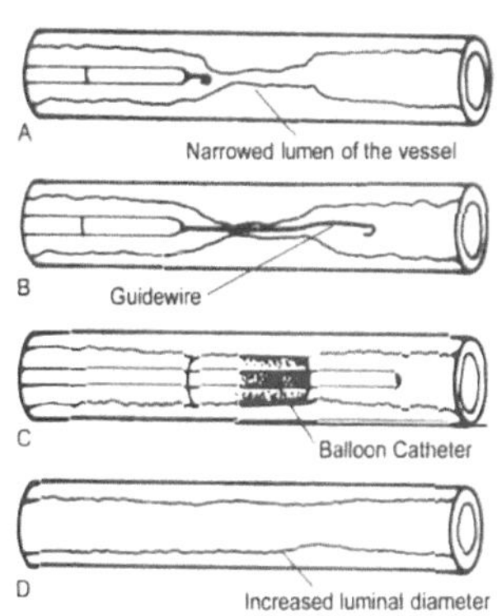

FIGURE 14.8 Balloon catheter angioplasty.

2. **Embolization:** It is defined as the introduction of various substances into the circulation to prevent hemorrhage and tumors by stopping their blood supply (Powsner et al., 2013) (Figure 14.9).

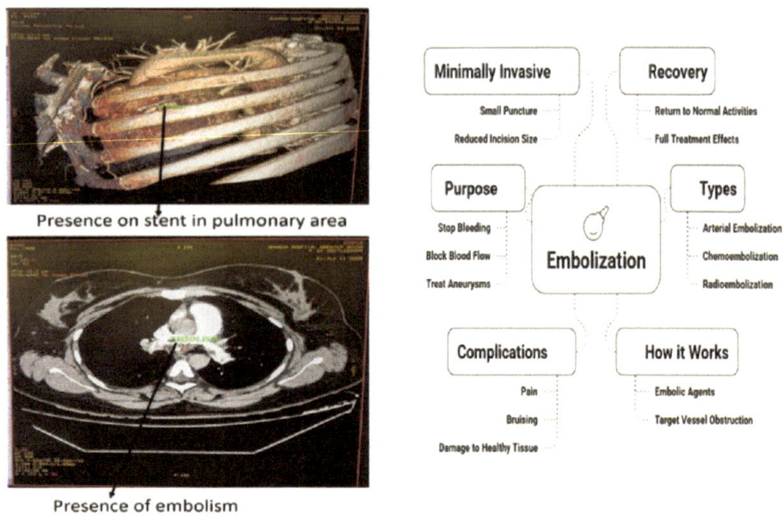

FIGURE 14.9 Bronchial vein embolism.

3. **Vertebroplasty:** It is a procedure performed to treat spinal compression fracture. In this procedure medical-grade bone cement is injected directly into the fractured vertebra (Powsner, et al., 2013). This cement hardens quickly and acts like an internal cast (Figure 14.10).

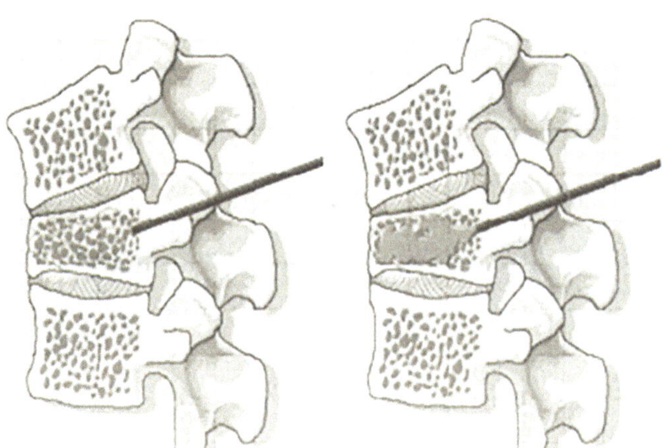

FIGURE 14.10 Cement injection in vertebrae.

4. **Biopsy:** It is a procedure of removing a piece of tissue or a sample of cells from a patient's body so that it can be tested in a laboratory (Powsner et al., 2013) (Figure 14.11).

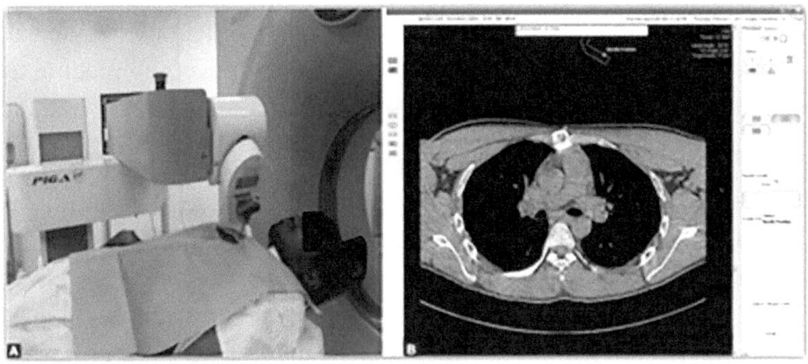

FIGURE 14.11 Sternal biopsy.

14.2.3 THERAPY RADIOGRAPHY

In therapy radiography, we do not try to create diagnostic images but use the biological effects of radiation to kill the tumor cells. At the same time, we try to cause as little damage as possible to the healthy cells in the body. Some distinct types of radiation treatment methods are teletherapy, brachytherapy, and radionuclide therapy (Graham and Paul, 2003) (Figure 14.12).

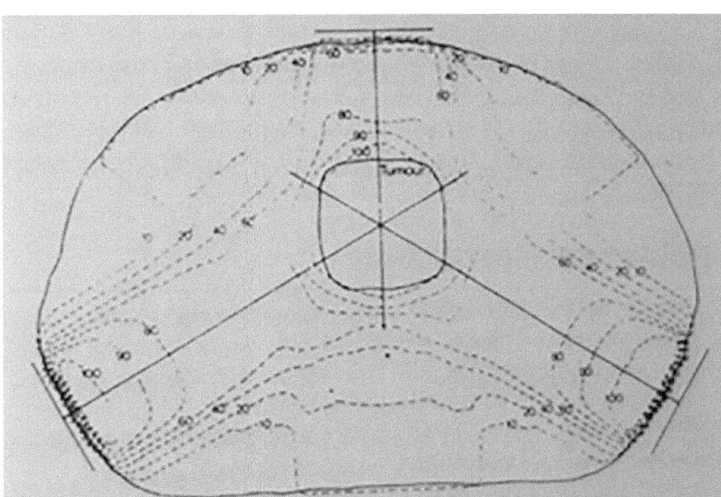

FIGURE 14.12 Examples of radiotherapy treatment plans.

1. **Teletherapy:** In this an external radiation source normally x-rays or gamma rays is directed at the tumor. This is often achieved by treating the tumor from a number of fields. When the treatment plan has been produced, the positions of the treatment fields on the patient are checked by a simulator where the treatment angles can be set up in accurate position and immobilization is achieved by placing the part in a specially prepared clear plastic shell (Graham and Paul, 2003).
2. **Brachytherapy:** When the external radiation beam directed to the tumor cells, the radiation also travel through the healthy tissues to reach the tumor. This technique means that a large dose can be delivered to the tumor while a much smaller dose strikes the surrounding tissues because of the effects of the Inverse Square law. This technique is often used in the treatment of pelvic cancers (Graham and Paul, 2003).
3. **Radionuclide Therapy:** A third possibility is that the radiation can be delivered to the tissue by allowing the tissues to absorb a certain radionuclide. If we take an example of the treatment of an overactive thyroid gland. The activity of the gland can be reduced by removing part of the gland surgically or some of its tissues may be destroyed using radiation. The patient is given an oral solution of sodium iodine where the iodine is in the form of I (a beta particle emitter) results in a radiation dose to the thyroid tissue which reduces its metabolic rate to normal. Some of these isotopes are taken up by the gland and the rest is secreted in the urine. Because of the limited range of beta particles produced, there is less radiation dose to the structures around the thyroid than there would be if we used an external radiation dose (Graham and Paul, 2003).

KEYWORDS

- **angioplasty**
- **computed tomography**
- **fluoroscopy**
- **interventional radiologist**
- **kyphoplasty**

- **magnetic resonance imaging**
- **nuclear medicine**
- **static images**
- **therapy radiography**
- **tube ablation**
- **uterine fibroids**

REFERENCES

Cherryman, G. (2005). Clark's positioning in radiography. *British Dental Journal, 199*(11), 752–752.

Graham, D. T., & Paul, C. (2003). *Principles of Radiological Physics.*

Gupta, A. K., Chowdhury, V., & Khandelwal, N. (2013). *Diagnostic Radiology: Recent Advances and Applied Physics in Imaging.*

Powsner, R. A., Palmer, M. R., & Powsner, E. R. (2013). *Essentials of Nuclear Medicine Physics and Instrumentation.* John Wiley & Sons.

CHAPTER 15

Interpretation of Imaging and Radiology Results

ANKUSH VERMA,[1,*] AMIT PRATAP SINGH CHOUHAN,[2] and VANDANA SINGH[3]

[1]*Department of Radiology, Sharda School of Allied Health Sciences, Sharda University, Greater Noida, Uttar Pradesh, India*

[2]*Department of Radiology, School of Allied Health Sciences, Galgotias University, Greater Noida, Uttar Pradesh, India*

[3]*Department of Microbiology, Sharda School of Allied Health Sciences, Sharda University, Greater Noida, Uttar Pradesh, India*

*Corresponding author

ABSTRACT

The interpretation of imaging and radiology results plays a pivotal role in modern healthcare, influencing diagnostic accuracy and treatment decisions. This chapter explores the significance of accurate interpretation, emphasizing the integration of advanced imaging technologies such as MRI, CT scans, and X-rays. It delves into the complexities faced by radiologists in deciphering subtle nuances and abnormalities, highlighting the evolving role of artificial intelligence (AI) in aiding diagnostics. The abstract also addresses the interdisciplinary collaboration required for comprehensive patient care, discussing challenges and advancements in communication between radiologists and clinicians. Ultimately, it underscores the critical impact of precise imaging interpretation on patient outcomes and the advancement of medical practice.

Allied Healthcare in Practice: An Introduction to Integrated Patient Care. Sally Lukose, Karuna Singh (Eds.)

DOI: 10.1201/9781998511037-18

15.1 INTRODUCTION

The process of interpreting medical images obtained through various imaging methods such as X-rays, CT scans, MRIs, and ultrasound (USG) is known as imaging and radiology results interpretation (Umar and Atabo, 2019). Radiologists and other healthcare professionals utilize these images to diagnose and treat a broad variety of diseases and conditions. The interpretation of imaging data comprises a detailed analysis of the pictures, which includes evaluating the size, shape, density, and texture of the tissues and organs that were studied (Lubner et al., 2017). Furthermore, radiologists examine the images for any abnormalities or irregularities that might indicate a medical issue. The radiologist will prepare a report summarizing their study of the images and providing a diagnosis. In most circumstances, the report will include detailed information on the images, any abnormalities or areas of concern, and recommendations for future testing or treatment. It's important to remember that interpreting imaging data requires broad knowledge and expertise and should only be performed by licensed healthcare professionals like radiologists (Waite et al., 2019). For an accurate diagnosis and efficient treatment of medical disorders, correct interpretation of imaging results is essential.

Interpreting imaging and radiology data is a crucial component of contemporary medicine since it enables medical practitioners to view the human body's interior components without undergoing any invasive procedures (Umar and Atabo, 2019). It is essential to the diagnosis, staging, and monitoring of many different illnesses and ailments, including cancer, heart disease, and neurological problems. There are several different imaging techniques used in medicine, each with advantages and disadvantages (Kasban et al., 2015). X-rays are frequently used to see bones and other hard tissues, whereas CT scans and MRI are better suited for imaging soft tissues like the brain, liver, and lungs (Lusic and Grinstaff, 2013). When pregnant, USG is frequently used to check the internal organs of the abdomen and to track the growth of the fetus. The interpretation of imaging and radiology data necessitates significant understanding of anatomy, physiology, and pathology, as well as skill in the imaging technology being employed (Van der et al., 2014). Radiologists and other healthcare professionals who specialize in imaging are educated to see tiny changes and variances in images that might signal a medical problem. Effective communication between radiologists and other healthcare physicians is essential for ensuring that imaging results are correctly reviewed and acted upon. Radiologists must provide non-specialists with clear and succinct findings, while healthcare professionals must be able to assess the data and use it to contribute to clinical decision-making.

The interpretation of imaging and radiography data is not a one-size-fits-all methodology, and the method may differ based on the patient's age, medical history, and symptoms (Tuena et al., 2020). A pediatric radiologist, for example, may consider various factors when interpreting imaging records in a child compared to an adult. The interpretation of imaging data may include some doubt or uncertainty, particularly if the imaging findings are ambiguous or do not conclusively point to a certain diagnosis (Harrison, 1999). Imaging tests or other diagnostic procedures may be essential in such circumstances to establish a more accurate diagnosis. The interpretation of imaging data is also highly susceptible to possible errors or constraints, such as methodological errors in imaging equipment or human error throughout the interpretation process. To reduce these risks, imaging services may have quality control procedures in place, such as routine radiologist peer reviews and imaging equipment calibration and repairs (Williamson et al., 2008). In recent years, the use of machine learning and AI algorithms to aid in the interpretation of imaging data has gained popularity. These technologies have the potential to increase the precision and efficacy of image interpretation while evaluating vast volumes of imaging data (Buchberger et al., 2018). Overall, the process of analyzing imaging and radiology data is vital and complex, necessitating specialized knowledge and experience (Sitapati et al., 2017). Radiologists and other healthcare practitioners can help improve patient outcomes and ensure that patients receive appropriate therapy for their medical concerns by delivering accurate and timely diagnoses (Langlotz et al., 2019).

15.2 IMAGING TECHNIQUES

Radiology is a medical specialty that uses imaging procedures to analyze and treat disorders. Imaging technologies are often used in health diagnostics. The interpretation of imaging and radiography data demands a detailed understanding of human anatomy and physiology. Here we will discuss some of the most often used imaging modalities aimed at diagnosing illnesses, as well as exactly how their outcomes are interpreted (Figure 15.1).

1. **Imaging with X-ray:** Radiologists use X-ray images to read anomalies for better treatment of patients, for instance, the presence of a tumor, change in the shape or size of an organ, and so forth (Mustapha et al., 2021). The interior organs are scanned by using the X-ray imaging technique, a non-invasive diagnostic approach. This instrument is often employed for the identification of diseases or disorders of the gastrointestinal tract, lungs, and bones.
2. **Using Computed Tomography (CT) Scanning:** Computed tomography produces detailed pictures of the inner anatomical structures by using a series of X-ray scans taken from various projections. This method is one of the best for the analysis of injuries, diseases, tumors, and so forth. This helps radiologists to better diagnose anomalies, such as the presence of a mass or a change in the shape or morphology of an organ (Irum et al., 2012).
3. **Imaging with Magnetic Resonance Imaging (MRI):** This is among the non-invasive diagnostic methods that create finely precise clinically important images of the human body's interior organs by using radio waves along with a strong magnetic field (Siddiq, 2020). This technique is frequently used for the detection of cancer, brain, and spinal cord diseases, injury to soft tissues, and so forth. This technique is among the key diagnostic tools for radiologists as it helps in the analysis of anomalies, such as the presence of malignant or benign cancer, or an anomaly in the shape or size of an organ.
4. **Imaging with Ultrasound:** Ultrasound imaging is also a non-invasive diagnostic procedure that applies high-frequency sound waves to generate images of internal organs. This scan is one of the most important tools for the diagnosis of pregnancy, heart disease, genital tract infection, calculus, intestinal difficulties, and so forth. This scan helps the radiologists in the analysis of deformities, such as the existence of a tumor or an alteration in the shape or size of an organ or body parts.
5. **Imaging with Nuclear Medicine:** Nuclear medicine imaging is a technique that produces images of the internal organs by using minute quantities of radioactive material such as FDG, iodine,

technetium, and so forth. This imaging technique is frequently used to identify oncogenic structures, heart disease, bone disorders, and so forth. This helps the radiologists to look up the regions of aberrant activity in nuclear medicine scans/images that might relate to the existence of a disease or sickness.

6. **Imaging with Positron Emission Tomography (PET) Scan:** PET scan imaging is a radiological diagnostic technique that uses radioactive material such as FDG and iodine to provide radiological images of the human body's metabolic activity. PET scan imaging is commonly done to identify cancer, heart disease, and brain disorders (Phelps, 2000). To interpret PET scan results, radiologists read out the areas of abnormal metabolic activity in the films that may indicate the presence of a disease or sickness.
7. **Imaging with Mammography:** Mammography is a kind of radiological imaging that is used to identify and diagnose breast cancer. Before depicting the findings of a mammography, radiologists analyze the breast tissues for detecting any kind of anomalous densities, lumps, or calcifications.
8. **Fluoroscopy Imaging:** Fluoroscopy is a type of radiological imaging procedure that uses continuous X-rays to diagnose any moving organs such as the circulatory and digestive systems. To check for anomalies in the data, radiologists assess the motion or form of the structures being inspected by fluoroscopy.
9. **Angiography:** Angiography is a radio-imaging procedure that uses X-ray imaging and contrast material to image the blood vessels in the human body through radiography. Angiography is generally used to diagnose and treat arterial disease of the cardiovascular system. Angiography imaging procedures are being imaged and examined by radiologists to see any kind of blockages, narrowing, or anomalies in the blood vessels (Weinreich et al., 2017).
10. **Dual-Energy X-ray Absorptiometry (DEXA):** DEXA is a diagnostic procedure that utilizes X-rays to assess bone density, detect abnormal anatomy, and identify pathologies like osteoporosis. Radiologists diagnose cases with low bone density, which may indicate a higher risk of bone fractures.

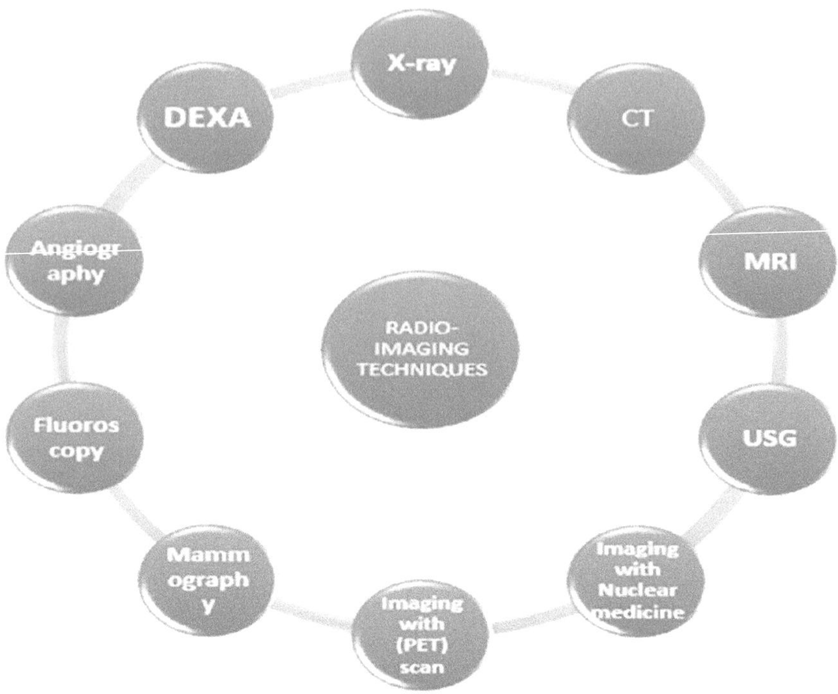

FIGURE 15.1 List of various radio imaging techniques used in patient care.

15.3 FINDINGS

Findings in imaging, diagnostics, and radiology are used as critical diagnostic tools by healthcare practitioners and radiologists to examine and treat a comprehensive range of medically related diseases (Makanjee et al., 2015). To interpret and diagnose the appropriate course of therapy for the patient, these imaged data from radiography must be carefully evaluated. Healthcare practitioners, such as radiologists, should keep the following important points in mind when assessing imaging and radiographic data (Hardy and Harvey, 2020):

1. **Location and Size of Pathologies/Anomalies:** The location and size of pathologies such as tumors, cysts, or lesions are assessed based on radio-imaging results. By examining and assessing the locations of these pathologies, healthcare workers can determine and identify the severity of the illness and the extent to which it has spread to other parts of the body. The severity of the anomalies

can help determine the stage of the disease, which can further provide the best therapeutic course.

2. **Shape and Appearance of Anomalies:** Anomalies in radio-imaging and radiography can be determined by their shape and exterior appearance, which can provide useful diagnostic information. The presence of an anomaly may assist medical practitioners in classifying different severities of illnesses or disorders.
3. **Density and Contrast of Tissues:** The final results of imaging and radiography show the body's various tissue densities based on X-ray attenuation. In X-ray imaging procedures, less dense tissues, such as muscle, appear darker than denser tissues, such as bone, which appears white. Some tissues or structures can be viewed more clearly during radio-imaging procedures by utilizing contrast media or dye.
4. **Blood Flow and Perfusion:** Radio-imaging procedures that can provide information on blood flow and perfusion to different body areas include CT scans and MRIs. This data, acquired after performing the perfusion procedure, can be used to analyze and assess disorders such as stroke or heart disease. For example, CT angiography can be used to diagnose any blood vessel disease and identify areas of occlusion or constriction.
5. **Structural Abnormalities:** The final outcomes of radio-imaging and radiography can reveal structural deformities such as bone fractures, dislocations, or herniation. This information from radio-imaging may be useful in identifying the best treatment options, such as surgery or immobilization.
6. **Presence of Fluid or Air:** Imaging technology investigations identify the presence of liquid or air in a patient's body. A radiological chest X-ray imaging, for example, can reveal the presence of air in the lungs, which may indicate the presence of pneumothorax or a collapsed lung. Radio-imaging investigations can also determine the presence of fluid in the abdomen, such as ascites or pleural effusion.
7. **Changes Over Time:** Radiology investigation outcomes are used to track and trace changes in the size or appearance of abnormalities

over time. This can be helpful in tracking, identifying, and analyzing the progression of a disease and the follow-up of the effectiveness of a therapy. Following therapy, different imaging scans may be undertaken to determine and analyze whether the pathologies have not resurfaced or grown in size.

8. **Calcifications:** Calcifications are calcium deposits that can be seen on radio-imaging procedures such as mammograms, X-rays, or CT scans. Soft tissue calcification is commonly seen and caused by a wide range of pathologies. The most commonly recommended procedures to identify calcifications are X-ray and CT.
9. **Inflammation:** Inflammation can be identified and analyzed on radio-imaging investigations such as MRIs or CT scans by the presence of edema, increased blood flow, or changes in tissue density. Inflammation in any body part can be a symptom of a more serious condition, such as an infection or an autoimmune disease.
10. **Functional Imaging:** PET scans and functional MRIs, for example, can be used to evaluate the function of numerous organs and tissues throughout the body, most commonly for neuro-imaging. These radio-imaging procedures can detect metabolic, blood flow, or oxygenation anomalies that may indicate the level of severity of a disease.

15.4 DIAGNOSIS

Radiology and imaging are used to detect and diagnose medical diseases. A thorough identification and assessment of medical images, including X-rays, CT scans, MRIs, and USGs, is required. These radiological images are analyzed by radiologists, who are medical experts with expertise in analyzing medical imaging, to detect abnormalities or changes in a patient's body (Hosny et al., 2018). Radio-imaging investigations also compare current and previous patient conditions to see how they evolve over time. A physician or specialist physician requests the necessary tests to begin the process of medical imaging diagnosis. Once the radio-imaging procedures have been completed and images are extracted, a radiologist identifies and examines the images to check for any abnormalities or changes in the patient's body. Radiologists analyze the images to look for any abnormal patterns, variations, and other pathologies that might help with diagnosis. Radio-imaging and radiological image interpretation are important measures in modern medicine, helping medical practitioners and healthcare workers identify and diagnose ailments ranging from shattered bone fractures to cancerous pathologies. A precise medical diagnosis using radio-imaging investigations requires the expertise and knowledge of a radiology physician who can identify and analyze minute or small anomalies and changes in the images that would otherwise go unreported. After identifying and analyzing the diagnosis, the specialist physician may prepare an appropriate treatment plan for the patient. In modern medicine, radio-imaging and radiology image interpretation are important techniques for both diagnostic and therapeutic planning. Specialized physicians can better understand what is going on within a patient's body with the help of medical imaging investigations. Radiological investigations also help in tracking therapeutic progress and detecting anomalies through which the patient is suffering. Besides identifying and analyzing abnormalities and changes in the patient's body, radiologists can also help physicians choose the best course of action against the abnormalities in the patient's body. A radiologist, for example, may recommend more radio-imaging tests, a biopsy, or surgery based on the results (Mitra and Shankar, 2014). Medical imaging investigations are used in a variety of medical specialties, such as neurology, oncology, cardiology, and orthopedics, to check for any major or minor pathologies. Advancements in medical imaging technology have resulted in the improvement of innovative imaging investigations that can create more detailed, enhanced images and improve diagnostic accuracy (Doi, 2006). 3D imaging, multi-planar imaging, SSD, and computer-assisted diagnosis (CAD), for example, have revolutionized radiology, allowing radiologists to view the body in more detail, across more planes, and with greater clarity than ever before.

Differential diagnosis plays a crucial role in radiology and radiological image interpretation. Radiologists must evaluate and analyze a wide range of probable illnesses before making a final decision on diagnosis based on previous and current medical images (Pesapane et al., 2018). The practice of comparing the patient's current symptoms and previous medical history through the results of medical images is known as differential diagnosis. During a medical diagnosis, radiologists must consider additional factors such as the medical history, patient's age, gender, and overall health. For example, if a patient complains of chest pain, the radiologist may request radio-imaging investigations, such as an X-ray or CT scan, to evaluate and analyze the chest region. Based on the radiological scans and investigations, the radiologist will consider a variety of possible diagnoses, such as pneumothorax, collapsed lung, pneumonia, or lung cancer. After analyzing the investigation results, the radiologist will use their knowledge and expertise to narrow down the number of probable diagnoses before making a final conclusion. In rare cases, further radio-imaging tests may be required to confirm a diagnosis or rule out other probable disorders. For example, if a patient's chest X-ray reveals a concerning lump, the radiologist may request a biopsy or additional radio-imaging tests, such as a PET scan, to determine and confirm whether the growth is cancerous or not. Differential diagnosis is a critical method of investigation for ensuring that patients receive the correct diagnosis and treatment for their disease. A mistake by a radiologist or specialist physician can have serious consequences for the patient's health; hence, radiologists must take a thorough approach to imaging and radiological image interpretation.

Differential diagnosis is especially important in radio-imaging and radiological image interpretation when the patient presents with non-specific symptoms or symptoms that might be caused by a range of disorders. For example, a patient suffering from stomach pain might be experiencing appendicitis, diverticulitis, or an ovarian cyst. The radiologist must carefully evaluate and analyze the imaging test results to determine the most probable diagnosis (Lumbreras et al., 2010). In other circumstances, imaging investigation findings may be imprecise or display contradictory signals, which makes a specific diagnosis more difficult to establish. In some severe situations, radiologists may communicate with medical specialists, such as a specialist or a multidisciplinary team, to ensure that the patient receives the most accurate medical diagnosis and appropriate treatment.

15.5 CLINICAL CORRELATION

Understanding radio-imaging investigations and radiographic results relies heavily on clinical correlation. Clinical correlation requires examining the patient's clinical history and presentation, as well as the imaging data, in order to arrive at an accurate radio-imaging diagnosis and treatment plan (Mitra and Shankar, 2015). Clinical correlation is the process of correlating imaging data with clinical complaint information such as symptoms, physical examination, and test findings to arrive at an accurate diagnosis. It requires physicians to consider the patient's medical history, age, gender, and any comorbidities.

For example, a patient with a medical history of lung cancer would undergo a chest X-ray or CT scan to track the progression of the lung cancer. If an X-ray or CT scan reveals a new lung nodule, the radiologist must decide whether it is a newly developed tumor or a metastasis from an earlier malignancy. Physicians and radiologists must also take into account the patient's symptoms, such as coughing or breathing difficulties, as well as any recent changes to their health (Gunderman et al., 2001).

15.5.1 IMPORTANCE OF CLINICAL CORRELATION

Clinical correlation is important for several reasons. First of all, it ensures that radio-imaging findings are interpreted and analyzed in the correct clinical perspective (Kuhl and Schild, 2000). Imaging investigation outcomes in some patients may be absolutely innocuous, while in others, they may be symptoms of a serious underlying condition. As a result, in order to determine if any radio-imaging findings are significant, a radiologist must have clear information about the patient's clinical history. Secondly, clinical correlation also assists in suggesting the avoidance of unnecessary diagnostic tests and procedures. For example, a patient with a prolonged history of back pain may undergo an MRI scan that may indicate a herniated disc or any other pathology. Third, clinical correlation of the patient's symptoms with radio-imaging also helps improve the chances of diagnostic accuracy and precision. When the extracted imaging data is unsatisfactory, clinical correlation may help identify and analyze additional diagnostic investigations that may be necessary and helpful to obtain an accurate conclusive diagnosis. Additionally, clinical correlation can also help prevent misdiagnosis or delayed diagnosis of any severe disease in the patient, both of which can have major consequences for patient outcomes if not diagnosed earlier. Clinical correlation is a crucial aspect of assessing radio-imaging and radiology results. For accurate diagnosis, imaging findings must be combined with clinical data (Mitra and Shankar, 2014). Clinical correlation is also essential for interpreting imaging data in the context of the patient, reducing unnecessary diagnostic investigations and therapies, and improving diagnostic accuracy. Radiologists and specialist physicians must be aware of the importance of clinical correlation, and both must work thoroughly together to provide the most accurate and useful diagnostic information for patient care (Chou et al., 2011).

15.6 CONCLUSION

Medical diagnosis and therapeutic planning for any pathologies rely heavily on the radiological interpretation of imaging and radiographic data. Radiology is a branch of medicine that uses different radio waves and magnetic properties to diagnose and treat diseases using radio imaging investigations such as X-rays, USG, MRI, CT scans, and PET scans. Interpreting imaging and radiology data requires specific expertise, experience, knowledge, and abilities to detect any anomalies in a patient's anatomy and physiological structure, as well as the interpretation of various imaging modalities. Radiologists are medical professionals who specialize in the interpretation, identification, and analysis of medical images from different modalities. When analyzing imaging and radiography data, radiologists must look for abnormalities or changes in any structure of a patient's organs, tissues, and bones. These anomalies seen in medical imaging may indicate the presence of a disease or injury. After identifying and analyzing imaging, radiologists may look for signs of inflammation, infection, or malignancies. In some cases, imaging and radiology data can provide a conclusive and accurate diagnosis; for example, a CT scan may indicate a kidney stone, and an MRI may reveal a herniated disc in the spine. A complete medical evaluation of a patient includes a medical history, physical examination, and laboratory tests, which play an essential role in establishing an accurate, precise diagnosis and creating an appropriate treatment plan.

Imaging and radiographic findings can provide radiologists, physicians, and other healthcare providers with essential information about a patient's condition. These interpreted data can help define the extent and severity of an injury or disease, follow the progression of any severe condition, or assess the success of a treatment approach. One advantage of imaging and radiology investigations is that they are non-invasive or minimally invasive procedures, which means they do not require surgery or other invasive treatments. Minimally invasive investigations make them a useful tool for diagnosis and therapy since they can provide important information without putting the patient's life at risk of complications. However, analyzing radio-imaging and radiography data requires specialist experience and competence. It is also important to understand that imaging and radiography findings can sometimes be misleading, resulting in false positives or false negatives. For example, a benign tumor may appear concerning on a CT scan, leading to more testing or even unnecessary surgery, which is a disadvantage. Similarly, cancer may not be clearly seen on imaging investigations until it has grown sufficiently, resulting in a delay in detection and treatment, leading to the severity of the disease.

In brief, interpreting imaging and radiology data is an essential part of medical diagnosis and therapeutic planning for any pathologies. Radiologists use their knowledge, expertise, and experience to detect any abnormalities or changes in the structure or function of organs, tissues, and bones. Overall, image interpretation and radiographic data involve a careful study, identification, and analysis of all relevant information, including the patient's medical history and physical exam. When radiographic data is used effectively and in conjunction with other diagnostic technologies, imaging and radiography may be powerful tools for improving patient outcomes and providing critical insights into the patient's condition.

KEYWORDS

- **computed tomography**
- **imaging modalities**
- **magnetic resonance imaging**
- **positron emission tomography**
- **radio imaging investigation**
- **radiographic data**
- **radiological interpretation**
- **therapeutic planning**

REFERENCES

Buchberger, A. R., DeLaney, K., Johnson, J., & Li, L. (2018). Mass spectrometry imaging: A review of emerging advancements and future insights. *Analytical Chemistry, 90*(1), 240–244.

Chou, R., Qaseem, A., Owens, D. K., Shekelle, P., & Physicians. (2011). Diagnostic imaging for low back pain: Advice for high-value health care from the American College of Physicians. *Annals of Internal Medicine, 154*(3), 181–189.

Doi, K. (2006). Diagnostic imaging over the last 50 years: Research and development in medical imaging science and technology. *Physics in Medicine & Biology, 51*(13), R5.

Gunderman, R. B., Phillips, M. D., & Cohen, M. D. (2001). Improving clinical histories on radiology requisitions. *Academic Radiology, 8*(4), 299–303.

Hardy, M., & Harvey, H. (2020). Artificial intelligence in diagnostic imaging: Impact on the radiography profession. *The British Journal of Radiology, 93*(1108), 20190840.

Harrison, P. J. (1999). The neuropathology of schizophrenia: A critical review of the data and their interpretation. *Brain, 122*(4), 593–624.

Hosny, A., Parmar, C., Quackenbush, J., Schwartz, L. H., & Aerts, H. J. (2018). Artificial intelligence in radiology. *Nature Reviews Cancer, 18*(8), 500–510.

Irum, I., Raza, M., & Sharif, M. (2012). Morphological techniques for medical images: A review. *Research Journal of Applied Sciences, Engineering and Technology, 4*(17), 2948–2962.

Kasban, H., El-Bendary, M., & Salama, D. (2015). A comparative study of medical imaging techniques. *International Journal of Information Science and Intelligent Systems, 4*(2), 37–58.

Kuhl, C. K., & Schild, H. H. (2000). Dynamic image interpretation of MRI of the breast. *Journal of Magnetic Resonance Imaging, 12*(6), 965–974.

Langlotz, C. P., Allen, B., Erickson, B. J., Kalpathy-Cramer, J., Bigelow, K., Cook, T. S., Flanders, A. E., Lungren, M. P., Mendelson, D. S., & Rudie, J. D. (2019). A roadmap for foundational research on artificial intelligence in medical imaging: From the 2018 NIH/RSNA/ACR/The Academy Workshop. *Radiology, 291*(3), 781–791.

Lubner, M. G., Smith, A. D., Sandrasegaran, K., Sahani, D. V., & Pickhardt, P. J. (2017). CT texture analysis: Definitions, applications, biologic correlates, and challenges. *Radiographics, 37*(5), 1483–1503.

Lumbreras, B., Donat, L., & Hernández-Aguado, I. (2010). Incidental findings in imaging diagnostic tests: A systematic review. *The British Journal of Radiology, 83*(988), 276–289.

Lusic, H., & Grinstaff, M. W. (2013). X-ray computed tomography contrast agents. *Chemical Reviews, 113*(3), 1641–1666.

Makanjee, C. R., Hoffmann, W. A., & Bergh, A. M. (2015). Healthcare provider and patient perspectives on diagnostic imaging investigations. *African Journal of Primary Health Care and Family Medicine, 7*(1), 1–10.

Mitra, S., & Shankar, B. U. (2014). Integrating radio imaging with gene expressions toward a personalized management of cancer. *IEEE Transactions on Human-Machine Systems, 44*(5), 664–677.

Mitra, S., & Shankar, B. U. (2015). Medical image analysis for cancer management in natural computing framework. *Information Sciences, 306*, 111–131.

Mustapha, M. T., Uzun, B., Ozsahin, D. U., & Ozsahin, I. (2021). A comparative study of X-ray based medical imaging devices. In *Applications of Multi-Criteria Decision-Making Theories in Healthcare and Biomedical Engineering* (pp. 163–180). Elsevier.

Pesapane, F., Codari, M., & Sardanelli, F. (2018). Artificial intelligence in medical imaging: Threat or opportunity? Radiologists again at the forefront of innovation in medicine. *European Radiology Experimental, 2*, 1–10.

Phelps, M. E. (2000). Positron emission tomography provides molecular imaging of biological processes. *Proceedings of the National Academy of Sciences, 97*(16), 9226–9233.

Siddiq, M. (2020). ML-based medical image analysis for anomaly detection in CT scans, X-rays, and MRIs. *Devotion Journal of Community Service, 2*(1), 53–64.

Sitapati, A., Kim, H., Berkovich, B., Marmor, R., Singh, S., El-Kareh, R., Clay, B., & Ohno-Machado, L. (2017). Integrated precision medicine: The role of electronic health records in delivering personalized treatment. *Wiley Interdisciplinary Reviews: Systems Biology and Medicine, 9*(3), 1378.

Tuena, C., Semonella, M., Fernández-Álvarez, J., Colombo, D., & Cipresso, P. (2020). Predictive precision medicine: Towards the computational challenge. In *P5 eHealth: An Agenda for the Health Technologies of the Future* (pp. 71–86).

Umar, A., & Atabo, S. (2019). A review of imaging techniques in scientific research/clinical diagnosis. *MOJ Anatomy & Physiology, 6*(5), 175–183.

Van der Gijp, A., Van der Schaaf, M., Van der Schaaf, I., Huige, J., Ravesloot, C., Van Schaik, J., & Ten Cate, T. J. (2014). Interpretation of radiological images: Towards a framework of knowledge and skills. *Advances in Health Sciences Education, 19*, 565–580.

Waite, S., Grigorian, A., Alexander, R. G., Macknik, S. L., Carrasco, M., Heeger, D. J., & Martinez-Conde, S. (2019). Analysis of perceptual expertise in radiology–Current knowledge and a new perspective. *Frontiers in Human Neuroscience, 13*, 213–215.

Weinreich, M., Litwok, Y., Mui, L. W., & Lau, J. F. (2017). Advanced vascular imaging. *Vascular Medicine, 22*(1), 73–76.

Williamson, J. F., Dunscombe, P. B., Sharpe, M. B., Thomadsen, B. R., Purdy, J. A., & Deye, J. A. (2008). Quality assurance needs for modern image-based radiotherapy: Recommendations from the 2007 interorganizational symposium on "Quality assurance of radiation therapy: Challenges of advanced technology." *International Journal of Radiation Oncology Biology Physics, 71*(1), S2–S12.

CHAPTER 16

Rehabilitation and Therapy: An Overview

MEENAKSHI VERMA,[1] PRAGYA DUTT,[2] and RACHNA[3]

[1]*Department of Physiotherapy, Sharda School of Allied Health Sciences, Sharda University, Greater Noida, Uttar Pradesh, India*

[2]*Select Rehabilitation Nursing Home, Southwood Heights Drive, Jamesville, New York, USA*

[3]*Department of Medical Laboratory Technology, Nims college of Allied and health care Sciences, NIIMS University, Jaipur, Rajasthan, India*

*Corresponding author

ABSTRACT

The idea of rehabilitation is one that is spoken about extensively worldwide. This is not unexpected, given that over a billion people globally—more than 15% of the population—live with a handicap. Furthermore, according to a recent report, 2.40 billion individuals globally experience conditions that hinder their capacity to carry out daily tasks and could potentially benefit from rehabilitation services. This implies that one in three individuals will require rehabilitation services at some point during their illness or injury.

There is a wide range of rehabilitation within a patient's course. It includes help with learning basic communication skills, exercise regimens to improve or maintain the best possible health, happiness, and career, and advanced neurological rehabilitation following a serious accident or CVA.

Giving people the skills they need to live life to the fullest is the goal of rehabilitation. It helps people recover knowledge, skills, or talents that

Allied Healthcare in Practice: An Introduction to Integrated Patient Care. Sally Lukose, Karuna Singh (Eds.)

DOI: 10.1201/9781998511037-19

may have been lost or damaged due to disease, accident, or handicap. This chapter deals with the role of the multidisciplinary team in rehabilitation, such as Physical Therapists, Occupational Therapists (OT's), and Speech Therapists.

16.1 INTRODUCTION

Rehabilitation and therapy play an important role in the recovery and improvement of individuals who have experienced physical, psychological, or cognitive impairments due to injury, illness, or other conditions. This chapter provides an overview of rehabilitation and therapy, exploring their goals, principles, and various approaches used to help individuals regain independence and quality of life. There is a lot of discussion about rehabilitation in various parts of the world. This is not at all unexpected considering that more than a billion people—more than 15% of the population—live with some form of disability. Additionally, a recent study indicated that 2.41 billion people, or one in three individuals, suffer from disorders that impair their capacity to perform daily activities and may be helped by rehabilitation therapies.

Maximizing a person's functional ability while concentrating on their present talents is the aim of rehabilitation. Combining and coordinating medical, social, educational, and occupational treatments achieves this. For the disabled person, it prolongs life by increasing productivity and purpose in their daily existence. After curative and preventative care, this is the third stage of medical treatment. By preventing interactions between an agent, a host, and an environment, a disease is initially avoided from arising through preventive medicine. The second stage of medicine, known as curative medicine, aims to treat the condition. Curative medicine is what most doctors practice. The disease-causing agent has been removed from the host in certain cases, like poliomyelitis, yet residual symptoms like paralysis still exist. Rheumatoid arthritis is one such ailment that has no known treatment. As a result, a third stage is required, called rehabilitation, which involves both medical care and social responsibilities.

The earliest possible start of rehabilitation is necessary for the greatest outcomes. It is administered in conjunction with a specific medication or surgical treatment for the underlying condition. Medical or social vocational rehabilitation are both options. Using medical and paramedical expertise to treat a patient is known as medical rehabilitation. The purpose of medical rehabilitation is to reduce impairment. Following medical rehabilitation, or occasionally given along with it, is social vocational rehabilitation. The purpose of social vocational rehabilitation is to limit handicaps.

The World Health Organization (WHO) lists the "enhancement of good health, prevention of diseases, treatment, and palliative care" as other crucial elements of universal health coverage (UHC) in addition to rehabilitation. The purpose of rehabilitation is to enable patients to engage in work, recreational, and educational activities, as well as play major roles in society and become functionally independent in their daily activities (ADL). Rehabilitation is unquestionably crucial to achieving the overall goal of universal health, which promotes the growth of an active and healthy global population, as well as benefits to one's own health.

In rehabilitation, in addition to the underlying medical issues, the user's objectives and preferences are taken into account. Rehabilitation is a very person-centered approach to healthcare. Information on functioning is essential for decision-making since the purpose of rehabilitation is to maximize functioning in the setting of impairments, injuries, and acute or chronic diseases. Throughout the healthcare system:

- Information on user functioning supports goal planning and outcome evaluation throughout the treatment stages of acute care, post-acute care, and long-term care, as well as across the continuum of rehabilitation care (primary, secondary, and tertiary).
- Data on user functioning can be gathered at the program or facility level to improve quality assurance, service planning, and therapy outcomes monitoring.
- Evidence is available for decision-makers to use when organizing healthcare and rehabilitation programs and evaluating their results in the form of aggregated clinical data on functioning.

16.2 REHABILITATION ELEMENTS

Preventive, restorative, supportive, and palliative are the four components of rehabilitation that Dietz (1980) identified in regard to persons with cancer, and which are currently used throughout rehabilitation for a variety of illnesses.

16.2.1 PREVENTIVE REHABILITATION

Preventing or delaying the onset of new impairments is the aim of education, counseling, and therapy, and preserving an individual's degree of proficiency. This kind of treatment is standard procedure for long-term illnesses like cancer, diabetes, chronic obstructive pulmonary disease (COPD), and many neurological problems. It also forms the basis for assisted self-management and can aid in the development of therapies that aim to maintain function for the longest period of time.

Handicap prevention does not simply begin at birth, with the commencement of a disease, or with the occurrence of a main handicap. When genetic counseling is used, it is sometimes possible to anticipate a child's potential for handicap owing to genetic abnormalities or blood type incompatibility before the child is even born. For Duchenne's muscular dystrophy, for instance, it is feasible to advise the parents against having further children in case they get the condition later.

Future population growth, especially among the elderly, will inevitably lead to a substantial rise in the population of people with impairments. The fact that more individuals are surviving potentially deadly conditions like brain damage is paradoxical given the great achievements that medical science has made in that area. Therefore, a decline in mortality must be accompanied by an increase in morbidity. Rehabilitation focuses on both morbidity and quality of life. Unfortunately, the gap between the number of medical and paramedical personnel needed to care for people with disabilities is growing.

Neurologists, orthopedic surgeons, and pediatricians have an increasingly important role in the area of medical rehabilitation in recent years. This situation demonstrates the respect and relevance that rehabilitation medicine is receiving from other professions. If additional effective prevention methods are not developed to shield individuals from main disability in the future, the recently diagnosed impaired persons would face a challenging situation.

Consider a nuclear family where both the husband and the wife are employed. This family would lose all of its joy, leisure, and free time if a disabled child or elderly member were present. Each of its members will have to make a lot of sacrifices on their own in order to care for the sufferer. In the same way that we can currently avoid communicable diseases, the medical community must take action to prevent epidemics of incapacity.

16.2.2 LEVELS OF PREVENTION

Preventive healthcare is any endeavor to stop a person from sliding down the health status scale, while therapeutic healthcare is any effort to bring it up towards the peak, or optimum, health. The WHO divides this entire range into three degrees of prevention (Figure 16.1).

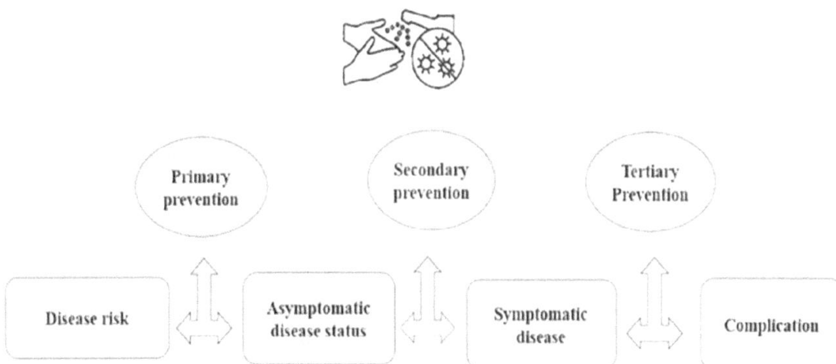

FIGURE 16.1 Different levels of prevention.

16.2.3 RESTORATIVE REHABILITATION

Restorative rehabilitation concentrates on therapies that repair deficits in order to achieve the maximum functional recovery possible, such as diminished respiratory capacity, diminished physical strength, and cognitive decline. Following surgery, illness, or acute events like a serious accident or stroke, this type of therapy is frequently used to help patients regain their fullest possible function.

16.2.4 SUPPORTIVE REHABILITATION

In order to improve a person's capacity for self-care and mobility, supportive rehabilitation uses strategies including teaching compensatory skills or alternative methods of accomplishing tasks, as well as providing self-help resources. This may mean providing assistive devices or making changes to the environment. The term "adaptive rehabilitation" also applies to this.

16.2.5 PALLIATIVE REHABILITATION

Palliative rehabilitation is a service that supports individuals with terminal diseases in living meaningful lives—both physically and socially—while respecting their desires. In order to maximize functional independence and enhance comfort and quality of life, it usually focuses on treating symptoms such as dyspnea, pain, and edema, preventing muscular shortening, providing breathing support, addressing mental health, promoting relaxation, or using assistive technology.

16.3 IMPAIRMENT, DISABILITY, AND HANDICAP

These terms are defined as follows by the International Classification of Impairments, Disabilities, and Handicaps (ICIDH, 1980) of the WHO:

1. **Impairment:** Any loss or deviation from normal anatomical, physiological, or psychological structure or function; for example, losing a finger, a heart's incapacity to pump blood, or certain chemicals that cause Parkinson's disease being absent. Not all impairments result in handicap; for instance, the removal of the pinna in the ear, while an impairment, would only result in an aesthetic deficit rather than hearing loss.
2. **Disability:** Any limitation or inability to perform an activity in a way that is considered typical for a person due to an impairment; walking difficulties after lower limb amputation are one example. It is crucial to emphasize that sports like windsurfing and rock climbing are not included in the list of activities that should be considered for handicap. To be considered handicapped, an individual must be unable to perform everyday tasks that are usual for their age, sex, or physical characteristics.
3. **Handicap:** A handicap is a social disadvantage resulting from an impairment or disability that limits an individual's capacity to fulfill a function that is typically expected of them. This is contingent upon the individual's age, gender, social milieu, and cultural heritage. When establishing handicap, a variety of socioeconomic factors are taken into account, including family background, skills attained, and financial stability. Many governments throughout

the world are becoming more inclusive in their approaches as a result of their recognition of the societal impact of disability.

A problem's expression at the tissue or organ level is impairment; an individual's level is disability; and a problem's manifestation at the societal level is handicap (Figure 16.2).

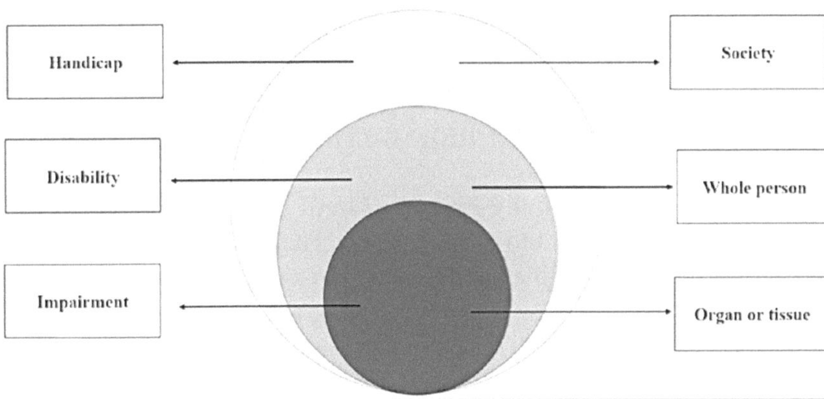

FIGURE 16.2 Impairment disability and handicap.

16.4 THE GOALS OF REHABILITATION AND THERAPY

The goal of providing therapy, counseling, and education is to delay or stop the onset of new impairments and preserve an individual's degree of proficiency. This kind of therapy is standard procedure for long-term diseases such as cancer, diabetes, COPD, and numerous neurological disorders. Additionally, it serves as the foundation for supported self-management and can help in the creation of treatments that seek to preserve function for as long as feasible (Mauk, 2011). People with disabilities struggle with:

1. **Orientation:** For a person with cerebral palsy or a brain injury, being oriented to his environment would make it difficult for him to do basic everyday tasks like dressing or using the washroom.
2. **Physical Independence:** Every person with a disability hopes to become less dependent on those who care for him.
3. **Mobility:** Mobility is significantly hampered by illnesses like poliomyelitis and paraplegia, making even routine chores like moving about the home exceedingly difficult.

4. **Occupational Integration:** Occupational integration involves employment training and placement.
5. **Integration Into Society:** No man is an island; thus, efforts must be taken to include disabled persons in society rather than isolate them.
6. **Financial Independence:** The position must provide a means of support.

16.5 SOCIO-VOCATIONAL REHABILITATION

No one is considered totally recovered until all of the aforementioned factors have been taken into consideration. The goal of social-vocational rehabilitation is to give the handicapped person a job, a home free from obstacles, and the appropriate social setting to lessen their disability. It should not be taken lightly that it is just another job agency. The "right to work" idea, which treats labor as more than just a method to make money but as a way of life and a means to give people dignity, is at the core of vocational rehabilitation. Thus, it serves as a channel for their ambitions and raises their sense of self as a self-sufficient member of society.

It gives people more power—not simply economically, but also in a more fundamental and significant way. It forces someone to stand up straight. They are freed from being tied to a job by it. Undoubtedly, not every person with a disability is able to stand on their own two feet. A more grounded and practical strategy is required.

Questions about the need for the disabled to work are understandably raised in a nation like ours where even the physically fit lack employment. We must remember, nevertheless, that every person has a fundamental right to self-realization through social integration.

The social worker primarily seeks to provide emotional support to the patient and their family members. They also raise awareness of disability and its limitations in the community. Socio-vocational rehabilitation is also responsible for putting the patient through employment training and ensuring that they are placed in a job paying a living wage. This is a collaborative endeavor involving experts like the trainer and vocational evaluator.

Employers must be incentivized to utilize the services of people with disabilities by offering rewards like tax benefits and social recognition. To achieve this goal, legislation will need to be passed in order to restore the differently abled to their proper status in society. A turning point in the lives of the disabled in that nation came with the passage of the Americans with Disabilities Act (ADA) in 1991. The PWD (Persons with Disabilities) Act 1995 was passed in India. There is no way to overstate the importance of the community. There must be awareness campaigns, and self-confidence must be built.

These days, community-based rehabilitation is the main focus, wherein knowledgeable personnel—ideally from the community—are made accessible even to rural locations and linked to the basic health care setup. Adults might receive training in a profession that fits their environment and community. For instance, it is possible to provide a device with a sickle and educate a grass cutter who has lost their right hand to return to their previous employment in their community. The fact that they are receiving training in the field of their choosing, where they have the contacts and reputation necessary to get a job, is another inherent benefit.

16.6 TYPES OF REHABILITATION AND THERAPY

An interdisciplinary method is frequently used to carry out therapy and rehabilitation, comprising a group of medical experts from several fields. Doctors, psychologists, social workers, OT's, speech-language pathologists (SLP), physical therapists, and other professionals might be a part of this team. Together, these professionals develop a comprehensive, all-inclusive treatment strategy that is tailored to the patient's requirements.

16.6.1 PHYSICAL THERAPY

Physical function and mobility are the main goals of physical therapy. It involves movements, stretches, and other methods designed to enhance coordination, balance, flexibility, and strength. Physical therapists assist patients who are recuperating from illnesses, operations, or chronic ailments so they may move more freely and have less discomfort. OT's analyze their patients' cognitive and physical capacities.

16.6.2 SPEECH THERAPY

Diagnosing and treating abnormalities of speech, language, communication, and swallowing are the main goals of speech therapy, commonly referred to as speech-language pathology. Speech therapists help those who struggle to swallow as well as those who have trouble articulating sounds, expressing themselves, or understanding language.

16.6.3 COGNITIVE REHABILITATION

Memory, attention, problem-solving, and executive functioning are just a few examples of the cognitive abilities that cognitive rehabilitation tries to enhance. People who are recuperating from strokes, severe brain injuries, or neurodegenerative diseases frequently use this form of therapy.

16.6.4 VOCATIONAL REHABILITATION

Following an illness or disability that limits their capacity to work, vocational rehabilitation helps people move back into the workforce or explore other employment prospects. Vocational therapists assist people in achieving their work objectives by offering vocational training, career counseling, and support.

16.6.5 PSYCHOLOGICAL THERAPY

Psychological treatment, usually referred to as psychotherapy or counseling, deals with a person's emotional and mental health. In order to manage stress, deal with emotional difficulties, and create methods for sustaining mental health, psychologists or counselors interact with patients (Figure 16.3).

16.7 REHABILITATION SETTINGS

Rehabilitation and therapy can be provided in various settings, including:

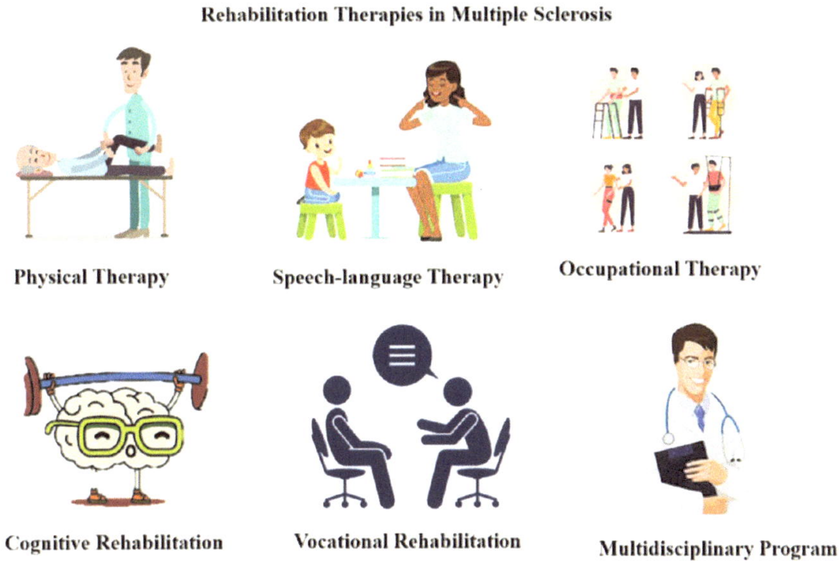
Rehabilitation Therapies in Multiple Sclerosis
Physical Therapy
Speech-language Therapy
Occupational Therapy
Cognitive Rehabilitation
Vocational Rehabilitation
Multidisciplinary Program

FIGURE 16.3 Rehabilitation therapies in multiple sclerosis.

16.7.1 IN-PATIENT REHABILITATION CENTERS

Individuals with significant rehabilitation requirements might receive comprehensive, interdisciplinary treatment at in-patient rehabilitation facilities. Patients receive daily therapy and medical oversight while residing in the institution.

16.7.2 OUT-PATIENT REHABILITATION CENTERS

For patients who do not require round-the-clock medical monitoring, out-patient centers offer rehabilitation treatments. When a person lives at home, they go to therapy at set times.

16.7.3 HOME-BASED REHABILITATION

Rehabilitation treatments can be provided to patients at home if they have mobility issues or live in a distant location. Home-based therapy allows individualized care in the patient's comfortable setting.

16.7.4 COMMUNITY-BASED PROGRAMS

Community-based rehabilitation programs work to integrate people with disabilities into their local communities by offering resources, support, and training in specific skills.

16.8 EMERGING TRENDS IN REHABILITATION AND THERAPY

New developments are influencing the field of treatment and rehabilitation as technology evolves. Wearable technology, telemedicine, and virtual reality (VR) are all being used more and more to improve accessibility and treatment efficiency.

16.9 COMMUNITY-BASED REHABILITATION (CBR)

Community-based rehabilitation (CBR) is a strategy that is utilized in the community to promote social inclusion, equality of opportunity, and rehabilitation for people with disabilities. The community as a whole, including the disabled individuals themselves, their families, friends, and the nearby health, educational, and socio-vocational facilities, collaborates with rehabilitation professionals to help the affected groups of people become self-sufficient.

In order to overcome flaws in earlier rehabilitation methods, the WHO published a guidebook in the 1980s called "Training in the Community for People with Disabilities." CBR originated from this concept. To acknowledge this, the Asia and Pacific Decade for the Handicapped was declared by the Economic and Social Commission for Asia and the Pacific (ESCAP) from 1993 to 2002.

The objectives of CBR are to ensure that the benefits outlined in the Rights of Persons with Disabilities Convention reach the majority by:

i. Assisting individuals with disabilities in making the most of their physical and mental capacities.
ii. Facilitating their access to regular services and opportunities.
iii. Encouraging patients to participate actively in their communities and society as a whole.
iv. Engaging communities to advocate for the inclusion of individuals with disabilities in society by reducing barriers to participation, raising public awareness of impairments, and promoting their rights.

These CBR principles have been successfully used by more than 90 nations worldwide. India is a sizable nation with a large rural population. According to Mahatma Gandhi, India's people reside in its villages. Professional assistance cannot be delivered to persons with disabilities at their doorsteps across the entire country. Therefore, we must choose a strategy that is straightforward and advantageous to a broader population. The general objectives of CBR programs are:

- Early disability identification and care.
- Prevention of disabilities.
- Recognition of high-risk fetuses and moms.
- An assessment of the family's and the disabled person's perceived requirements.
- Neighborhood-based or at-home programs.
- Parental participation.
- Children's play groups and integrated education.
- Organizations run by and for disabled persons.

The core concept of the multi-layered approach to CBR is the decentralization of accountability and resources, both financial and human, to community-level groups. The opportunity to fully participate in the social, political, and economic life of the community is provided to those with disabilities. For handicapped people living in rural areas, CBR is the best rehabilitation program since it is delivered right to their door and is supported by locals and resources.

CBR is community-based rehabilitation that is carried out at the community level with the help of the community. Disability-related individuals and their families actively participate in decision-making, as do community members.

CBR is an initiative for self-help based on:

- Understanding and concern of the community.
- Proposals from the community.
- Designing from the community.
- Funds from the community.
- Application by the community.
- Evaluation by the community.
- Changes by the community.
- Satisfaction to and from the community.

16.9.1 CRITERIA

CBR programs must coordinate service delivery at the local level, and people with disabilities must be included in CBR programs; at all stages, they must have distinct decision-making roles.

16.9.2 ASPECTS OF COMMUNITY-BASED REHABILITATION (CBR)

CBR has 4 key components:

- Medicative Academic
- Economical Communal

The medical component often begins with a professional group evaluating the impairment. A thorough program is laid out, and devoted, trained staff at the local level implement it. Typically, the patient's family members receive training as well. Education is provided to people who require fundamental information and skills whenever it is necessary. This becomes increasingly important for kids with cerebral palsy. The patient will be given the educational, occupational, and extracurricular skills necessary to apply for jobs, start their own businesses, and improve their financial situation.

16.9.3 SOCIETY NEEDS TO BE INVOLVED IN COMMUNITY-BASED REHABILITATION (CBR)

Any CBR program's success depends on elements including cost efficiency, personal values, and societal acceptance.

16.9.4 MEMBERS OF THE (COMMUNITY-BASED REHABILITATION) CBR TEAM

Being the beneficiary of the services, the patient must be first and foremost involved in all decision-making processes. As role models and mentors for other people with disabilities, individuals with disabilities are often more successful than persons without impairments. The idcal persons to administer the program are those who live nearby, such as members of the community and families of disabled people who are familiar with the area's geography, economics, and environmental circumstances. Governments (local, regional, and national) as well as non-governmental groups and medical experts will provide support. In their position as educators, social scientists, and other professionals are frequently employed.

The phrase "corporate social responsibility" (CSR), which refers to a commitment to return part of the advantages of one's activities to the society in which one works, was recently created by the corporate sector, which is made up of successful businesses and industries.

A schoolteacher who volunteers her spare time to help children with special needs, a multipurpose rehabilitation worker (a trained individual who can identify disability, give basic physiotherapy (PT), and prescribe orthotics), and Primary Health Care (PHC) staff are the other members. Locally available skilled workers comprise carpenters with training in the fabrication of aids and equipment, local leaders who can try to create barrier-free environments, and school teachers. It is necessary to teach the PHC's medical officers and staff in handicap management. The Rehabilitation Council of India launched one of the biggest orientation programs of its type for PHC doctors throughout India to help them become more aware of rehabilitation.

16.10 CONCLUSION

To help people with a variety of physical, psychological, and cognitive issues regain their functional abilities, increase their independence, and generally improve their well-being, rehabilitation and therapy are crucial components of healthcare. Recovery and therapy experts collaborate and use an interdisciplinary approach to deliver individualized and successful treatment to assist people in achieving their recovery objectives and leading satisfying lives.

KEYWORDS

- **corporate sector**
- **corporate social responsibility**
- **disability physical therapist**
- **environmental circumstances**
- **non-governmental groups**
- **occupational therapist**
- **physical exercise**
- **rehabilitation**
- **social scientists**
- **speech therapist**

REFERENCES

Benson, D. (1979). *Aphasia, Alexia and Agraphia*. Churchill Livingstone.

Bromley, I. (2006). *Tetraplegia and Paraplegia: A Guide for Physiotherapists*.

Clayton's electrotherapy: Theory and practice. (1999). AITBS.

DeLisa, J. A., Gans, B. M., & Nicholas, E. (2004). *Physical Medicine and Rehabilitation: Principles and Practice*.

DeLorme, T. L., & Watkins, A. L. (1993). *Progressive Resistance Exercise*. Appleton-Century-Crofts.

Dietz, J. H. Jr. (1980). Adaptive rehabilitation in cancer: A program to improve quality of survival. *Postgraduate Medicine, 68*(1), 145–153.

Gardiner, D. M. (n.d.). *Principles of Exercise Therapy*. CBS.

Hollis, M., & Fletcher-Cook, P. (2003). *Practical Exercise Therapy*.

Kottke, F. J., Stillwell, G. K., & Lehmann, J. F. (1982). *Krusen's Handbook of Physical Medicine and Rehabilitation* (3rd ed.). W. B. Saunders.

Low, J., & Reed, A. (2002). *Electrotherapy Explained: Principles*. Butterworth-Heinemann.

Maitland, G. D. (1997). *Maitland's Vertebral Manipulation*. Butterworth-Heinemann.

Voss, D. (1989). *Proprioceptive Neuromuscular Facilitation*. Lippincott.

World Health Organization. (1995). *Disability Prevention and Rehabilitation: Primary Health Care–Guide for District Health and Rehabilitation Managers*.

Wright, J. (2000). The Functional Assessment Measure: The Center for Outcome Measurement in Brain Injury.

CHAPTER 17

Physical Therapy Techniques and Interventions

ARCHANA KHANNA

Department of Physiotherapy, Sharda School of Allied Health Sciences, Sharda University, Greater Noida, Uttar Pradesh, India

ABSTRACT

Nowadays, people suffer from multiple problems such as low backache and poor posture. Physical therapy has been one of the oldest techniques that play an important role in the rehabilitation of any musculoskeletal, neurological, cardiopulmonary, and sports-related condition. Physiotherapy (PT) consists of a vast range of interventions and techniques that can be used for rehabilitation purposes. These can range from the use of electrotherapeutic modalities (such as ultrasound (USG), interferential therapy, TENS), simple exercises (such as active or passive range of motion exercises), to specialized techniques such as joint mobilization, the Bobath technique, myofascial release, taping, and so forth. These interventions have been used extensively in conditions such as stroke, knee replacement, muscle injuries, and many other conditions. PT not only aids in healing and recovery but also reduces rehabilitation time. It helps to reduce pain and inflammation in both acute and chronic conditions. If used effectively, it can prevent or delay surgeries like joint replacement; hence, it is very beneficial for the athletic population as well. The present chapter deals with the different physical therapy interventions available for rehabilitation purposes.

Allied Healthcare in Practice: An Introduction to Integrated Patient Care. Sally Lukose, Karuna Singh (Eds.)

DOI: 10.1201/9781998511037-20

17.1 INTRODUCTION

A healthcare system is composed of a team comprising physicians, medical experts, and physiotherapists. Physiotherapists play a vital role not only in rehabilitating patients according to their needs but also in educating them about disease and injury prevention. A skillful approach combined with recent evidence-based practice enables physiotherapists to provide quality healthcare to patients suffering from a wide range of musculoskeletal, neurological, cardiopulmonary, or sports-related injuries (Howick et al., 2011). Their knowledge and clinical decision-making skills for applying therapeutic interventions help to reduce rehabilitation time and bring the patient back to his or her normal optimal functioning (Mohanakrishnan, 2015). Physical therapy is not only effective for injuries or general musculoskeletal complaints but also following surgeries such as ligament repair or reconstruction and joint replacement surgeries.

Recently, physiotherapy (PT) came into the picture following the COVID-19 pandemic, where patients suffered from severe chest problems, and PT interventions in the form of chest physical therapy helped patients restore their normal breathing patterns and oxygenation levels. The therapeutic interventions applied by physiotherapists help patients reduce their pain, regain or improve their range of motion, strength, and restore their movement and function (Stephensen et al., 2017). Any disability and loss of function that can develop in the future can be prevented by re-educating patients and applying the best evidence-based physiotherapeutic interventions.

17.2 THERAPEUTIC INTERVENTIONS

Physiotherapeutic interventions include a vast range of methods and techniques, including electrotherapeutic modalities as well as exercises and manual therapy. It involves the application of the interventions (e.g., modalities, exercises) along with a properly coordinated plan of care, including documentation as well as patient and family re-education about the condition and instructions to be followed before the next follow-up (Yamato et al., 2016). The direct interventions can be provided in the form of therapeutic exercise, functional re-education, specialized techniques of manual therapy, usage of orthotics or prosthetics, and electrotherapeutic modalities.

The application of direct interventions is based on the goals planned for the patient as per specific impairment, disability, or functional limitations. The use of therapeutic exercises and functional re-education at different levels constitutes the core elements for the plan of care by a physiotherapist. The intervention selected should be based on the findings of proper assessment, diagnosis, and evidence-based practice. Regular follow-up of the patient's condition ensures that alterations in intervention can be made if required. Change may be desirable if the patient's condition does not improve or the clinical outcome is not as expected. Common direct interventions include the following.

17.2.1 THERAPEUTIC EXERCISE

A systematically planned body movement done to improve, restore, and/or enhance physical function can be termed therapeutic exercise. These include exercises for improving muscle strength, power, endurance, stretching techniques, postural re-education, breathing exercises, ventilatory muscle training, relaxation exercises, and so forth. The exercises can be performed actively or passively (Bielecki and Tadi, 2022).

17.2.2 ELECTROTHERAPY

Electrotherapy has been widely used as a method to relieve pain and improve function. It involves the application of electric current to the affected area to aid in pain reduction, functional training, assist in the force generation capacity of muscles, maintain strength following injury or surgery, increase blood flow, reduce edema, and help in wound healing. It includes multiple modalities such as Transcutaneous Electrical Nerve Stimulation (TENS), USG, LASER, neuromuscular electrical stimulators, shortwave diathermy, and so forth (Watson, 2000). These modalities involve the application of heat, which may be applied at the superficial or deeper level to achieve the desired physiological effect. Modalities providing superficial heat include paraffin wax baths, hydrocollator packs, whirlpools, and infrared radiation. Deep heating modalities include shortwave diathermy, microwave diathermy, and USG therapy. These modalities lead to improved circulation via vasodilation, decreased pain, relaxed muscles, and increased extensibility of soft tissues (Ahmed et al., 2021).

17.2.2.1 ULTRASOUND

Ultrasound is a deep-penetrating modality that causes tissue changes through thermal and non-thermal (mechanical) mechanisms. USG includes mechanical vibrations similar to sound waves but at a higher frequency. The commonly used frequencies include 1 MHz and 3 MHz. USG may be applied in a continuous mode or pulsed mode depending on whether the condition is acute or chronic. It affects all the phases of tissue healing, thereby affecting the activity of phagocytic cells and the release of inflammatory mediators, hence activating fibroblasts to stimulate the production of collagen. The deep heating effects of USG, such as the piezoelectric effect, acoustic streaming, and cavitation, are used for various musculoskeletal conditions. The application of USG helps to increase blood flow, tissue extensibility, and pain and spasm reduction, thereby increasing the rate of tissue repair (Wagai, 2007). USG therapy has been reported to decrease the pain intensity in patients with chronic non-specific low back pain (Haile et al., 2021).

17.2.2.2 LASER

Laser refers to Light Amplification by Stimulated Emission of Radiation. Lasers differ from ordinary light due to their properties of monochromaticity, coherence, and collimation. Commonly used lasers include ruby laser, helium-neon laser, and diode laser. The low-power or cold laser has no or minimal thermal effects, but it is effective for soft tissue healing and pain reduction (Herrmann et al., 2012). High-intensity laser therapy involves high-intensity power to irradiate deeper tissues in a shorter time span (Boyraz et al., 2015; Conforti and Fachinetti, 2013; Ezzati et al., 2019). Cotler et al. concluded that low-power laser therapy is an economic treatment option for reducing pain and improving quality of life. It is readily absorbed by the soft tissues (2015). Low-power laser therapy is reported to decrease acute and chronic pain, induce recovery of damaged nerves, enhance peripheral circulation and metabolism, and reduce joint inflammation (Cotler et al., 2015). On the contrary, high-intensity laser is reported to be beneficial in reducing musculoskeletal pain (Taradaj et al., 2017).

17.2.2.3 CRYOTHERAPY

It involves the application of ice to obtain therapeutic effects. Cryotherapy has been identified as an integral part of PT, especially among sports physiotherapists (Belanger, 2015). It can be applied using massage, whirlpool, spray, contrast baths, ice immersion, and cold compression. The application of cryotherapy is indicated for conditions such as acute soft tissue injuries (e.g., ankle sprain, muscle strain), tenosynovitis, bursitis, and so forth. Cryotherapy results in a reduction of pain and inflammation due to physiological effects like vasoconstriction and decreased metabolic rate. With reduced blood flow to the affected part, the tendency for the development of edema is delayed. In addition, the slow metabolic rate leads to lesser production of inflammatory mediators, hence causing a reduction in pain and edema (Ni et al., 2015). It has been found that cryotherapy benefits patients with musculoskeletal and neurological conditions.

17.2.2.4 TRANSCUTANEOUS ELECTRICAL NERVE STIMULATION (TENS)

It is a non-invasive method primarily used to decrease pain levels. It acts by causing electrical stimulation of the A delta and C fibers, hence activating the pain gate mechanism and/or the release of beta-endorphins and encephalins, leading to the inhibition of pain transmission. TENS can be high or low TENS based on the frequency used (Wu et al., 2017). The application of TENS has been found to be effective in a number of conditions such as osteoarthritis, postoperative pain, and acute painful conditions. Positive results of TENS have been suggested in primary dysmenorrhea (Elboim et al., 2020). Highly beneficial effects of TENS have been reported in cases of chronic pain due to neuralgia, radiculopathy, phantom limb, cancer-related pain, and any kind of chronic musculoskeletal pain (Johnson and Martinson, 2007).

17.2.3 BIOFEEDBACK

It is a technique that applies feedback in the form of visual, physical, and auditory cues to control body functions and improve patients' performance (Onate et al., 2001). Different types of biofeedback are available, such as EMG, EEG, and GSR biofeedback. Recently, virtual reality (VR) exercise gaming is also being used as a feedback method during rehabilitation. With this method, the patient performs activities using the graphical or audio-visual feedback provided by the VR environment (Riener et al., 2006). Physiological feedback, such as that given by EMG, has been found to be more effective than electrical stimulation for improving the peak torque of the quadriceps femoris muscle following reconstruction of the anterior cruciate ligament (Draper and Ballard, 1991). EMG biofeedback has also been found to be effective in improving hand function and gait in hemiplegic patients following a cerebrovascular accident (Aiello, 2005; Armagan et al., 2003).

17.2.4 HYDROTHERAPY

Hydrotherapy, or aqua therapy, refers to any activity performed in water to assist in rehabilitation and recovery from hard training or serious injury (Bartels et al., 2007; Brody and Geigle, 2009). It involves different exercises being performed in warm water and is a popular treatment for patients with neurologic and musculoskeletal conditions (Kamioka et al., 2010). The goals of this therapy are muscle relaxation, improving joint motion, and reducing pain (Eversden et al., 2007). Hydrotherapy has been found to be effective in improving pain, function, joint mobility, strength, and balance, particularly among older adults, subjects with rheumatic conditions, and those with chronic low back pain (Geytenbeek, 2002). Hydrotherapy is found to be beneficial for chronic low back pain (Ma et al., 2022). It has been suggested that monitored aquatic-based exercises effectively improve muscle strength, fatigue, quality of life, and skin disease activity more than land-based exercises in children with juvenile dermatomyositis (Samhan et al., 2020).

17.2.5 MANUAL THERAPY

Apart from the conventional PT comprising electrotherapy and therapeutic exercises, manual PT also plays a very essential role in the rehabilitation of individuals. The commonly used manual therapy techniques include methods like Cyriax, Mulligan's, McKenzie, Maitland, and Kaltenborn, and so forth. Manual therapy involves the application of different skilled techniques on the patient. These techniques can be used for assessment, diagnosis, and treatment. Manual therapy techniques include the following:

- Manipulation.
- Mobilization.
- Stretching.
- Muscle energy techniques.

17.2.5.1 MAITLAND'S MOBILIZATION TECHNIQUE

Maitland's mobilization involves the application of skilled manual therapy techniques using physiological or accessory motion. These are applied at different speeds and amplitudes, which can range from a small-amplitude force applied at high velocity to a large-amplitude force applied at slow velocity. By applying the concave-convex rule, these can be performed to achieve therapeutic effects such as pain reduction and improved range of motion. It can be applied to peripheral joints as well as the spine. The different glides used to achieve these therapeutic effects include antero-posterior, posteroanterior, longitudinal caudal, longitudinal cephalic, joint distraction, and medial and lateral glide (Shabbir et al., 2021). Grades I–IV of mobilization are reported to be effective for pain reduction and improving function and range of motion at the cervical spine in chronic neck pain patients. For adhesive capsulitis, the addition of Maitland mobilization to exercises has proven to be effective in relieving pain, range, and shoulder function (Kumar et al., 2012).

17.2.5.2 MCKENZIE METHOD

This technique was introduced by Robin McKenzie in 1981 for the treatment of spinal and extremity musculoskeletal disorders. McKenzie's system involves repeated or sustained movements to reduce and eliminate the symptoms for restoring function. The technique is used primarily for the spine and peripheral joints. Based on a thorough assessment, the symptoms are classified into syndromes relating to derangement, dysfunction, and posture (Abady et al., 2017). McKenzie's method is based upon the direction of movement that leads to reduction, centralization, or abolition of the symptoms. It aims to maintain these improvements while the patient returns to normal activity. A combination of McKenzie and stabilization exercises has been found to be more effective than conventional exercises for reducing functional disability in chronic nonspecific low back pain patients (Alhakami et al., 2019). These are also reported to be beneficial in improving forward head posture and respiratory function, as reported by Kim et al. (2019). For neck pain of any severity, the McKenzie method has proven to provide a statistically significant improvement when compared with control intervention (Baumann et al., 2023).

17.2.5.3 MULLIGAN'S TECHNIQUE

It involves the use of joint mobilization or glides. If a restriction in the joint, decreased range of motion, or pain is observed during examination, the joint is repositioned using hands or a belt. The glides used under Mulligan's method include Natural Apophyseal Glides (NAGs) and Sustained Natural Apophyseal Glides (SNAGs). With NAGs, the joints are mobilized mid-way through the range. A SNAG is then applied to take the joint through the full range of motion without any pain. NAGs can be applied to the cervical and upper thoracic spine. SNAGs can be used at the neck, thoracic and lumbar regions, ribs, and sacroiliac joints (Mulligan, 2004). Mulligan's techniques have been found to be effective in improving pain and functional mobility in individuals with knee osteoarthritis and rotator cuff syndrome (Bhagat et al., 2020; Menek et al., 2019). For rotator cuff syndrome, it also improved the DASH score and a few parameters of the SF-36 when compared with conventional treatment.

17.3 APPLICATIONS OF PHYSICAL THERAPY INTERVENTIONS

Pain is the most common symptom experienced in any condition. It can arise due to common musculoskeletal problems or due to any underlying pathophysiological condition. Post-surgical pain is a common symptom following surgery that persists over a period of time, thus affecting the quality of life of an individual. Though medications are prescribed to alleviate the pain, PT has also shown a positive response in reducing the pain in such cases. The application of PT has been reported to improve pain, quality of life, physical function, and depression (Robinson et al., 2019). PT has also been found to be effective in managing central neuropathic pain due to any underlying cause, as reported in research where authors found TENS and mirror therapy to be effective in a significant reduction of pain among stroke patients (Kannan et al., 2022).

Physiotherapy has been found to be very effective in neurological conditions such as stroke, Parkinson's disease, Guillain-Barré syndrome, multiple sclerosis, cerebral palsy, and so forth (Dua et al., 2006; Yang et al., 2023). It plays an important role in the management of functional motor disorders among patients (Nielsen et al., 2015). In Parkinson's disease, different PT applications such as conventional PT, resistance training, VR exergaming, and hydrotherapy significantly improved motor symptoms, balance, gait, and quality of life (Radder et al., 2020).

Multiple types of PT techniques and procedures have been found to be effective for neurological conditions such as Parkinson's disease, stroke, polyneuropathy, and so forth (Spanakis et al., 2022). These include the application of balance and coordination training, robot-assisted therapy, and treadmill training. The application of aquatic therapy in combination with conventional PT was found to be effective among stroke patients (Moritz et al., 2019). Musculoskeletal conditions are a major cause of pain, disability, and expenditure on health (WHO, 2003).

Musculoskeletal disorders in occupational environments are also a major public health issue in the world. Due to the significant demands of the job, these disorders affect work habits, quality of work, and quality of life of an individual, with health professionals being at higher risk due to their varied interventions requiring significant loads (Davis and Kotowski, 2015; Epstein et al., 2017; Vieira et al., 2016).

A multimodal PT program has been found to relieve work-related musculoskeletal pain in office workers (Fortún et al., 2021). Physical therapy interventions, including ergonomic advice, can prevent and manage musculoskeletal disorders (Chen et al., 2017; Prall and Ross, 2019). Physical therapy-based exercise plans for office workers can help to improve their body awareness and pain, hence increasing their work efficiency (Moreira Silva et al., 2014; Shariat et al., 2017).

Low back pain is commonly experienced by most individuals, and physical therapy interventions have been found to be effective in reducing chronic low back pain (Lewis et al., 2008). These have been known to be a first-line treatment for relieving chronic backache (Shipton, 2017). There is strong evidence for the use of PT among children and adolescents suffering from non-specific low back pain (García et al., 2022). Exercise induces pain relief by the activation of central inhibitory pathways (Chou et al., 2017). Exercise induces pain relief caused by several mechanisms, including opioids, serotonin, and so forth (Da Silva and Galdino, 2017).

Following spinal cord injury, PT plays an integral role in rehabilitation. It aims at applying different interventions to improve body structure and function. For such patients, physical interventions are focused on improving quality of life, interpersonal relationships, and increasing participation in the community (Harvey, 2008; Stack and Stokes, 2012). Cardiopulmonary conditions such as chronic obstructive pulmonary disease (COPD) are among the major causes of disability and mortality around the world and are expected to increase in the coming years (Murray and Lopez, 1997). COPD is characterized by symptoms such as worsening cough and shortness of breath. These patients require an improvement in lung function through adequate removal of airway secretions (Vestbo et al., 2013). PT interventions used to achieve these goals include percussion, vibration techniques, postural drainage, active cycle of breathing, thoracic expansion exercises, and so forth (Pryor, 2008). When compared with standard care, multiple PT modalities have reportedly improved the function of hospitalized COPD patients with acute exacerbation in addition to other outcome measures (Torres et al., 2017). For multiple cardiorespiratory conditions, breathing exercises have been found to be beneficial for improving health-related quality of life. In addition, inspiratory muscle training improved the inspiratory muscle strength, and chest therapy aided in the clearance of sputum (Tang et al., 2010). Physical therapy interventions also improve exercise tolerance and mobility, and reduce dyspnea in conditions such as bronchitis and asthma (Dimitrova et al., 2016; Grigorova et al., 2014). Supervised chest PT, given as a combination of relaxation exercises, pursed lip breathing, and active expiration, led to more improvement in anxiety, depression, and dyspnea in comparison to those who received usual care (Valenza et al., 2014).

Physiotherapy played a key role in the rehabilitation of COVID-19 patients as well. Abdullahi (2020) reported that chest physiotherapy given to COVID-19 patients after discharge in the form of respiratory muscle training, diaphragmatic breathing, stretching exercises, and home exercises led to improved FEC1, FEV1/FVC%, endurance, and quality of life, as well as a reduction in anxiety and depression symptoms (2020). As an integral part of the sports medicine team, PT plays a major role in managing sports injuries (Chang et al., 2021; Macedo et al., 2019). Sports physiotherapists prevent and manage sports injuries at all ages and levels and work with all athletes for injury prevention, restoring optimal function during rehabilitation, and enhancing sports performance (Bulley and Donaghy, 2005; Caparros et al., 2017). It has been reported that in phase I of rehabilitation, the use of electrophysiology modalities, joint mobilization grade I-II, massage, relaxation therapy, and exercise therapy have been found to be effective for pain reduction (Anderson et al., 2009; Jones and Wilson, 2019).

Sports injuries often result in reduced range of motion and flexibility due to contraction of the wound and fibrosis (Frontera, 2003). Flexibility training incorporated into rehabilitation programs helps to improve the joint range of motion. Stretching techniques such as static, ballistic, and Proprioceptive neuromuscular facilitation (PNF) are commonly used to improve range of motion. Sports injuries can result in muscle weakness, lack of muscle strength, and endurance. Following a sports injury, rehabilitation incorporating aerobic and resistance/strength training helps to restore the optimal physical function required for a return to sports. Sports injuries to ligaments, tendons, or joints can result in loss of proprioception and coordination, which are very essential and important components for any sport (Buschbacher et al., 2009). Specific training is available to restore these functions.

17.4 CONCLUSION

Physical therapy has been used extensively for managing multiple musculoskeletal, neurological, cardiorespiratory, and sports-related injuries. When used properly, these interventions cause remarkable improvement in the function of an individual undergoing rehabilitation. Physical therapy can be very beneficial in reducing rehabilitation time, restoring optimal structure and function, thus leading to an improved quality of life.

KEYWORDS

- **central neuropathic pain**
- **exercise**
- **inflammation**
- **mirror therapy**
- **musculoskeletal problems**
- **neurological conditions**
- **physical therapy**
- **rehabilitation**

REFERENCES

Abady, A. H., Rosedale, R., Chenworth, B. M., Rotondi, M. A., & Overend, T. J. (2017). Application of the McKenzie system of Mechanical Diagnosis and Therapy (MDT) in patients with shoulder pain: A prospective longitudinal study. *Journal of Manual & Manipulative Therapy, 25*(5), 235–243.

Abdullahi, A. (2020). Safety and efficacy of chest physiotherapy in patients with COVID-19: A critical review. *Frontiers in Medicine, 7*, 454.

Ahmed, Y. A., Shafeek, M. M., & El-Kasem, S. T. A. (2021). Effect of cold versus heat modalities on dynamic balance in healthy adolescents. *Physiotherapy Quarterly, 29*(2), 56–61.

Aiello, E., Gates, D. H., Patritti, B. L., Cairns, K. D., Meister, M., Clancy, E. A., & Bonato, P. (2005). Visual EMG biofeedback to improve ankle function in hemiparetic gait. *Conference Proceedings IEEE Engineering in Medicine and Biology Society, 2005*, 7703–7706.

Alhakami, A. M., Davis, S., Qasheesh, M., Shaphe, A., & Chahal, A. (2019). Effects of McKenzie and stabilization exercises in reducing pain intensity and functional disability in individuals with nonspecific chronic low back pain: A systematic review. *Journal of Physical Therapy Science, 31*(7), 590–597.

Alneyadi, M., Drissi, N., Almeqbaali, M., & Ouhbi, S. (2021). Biofeedback-based connected mental health interventions for anxiety: Systematic literature review. *JMIR Mhealth Uhealth, 9*(4), e26038.

Anderson, M. K., Parr, G. P., & Hall, S. J. (2009). *Foundations of Athletic Training: Prevention, Assessment, and Management*. Lippincott Williams & Wilkins.

Armagan, O., Tascioglu, F., & Oner, C. (2003). Electromyographic biofeedback in the treatment of the hemiplegic hand: A placebo-controlled study. *American Journal of Physical Medicine & Rehabilitation, 82*(11), 856.

Bartels, E. M., Juhl, C. B., Christensen, R., Hagen, K. B., Danneskiold-Samsøe, B., Dagfinrud, H., & Lund, H. (2016). Aquatic exercise for the treatment of knee and hip osteoarthritis. *The Cochrane Database of Systematic Reviews, 3*(3), CD005523.

Baumann, A. N., Orellana, K., Landis, L., et al. (2023). The McKenzie Method is an effective rehabilitation paradigm for treating adults with moderate-to-severe neck pain: A systematic review with meta-analysis. *Cureus, 15*(5), e39218.

Belanger, A. Y. (2015). *Therapeutic Electrophysical Agents: Evidence Behind Practice* (3rd ed.). Lippincott Williams & Wilkins.

Bhagat, M., Neelapala, Y. V. R., & Gangavelli, R. (2020). Immediate effects of Mulligan's techniques on pain and functional mobility in individuals with knee osteoarthritis: A randomized control trial. *Physiotherapy Research International, 25*(1), e1812.

Bielecki, J. E., & Tadi, P. (2022). Therapeutic exercise. In *StatPearls*. Treasure Island Publishing.

Boyraz, I., Yildiz, A., Koc, B., & Sarman, H. (2015). Comparison of high-intensity laser therapy and ultrasound treatment in patients with lumbar discopathy. *Biomedical Research International, 2015*, 304328.

Brody, L. T., & Geigle, P. R. (2009). *Aquatic Exercise for Rehabilitation and Training*. Human Kinetics.

Bulley, C., & Donaghy, M. (2005). Sports physiotherapy competencies: The first step towards a common platform for specialist professional recognition. *Physical Therapy in Sport, 6*(2), 103–108.

Buschbacher, R., Prahlow, N., & Dave, S. J. (2009). *Sports and Medicine Rehabilitation: A Sport-Specific Approach* (2nd ed.). Lippincott Williams & Wilkins.

Caparrós, T., Pujol, M., & Salas, C. (2017). General guidelines in the rehabilitation process for return to training after a sports injury. *Apunts Medicina de l'Esport, 52*(196), 167–172.

Chang, J. Y., You, S. J. H., Grant, M. E., Lee, J. H., Kim, T. G., Kim, K. S., Chang, J. S., Choi, J. Y., Lee, Y. H., & Kong, I. D. (2021). Review of physiotherapy service for athletes of the 2018 Olympic Winter Games: Consideration of preparation for two polyclinics. *Physical Therapy in Sport, 49*, 106–111.

Chen, X., Coombes, B. K., Sjøgaard, G., Jun, D., O'Leary, S., & Johnston, V. (2018). Workplace-based interventions for neck pain in office workers: Systematic review and meta-analysis. *Physical Therapy, 98*(1), 40–62.

Chou, R., Deyo, R., Friedly, J., Skelly, A., Hashimoto, R., Weimer, M., Fu, R., Dana, T., Kraegel, P., Griffin, J., Grusing, S., & Brodt, E. D. (2017). Nonpharmacologic therapies for low back pain: A systematic review for an American College of Physicians Clinical Practice Guideline. *Annals of Internal Medicine, 166*(7), 493–505.

Conforti, M., & Fachinetti, G. P. (2013). High-power laser therapy treatment compared to simple segmental physical rehabilitation in whiplash injuries (1° and 2° grade of the Quebec Task Force classification) involving muscles and ligaments. *Muscles, Ligaments and Tendons Journal, 3*(2), 106–111.

Cotler, H. B., Chow, R. T., Hamblin, M. R., & Carroll, J. (2015). The use of low-level laser therapy (LLLT) for musculoskeletal pain. *MOJ Orthopedics & Rheumatology, 2*(5), 00068.

Da Silva Santos, R., & Galdino, G. (2018). Endogenous systems involved in exercise-induced analgesia. *Journal of Physiology and Pharmacology, 69*(1), 3–13.

Davis, K. G., & Kotowski, S. E. (2015). Prevalence of musculoskeletal disorders for nurses in hospitals, long-term care facilities, and home health care: A comprehensive review. *Human Factors, 57*(5), 754–792.

Dimitrova, A., Lyubenova, D., & Grigorova-Petrova, K. (2016). Kineziterapiya pri belodrobni bolesti. In Kostov, K. (Ed.), *Belodrobni bolezni*. Spiro.

Draper, V., & Ballard, L. (1991). Electrical stimulation versus electromyographic biofeedback in the recovery of quadriceps femoris muscle function following anterior cruciate ligament surgery. *Physical Therapy, 71*(6), 455–461.

Dua, T., Garrido-Cumbrera, M., Mathers, C., & Saxena, S. (2006). Global burden of neurological disorders: Estimates and projections. In *Neurological Disorders: Public Health Challenges*. WHO Press.

Elboim-Gabyzon, M., & Kalichman, L. (2020). Transcutaneous electrical nerve stimulation (TENS) for primary dysmenorrhea: An overview. *International Journal of Women's Health, 8*(12), 1–10.

Epstein, S., Sparer, E. H., Tran, B. N., Ruan, Q. Z., Dennerlein, J. T., Singhal, D., & Lee, B. T. (2018). Prevalence of work-related musculoskeletal disorders among surgeons and interventionalists: A systematic review and meta-analysis. *JAMA Surgery, 153*(2), e174947.

Eversden, L., Maggs, F., Nightingale, P., & Jobanputra, P. (2007). A pragmatic randomised controlled trial of hydrotherapy and land exercises on overall well-being and quality of life in rheumatoid arthritis. *BMC Musculoskeletal Disorders, 8*(1), 23.

Ezzati, K., Fekrazad, R., & Raoufi, Z. (2019). The effects of photobiomodulation therapy on post-surgical pain. *Journal of Lasers in Medical Sciences, 10*(2), 79–85.

Fortún-Rabadán, R., Jiménez-Sánchez, C., Flores-Yaben, O., & Bellosta-López, P. (2021). Workplace physiotherapy for musculoskeletal pain-relief in office workers: A pilot study. *Journal of Education and Health Promotion, 27*(10), 75.

Frontera, W. R. (2003). Rehabilitation of sports injuries: Scientific basis. In *Encyclopaedia of Sports Medicine* (Vol. X). Blackwell Science Ltd.

García-Moreno, J. M., Calvo-Muñoz, I., Gómez-Conesa, A., & López-López, J. A. (2022). Effectiveness of physiotherapy interventions for back care and the prevention of non-specific low back pain in children and adolescents: A systematic review and meta-analysis. *BMC Musculoskeletal Disorders, 23*, 314.

Geytenbeek, J. (2002). Evidence for effective hydrotherapy. *Physiotherapy, 8*(9), 514–529.

Grigorova-Petrova, K., Lubenova, D., Dimitrova, A., Baldaranov, D., & Lozeva, J. (2014). Feasibility of early physical therapy program in-hospital patients with acute ischemic stroke. *Open Access Macedonian Journal of Medical Sciences, 2*(3), 452–455.

Haile, G., Hailemariam, T. T., & Haile, T. G. (2021). Effectiveness of ultrasound therapy on the management of chronic non-specific low back pain: A systematic review. *Journal of Pain Research, 17*, 1251–1257.

Harvey, L. (2008). *Management of Spinal Cord Injuries: A Guide for Physiotherapists*. Elsevier Health Sciences.

Herrmann, T. R. W., Liatsikov, E. N., Nagele, U., Traxer, O., & Merseburger, A. S. (2012). EAU guidelines on laser technologies. *European Urology, 61*(4), 783–795.

Howick, J., Chalmers, I., Glasziou, P., et al. (2011). *The Oxford Levels of Evidence*. Oxford Centre for Evidence-Based Medicine.

Johnson, M., & Martinson, M. (2007). Efficacy of electrical nerve stimulation for chronic musculoskeletal pain: A meta-analysis of randomized controlled trials. *Pain, 130*(1, 2), 157–165.

Jones, G., & Wilson, E. (2019). *Everyday Sport Injuries: The Essential Step-by-Step Guide to Prevention, Diagnosis, and Treatment*. DK Publishing.

Kamioka, H., Tsutani, K., Okuizumi, H., Mutoh, Y., Ohta, M., Handa, S., Okada, S., Kitayuguchi, J., Kamada, M., Shiozawa, N., & Honda, T. (2010). Effectiveness of aquatic exercise and balneotherapy: A summary of systematic reviews based on randomized controlled trials of water immersion therapies. *Journal of Epidemiology, 20*(1), 2–12.

Kannan, P., Bello, U. M., & Winser, S. J. (2022). Physiotherapy interventions may relieve pain in individuals with central neuropathic pain: A systematic review and meta-analysis of randomized controlled trials. *Therapeutic Advances in Chronic Disease, 13*.

Kim, S., Jung, J., & Kim, N. (2019). The effects of McKenzie exercise on forward head posture and respiratory function. *Journal of Korean Physical Therapy, 31*, 351–357.

Kumar, A., Kumar, S., Aggarwal, A., Kumar, R., & Das, P. G. (2012). Effectiveness of Maitland techniques in idiopathic shoulder adhesive capsulitis. *International Scholarly Research Notices, 8*.

Lewis, A., Morris, M. E., & Walsh, C. (2008). Are physiotherapy exercises effective in reducing chronic low back pain? In *Database of Abstracts of Reviews of Effects (DARE): Quality-Assessed Reviews*. Centre for Reviews and Dissemination (UK).

Ma, J., Zhang, T., He, Y., et al. (2022). Effect of aquatic physical therapy on chronic low back pain: A systematic review and meta-analysis. *BMC Musculoskeletal Disorders, 23*, 1050.

Macedo, C. S. G., Tadiello, F. F., Medeiros, L. T., Antonelo, M. C., Alves, M. A. F., & Mendonça, L. D. (2019). Physical therapy service delivered in the polyclinic during the Rio 2016 Paralympic Games. *Physical Therapy in Sport, 36*, 62–67.

Meṇek, B., Tarakci, D., & Algun, Z. C. (2019). The effect of Mulligan mobilization on pain and life quality of patients with rotator cuff syndrome: A randomized controlled trial. *Journal of Back and Musculoskeletal Rehabilitation, 32*(1), 171–178.

Mohanakrishnan, J. (2015). Role of physical therapist in rehabilitation. *Conference Paper*.

Moreira-Silva, I., Santos, R., Abreu, S., & Mota, J. (2014). The effect of a physical activity program on decreasing physical disability indicated by musculoskeletal pain and related symptoms among workers: A pilot study. *International Journal of Occupational Safety and Ergonomics, 20*, 55–64.

Moritz, T. A., Snowdon, D. A., & Peiris, C. L. (2020). Combining aquatic physiotherapy with usual care physiotherapy for people with neurological conditions: A systematic review. *Physiotherapy Research International, 25*(1), e1813.

Mulligan, M. R. (2004). *Manual Therapy NAGS, SNAGS, MWMS, etc.* (5th ed.).

Murray, C. J., & Lopez, A. D. (1997). Alternative projections of mortality and disability by cause 1990–2020: Global burden of disease study. *The Lancet, 349*(9064), 1498–1504.

Ni, S. H., Jang, W. T., Guo, L., Jin, Y. H., Jiang, T. L., Zhao, Y., & Zhao, J. (2015). Cryotherapy on postoperative rehabilitation of joint arthroplasty. *Knee Surgery, Sports Traumatology, Arthroscopy, 23*, 3354–3361.

Nielsen, G., Stone, J., Matthews, A., Brown, M., Sparkes, C., Farmer, R., Masterton, L., Duncan, L., Winters, A., Daniell, L., Lumsden, C., Carson, A., David, A. S., & Edwards, M. (2015). Physiotherapy for functional motor disorders: A consensus recommendation. *Journal of Neurology, Neurosurgery & Psychiatry, 86*(10), 1113–1119.

Onate, J. A., Guskiewicz, K. M., & Sullivan, R. J. (2001). Augmented feedback reduces jump landing forces. *Journal of Orthopaedic & Sports Physical Therapy, 31*(9), 511–517.

Prall, J., & Ross, M. (2019). The management of work-related musculoskeletal injuries in an occupational health setting: The role of the physical therapist. *Journal of Exercise Rehabilitation, 15*, 193–199.

Pryor, J. A., Webber, B. A., Bethune, D. D., et al. (2008). *Physiotherapy Techniques* (2nd ed.). Churchill Livingstone.

Radder, D. L. M., Silva de Lima, A. L., Domingos, J., Keus, S. H. J., Van Nimwegen, M., Bloem, B. R., & de Vries, M. (2020). Physiotherapy in Parkinson's disease: A meta-analysis of present treatment modalities. *Neurorehabilitation and Neural Repair, 34*(10), 871–880.

Riener, R., Colombo, G., & Lunenburger, L. (2006). Overview of robot-aided gait biofeedback and assessment. In *Proceedings of the First International Conference on Biomedical Robotics and Biomechatronics*. IEEE.

Robinson, A., McIntosh, J., Peberdy, H., Wishart, D., Brown, G., Pope, H., & Kumar, S. (2019). The effectiveness of physiotherapy interventions on pain and quality of life in adults with persistent post-surgical pain compared to usual care: A systematic review. *PLoS One, 14*(12), e0226227.

Samhan, A., Mohamed, N., Elnaggar, R., & Mahmoud, W. (2020). Assessment of the clinical effects of aquatic-based exercises in the treatment of children with juvenile dermatomyositis: A 2 × 2 controlled crossover trial. *Archives of Rheumatology, 35*(1), 97–106.

Shabbir, M., Arshad, N., Naz, A., & Saleem, N. (2021). Clinical outcomes of Maitland mobilization in patients with myofascial chronic neck pain: A randomized trial. *Pakistan Journal of Medical Sciences, 37*(4), 1172–1181.

Shariat, A., Cleland, J. A., Danaee, M., Kargarfard, M., Sangelaji, B., & Tamrin, S. B. (2018). Effects of stretching exercise training and ergonomic modifications on musculoskeletal discomforts of office workers: A randomized controlled trial. *Brazilian Journal of Physical Therapy, 22*, 144–153.

Shipton, E. A. (2018). Physical therapy approaches in the treatment of low back pain. *Pain and Therapy, 7*(2), 127–137.

Spanakis, M., Xylouri, I., Patelarou, E., & Patelarou, A. (2022). A literature review of high-tech physiotherapy interventions in the elderly with neurological disorders. *International Journal of Environmental Research and Public Health, 19*(15), 9233.

Stack, E., & Stokes, M. (2012). *Physical Management for Neurological Conditions*. Elsevier Churchill Livingstone.

Stephensen, D., Bladen, M., & McLaughlin, P. (2018). Recent advances in musculoskeletal physiotherapy for haemophilia. *Therapeutic Advances in Hematology, 9*(8), 227–237.

Tang, C. Y., Taylor, N. F., & Blackstock, F. C. (2010). Chest physiotherapy for patients admitted to hospital with an acute exacerbation of chronic obstructive pulmonary disease (COPD): A systematic review. *Physiotherapy, 96*(1), 1–13.

Taradaj, J., Rajfur, K., Shay, B., Rajfur, J., Ptaszkowski, K., Walewicz, K., Dymarek, R., Sopel, M., & Rosińczuk, J. (2018). Photobiomodulation using high- or low-level laser irradiations in patients with lumbar disc degenerative changes: Disappointing outcomes and remarks. *Clinical Interventions in Aging, 13*, 1445–1455.

Torres-Sánchez, I., Cruz-Ramírez, R., Cabrera-Martos, I., Díaz-Pelegrina, A., & Valenza, M. C. (2017). Results of physiotherapy treatments in exacerbations of chronic obstructive pulmonary disease: A systematic review. *Physiotherapy Canada, 69*(2), 122–132.

Valenza, M. C., Valenza-Peña, G., Torres-Sánchez, I., González-Jiménez, E., Conde-Valero, A., & Valenza-Demet, G. (2014). Effectiveness of controlled breathing techniques on anxiety and depression in hospitalized patients with COPD: A randomized clinical trial. *Respiratory Care, 59*(2), 209–215.

Vestbo, J., Hurd, S. S., Agustí, A. G., Jones, P. W., Vogelmeier, C., Anzueto, A., Barnes, P. J., Fabbri, L. M., Martinez, F. J., Nishimura, M., Stockley, R. A., Sin, D. D., & Rodriguez-Roisin, R. (2013). Global strategy for the diagnosis, management, and prevention of chronic obstructive pulmonary disease: GOLD executive summary. *American Journal of Respiratory and Critical Care Medicine, 187*(4), 347–365.

Vieira, E. R., Schneider, P., Guidera, C., Gadotti, I. C., & Brunt, D. (2016). Work-related musculoskeletal disorders among physical therapists: A systematic review. *Journal of Back and Musculoskeletal Rehabilitation, 29*(3), 417–428.

Wagai, T. (2007). Studies on the foundation and development of diagnostic ultrasound. *Proceedings of the Japan Academy, Series B: Physical and Biological Sciences, 83*(8), 256–265.

Watson, T. (2000). The role of electrotherapy in contemporary physiotherapy practice. *Manual Therapy, 5*(3), 132–141.

WHO Scientific Group on the Burden of Musculoskeletal Conditions at the Start of the New Millennium. (2003). The burden of musculoskeletal conditions at the start of the new millennium. *World Health Organization Technical Report Series, 919*, i–x, 1–218.

Wu, L. C., Weng, P. W., Chen, C. H., Huang, Y., Tsuang, Y. H., & Chiang, C. J. (2018). Literature review and meta-analysis of transcutaneous electrical nerve stimulation in treating chronic back pain. *Regional Anesthesia & Pain Medicine, 43*(4), 425–433.

Yamato, T. P., Maher, C. G., Saragiotto, B. T., Hoffmann, T. C., & Moseley, A. M. (2016). How completely are physiotherapy interventions described in reports of randomised trials? *Physiotherapy, 102*(2), 121–126.

Yang, Y., Wang, Y., Gao, T., Reyila, A., Liu, J., Liu, J., & Han, H. (2023). Effect of physiotherapy interventions on motor symptoms in people with Parkinson's disease: A systematic review and meta-analysis. *Biological Research for Nursing, 25*(4), 586–605.

CHAPTER 18

Occupational Therapy Techniques and Interventions

MEENAKSHI VERMA

Department of Physiotherapy, Sharda School of Allied Health Sciences, Sharda University, Greater Noida, Uttar Pradesh, India

ABSTRACT

The goal of occupational therapy, a client-centered health profession, is to improve health and well-being via occupation, which is defined as worthwhile and purposeful activities that offer people a sense of self and allow them to live freely. The main objective of occupational therapy is to enable patients to engage in activities that are a part of daily life, such as employment, pleasure, or self-care. By altering the job and/or surroundings to more effectively encourage occupational engagement, occupational therapists (OT's) work with individuals and communities to strengthen their capacity to engage in the professions they want to, need to, or are obliged to perform.

A "whole-person approach" to a person's physical and mental health is taken by occupational therapy in order to enhance function and assist people in realizing their full potential. The several strategies and tactics used to ensure that each patient is getting closer to the goals they have set for themselves are covered in this chapter.

18.1 INTRODUCTION

Using intentional activities and treatments, occupational therapy is a specialty in healthcare that helps people achieve independence, functioning,

Allied Healthcare in Practice: An Introduction to Integrated Patient Care. Sally Lukose, Karuna Singh (Eds.)

DOI: 10.1201/9781998511037-21

and a higher quality of life. Occupational therapists (OT's) assist individuals of all ages with a range of developmental, mental, emotional, and physical difficulties. As a client-centered health profession, occupational therapy seeks to enhance health and well-being via employment. When we talk of occupation, we mean the worthwhile and satisfying pursuits that allow people the ability to live freely and authentically.

Making it feasible for patients to engage in activities that are part of everyday living, such as self-care, work, or leisure, is the primary goal of occupational therapy (Baum and Christiansen, 1897). Occupational therapists work with individuals and communities to increase their ability to engage in the professions they want to, need to, or are expected to do by modifying the occupation and/or environment to better foster occupational engagement.

This chapter explores a comprehensive overview of occupational therapy techniques and interventions, showcasing the diverse approaches employed to address specific goals and enhance overall well-being (Figure 18.1).

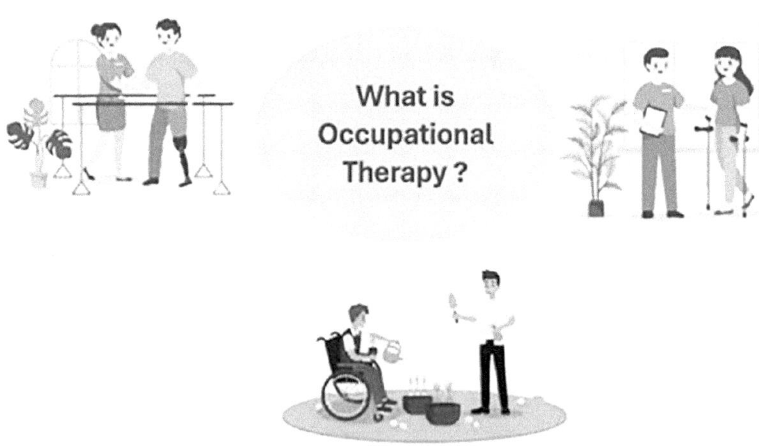

FIGURE 18.1 Occupational therapy.

Occupational therapy is described by the WHO as "the art and science of guiding man's participation in certain activities to repair, strengthen, and increase function." The occupational therapist is engaged to maximize independence; it is his responsibility to assess the patient and teach him how to take care of himself in ways such as dressing, eating, bathing, and maintaining personal hygiene.

OT's support preserving and enhancing joint range of motion, muscular strength, endurance, and coordination, often of the upper limbs, during the duration of the treatment. This aids the patient in examining their vocations and extracurricular pursuits. Therefore, when a change in job is expected, the occupational therapist needs to collaborate with the vocational counselor. He offers comprehensive instruction in home management skills to those who are housebound, employing basic self-care techniques to reduce exhaustion and save energy.

The occupational therapist assesses the house, makes recommendations for changes to create a barrier-free environment, and teaches the patient to compensate for sensory and perceptual limitations while taking into account individual social and cultural preferences. In addition to instructing the patient on how to utilize orthoses, self-help tools, or adaptive equipment as needed, he also shows the patient's family how to retain the patient's independence and reduce overprotection.

In patients with severe disabilities and upper limb amputations, he teaches the functional use of a prosthesis or environmental control systems. He collaborates with physiotherapists to achieve predetermined goals by employing "activities" rather than motions and works with orthotists to create splints. In order to optimize function and assist individuals in reaching their maximum potential, occupational therapy takes a "whole-person approach" to a person's mental and physical well-being (Clark et al., 1891). This is achieved by emphasizing activities of daily living (ADLs), which are the cornerstone of independent living, and by providing the individual with the means to remove barriers that prevent them from participating in the activities that are meaningful to them. OT's believe that an individual's abilities—physical, emotional, or cognitive—as well as the characteristics of their job and the physical, social, cultural, attitudinal, and governmental environments may all influence how involved a person is or is not. To improve occupational involvement, people can change their settings, occupations, or any combination of these with the assistance of OT's.

The WFOT, which serves as the profession's worldwide voice and establishes best practices, is in charge of overseeing occupational therapy on a global scale. OT's can work as independent practitioners or as members of healthcare organizations or rehabilitation teams. They can also accept referrals from a variety of sources, including from the patient themselves (self-referral) or from other individuals connected to the patient.

The Occupational Therapist's key Roles are as follows (Figure 18.2).

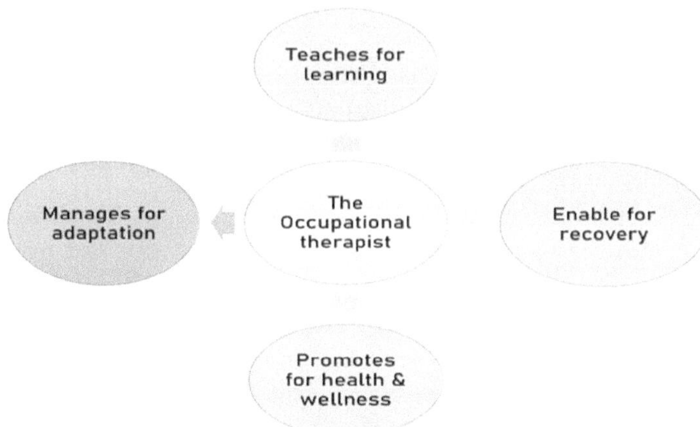

FIGURE 18.2 The occupational therapist's roles.

1. Working together with the client to achieve the goal of engaging in meaningful and purposeful ADL is the therapist's responsibility.
2. Working alongside other medical professionals in social welfare, geriatric, or rehabilitation teams, a team member's role is to assist clients in achieving their desired health goals.
3. The consulting job entails working in tandem with the client's friends, family, coworkers, and other relevant parties (such as architects and landlords) to assist them in achieving their objectives. These positions require the OT's management and collaboration in interpersonal connections (Yerxa, 2001). As a result, OTs counsel, advise, recommend, and coach clients to address difficulties (Glanz and Richman, 1897).

18.2 SKILLS AND KNOWLEDGE RELATING TO CLINICAL PRACTICE

Occupational therapists have a thorough education in the medical, social behavioral, mental health, and occupational sciences, which gives them the attitudes, skills, and knowledge necessary to work cooperatively with individuals, whether they are working one-on-one, in groups, or in communities. All persons, including those who have a physical structure or function limitation brought on by a medical condition, are restricted in their involvement, or are socially excluded because they belong to social or cultural minority groups, can receive occupational therapy. OT's work in collaboration with the patient and their support systems to identify what is restricting a patient's movement and function. They do this by recognizing the effects of social, physical, psychological, and environmental factors and assisting the patient in deciding how to best address their needs.

1. Pay close attention to a person's line of work. The term "occupation" is used by OT's to refer to all the activities we engage in to take care of ourselves and others, socialize and enjoy, and work hard and give back to our communities and cultures.
2. Our jobs are the things we do to fill our days with activities that have value and a purpose. OT's are masters in empowering you to enjoy life to the fullest despite obstacles, restrictions, and disabilities because they recognize how crucial these daily tasks are to all of us.
3. For kids, encouraging involvement in activities like play and school, as well as fostering growth and emerging autonomous skills, will be the main points of attention.
4. OT's know how to help people achieve their highest degree of independence and autonomy because they are aware of how disease, injury, disability, or difficult life experiences might influence their capacity to carry out the daily tasks that are essential to them.
5. OT's are specialists in determining how various medical illnesses might impair people's skills and assisting them in overcoming or navigating the challenges that are interfering with their everyday tasks.
6. Occupational therapy emphasizes a person's abilities, and the treatment is always determined by the client's choices (or, in the case of children, those of their family).
7. By creating a program that is specific to each person's situation and requirements, occupational therapy is person-centered and supports people in leading fulfilling lives.

18.3 ASSESSMENT AND EVALUATION

Occupational therapy is predicated on both baseline and ongoing evaluations. Together, the occupational therapist and the client focus on obstacles pertaining to everyday tasks as well as individual and environmental abilities. Standardized methods, interviews, observations in various situations, and correspondence with important persons in the individual's life are all part of the evaluation process.

Following the evaluation, the patient and the occupational therapist will work together to determine the objectives that occupational therapy may assist the patient in achieving. They'll concentrate on the essentials and work to design a fresh strategy to accomplish their goals or assist them in returning to their previous level of daily function.

18.4 OCCUPATIONAL THERAPY TECHNIQUES AND INTERVENTIONS

Occupational therapy methods and strategies encompass a range of approaches designed to improve functional abilities, foster independence, and enhance the overall quality of life for persons dealing with a variety of issues. These methods are designed to improve a person's physical, mental, emotional, and social well-being. Below are some commonly used occupational therapy techniques and interventions:

18.4.1 ACTIVITY ANALYSIS AND GRADING

- Occupational therapists analyze activities to understand the demands and challenges they present for the individual.
- Activities are graded or adjusted in difficulty to match the person's current abilities, gradually increasing as progress is made.

18.4.2 THERAPEUTIC EXERCISE

- Exercise programs are designed to enhance coordination, flexibility, strength, and endurance.

- Therapists use various exercise modalities, such as resistance training, range of motion exercises, and balance activities.

18.4.3 SENSORY INTEGRATION

- This technique is used for individuals with sensory processing difficulties.
- Therapists create sensory-rich environments and engage clients in activities that help regulate sensory input.

18.4.4 COGNITIVE REHABILITATION

- Cognitive exercises and strategies are employed to address memory, attention, problem-solving, and executive functioning difficulties.
- Memory aids and compensatory techniques are taught to support daily tasks.

18.4.5 ADAPTIVE EQUIPMENT AND ASSISTIVE TECHNOLOGY

- Occupational therapists assess and prescribe assistive devices, such as mobility aids (wheelchairs, canes) and adaptive tools to enhance independence.
- Assistive technology, like voice-activated devices or computer software, may be used to aid communication and daily tasks.

18.4.6 ACTIVITIES OF DAILY LIVING (ADL) TRAINING

- Activities of daily living interventions focus on improving self-care skills, such as dressing, grooming, eating, and bathing.
- Therapists use task-specific training to facilitate independence in these activities.

18.4.7 ENVIRONMENTAL MODIFICATIONS

- In order to meet each person's unique requirements and ensure safety and accessibility, occupational therapists (OT's) evaluate the physical environment and make necessary adjustments. These adjustments may involve moving furniture to improve navigation or adding grab bars or ramps.
- The initial step in housing adaptation treatments is the methodical gathering of data to determine the client's issue. Preferably, the basis for this identification should be person-environment-occupational exchanges. After the data is analyzed, the house adaptation is planned, and this process calls for the client and his or her family to be actively involved. Actions including removing thresholds, installing shower stalls in place of bathtubs, and setting up ramps, grab bars, and handrails (Figure 18.3) are among the most common.

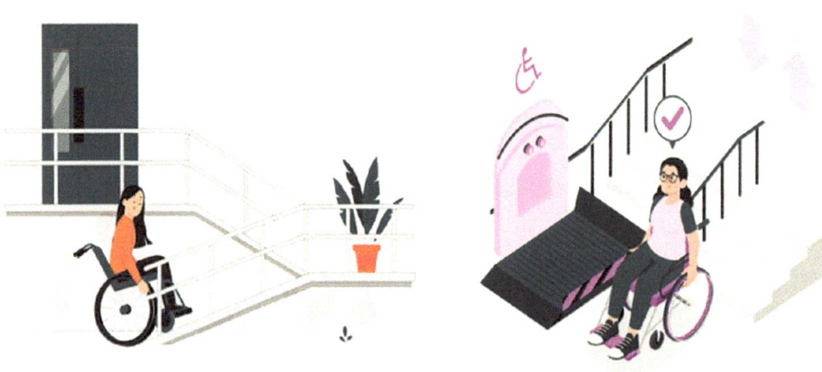

FIGURE 18.3 Installation of ramps at entrance.

For clients who have official or informal assistants, the ergonomic features of their work environment must be taken into account. Occupational therapists (OTs) face significant challenges when implementing housing adaptation interventions, as they are addressing one of the most intimate aspects of a person's life. There is an inherent risk of conflicts of interest throughout the process.

18.4.8 PAIN MANAGEMENT INTERVENTIONS

Modalities like heat, cold, electrical stimulation, or relaxation techniques are used to manage pain and discomfort.

18.4.9 SOCIAL SKILLS TRAINING

- Social interventions are employed to improve communication and interpersonal skills.
- Group therapy sessions may be utilized for social engagement practice.

18.4.10 WORK-RELATED INTERVENTIONS

- Vocational rehabilitation focuses on helping individuals return to work or engage in meaningful employment.
- Job coaching, workplace accommodations, and vocational training are provided.

18.5 ROLE OF OCCUPATIONAL THERAPIST IN PEDIATRIC INTERVENTIONS

Occupational therapy techniques and interventions in pediatrics are designed to address the unique developmental needs of children and help them participate in activities that are essential for their growth, learning, and socialization. Pediatric occupational therapists work with children of all ages, from infants to adolescents, and tailor their interventions to suit each child's specific challenges and abilities. Below are a few typical occupational therapy methods and interventions used in pediatric settings:

1. **Sensory Integration Therapy:**

   i. Sensory integration activities help children process and respond appropriately to sensory information from their environment.

   ii. Therapists use sensory-rich play activities to address sensory processing difficulties and enhance self-regulation.

2. **Play-Based Therapy:**
   i. Play is the natural way children learn and develop essential skills.
   ii. Occupational therapists use play-based interventions to improve fine motor skills, social skills, communication, and problem-solving abilities.
3. **Fine Motor Skill Development:**
   i. Activities that target hand strength, dexterity, and hand-eye coordination are used to improve fine motor skills.
   ii. These interventions help with tasks like handwriting, using utensils, and manipulating small objects.
4. **Gross Motor Skill Training:**
   i. Gross motor interventions focus on enhancing large muscle movements, balance, and coordination.
   ii. Therapists use games and activities to improve skills like running, jumping, and climbing.
5. **Visual Perception and Visual Motor Integration:**
   i. Interventions to develop visual perception skills help children process and interpret visual information.
   ii. Visual-motor integration activities improve hand-eye coordination for tasks like writing and drawing.
6. **Self-Care Training:**
   i. Occupational therapists work with children on ADLs like dressing, grooming, and feeding.
   ii. Self-care interventions promote independence in self-care tasks appropriate for a child's age.
7. **Social Skills Training:** Therapists use group sessions and role-playing activities to help children improve social interactions, empathy, and communication with peers and adults.
8. **Handwriting and Pre-writing Skills:**

i. Interventions focus on pre-writing activities to develop foundational skills required for handwriting.
   ii. Therapists work on pencil grasp, letter formation, and writing speed.

9. **Behavior Management:** Occupational therapists may employ behavior modification techniques to address challenging behaviors and support self-regulation.
10. **Assistive Technology and Adaptive Equipment:** Therapists assess and recommend assistive technology or adaptive equipment to help children participate in activities at home, school, or play.
11. **Parent and Caregiver Education:** Occupational therapists educate parents and caregivers on strategies to support their child's development and generalize therapy gains into daily routines.
12. **School-Based Interventions:** Occupational therapists collaborate with teachers to implement strategies and accommodations to support a child's learning and grasping in the classroom.
13. **Environmental Modifications:** Therapists may suggest modifications in the home or school environment to enhance accessibility and safety for the child.
14. **Feeding Therapy:** For children with feeding difficulties, occupational therapists use specialized interventions to address sensory aversions and improve oral motor skills.

18.6 NEUROMUSCULAR AND MOVEMENT RELATED LEARNING

1. **Constraint-Induced Movement Therapy for Restoration of Upper-Limb Function:** Constraint-Induced Movement Therapy (CIMT), a behavioral strategy developed via research, is used to restore limb function after neurologic injury. The intervention makes use of both motor training techniques and psychological ideas to promote better movement quality and control, as well as enhanced use of the afflicted limb. Importantly, CIMT is created to produce improvements in real-world situations using behavioral techniques that make it easier for people to incorporate their recovered talents into their natural behavior.

   Constraint-Induced Movement Therapy has three main aspects:

   i. Repetitive, unilateral training procedures (such as practicing tasks and shaping);

   ii. A collection of behavioral strategies called the "transfer package," which encourages the transfer of therapeutic gains to real-world situations; and
   iii. Constraining the hand that is not affected by the constraint using one of several methods. Evidence suggests that CIMT enhances the more afflicted upper extremity's functional usage and occupational performance by backward learned inactivity and promoting use-dependent brain plasticity.

2. **Joint Protection:** Facilitating Modifications in Musculoskeletal Conditions – Applying ergonomic concepts to daily activities, changing working practices, adopting assistive technology, and changing settings are all part of joint protection. People who have musculoskeletal disorders such as rheumatoid arthritis (RA), osteoarthritis, and soft tissue rheumatisms are taught it. The distribution of weight over a number of joints, the use of assistive devices to lessen effort, the pacing of activities, the application of orthotics, and regular exercise are all common practices. Self-efficacy, motor learning, and cognitive-behavioral techniques are used. Trials show that using these strategies dramatically improves function, decreases pain, and changes joint-protection behavior in both the beginning and end stages of RA. This is in comparison to advice and demonstration alone. There is evidence that joint protection coupled with hand exercises increases grip strength in people with hand OA, but there is still conflict over its efficacy in those with soft-tissue rheumatisms.

3. **Neurodevelopmental Therapy:** Intervention for children with mental retardation using sensory integration and vestibular stimulation: Significant impairments in intellectual functioning and adaptable behavior, as shown by conceptual, social, and practical adaptation abilities, are characteristics of mental retardation, a disability. The brain organizes sensory input through a process called sensory integration. A broad spectrum of postural control and sensory integration dysfunctions are seen in mentally retarded children. Learning requires that children be able to take in sensory data from their environment and use it in purposeful activities. The goal-oriented play that the children actively participate in is the main emphasis of neurodevelopmental treatment.

Children with mental retardation, such as Down syndrome, cerebral palsy, delayed development, schizophrenia, abnormalities of a non-developed central nervous system (CNS), such as those in some premature infants, a specific learning disability, speech and receptive language difficulties, and behavior issues are the target population for NDT based on sensory integration or vestibular rehabilitation. Adults who have experienced brain injury leading to hemiplegia are also suitable candidates for these programs. Active play focused on promoting the child's adaptive responses is essential. Examples include the controlled multi-sensory stimulation rooms, or snoezelen, found in occupational therapy units, daycare, inpatient and outpatient centers, special education settings, inpatient/outpatient day centers, or homes.

The child's self-care, play, and academic abilities are all developed through the utilization of the environmental stimuli that are enabled and planned for by the OT. The OT positions the child and employs passive movement schema as well as oral, supporting, or visual cues to help the child develop motor skills. Instead of concentrating on the particular motor elements of the task, the child focuses on the objective.

18.7 CONCLUSION

Occupational therapy techniques and interventions are diverse and tailored to meet the new requirements and goals of each individual client. By addressing physical, cognitive, emotional, and environmental factors, occupational therapists strive to empower their clients to lead fulfilling and meaningful lives. The client-centered approach, coupled with evidence-based practices and innovative interventions, positions occupational therapy as a pivotal discipline in enhancing functional outcomes and promoting overall well-being for individuals of all ages and abilities.

KEYWORDS

- **activity of daily living**
- **client-centered approach**
- **evidence-based practices**
- **functional outcomes**

- **intervention**
- **mental well-being**
- **occupational therapy**
- **physical health**
- **physical well-being**
- **social well-being**
- **techniquess**

REFERENCES

Baum, C., & Christiansen, C. (1997). The occupational therapy context: Philosophy, principles, and practice. In C. Christiansen & C. Baum (Eds.), *Occupational Therapy: Enabling Function and Well-Being* (pp. 33–35). Slack.

Bobath, K., & Bobath, B. (1967). The neurodevelopmental intervention of cerebral palsy. *Developmental Medicine & Child Neurology, 9*, 373–390.

Bowman, M. H., Taub, E., Uswatte, G., et al. (2006). A treatment for a chronic stroke patient with a plegic hand combining CI therapy with conventional rehabilitation procedures: Case report. *NeuroRehabilitation, 21*, 167–176.

Candia, V., Elbert, T., Altenmüller, E., et al. (1999). Constraint-Induced Movement Therapy for focal hand dystonia in musicians. *The Lancet, 353*, 42.

Carroll, D. (1962). The disability in hemiplegia caused by cerebrovascular disease: Serial studies of 98 cases. *Journal of Chronic Diseases, 15*, 179–188.

Dromerick, A. W., Edwards, D. F., & Hahn, M. (2000). Does the application of Constraint-Induced Movement Therapy during acute rehabilitation reduce arm impairment after ischemic stroke? *Stroke, 82*, 2984–2988.

Noser, E. A., Ro, T., et al. (2007). Constraint-Induced Movement Therapy during early stroke rehabilitation. *Neurorehabilitation and Neural Repair, 21*, 14–24.

CHAPTER 19

Speech Therapy Techniques and Interventions

MEENAKSHI VERMA

Department of Physiotherapy, Sharda School of Allied Health Sciences, Sharda University, Greater Noida, Uttar Pradesh, India

ABSTRACT

Speech and dialect pathologists, often called speech and language therapists, are specialists in speech, language, voice, speaking, hearing, eating, and swallowing. They also specialize in the social and cognitive aspects of communication. They provide assessment, diagnosis, treatment, and support to help those who have difficulty with eating, swallowing, or interacting with others so they can realize their full potential. Within this framework, "human communication" encompasses all cognitive processes related to comprehending and utilizing spoken and written language, in addition to nonverbal and/or other modes of communication.

Speech and language therapists enhance people's capacity for speaking and swallowing, hence improving quality of life, by developing and implementing a treatment plan to address the symptoms or concerns of a communication or swallowing difficulty or related functional problems. Enhancing a person's effective results through written language, nonverbal communication, and/or alternative forms of communication is the final aim of counseling.

Allied Healthcare in Practice: An Introduction to Integrated Patient Care. Sally Lukose, Karuna Singh (Eds.)

DOI: 10.1201/9781998511037-22

19.1 INTRODUCTION

The confirmatory diagnosis and treatment of diverse speech and language impairments are the primary aim of speech therapy, a specialist profession within the subject of communication disorders. This chapter explores the foundational ideas of speech therapy and communication and presents a variety of methods for improving communication abilities in people with speech impairments.

The term "communication" refers to all of the actions, including speech and language functions, that people employ to connect with one another and transfer information. The capacity for language use and comprehension is vital to human existence, both in social interactions and in one's own intellectual pursuits. Although speech and language have many similarities, they are not exactly the same thing. Language functions include understanding formation, idea and emotion transmission through the use of standardized signs, markings, sounds, gestures, and their sequential arrangement in accordance with agreed grammatical rules. On the other hand, speech focuses more on the phonetic and articulatory components of verbal communication.

As a separate profession, speech-language pathologists can operate alone or in conjunction with experts in the fields of audiology, medicine, nursing, dietetics, education, physiotherapy (PT), occupational therapy, psychology, child care, and social work. In addition, they are able to take referrals from a range of sources, including the patient.

Language dysfunction is usually an indication of a brain disorder, more specifically of the dominant or working cerebral hemisphere. A speech issue may have a similar etiology. It may result from abnormalities in distinct brain regions or from extra cerebral mechanisms. Speech and language impairments are present in 10.8% of the population over the age of 65, but only 9.9% of people below 45 years of age. Children with articulation abnormalities (32.1%) and language disorders (43.7%) make up the majority of those who have communication problems. 15% of adults with speech and language impairments have aphasia (Figure 19.1).

Depending on the area that is damaged, speaking clearly may be completely or partially impossible. The following things will occur:

i. Reception of sound impulses that encode words in the main auditory area.

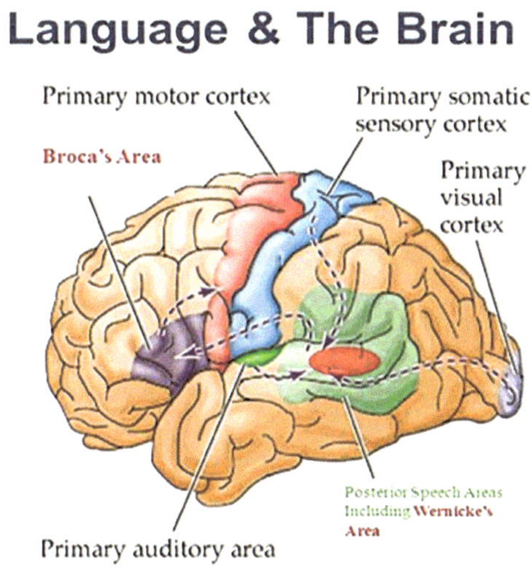

FIGURE 19.1 Language areas.

ii. Interpretation of words in Wernicke's area.
iii. Determination is also present in Wernicke's thoughts and spoken words.
iv. Signal transmission via the arcuate fasciculus from Wernicke's area to Broca's area.
v. The Broca's area skilled motor program is activated to govern word creation, transferring signals into the motor cortex to command the muscles used for speaking (Figures 19.2; 19.3).

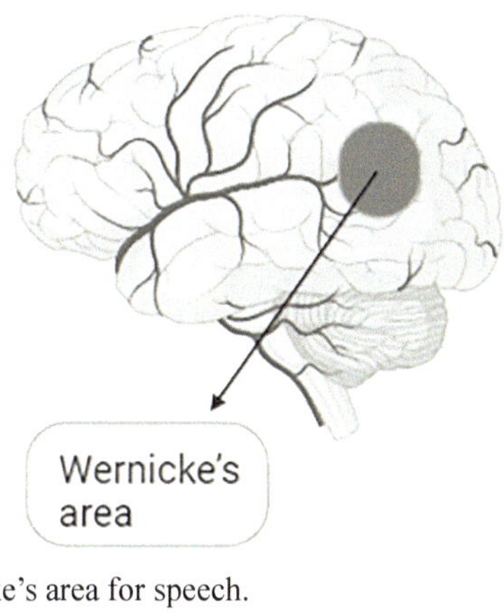

FIGURE 19.2 Wernicke's area for speech.

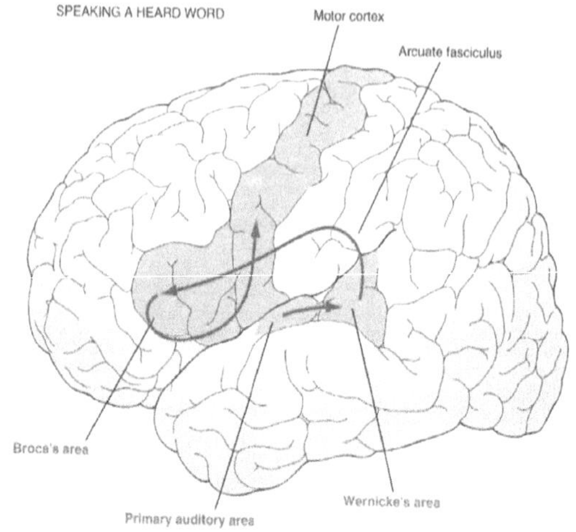

FIGURE 19.3 Broca's area process.

Rather than the major auditory area, the primary visual area is where words are first processed. Then, information goes through the initial stages of interpretation in the angular gyrus region before eventually reaching Wernicke's area, where it is fully recognized. The process continues in the same order as when speaking in response to the spoken word (Figure 19.4).

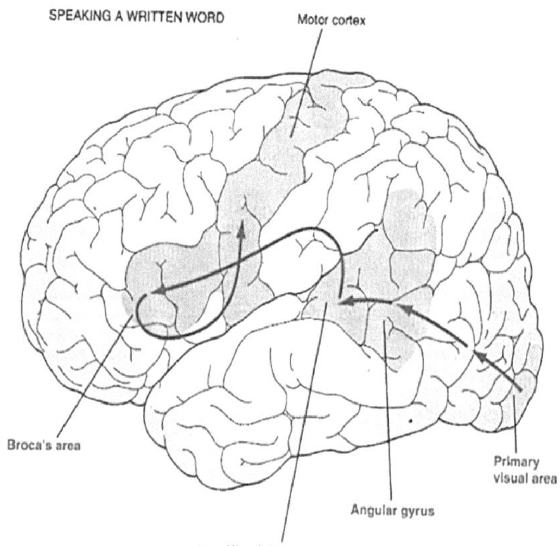

FIGURE 19.4 Process of Wernicke's area.

19.2 A LANGUAGE'S ORGANIZATION

Speech sounds, also known as phonemes, are the building blocks of words and are frequently classified as vowels or consonants. The study of a language's sound system is known as phonology.

- Phonemes are the fundamental linguistic building blocks of words.
- The vocabulary or lexicon of a language is made up of words.
- Consonants and vowels are joined to form bigger components known as syllables.
- The grammar or syntax of a language establishes the permissible order of words in sentences.
- The area of linguistics that studies word meanings is called semantics.
- Prosody uses stress and intonation to distinguish between questions, assertions, emotional expressions, astonishment, exclamations, and other speech patterns.

19.3 SPEECH AND LANGUAGE DISORDERS DUE TO DISEASE

A disorder called aphasia impairs one's capacity to utter words and/or comprehend written or spoken languages. Speech and language disturbances are associated with disorders affecting higher-order mental functioning, such as dementia, delirium, and confusion.

Speech and language functions are seldom lost in these conditions but are damaged as part of the general impairment of perceptual and intellectual functions, for example, extreme perseveration (palilalia) and echolalia, in which the patient repeats, parrot-like, words and phrases that he hears. An articulation deficit is concomitant with normal cognition, word memory, and brain function; this is a pure motor disorder of the articulatory muscles and can be caused by recurring spasms, stiffness, ataxia, or flaccid or spastic paralysis. Some of these disorders have been referred to as dysarthria's or anarthria's. Aphonia or dysphonia—loss of voice brought on by a laryngeal disease or its innervations. Language and articulation are unaltered.

19.4 CLINICAL PICTURES OF APHASIA

- **Broca's Aphasia:** Motor expressive and non-fluent.

- **Wernicke's Aphasia:** Sensory , receptive and fluent.
- **Global Aphasia:** Both types.

19.5 DISSOCIATIVE LANGUAGE SYNDROMES

- Conduction aphasia.
- Word deafness (auditory verbal agnosia).
- Word blindness (visual verbal agnosia or alexia).
- Various types of mutism.
- Anomia (nominal or amnesic aphasia).
- Transcortical aphasias.

19.6 BED SIDE LANGUAGE EXAMINATION

Start by asking about the patients' native tongue, prior literacy level, education, and handedness. The first step in any bedside language test is to observe the patient's speech and understanding during a clinical interview. Examiners can gain a lot of insight about a patient's speech function if they intentionally observe the patient's speech patterns and responses to queries. The majority of informal interviews are used to identify mild word-finding difficulties, sporadic paraphasic mistakes, and higher-level deficiencies in discourse planning and communication pragmatics, such as the use of humor and irony.

1. Alexander and Benson (1997) revised the six-part bedside language exam that was made popular by Frank Benson and Norman Gash Wind. Speaking spontaneously, naming, understanding auditorily, repeating, and perusing: (i) reading aloud; (ii) writing and reading comprehension: (i) unplanned phrases; (ii) copying and writing to dictation.
2. The description of spontaneous speech is the first section of the examination. One way to get a speech sample from the patient is to ask them to describe the weather or why they are seeing the doctor. Reciting lists, such as a counting list or a list of the days of the week, might be beneficial if speech is lacking or non-existent. Fluency is the most crucial factor in spontaneous speaking. Speech that is fluid moves quickly and naturally. Speech that is not fluid is

delivered in brief bursts or in single words, sometimes with hesitation and pauses in between. Primary features such as difficulty of commencement, articulation, phonation or voice loudness, speech tempo, prosody or melodic intonation, and phrase length should be addressed initially.

3. Secondly, spoken utterance content should be examined for word-seeking pauses, circumlocutions, and mistakes such as neologisms and literal and verbal paraphasia's. In the second section of the bedside examination, the patient is asked to name items, pieces of objects, photographs, colors, or body parts that they are confronted with. Testing a few things from each category is recommended since anomia might be word class specific. People's proper names are frequently negatively impacted. To make sure the patient recognizes the objects or individuals that they are unable to name, the examiner should probe with inquiries.

19.7 AUDITORY COMPREHENSION

To test this, the patient is initially asked to follow a series of instructions that comprise one, two, and three steps. To give an order in one step would be to thrust out your tongue. The instructions are to raise your left thumb and close your eyes in two steps. At least at this basic level, successfully following instructions guarantees sufficient comprehension; nonetheless, failing to follow instructions does not always imply a lack of comprehension. Exercises such as yes-or-no questions or orders that just demand a pointing answer are ideal for testing understanding because they don't involve a motor act. The patient has to be able to direct, comprehend the language used by the examiner, and possess the necessary motor skills to do the task without experiencing any apraxia. Posing absurd queries, such as "Do you vomit every day?" and receiving prompt responses revealed whether or not the patient comprehended. Unexpected results are sometimes derived from absurd questions, given that many aphasics mask their communication difficulties with humor.

19.7.1 REPETITION

Word and phrase repetition should be carefully considered. Patients with dysarthria struggle with fast consonant sequences, such as "Methodist

Episcopal," while aphasics struggle more with sentences that are highly structured. For aphasics, the statement "No, ifs, ands, or buts" is very difficult. Aphasics frequently reproduce well-known or "high probability" words far more accurately than unknown ones. Aphasics frequently reproduce well-known or highly probable sentences far more accurately than unknown ones. Tests on reading comprehension and spoken aloud should be administered. The examiner should have a few printed instructions with them so they may quickly compare reading and auditory understanding. Of course, the premorbid reading level of the patient must be known to the examiner.

19.7.2 WRITING

Not only do the sometimes-overlooked components of the bedside examination offer a further example of expressive language, but they also enable a spelling analysis that is not feasible with spoken language. Sentences that explain the patient's reason for visiting for an examination, for example, are examples of spontaneous writing that is particularly sensitive to language difficulties. If this doesn't work, you could also attempt copying and writing to dictation. Evaluations of language at the bedside are integrated with standard neurological and mental status evaluations.

19.8 EXAMINATIONS OF APHASIA

19.8.1 TOKEN TEST

The goal of this highly discriminating test is to identify even the slightest deficiencies in auditory comprehension. Token tests are straightforward and need little preparation. In order to represent every conceivable combination, the test calls for 19 tokens, which vary in form (circle and square), size (small-large), and color (red, yellow, green, blue, and white). The tokens are set in front of the patient, who is given more detailed instructions to manipulate them. Test commands total 62.

19.8.2 APHASIA LANGUAGE PERFORMANCE SCALES (ALPS)

Four 10-part subtests cover the modalities of listening, talking, reading, and writing. Each subtest permits scaling of performance within the modality from 1 to 10, different levels of performance being defined in terms of message length and complexity (single words, phrases, sentences, multi-sentence groups).

19.8.3 FUNCTIONAL COMMUNICATION PROFILE (FCP)

In informal interaction with the patient in a conversational situation, the clinician rates his ability to use residual communication skills in 45 activities. Ratings are made on a 9-point scale; a percentage score can be derived to indicate the general language ability of the patient.

19.8.4 CAPABILITY OF COMMUNICATION IN DAILY LIVING (CADL)

The examiner assesses the patients' capacity to do 68 distinct communication activities, comprising varying degrees of speaking, listening, reading, and writing, through interviews and role-playing. Reactions are graded utilizing a 3-point rating: 0 = Communication breakdown; 1 = Communication with some degree of success; 2 = Interaction.

19.8.5 WESTERN APHASIA BATTERY (WAB)

WAB has four oral language subtests (spontaneous speech, comprehension, repetition, and naming) upon which the aphasia quotient (AQ) is based. Additional tests of reading, writing, praxis, drawing, block design, and calculation can be combined to yield a performance quotient (PQ). AQ and PQ combined provide a cortical quotient (CQ) as a summary of cognitive function.

19.9 MANAGEMENT

Speech-language pathologists (SLPs), speech-language therapists (SALTs), and occasionally speech therapists work in the discipline of speech-language pathology. A university-trained practitioner with expertise in swallowing and communication disorders is known as a SLP. Additionally, SLPs are crucial in the detection, diagnosis, and management of autism spectrum disorders, frequently working in tandem with psychologists and pediatricians.

SLPs are experts in the assessment, diagnosis, treatment, and prevention of swallowing difficulties, voice disorders, cognitive-communication disorders, and communication disorders (i.e., speech and language impairments). SLPs are crucial in the diagnosis and management of autism spectrum disorder, frequently working in conjunction with psychologists and pediatricians.

The main premise of aphasia therapy is that language is not lost in the brain; rather, language retrieval of its constituent parts is compromised. Therapy for aphasia has often been approached using one of two paradigms. Either a direct treatment model or a substitute skill model is predicated on the idea that understanding the mechanism that underlies normal performance is essential to its success. Deaf people who use speech reading, a visual input rather than an aural one, as a tool to understand spoken language are an example of a substitution skill model.

The two principles that underlie most treatment methods reflect contrasting views of aphasia as either impaired access to language or a loss of language. The stimulation methods generally follow an impaired access theory, and pedagogic approaches are based on a theory of aphasia as a language loss.

However, in reality, a large portion of aphasia treatment focuses on the performance side of language, with the idea that task-oriented approaches and repeated practice might help recover damaged abilities (e.g., naming practice). Self-cueing and repetition activities that modify vocabulary and grammatical rules are two often employed strategies. Another strategy is to encourage residual language usage in the patient by facilitating discussion in a permissive environment where the patient's answers are welcomed and the subjects are relevant to the staff.

19.9.1 PROMOTING APHASICS' COMMUNICATIVE EFFECTIVENESS (PACE THERAPY)

This approach incorporates components of face-to-face conversation and is based upon a pragmatic approach to language, pragmatics being the study of how language is used in context. PACE is based upon a few principles; there is a change of new messages between clinician and patient. Messages are represented by pictures of familiar objects, actions, and stories.

A stack of such pictures is available to the patient and clinician, who alternatively draw from them and engage in transmitting messages to each other. The listener is unaware of the nature of the message before it is conveyed by the speaker. The speaker has a free choice of communicative channels to use in conveying new information.

Aphasic patients may use whatever oral language is available to them, or they may write messages, use natural and conventional gesturing, pantomime, drawing, and pointing to pictures, printed words, or objects in the room. These channels can be used singly or in combinations in any way the speaker chooses to convey the message as best they can.

The clinician and patient both participate as senders and receivers of messages. They take turns in conversation, alternately selecting a message from the stack of pictures. When the clinician speaks, they present a kind of model showing the patient how to use different channels as well as different types of communicative behavior within a particular channel. The clinician determines whether the patient has comprehended the message. Then roles are reversed, and the patient conveys the message, determining whether the clinician has received their message.

Feedback is provided by the clinician in response to the patient's success in conveying a message. Emphasis is not on trying to improve the patient's nicety of verbalization but rather on their accomplishing adequate conveyance of messages. The developer of PACE indicates that it can be readily modified to deal with different degrees of severity of aphasia and different special problems in communication.

19.9.2 VISUAL ACTION THERAPY

Helm and Benson (1978) describe a method in which patients are taught to understand and produce symbolic gestures as a precursor to language treatment. A group of objects (razor, screwdriver, cup, etc.) that can be readily manipulated with one hand and are capable of being symbolized by a single gesture is selected. Large and small line drawings of these objects are also used, as well as line drawings of the objects being manipulated by a person. The patient is taught to match real objects with large drawings, then with small drawings. They are then taught to manipulate the objects while looking at action drawings. The patients become able to select the appropriate object from a group of objects and pretend to use it after being shown a selected action drawing. The patient is then trained to recognize and produce a distinctive pantomime gesture in association with each object. By the time the program ends, the patient can produce representational gestures to represent small line drawings. The designers of this program have reported that globally aphasic patients exposed to this regimen have demonstrated an increase in auditory comprehension, the ability to communicate by gesture, and in the use of oral language as well.

Helm and Barresi (1980) have suggested another procedure for severely aphasic patients, which involves their developing voluntary control over involuntary utterances. The patient is shown printed words that he has been heard to say (even his stereotypical "no," "oh," "I don't know," or obscenities) and emotionally laden words likely to express some sort of result. If the patient is able to read a word aloud, it is printed on an index card to be used in self-monitored drills. If, instead of uttering the printed words, the patients utter some other real word, the original word is discarded, and the substituted words are printed on an index card instead. The patient's real word errors thus become correct responses. Subsequent practice in oral reading is done with these target words, using them in naming and other activities. Since only the patients' real word utterances are used, they seem to struggle less in processing them. They can practice their words with other patients or with family and gradually develop more verbal skills.

An approach suggested by Towey and Pettit (1980) emphasizes communication competencies in nonlinguistic areas. It promotes a patient's ability to take in all available communicative behaviors, nonverbal as well as verbal, and to make appropriate selections from among the possible responses. They suggest nine important areas for improving communication competence in global aphasia.

There are three important verbal behaviors.

1. The use of the patient's name or title in such a way as not to offend him, but to establish a good relationship, avoiding first names if the use of titles would be more appropriate.
2. Verbal responses used by the clinician, such as expressions of understanding of and feeling for the patient's affect (e.g., "I know that you are very angry").
3. Avoiding interruptions of the speaker, allowing the patient to try to communicate and to avoid rejection and frustration that result from interrupting his perhaps unintelligible message.

Four nonverbal behaviors are emphasized.

1. Eye contact, encouraged in both the patient and clinician, as lack of it might signify anxiety, poor self-image, or rejection.
2. Head nodding, indicating participation, understanding, and desire to respond within an interaction.
3. Pleasantness and appropriateness of facial expressions, reflecting support, empathy, and concern.
4. Reciprocity of affect displays—smiling, laughing, frowning, scowling, and other cues are responded to in a reflection of the patient's affect, indicating empathy and understanding of what the patient is feeling.

19.9.3 VISUAL COMMUNICATION THERAPY (VIC)

This is a method of experimentation intended for worldwide aphasia. VIC uses an index card system with random symbols that stand in for lexical and syntactic elements that the patient learns to manipulate in order to:

(i) Comply with an instruction; (ii) Describe your wants, desires, and other feelings.

The approach aims to avoid the patient with global aphasia using their native speech language, which is significantly degraded and frequently unavailable. Steel et al. and Weinrich et al. (1906) presented an application and adaptation of the VIC system called Computer-Aided Visual Communication (C-VIC), which showed that C-VIC training may enhance spoken language.

19.9.4 FUNCTIONAL COMMUNICATION TREATMENT

Developed by Aten et al., this approach focuses on reestablishing communication in its widest meaning. The goal of treatment is to enhance information processing in activities of daily living (ADL), social engagement, and self-expression of psychological and physical needs. Calendars, neighborhood maps, and grocery store products were among the materials utilized in treatment. The emphasis of the non-modality-bound treatment is on the regular application of daily activities that are individually relevant.

In order to promote efficient communication, patients are instructed to gesture in response to the majority of spoken words.

Syndromes of aberrant articulation, or the motor production of speech, without defective language function are known as motor speech disorders. It should be possible for a patient with a motor speech problem to write in a typical expressive manner and to understand written and spoken language. When someone with a motor speech impairment records a patient's speech and types it into a text document, the text ought to appear in normal language.

19.10 DYSARTHRIA

When the oromandibular pharyngeal muscles are not activated normally, sounds or phonemes are articulated abnormally, resulting in dysarthria. This can impact the range, accuracy, timing, strength, and speed of speech. While sensory deficiencies may occasionally play a role, dysarthria is mostly neurogenic, linked to malfunctioning of the central nervous system (CNS), nerves, neuromuscular junction, and muscle. Local anatomical issues with the tongue, palate, or larynx can also contribute to atypical speech patterns. In addition to articulation, dysarthria can also impact respiration, phonation, and prosody (emotional tone) of speech. Anarthria is the complete loss of the capacity to speak, whereas dysarthria typically results in consonant sound distortion.

- **The Analysis of Dysarthria:** Proper bilateral coordination of the tongue, lips, palate, larynx, and breathing muscles is necessary for accurate articulation. These may be affected by lesions in the motor neurons of the upper and lower limbs, the coordinating effect of the extrapyramidal and cerebellar systems, or the muscles themselves. Ask the patient to repeat certain words during the evaluation. Although there are a lot of tongue twisters, it is best to start with simpler terms because the average individual could have a lot of trouble understanding some of the typical exam phrases. Among these are Methodist Episcopal "British Constitution" churches (The Devonshire County Council). Peter Piper took a pickled pepper peck. Request that the patient read a passage from an easy-to-read book.

To assess whether the patient's muscles are fatigued, have them count backward from 30 or higher. Listen to the words to see if they blend together awkwardly, if the rhythm is abrupt, erratic, or monotonous, if the speech is excessively loud or soft, if any specific letters are difficult to pronounce and which ones they are, if the speech has a nasal tone, and if the disruption is continuous, variable, or increases toward the end of each sentence or during extended counting.

19.11 BED SIDE FEATURES OF DYSARTHRIA

1. **Type Flaccid:** Auditory signs: Breathy nasal voice, imprecise consonants. Diseases: Stroke, myasthenia gravis.
2. **Spastic Type:** Location: Upper motor neurons on both sides, small and spastic tongue; excessive gag reflex and jaw jerk; letters b, p, d, and g suffer especially. Illnesses: tumor, stroke.
3. **Type Ataxic:** Cerebellum is the location. Auditory symptoms include: Excessive and uniform tension; irregular articulatory breakdowns. Diseases: degenerative disease, stroke.
4. **Hypokinetic:** Extra pyramidal localization. Signs of the ears: Quick speed, decreased volume, single pitch and single loudness; Parkinson's disease is one illness.
5. **Hyperkinetic Type:** Localization: Extra pyramidal. Auditory signs: Prolonged phonemes, variable rate, inappropriate silences, voice stoppages. Diseases: dystonia, Huntington's disease..

19.12 MANAGEMENT OF DYSARTHRIA

19.12.1 STRENGTHENING

Jaw opening/closing/lateralization and provide resistance. Lips can be closed isometrically with or without effort, puffed, spread, and rounded. The tongue can be lateralized and thrust out in response to opposition.

19.12.2 RELAXATION

To increase the tone of the muscles in individuals who are stiff and spastic. Shaking the head and opening the jaw to create lateral movement of the jaw. Chewing movements (decrease mild muscle hypertonus in the jaw and tongue).

19.12.3 STRETCHING

Maximal jaw opening maintained. Maximum lateralization, retraction, or protrusion of the tongue. Maximal sustained lip retraction, pursing, and puffing (to improve range of motion and reduce stiffness).

19.12.4 POSTURAL ADJUSTMENT

Important for maintaining adequate physiological support for respiration. Provided by adjustable beds, wheelchairs, and chairs with adjustable backs (Yorkston, 1988). Hixon, Putnam, and Sharp (1983) have discussed two compensatory modes of breathing for speech (useful for flaccid paralysis of the rib cage, diaphragm, and abdomen).

19.12.5 NECK BREATHING

In which SCM, scalene, and trapezius muscles of the neck are used to bring about to-and-fro displacement of the rib cage for inspiration.

19.12.6 GLOSSOPHARYNGEAL BREATHING (FROG BREATHING)

It is a self-generated positive pressure technique in which the upper airways and larynx are utilized to gradually pump small amounts of air into the lungs.

19.12.7 PROSTHETIC MANAGEMENT

Devices such as pacing boards, a tool that can be used by SLPs to target a variety of skills (Figure 19.5).

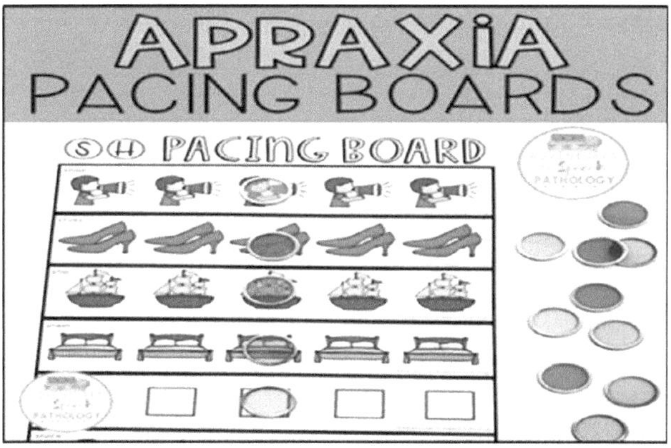

FIGURE 19.5 Apraxia pacing boards.

Source: https://www.teacherspayteachers.com/Product/Apraxia-Pacing-Boards-3762631

1. **Palatal Lift:** Consists of a palatal part that is attached to the teeth and a lift portion that extends posteriorly. It is useful for reducing hypernasality.
2. **Amplifiers:** To boost vocal intensity.
3. **Communication Boards:** To encourage participants to point to images.

   Augmentative communicative devices: For patients who are unable to communicate.
4. **Prosthesis:** That provides postural support during respiration or helps control expiration can be useful during speech.

In particular, those with spinal cord injuries who have intact diaphragmatic function but weak respiratory muscles can benefit from abdominal binders, often known as corsets, since they help improve posture, support weak stomach muscles, and increase respiratory support and airflow with less effort.

19.13 CONCLUSION

In order to improve communication skills for those with speech and language impairments, speech therapy is essential. Through systematic assessment and the application of various therapeutic techniques, SLPs empower individuals to overcome communication challenges and achieve effective communication.

KEYWORDS

- **communication**
- **evaluation**
- **interpersonal contact**
- **motor speech disorders**
- **motor speech impairment**
- **neighborhood maps**
- **non-modality-bound treatment**
- **speech and language therapists**
- **speech production**
- **swallowing**
- **therapy**

REFERENCES

Alexander, D. N., & Benson, D. F. (1997). Ideomotor apraxia: Behavioural dimensions and neuroanatomical basis. In *Neuropsychological Studies in Apraxia and Related Disorders* (pp. 125–136).

Aten, J. L., Caligiuri, M. P., & Holland, A. L. (1982). The efficacy of functional communication therapy for chronic aphasic patients. *Journal of Speech and Hearing Disorders, 47*, 93–96.

Helm, N. A., Butler, R. B., & Benson, D. F. (1978). Clinical aspects of aphasia. *Neurology, 28*, 113–121.

Hixon, T. J., Putnam, A. H. B., & Sharp, J. T. (1983). Speech production with flaccid paralysis of the rib cage, diaphragm, and abdomen. *Journal of Speech and Hearing Research, 26*, 315–327.

Lincoln, N. B., Mulley, G. P., Jones, A. C., & McGuirk, E. (1984). Effectiveness of speech therapy for aphasic stroke patients: A randomized controlled trial. *Lancet, 1*(8398), 1197–1200.

Towey, M. P., & Pettit, J. M. (1980). Improving communicative competence in global aphasia. *Journal of Speech and Hearing Disorders, 45*, 139–146.

Yorkston, K. M., & Beukelman, D. R. (1988). Articulatory adequacy in dysarthric speakers: A comparison of judging formats. *Journal of Communication Disorders, 21*, 351–361.

CHAPTER 20

Principles of Nutrition and Dietetics

BUSHRA SHAIDA,[1] ZOOBIYA ISLAM,[2,*] MUSKAN CHADHA,[3] and SHASTA ARZOO[4]

[1]*Department of Food Technology, Jamia Hamdard, New Delhi*

[2]*Department of Food and Nutrition, Jamia Hamdard University, New Delhi, India*

[3]*Department of Nutrition and Dietetics, Sharda School of Allied Health Sciences, Sharda University, Greater Noida, Uttar Pradesh, India*

[4]*Department of Nutrition, King Khalid University, Saudi Arabia*

*Corresponding author

ABSTRACT

Media reports suggesting particular meals or diet plans can affect a person's metabolism and energy expenditure, helping them lose weight, are becoming more commonplace among the general public. Nutrients include vitamins, minerals, proteins, carbohydrates, fats, fiber, and water. A person's chance of getting certain health disorders rises if their diet does not contain the proper balance of nutrients. This chapter aims to assess the available data regarding the roles of food, nutrients, and dietary habits in energy intake and energy expenditure. It looks into a number of intriguing aspects of how food affects health and illness. Food is significant because it is a source of some nutrients that are vital for our bodies. It was found that the use of certain nutrients and foods as a type of therapy. In other words, certain diseases necessitate the use of food and nutrients for their treatment. This chapter explores more insight about the underlying principles of different nutrients and their role in maintaining good health. The objectives of this unit are to provide an overview of the clinical relationship between food and health.

Allied Healthcare in Practice: An Introduction to Integrated Patient Care. Sally Lukose, Karuna Singh (Eds.)

DOI: 10.1201/9781998511037-23

20.1 INTRODUCTION

Food is a person's most basic necessity since it provides the body with fuel. It is packed with nutrients, including lipids, proteins, carbohydrates, vitamins, and minerals. These nutrients are essential for an individual's growth, development, and long-term maintenance of good health (Lennon et al., 2022). They play a crucial role in meeting the particular needs of women who are pregnant or nursing, as well as patients who are recuperating from illness.

Any solid or liquid that, when ingested, broken down, and absorbed by the body, gives it vital components known as nutrition and maintains it healthy is considered food. It is a basic requirement for survival. Food provides energy, which permits organ and tissue growth and repair. It also controls bodily systems and shields the body from illness.

20.1.1 FUNCTIONS OF FOOD

- **Physiological Function**

1. **Foods that Provide Energy:** Foods high in lipids and carbohydrates are referred to as foods that provide energy. They supply the energy needed to maintain the involuntary processes necessary for life to continue, to perform a variety of domestic, professional, and recreational tasks, and to transform food into nutrients the body can consume. The food that is consumed oxidizes to provide the necessary energy. Good sources of energy include cereals, dried fruits, oils, butter, ghee, roots and tubers, and nuts.
2. **Foods That Develop Muscle:** Foods high in protein are referred to as body-building foods. Rich sources of premium proteins include milk, beef, eggs, and seafood. Although the protein in pulses and nuts is good, it is not of very high quality. These foods support growth and help to sustain life. They provide energy as well.
3. **Foods That Are Protective and Regulatory:** Foods high in protein, vitamins, and minerals fall into this category. They are vital to health because they manage essential functions like blood coagulation, waste product elimination from the body, muscular

contraction, temperature regulation, and heart rate maintenance. Foods that are protective include milk, eggs, liver, fruits, and vegetables (Lennon et al., 2022).

20.1.2 FOOD'S SOCIAL FUNCTION

Our community's social, cultural, religious, and culinary lives have traditionally revolved around food. It has been used to convey affection, camaraderie, and joy during social, religious, and familial gatherings (Dornhorst et al., 2022).

20.1.3 PSYCHOLOGICAL FUNCTIONS OF FOOD

Foods not only meet people's bodily and social needs but also some of their emotional needs. Among these are feelings of affection, acceptance, and security (Dornhorst et al., 2022). Making delectable meals for family members, for instance, is a sign of love and affection.

20.1.4 FOOD AS NUTRIENT

The components of food that the body needs to receive in appropriate levels are known as nutrients. These consist of water, fiber, minerals, vitamins, proteins, lipids, and carbohydrates. It takes a variety of nutrients to become healthy. Most foods contain many nutrients, such as proteins, lipids, and other ingredients found in milk. Depending on how much of each type of nutrient we need to eat each day, they can be divided into macronutrients and micronutrients (Tappenden et al., 2015). The difference between macronutrients and micronutrients is illustrated in the figure on the following page.

20.1.5 NUTRIENT CATEGORY

The six primary classes of vital nutrients are water, vitamins, minerals, proteins, fats, and carbohydrates (Figure 20.1).

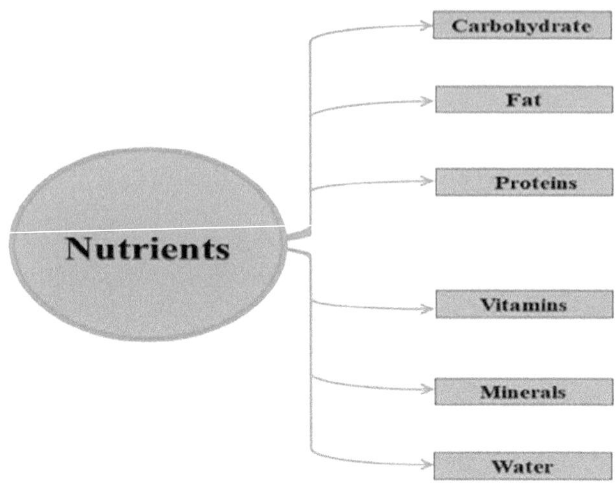

FIGURE 20.1 Nutrient categories.

On the other hand, the body only needs considerably lesser amounts of micronutrients. Micronutrients include things like vitamins and minerals. Some vitamins have requirements that are expressed in milligrams and micrograms (Rozga et al., 2020). A milligram is one thousandth of a gram. A microgram is one millionth of a gram (Table 20.1).

TABLE 20.1 Nutrient Categories and Their Examples

Nutrient Categories	Examples
Carbohydrates	Glucose, galactose, fructose, sucrose, dextrins, starches
Fats	Triglycerides, fatty acids, cholesterol
Proteins	Casein (Milk protein), albumins (egg, gluten (wheat)
Vitamins	Water-soluble: Vitamin C or ascorbic acid, B1 or B2 Or riboflavin, B12, niacin, folic acid, B6, Fat soluble: Vitamin A (B Carotene, Retinol) Vitamin D (Calciferol), Vitamin E (Tocopherol), Vitamin K
Minerals	Sodium, Potassium, chloride, magnesium, iodine, calcium, phosphorus, iron
Water	Soft water, rain water
Fibers	Cellulose, hemicellulose, pectin, lignin are not nutrients but needed as roughage and consumed with Nutrients

20.1.6 CARBOHYDRATES

Sugars, starches, and fiber are the three main forms of carbohydrates found in food. The body can digest sugars and starches, and it absorbs the by-products of that digestion. They are consequently "available" to the body in the sense that they can be used (Rozga et al., 2020). They are referred to as accessible carbohydrates for this reason. The main purpose of readily available carbohydrates is to provide the energy required for daily activities and maintaining biological processes. One gram of carbohydrates provides energy for carrying out tasks and supporting bodily functions. Four kilocalories (4 Kcal) are provided by one gram of carbohydrates. Kcal are used to quantify energy. One kilocalorie of heat is needed to raise the temperature of one kilogram of water by 1°C (Spiker et al., 2020). Carbohydrates function by saving proteins. Proteins won't be used for their ability to create muscle if the diet has enough carbohydrates. If not, energy will be released by destroying them. Carbohydrates are necessary for the proper breakdown of fat or fat catabolism. Lack of adequate carbs results in excessive fat breakdown, which causes by-products of fat metabolism to accumulate. These food scraps are hazardous. On the other hand, insoluble fiber is unavailable since it cannot be digested. "Fiber is made up of complex carbohydrate molecules like cellulose. This does not imply, however, that fiber is not valuable in any way. In the intestine, fiber expands by soaking up water. This facilitates easy stool transit and thus helps to avoid constipation (Martin et al., 2019). It's possible that you are already familiar with this feature. According to a new study, some fiber types may help control cholesterol and blood sugar levels. Furthermore, it has been found that a low intake of fiber is linked to the development of a number of illnesses, including obesity, diabetes, and cardiovascular disease (Marsh et al., 2022).

20.1.7 FATS

Compared to carbs, fat has more than double the energy density (9 kcal/gram). Fats are hence concentrated energy sources. Foods with a lot of fat satisfy hunger and taste better. A certain kind of tissue called adipose tissue is responsible for storing body fat that is not being used by the body. Under the skin and surrounding important organs like the kidney and heart, adipose tissue can be discovered. The body is kept warm by the layers of fat that lie beneath the skin. The vital organs are protected from damage by the padding that surrounds them, though. In addition to these functions, one of the primary functions of fats is to provide essential fatty acids. Saturated and unsaturated fatty acids are the two primary categories of fatty acids (Radford et al., 2022). The body cannot generate saturated fatty acids, therefore it must get them from the diet; this is why it considers them to be "essential." Important unsaturated fatty acids are linoleic and linolenic acids. Moreover, fatty acids are classified as n-3 or n-6 according to where their double bonds are located in their molecules. As an n-3 fatty acid, linolenic acid is categorized differently from linoleic acid, which is an n-6 fatty acid. As essential transporters of fat-soluble vitamins, lipids facilitate the absorption of these nutrients. The body cannot produce saturated fats, although they are necessary (Mitchell et al., 1968).

20.1.8 PROTEIN

The body is unable to produce certain amino acids, which are necessary for the creation of proteins. These amino acids are also known as essential amino acids.

All of the amino acids listed below are essential:

- Isoleucine.
- Leucine.
- Lysine.
- Methionine.
- Phenylalanine.
- Thyronine.
- Tryptophan.
- Valine.
- Histidine (vital for newborns only).

The body may create an additional category of amino acids. Many times, these amino acids are referred to as "non-essential," which may be deceptive. It's doubtful that their presence is random given their importance to the body. The body may produce a different class of amino acids. These amino acids are the ones that are optional. It seems unlikely that these amino acids are there by accident given the vital role they serve in the body. The non-essential amino acids are alanine, aspartic acid, cystine, cysteine, glutamic acid, glutamine, glycine, hydroxyproline, hydroxylysine, proline, serine, and tyrosine (Martin et al., 2019).

Proteins are essential for the growth and maintenance of bodily tissues, as was previously mentioned. But they can also be used for a variety of other bodily purposes. They facilitate digestion by functioning as digestive enzymes. They control the body's chemical reactions since they are metabolic enzymes. Furthermore, proteins are the building blocks of many other hormones. They also support defensive systems since proteins make up antibodies, which are essential parts of the immune system. Besides performing all these various roles, proteins also act as transporters, moving materials throughout the body, frequently via the bloodstream (Radford et al., 2022).

When the diet is deficient in the primary energy sources (carbohydrates and lipids), proteins are forced to act as an energy source. In these circumstances, proteins are compelled to act as the body's primary energy sources because carbs and fats are absent from the diet. In these situations, the body converts proteins into 4 Kcal per gram of protein.

20.1.9 VITAMINS

Vitamins: The body needs significantly less of vitamins and minerals than it does of carbohydrates, lipids, and proteins. Vitamins and minerals are referred to as micronutrients for this reason. In contrast, as we just established, because they are required in greater amounts, proteins, lipids, and carbohydrates collectively are referred to as macronutrients.

They either dissolve in fat or in water. The B-complex vitamins, which are water-soluble, are essential for the metabolism of proteins, lipids, and carbohydrates. Coenzymes include vitamins such as thiamine, riboflavin, niacin, and folic acid. Together with enzymes, these coenzymes support more rapid and effective metabolic reactions (Carlson et al., 2022). In order for healthy red blood cells to develop normally in the bone marrow, folic acid and vitamin B12 are essential. B12 and B6 must be consumed in appropriate amounts for the brain and digestive systems to work properly. Another water-soluble vitamin is vitamin C. The body produces the two stress chemicals adrenaline and norepinephrine, and ascorbic acid, or vitamin C, assists in their release (Murphy et al., 2022). Another theory is that vitamin C may aid in a person's ability to cope with stressful circumstances. This vitamin reduces oxidative stress. You may be aware that the process of oxidation results in the destruction of a number of components in the body, including unsaturated fatty acids. Vitamin C stops or slows down this process.

Four unique fat-soluble vitamins are required by the body. These include vitamins A, D, E, and K. Retinol is another name for vitamin A in general. The prefix "ol" denotes that it is an alcoholic beverage. Animal foods contain retinol (Vitamin A), which is absent from plant diets. However, plants do contain beta-carotene (b-carotene), an orange-yellow-green carotenoid pigment that is soluble in fat. The intriguing thing about the pigment is that it can be converted by the body into retinol or vitamin A. Naturally, beta-carotene is not the only type of carotenoid found in the diet (Spiker et al., 2020).

More carotenes can be converted to vitamin A in the body, albeit to a lesser extent. Vitamin A: This vitamin is required for the growth of skeletal and soft tissues as well as the preservation of healthy epithelial tissues. Meanwhile, the history of vitamin D is fascinating. It is the only vitamin that the body can produce on its own. The body must be exposed to sunlight for this to happen. The biological effects of vitamin D depend critically on the effective utilization of the two minerals calcium and phosphorus. Calcium and phosphorus can be absorbed more easily with the help of vitamin D (Dornhors et al., 2002). Additionally, it is necessary for the phosphate and calcium deposits in bones. Vitamin E performs a protective effect. By shielding them from oxidative and other deteriorating processes, it is believed to help maintain the strength of cell membranes. Vitamins A and C, as well as unsaturated fatty acids, are shielded from oxidation by these vitamins. The preventive properties of vitamin C were previously described (Freeland et al., 2013). Today, we know that vitamin E protects vitamin C from oxidation. Now, let's quickly go over the functions that vitamin K serves in the body. The synthesis of prothrombin depends on this vitamin.

20.1.10 MINERALS

Several of the minerals needed by the body have already been mentioned. Minerals are elements, as opposed to vitamins, which are molecules with a wide range of chemical characteristics. Some of the minerals included in the table, such as iron and iodine, are just marginally necessary (Choda et al., 2016). These minerals are also known as trace elements because of this. Copper and zinc are included in this group as well (Figure 20.2).

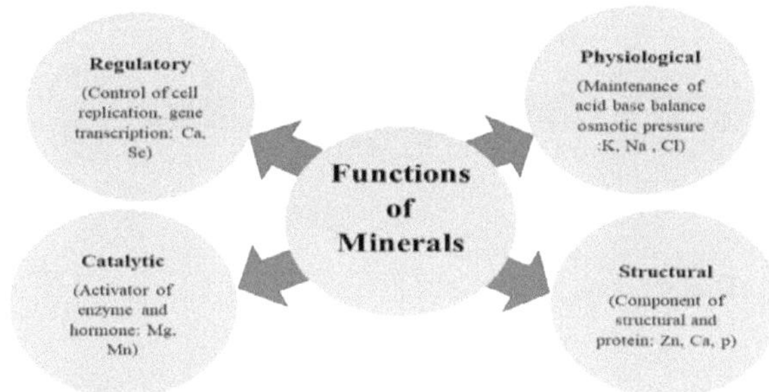

FIGURE 20.2 Functions of minerals.

20.2 FOOD AS MEDICINE

Food and nutrients are both employed as medicines in the form of oils, syrups, capsules, and tablets. It is important to remember that there are three categories of diseases: (i) Conditions or illnesses brought on by nutritional deficiencies; (ii) Diseases with multiple causes, some of which are connected to nutrition and food; (iii) Diseases that are not directly caused by food or nutrients.

Giving concentrated foods and nutrients is an effective treatment for the disorders we listed in the first category. Diet and food play a significant role in many illnesses. Examples of the second category of disorders include diabetes and coronary heart disease (CHD). Overindulging in refined carbohydrates and sugars can hasten the onset of diabetes in people who are already genetically prone to the disease. Similarly, eating diets high in fat (especially saturated fats and cholesterol) is thought to contribute to the fat accumulation in the arteries of the blood vessels, which results in vessel narrowing, also known as atherosclerosis, a major cause of cardiovascular and heart disease.

With respect to these illnesses, nutrition cannot treat the illness. It can only aid in preventing complications and monitoring the progression of the disease process. Therefore, diet therapy enables people to live life in better ways (Figure 20.3).

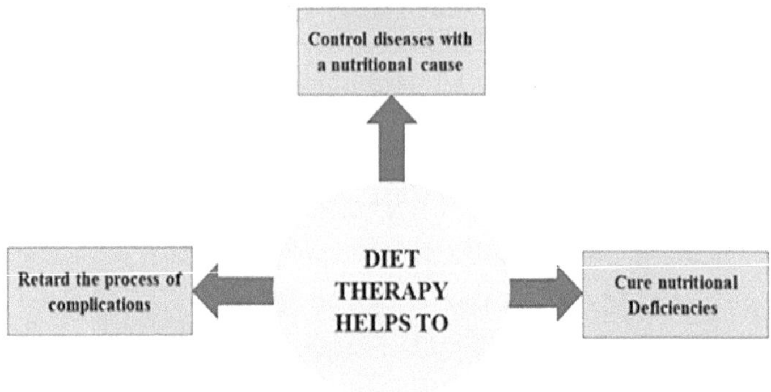

FIGURE 20.3 Diet therapy.

The third category includes illnesses that are contagious. Some of these might be spread by eating certain foods. Food is not the direct reason, though. Most often, dietary treatment is used in some capacity to treat these conditions. For instance, a patient would need to be provided with extra energy and foods high in protein in the appropriate form if they had a febrile infectious disease (a disease known to be accompanied by fever). Whether the fever is acute from typhoid or chronic from TB would determine this.

20.3 FOOD IN THE PREVENTION OF DISEASE

A dietitian or medical nutrition therapist's job is to guide patients and convert scientific information into dietary recommendations. From prenatal to geriatric care (which includes pregnancy, childbirth, and old age), they provide guidance and, when required, recommend dietary changes to preserve ideal nutrition and general well-being in healthy people. Furthermore, nutrition and diet therapy are essential for improving the health of individuals suffering from a variety of ailments. According to Lanham-New et al. (2019), this covers conditions like anemia, fever, typhoid, tuberculosis, ulcers, hyperacidity, heartburn, epilepsy, AIDS, hypertension, cancer, osteoporosis, obesity, burns, metabolic diseases (including diabetes), and disorders of the kidney, liver, and pancreas.

Patients undergoing treatments require nutritional assistance or intervention both prior to and following surgery. Therefore, in order to meet the nutritional needs of patients with a variety of illnesses and prescribe appropriate diets to maximize their health outcomes, clinical nutrition and dietetics are essential.

Diet therapy's goals include the following:

i. Encouragement of recovery; the diet is created to fulfill the patient's needs while taking into account their eating habits;
ii. Altering current diets to improve disease symptoms and keep them under control;
iii. Addressing nutritional deficiencies;
iv. Preventing both short- and long-term complications in the case of chronic diseases; and
v. Educating and counseling the patient about the importance of following the recommended diet (Figure 20.4).

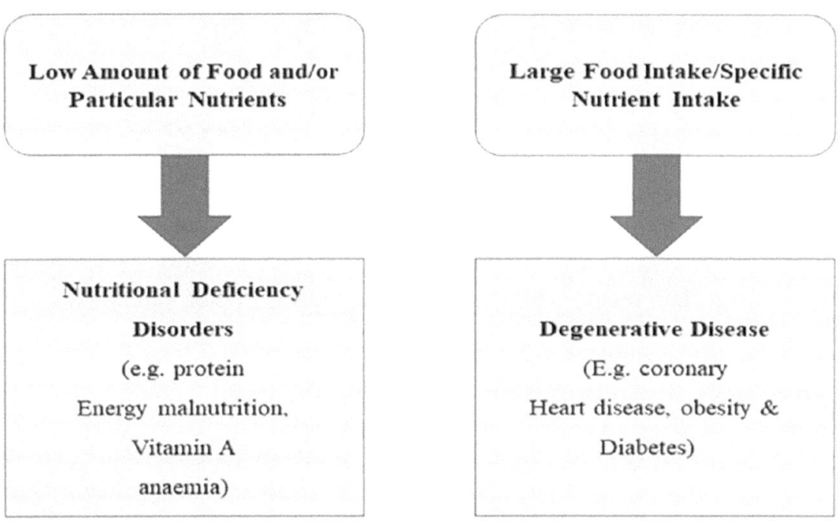

FIGURE 20.4 Effects of dietary intake, both high and low.

Dietitians also need to take into account how disease affects a person's acceptance and intake of food. Among the factors taken into account are (i) nutritional stress; (ii) psychological stress; (iii) the influence of disease on food acceptance; and (iv) the acceptability of modified therapeutic diets. Consequently, nutritional care during sickness is a structured set of tasks that includes:

- Assessing nutritional status.
- Diagnosing nutritional issues.
- The procedure of providing nutritional treatment entails.
- To address nutritional needs, nutrition interventions should be planned and prioritized observing, evaluating, and making necessary adjustments to the nutritional treatment's results.

This procedure is used with people or groups in a variety of contexts, such as:

- People in good health who use fitness/wellness programs/centers.
- Expectant mothers.
- Senior citizens.
- Patients in private practice settings obtaining medical care.
- Hospitalized patients receiving care in public, private, charitable, or municipal facilities.

To learn more about the patient's dietary needs and status, a nutritional assessment is necessary. It entails:

- Obtaining thorough records of one's medical, dietary, personal, and prescription history.
- Anthropometric evaluations
- Interpreting any potential nutritional deficiencies and future deficiencies by relating the data from laboratory and physical measurements with the foregoing and the doctor's diagnosis.

20.4 KEY PRINCIPLES OF FOOD AND HEALTH

1. **Principle 1:** Food nutrition is combined with numerous bioactive compounds, emphasizing a holistic dietary intake approach. There is a well-coordinated chemistry sequence in our bodies, which begins with whatever we eat in order for us to remain fit. These complex biochemical processes involve our cells as well as whole-body physiology. These controls are arranged with respect to the number of nutrients required for various biochemical reaction participants over time. Our body undergoes a complicated system of processes that take the largest advantage of whole food, which is as fresh as possible. Our bodies have developed specialized "biological systems" that only select a few components of mixed

molecules existing inside different foods (Liu, 2013; Shashirekha et al., 2015).

2. **Principle 2:** Vitamin supplements should not be considered a universal remedy for optimal health. The concept that chemical nutrients taken in supplement form are sufficient as a substitute for whole food is unscientific in terms of the complex and myriad aspects nutrition entails. It would probably provide only short-term benefits for sustained health and can even develop unexpected negative results. However, their ideal effect is achieved by deriving them in the form of whole foods and not isolated supplements. They attempt to extract benefits obtained from whole food by isolating some nutrients in the body, but this is not a proper understanding of the entire digestive system of the body (Binns et al., 2018).

3. **Principle 3:** All nutrients found in animal-based foods are more effectively provided by plant-based foods. Diets consisting of animal products are very distinct compared to the nutrition provided by plant-based food. Plant foods have more antioxidants, fibers, and minerals than animal ones. In addition, animal products contain relatively high levels of cholesterol and fat. Animal food supplies slightly more protein, vitamin B12, and vitamin D (frequently included in the product). However, one should consider that these positive aspects also have disadvantages, such as an increase in cholesterol, and consequently, appreciating the individual nutrient constituents of vegetable and non-vegetable foods is fundamental when adopting an appropriate eating regimen. Lastly, plant-based food sources are environmentally sustainable (Bryant, 2022).

4. **Principle 4:** Disease outcomes are not solely determined by genes. Nutrition also plays a pivotal role in influencing the activation of genes and genetic traits. One can safely state that every disease has a genetic basis. Genes are intricate codes controlling all our physiological processes, ranging from beneficial to disadvantageous. There are diseases like cancer, obesity, and diabetes that arise through gene transcription, whereas one's genesis is based on these genes. The importance of identifying specific genetic associations in the context of halting harmful genes is reflected in the significant amounts of money being poured into efforts at

untangling gene-disease linkages. The major factor is nutrition, as it plays a great role in the gene expressions that occur in the body. Nutrients that we ingest regulate gene activation and expression, resulting in cellular responses. Good genes can only be expressed if one has a healthy diet that is rich in all types of nutrients, thus enabling the body to survive and fight off diseases (Paoloni et al., 2003; Rucker and Tinker, 1986).

5. **Principle 5:** Nutrition has the capacity to significantly mitigate the adverse effects of toxic chemicals on the body. Numerous studies often focus on cancer-causing chemicals such as acrylamide, artificial sweeteners, nitrosamines, nitrites, alar, heterocyclic amines, and aflatoxin. The promotion stage involves nutrition that is crucial in either speeding up or delaying the disease's development. Essentially, dietary habits influence whether this disease will have long-term consequences on our health or not.
6. **Principle 6:** Nutrition prevents disease in early stages and can also effectively halt or reverse it in later stages. Optimal nutrition can also prevent, hinder, or even reverse established but not yet metastasizing (after initiation) cancer in experimental animals. These same nutritional practices help in achieving health throughout every stage of a disease. Clinical studies conducted on humans have also shown that a move to a whole food, plant-based diet could help individuals with cardiovascular disease reverse its occurrence, facilitate weight loss in obese individuals, and enable diabetics to reduce or discontinue medication, returning them to a more typical, pre-diabetic lifestyle (Venter et al., 2020).
7. **Principle 7:** Nutrition beneficial for one chronic disease supports overall health. This implies that the same optimal nutrition is beneficial for health and can act as a prevention of all diseases with common features in each case. The health benefits of a wholesome plant-based diet are more pronounced in some ailments, for example heart diseases, rather than in brain cancers; yet this regime is very effective in preventing different diseases. The health-promoting diet has no harmful side effects and does not cause a disease that promotes one disease while fighting another. Essentially, this will be a universally constructive diet for all health aspects (Kimokoti and Millen, 2016).

8. **Principle 8:** Good nutrition promotes interconnected health in every aspect. Since eating entails integrating what we eat into our bodies, it is among our most personal connections with our surroundings. However, there are other dimensions of our experiences that are just as important: physical, mental, emotional health, and environment. These several domains are inherently interconnected and represent a holistic idea; it is imperative that we include them in our understanding of health. It is astonishing to learn that following a diet that promotes overall health also benefits the health of the earth. A diet high in whole foods and plant-based nutrition results in less use of water and land, less use of resources, less pollution, and less suffering for farm animals. The close connections between these apparently separate domains highlight how deeply our decisions and their effects are related (Tiffon, 2018; Zavitsanou and Drigas, 2020).

20.5 DIET AND ITS TYPES

Any nutritional care plan must ensure that the appropriate amounts of all nutrients are consumed in relation to the needs determined by factors such as age, sex, physiological condition, occupation, and health status (Braakhuis et al., 2020).

- **Standard Diet:** A normal diet provides all the nutrients that a healthy person requires while including foods from every food group. However, sweets, spices, sauces, fried foods, and fatty foods are generally limited in hospital diets (Carlson et al., 2022).
- **Modified Diet:** A modified diet is customized to a patient's unique medical needs and may include one or more of the following changes: (i) Modifying the texture or consistency (such as fluid or soft diets); (ii) Modifying energy intake by adding or removing energy.

Among other things, Spiker et al. (2020) suggest modifying the amount of specific nutrients (e.g., increasing protein intake prior to surgery, lowering protein intake following kidney failure), adjusting fiber content, lowering fat intake, limiting sodium or fluid intake, and avoiding foods high in non-nutritive dietary constituents.

1. **Changes in Consistency:** Patients may be encouraged to follow a liquid, soft, or regular diet depending on their condition. At room temperature, (i) liquid diets have a largely fluid nature. These diets, also referred to as complete fluid diets, comprise foods that are nutritious but devoid of fiber. The benefit is that if the digestive system is healthy, nutrients can be absorbed quickly. People who can't chew or swallow normally are encouraged to follow this diet. For instance, milk, buttermilk, soup, coconut water, fruit juice, milkshakes, and so forth. This can be changed to a clear liquid diet, which has an even thinner consistency. Clear soups, strained juices, extremely light tea, and other things are examples of this kind of diet. After surgery, it is usually advised to follow a clear liquid diet. However, because of the limitations, it can be difficult to entirely satisfy an individual's dietary needs. Foods on a soft diet should be semi-solid, mildly seasoned, low in fiber, and free of substances that cause flatulence. It's simple to chew and digest these diets. Soft diets sometimes contain foods like khichdi and sago kheer. The foods chosen should lessen the chance of experiencing cramps, motion sickness, heartburn, stomach bloating, or other gastrointestinal problems (Gibney et al., 2013). Even for normal persons in the elder age group, we make certain changes. This type of diet, known as a mechanical soft diet, consists of mashed, pureed, and soft foods for older people who have difficulty chewing. On the other hand, a soft diet is a therapeutic adjustment. It has a gentle texture and only simple, readily digestible foods; no hard fiber, high-fat, or spicy foods are present. Such diets are prescribed when it is advised to give the digestive system a break.

2. **Feeding Techniques:** The most common and efficient way to feed patients is usually oral intake, or by mouth. However, some people, like those who are unconscious or have esophageal disorders, may have trouble swallowing or chewing. Alternatives such as intravenous feeding or tube feeding—which administers nutrition by means of a tube put into the nose and directed toward the stomach—are taken into consideration in such circumstances. Providing nutrient-complete meals via a tube is known as tube feeding. When the gastrointestinal tract is healthy and able to break down and absorb food, tube feeding is the way to go rather

than intravenous feeding, which is a drip-based method of delivering specific solutions into a vein (Martin et al., 2019).

3. **Chronic Disease Prevention:** Not only is it important for people who are already affected, but we can also control and postpone the onset of chronic diseases through diet and correct nutrition in conjunction with a healthy lifestyle. The food options of today, especially processed meals, are typically high in fat and/or sugar, loaded with additives, and manufactured from refined components, which leaves us lacking in fiber and other vital nutrients that are critical to our health (Lanham et al., 2019). This emphasizes how important it is to have assistance when making decisions. For example, rising rates of obesity and diabetes are a result of increasing intake of sugar and fat, decreased intake of fiber, and decreasing physical activity. Additionally, studies have demonstrated that regular use of processed foods with high sodium content and convenience foods rich in salt can contribute to these health issues. By offering appropriate food advising and assistance, clinical nutritionists can play a significant role in preventing the development of such problems. They may also be chosen to provide advice to other organizations, like schools, colleges, and others.

KEYWORDS

- **chewing difficulties**
- **chronic diseases**
- **clinical nutritionists**
- **complete fluid diets**
- **convenience foods**
- **diabetes**
- **diet consistency**
- **modified diet**
- **non-nutritive dietary constituents**
- **nutritional care plan**
- **obesity**
- **refined components**

REFERENCES

Binns, C. W., Lee, M. K., & Lee, A. H. (2018). Problems and prospects: Public health regulation of dietary supplements. *Annual Review of Public Health, 39*, 403–420.

Braakhuis, A., Monnard, C. R., Ellis, A., & Rozga, M. (2021). Consensus report of the Academy of Nutrition and Dietetics: Incorporating genetic testing into nutrition care. *Journal of the Academy of Nutrition and Dietetics, 121*(3), 545–552.

Bryant, C. J. (2022). Plant-based animal product alternatives are healthier and more environmentally sustainable than animal products. *Future Foods, 5*, 100174.

Carlsson, L., & Callaghan, E. (2022). The social license to practice sustainability: Concepts, barriers, and actions to support nutrition and dietetics practitioners in contributing to sustainable food systems. *Journal of Hunger & Environmental Nutrition*, 1–19.

Choda, S. (2016). Principle of nutrition and dietetics in Sowa Rigpa. *Bhutan Health Journal, 2*(1), 44–46.

Dornhorst, A., & Frost, G. (2022). The principles of dietary management of gestational diabetes: Reflection on current evidence. *Journal of Human Nutrition and Dietetics, 15*(2), 145–156.

Freeland-Graves, J. H., & Nitzke, S. (2013). Position of the Academy of Nutrition and Dietetics: Total diet approach to healthy eating. *Journal of the Academy of Nutrition and Dietetics, 113*(2), 307–317.

Gibney, M. J., Margetts, B. M., Kearney, J. M., & Arab, L. (2013). *Public Health Nutrition* (2nd ed.). John Wiley & Sons.

Kimokoti, R. W., & Millen, B. E. (2016). Nutrition for the prevention of chronic diseases. *Medical Clinics of North America, 100*(6), 1185–1198.

Lanham-New, S. A., Hill, T. R., Gallagher, A. M., & Vorster, H. H. (2019). *Introduction to Human Nutrition* (2nd ed.). John Wiley & Sons.

Lennon, S. L., Kazaks, A., McDermid, J. M., Murphy, M., Lawrence, J. C., & Proaño, G. V. (2022). An update to scientific decision making: The Academy of Nutrition and Dietetics' scientific integrity principles. *Journal of the Academy of Nutrition and Dietetics, 122*(12), 2346–2355.

Liu, R. H. (2013). Dietary bioactive compounds and their health implications. *Journal of Food Science, 78*(s1), A18–A25.

Martin-McGill, K. J., Lambert, B. A. R. N., Whiteley, V. J., Wood, S., Neal, E. G., Simpson, Z. R., & Ketogenic Dietitians Research Network (KDRN). (2019). Understanding the core principles of a 'modified ketogenic diet': A UK and Ireland perspective. *Journal of Human Nutrition and Dietetics, 32*(3), 385–390.

Mitchell, H. S., Rynbergen, H. J., Anderson, L., Dibble, M. V., & Cooper, L. F. (1968). *Nutrition in Health and Disease* (15th ed.). Macmillan.

Murphy, M., Lawrence, J. C., & Proaño, G. V. (2022). An update to scientific decision making: The Academy of Nutrition and Dietetics' scientific integrity principles. *Journal of the Academy of Nutrition and Dietetics, 122*(12), 2346–2355.

Paoloni-Giacobino, A., Grimble, R., & Pichard, C. (2003). Genetics and nutrition. *Clinical Nutrition, 22*(5), 429–435.

Radford-Smith, G., Banks, M., Lord, A., & Chachay, V. (2019). Dietary intake of patients with inflammatory bowel disease aligns poorly with traditional Mediterranean diet principles. *Nutrition & Dietetics, 79*(2), 229–237.

Rozga, M., Latulippe, M. E., & Steiber, A. (2020). Advancements in personalized nutrition technologies: Guiding principles for registered dietitian nutritionists. *Journal of the Academy of Nutrition and Dietetics, 120*(6), 1074–1085.

Rucker, R., & Tinker, D. (1986). The role of nutrition in gene expression: A fertile field for the application of molecular biology. *The Journal of Nutrition, 116*(2), 177–189.

Shashirekha, M., Mallikarjuna, S., & Rajarathnam, S. (2015). Status of bioactive compounds in foods, with focus on fruits and vegetables. *Critical Reviews in Food Science and Nutrition, 55*(10), 1324–1339.

Spiker, M., Reinhardt, S., & Bruening, M. (2020). Academy of Nutrition and Dietetics: Revised 2020 standards of professional performance for registered dietitian nutritionists (competent, proficient, and expert) in sustainable, resilient, and healthy food and water systems. *Journal of the Academy of Nutrition and Dietetics, 120*(9), 1568–1585.

Tappenden, K. A., Elliott, C. H., Emenaker, N., Fogli, J., Kuehneman, T., Lewis, N., & Wright, L. E. (2015). A unifying vision for scientific decision making: The Academy of Nutrition and Dietetics' scientific integrity principles. *Journal of the Academy of Nutrition and Dietetics, 115*(9), 1486–1490.

Tiffon, C. (2018). The impact of nutrition and environmental epigenetics on human health and disease. *International Journal of Molecular Sciences, 19*(11), 3425.

Venter, C., Eyerich, S., Sarin, T., & Klatt, K. C. (2020). Nutrition and the immune system: A complicated tango. *Nutrients, 12*(3), 818.

Zavitsanou, A., & Drigas, A. (2021). Nutrition in mental and physical health. *Technium Social Sciences Journal, 23*, 67–78.

CHAPTER 21

Food and Nutrition Requirements

ADITI RIKHARI, SHALVIKA TRIPATHI, PRATISHTHA KESARWANI, and AKANSHA*

Department of Nutrition and Dietetics, Sharda School of Allied Health Sciences, Sharda University, Greater Noida, Uttar Pradesh, India

*Corresponding author

ABSTRACT

Nutrition can enhance strong immune systems, which helps to decrease the risk of communicable and non-communicable diseases. Longer life spans are all associated with good nutrition. Throughout a person's life, their body continuously develops and evolves, and food serves as the fuel for those changes. Pregnancy, infancy, toddlerhood, childhood, puberty, adolescence, adulthood, and elder years are the main phases of the human life cycle. At every stage of the human life cycle, health and wellness are assured by proper nutrition and exercise. The nutritional requirements of an individual depend on age, physical activity, and gender. The Food and Nutrition Board has determined the levels of essential nutrient intake known as Recommended Dietary Allowances (RDA). Through RDA, a person can take a sufficient amount of all macro and micro nutrients to meet their nutrient needs. One of the easiest ways to lessen the burden of various diseases and their risk factors, such as obesity, can be prevented by taking a balanced diet. This chapter will help to understand the requirement of nutrients in different stages of life, the interrelationship between nutrition and health, and shed light on the idea of a balanced diet.

Allied Healthcare in Practice: An Introduction to Integrated Patient Care. Sally Lukose, Karuna Singh (Eds.)

DOI: 10.1201/9781998511037-24

21.1 INTRODUCTION

An individual must be well-nourished in order to live a healthy life. From the very beginning of life, a healthy diet is necessary for appropriate growth, development, and continued activity. The consumption of food is mostly influenced by production and distribution, which establishes the population's dietary and health conditions. The recommended dietary allowances (RDA) are technical and centered on nutrients. Foods provide many more benefits besides just supplying nutrients (phytochemicals that are not nutrients) that are good for health. Considering what people eat, it's important to promote food-based nutrition rather than just focusing on nutrients (Jauncey, 2000). Therefore, the focus has shifted from a nutritional emphasis to the use of food as a primary means of achieving ideal nutritional status. The scientific understanding of nutrients is translated into precise dietary recommendations by dietary guidelines. They represent the suggested dietary allowances of nutrients in terms of diets that the general public ought to eat. The recommendations support the idea of eating a diet sufficient in nutrients and leading a healthy lifestyle from the moment of conception until old age. The main dietary concerns are an inadequate or unbalanced intake of foods and/or nutrients (Shetty, 2002). Low birth weight, childhood protein-energy deficiency, chronic energy micronutrient malnutrition, adult deficiencies, and non-communicable illnesses are linked to food. However, illnesses on either extreme of the spectrum of malnutrition, both excessive and insufficient, are significant. Current evidence suggests that chronic diet-related diseases may be accelerated by undernutrition during pregnancy, leading to illnesses later in life. Population growth, shifting demographics, and rapid changes in customs and urbanization are factors in the emergence of certain unhealthy eating habits and inactivity, which lead to diet-related long-term illnesses (Robinson, 2015).

21.2 ESSENTIAL NUTRIENTS

21.2.1 ENERGY

In every human diet, carbohydrates—which can be simple or complex—are a primary source of energy. They yield 4 Kcal/g of energy. Fruits, vegetables, and honey include the simple carbohydrates glucose and fructose, while sugar contains sucrose and lactose in milk, whereas starches in cereals are the complex polysaccharides. Grains, legumes, root crops, and animal products contain glycogen (Bour Bour et al., 2023). The additional complex carbohydrates that are difficult for the human digestive system to break down are cellulose found in whole grains and vegetables, as well as the gums and pectins that make up the dietary fiber component in fruits, vegetables, and cereals. In India, carbohydrates found in plants account for 70–80% of total calorie intake, such as cereals, pulses, and millets. Dietary fiber raises the satiety value and slows down the absorption of fats and carbohydrates. Fiber-rich diets increase the volume of stools and lower blood levels of fat and glucose. Diets high in complex carbohydrates are considered healthier than low-fiber diets that mostly consist of processed and refined foods (Kirkby, 2023).

The total energy requirements for Indians, as per the ICMR 2020 guidelines, differ for all age groups depending on their physical activity level. For adult men, in sedentary, moderate, and heavy categories, the requirements are 2110, 2710, and 3470 Kcal/day, respectively. For adult women, in sedentary, moderate, and heavy categories, the requirements are 1660, 2130, and 2720 Kcal/day, respectively. For pregnant women, the additional calorie requirements are +350, and for lactating women, during the first 6 months, the additional calorie requirements are +600, and during (7–12 months), it is +520 Kcal/day. For infants, during (0–6) months and (7–12) months, the calorie requirements are 530 and 660 Kcal/day, respectively. For children aged (1–3) years, (4–6) years, and (7–9) years, the calorie requirements are 1110, 1360, and 1700 Kcal/day, respectively. For boys aged (10–12) years, (13–15) years, and (16–18) years, the calorie requirements are 2220, 2860, and 3320 Kcal/day, respectively. For girls aged (10–12) years, (13–15) years, and (16–18) years, the calorie requirements are 2060, 2400, and 2500 Kcal/day, respectively (ICMR, 2020).

21.2.2 PROTEIN

The fundamental structural and functional elements of all living cells are proteins. Our bodies contain almost half of their protein as muscle, with the remaining portion found in bone, cartilage, and skin. Different amino acids combine to form complex molecules known as proteins. Because the human body is unable to produce some amino acids, they are considered "essential" and must be obtained from the diet. These amino acids are found in proteins. To create proteins, the body can synthesize additional non-essential amino acids. In addition to their many uses, proteins are an excellent source of energy (4 Kcal/g). The amount of protein needed varies with age, physiological state, and stress level. Growing children and babies, expectant mothers, and people who are ill or under stress all need more protein. Rich sources of protein include plant foods like pulses and legumes, as well as animal foods like milk, meat, fish, and eggs (Bour et al., 2023).

Because they include all of the required amino acids in the proper amounts, animal proteins are of the highest quality; in contrast, plant or vegetable proteins are of lower quality due to the low concentration of some important amino acids. The majority of the amino acids, however, are found in grains, millets, and pulses; these nutrients work in concert to produce higher-quality proteins (Bray, 2011). For people consuming a cereal-based diet with low-quality protein, the protein requirements are 1 g/kg per day. Note: The cereal-legume-milk composition of the diet should be 3:1:2.5 for good protein quality.

The human protein requirement for different age groups is defined by the ICMR 2020. For adult men, in sedentary, moderate, and heavy categories, the RDA requirement is 54 g/day, respectively. For adult women, in sedentary, moderate, and heavy categories, the requirement is 46 g/day, respectively. For pregnant women, the additional protein requirements during the 2nd and 3rd trimesters are +7.6 and +17.6 g/day, and for lactating women, during the first 6 months, the additional protein requirements are +13.6, and during (6–12 months), it is +10.6 g/day. For infants, during (0–6) months and (6–12) months, the protein requirements are 8.0 and 10.5 g/day, respectively. For children, of age (1–3) years, (4–6) years, and (7–9) years, the protein requirements are 12.5, 16.0, and 23.0 g/day, respectively. For boys, of age (10–12) years, (13–15) years, and (16–18) years, the protein requirements are 32.0, 45.0, and 55.0 g/day, respectively. For girls, of age (10–12) years, (13–15) years, and (16–18) years, the protein requirements are 33.0, 43.0, and 46.0 g/day, respectively (ICMR, 2020).

21.2.3 FAT

Dietary visible fats are oils and fats like butter, ghee, and vanaspati. As a concentrated source of energy with 9 Kcal/g, fats are composed of various ratios of fatty acids. Dietary fats come from two sources: visible or added fats and oils (cooking oil) and the invisible fat included in plant and animal diets. Carotenoids and fat-soluble vitamins (A, D, E, and K) are transported and better absorbed by fats. Additionally, they are important sources of polyunsaturated fatty acids. To meet the requirements of essential fatty acids, the diet must contain enough good-quality fat in the right amounts, together with enough polyunsaturated fatty acids in the right ratios. Blood levels of triglycerides and cholesterol are influenced by the kind and amount of fat consumed daily (Bray, 2011).

A sufficient amount of fat should be included in diets, especially for babies and kids, as their energy requirements per kilogram (kg) of body weight are almost twice as high as those of adults. Adults should be advised to limit their intake of cholesterol (found in red meat, eggs, and organ meat) and saturated fat (found in butter, ghee, and hydrogenated fats). Overindulgence in these substances may result in cancer, diabetes, heart disease, and obesity (Abbott et al., 2012).

21.2.4 VITAMINS AND MINERALS

Vitamins are needed in small quantities, and chronic nutritional deficiencies cause a number of illnesses. Sometimes vitamins must be taken as medicines or tonics in order to remedy this situation. While vitamins do not provide energy in and of themselves, they do aid in the breakdown of fats and carbohydrates into energy. Food must therefore have the necessary quantity of vitamins. Different kinds of vitamins exist. A specific vitamin, or a combination of two or more vitamins, supports the function of a certain body organ and safeguards health. Every vitamin has a distinct purpose and cannot be substituted for another (Singh, 2004). Table 21.1 explains the function and sources of various vitamins.

Calcium is present in substantial levels in our teeth and bones. A baby's bones contain roughly 30g of calcium, but an adult's bones contain about 1 Kg of calcium overall. Therefore, the bones need to be supplemented with a significant amount of calcium during the stage of growth from baby to adult. For this reason, pregnant women and toddlers are prescribed calcium tablets by doctors. The body constantly contains calcium together with another mineral, phosphorus. Green leafy vegetables and milk are excellent sources of calcium. It is also necessary for blood clotting and for the healthy operation of muscles (Quintaes and Diez, 2015).

TABLE 21.1 Vitamins and Their Function and Sources

Vitamins	Functions	Sources	References
Vitamin A	Allows for our vision in low light. Essential for shiny hair, smooth skin, and healthy eyes, Necessary for appropriate skeletal structure	Dark leafy vegetables, Butter, ghee, milk, egg-yolk, Fatty fish yellow vegetable, fruits	McCauley et al. (2015)
Vitamin B complex	Vital to the nerves, provides ability to function like functioning of heart, brain, and other essential organs. Needed for healthy development and growth. Aids in the prevention of anemia	Egg, liver, brain, kidney, milk, whole cereals, pulses, sprouted pulses	William (2022)
Vitamin D	Aids with the intestinal absorption of calcium and phosphorus necessary for the healthy development of bones	Exposure to sunlight, milk, Egg, fish liver oil, Chicken, Butter, ghee	Shirvani et al. (2019)
Vitamin C	Facilitates the quick healing of wounds, aids in iron uptake, Daily consumption increases immunity to infections	Citrus fruits, Amla, guava, papaya, and Green leafy vegetables	Coker et al. (2023)
Vitamin E	Keeps vitamin A from being destroyed	All types of Vegetable oils and Cereals, cereal germ oil, Nuts, Legumes	Lokhande et al. (2023)
Vitamin K	Stops bleeding from wounds by causing the blood to clot.	Green leafy vegetables	Dolin et al. (2024)

Iron is another essential mineral that the blood needs to produce hemoglobin. The red color of blood is attributed to hemoglobin. The entire quantity of iron in the body is roughly 3 g, compared to 1 kg of calcium. Pregnant mothers and developing children both require iron. Women require more iron since they lose it during the menstrual cycle (Quintaes and Diez, 2015).

Our bodies require about 17 distinct minerals to function properly, yet their quantity is negligible when compared to the majority of the food we eat. Thus, the term "micronutrients" is frequently used to describe these minerals. Certain minerals participate in chemical reactions within the cells since they are components of bodily fluids and cells. Are you familiar with toothpastes that contain fluoride? For teeth to grow robust and resistant to decay, fluoride is necessary. For this reason, fluoride-containing toothpastes are being advertised these days. However, too much fluoride can also be hazardous. There is too much fluoride in the water in certain parts of Andhra Pradesh and Punjab. When this water is consumed, teeth become discolored and lose their shine (Dary and Hurrell, 2006).

Everyone uses the same salt at every meal. It is necessary for the body to function properly. Sodium chloride is what common salt is. A tiny quantity of iodine plays a significant role in the hormone that the thyroid gland in the neck produces. Its absence results in the swelling of the thyroid gland, which is known as goiter. There is now iodized salt on the market that can supply us with iodine (Shenkin, 2006).

Water is a part of every bodily fluid, including digestive juices, blood, and so forth. Between 50 and 70% of body weight is made up of water. It is necessary for a number of metabolic processes. Actually, no material can be used by our body unless it is first converted into a water-soluble form. Food becomes liquid during digestion, making it easily absorbed and transported to the required locations by the blood. The leftover items, such as urea, are transported by blood to the kidneys, where they are eliminated. Water also contributes to controlling body temperature through sweating. The body's daily water requirements vary depending on the type of food, exercise level, and climate (Pathan et al., 2023).

21.3 NUTRITIONAL REQUIREMENT

21.3.1 NUTRITIONAL REQUIREMENTS OF AN INFANT

The initial year of life is a time of rapid development that lays the foundation for the child's future growth. During infancy, an infant's energy requirements per kg of body weight are over two times the amount of an adult's energy requirements per kg of body weight. You may be asking how we arrived at this relationship. According to the RDA table, a sedentary man's daily energy intake is 2110 Kcal. When we express the energy need per kilogram of body weight, we get an estimated number of 32.46 Kcal/kg body weight (i.e., if the reference weight is 65 kg, 65 x 32.46 = 2109 Kcal). When compared to an infant, it is apparent that the infant's demands (per kg of body weight) are significantly higher. This means that the overall value for an adult is higher, but the figure per kg of body weight is lower. The infant's requirement for proteins, vitamins, and minerals (per kg of body weight) is also several times that of an adult (Patel and Rouster, 2020).

1. **Energy Requirement:** Infants have a limited stomach capacity and an energy need per kilogram of body weight that is approximately three times that of adults. Carbohydrate is essential for newborn nutrition and development. Carbohydrates allow proteins to be fully used for muscular growth and tissue repair. Infants less than 6 months need 110–120 kcal/kg/day of calories, while a 1-year-old requires 100 kcal/kg/day. The energy is taken from mature human milk, the carbohydrate is estimated as lactose, and the mineral elements are expressed as ash at 0.2%. It has 60–75 kcal/100 mL of energy. Protein: 3–5%, fat: 6.9–7.2%, carbohydrate: 0.8%–0.9% (Maurya et al., 2020).
2. **Nutrient Profiles:** Macronutrients: According to the latest meta-analysis, the average amount of protein in term infant mothers' breast milk is around 1.17 g/100 mL in the first month after childbirth and 1.0 g/100 mL in the subsequent two months. After accounting for non-protein nitrogen (NPN), which is estimated to be 25%, the average amount of protein in breast milk in the first month after birth is 1.36 g/100 mL, and 1.17 g/100 mL in the following two and three months. The protein intake for all three age groups is 8 g/day, with average daily breastfeeding milk intakes ranging from 600 mL/day (0 to under 1 month), 694 mL/day (1 to under 2 months), and 723 mL/day (2 to under 4 months) (Richter et al., 2019).
3. **Fats, Lipids Requirement:** Dietary fats account for a sizable amount of the nutrients received through food. They provide vital fatty acids, energy, and fat-soluble vitamins such as A, D, E, and K to newborns and young children. Triglycerides, composed of three fatty acids esterified to a glycerol backbone, make up the majority of the lipids in human milk and infant formulas (>95%). Lipids are the main supplier of energy, accounting for almost 90% of the energy required by newborns in their first six months of life. Lipids are also an efficient means of storing energy: the energy cost of synthesizing and storing fat from glucose is 25%, while when lipid is the substrate, it is just 1% to 4%. Breast-fed neonates appear to have higher fat mass than formula-fed infants at three to six months of age, while they have a smaller proportion of fat later in life (Delplanque et al., 2015).

4. **Carbohydrates (Energy):** Glucose is the brain's principal source of carbohydrates. Carbohydrates provide the majority of calories, accounting for 40–55% of daily requirements. While carbohydrates are consumed in the form of disaccharides, oligosaccharides, and polysaccharides, lactose is the predominant enteral source of glucose in human milk and normal infant formula. The amount of carbohydrate required is based on the total estimated energy requirement, which includes energy from non-carbohydrate sources (Patel and Rouster, 2020).

21.3.2 THE WEANING PROCESS

In comparison to breastfeeding studies, the entire procedure of weaning, that is, the gradual transition from a milk-based diet to a nutrition based on solid foods, is unclear. The age and kind of first solid food are commonly documented, but analyzing food and nutrient intake throughout weaning is less usual. This could be due to the difficulties of estimating intake in newborn infants; nevertheless, because nutritional habits and intakes fluctuate rapidly in late infancy, defining the time and important exposures that must be characterized could be difficult. As a result, there is currently no evidence to examine the possible long-term repercussions of variation in weaning techniques on adult health outcomes; however, younger cohorts formed in recent years will begin to provide such data in the future (Robinson, 2015).

21.3.3 NUTRITIONAL NEEDS OF CHILDREN AND ADOLESCENTS

Adolescent growth and development are transformational and have huge consequences for an individual's health throughout their life, in addition to the health of their future children. Adolescents nowadays are growing up through an unprecedented period of change in food environments, with nutritional concerns such as deficiency of micronutrients and food scarcity persisting, while obesity and overweight are on the rise. In a period of pervasive policy misuse, research on nutrition during adolescence has been underinvested in contrast to research on nutrition during other age groups, limiting the development of adolescent-responsive nutritional policies. As a result, there is a dearth of a comprehensive perspective on teenage development and growth, as well as the importance of nutrition. Nutrition has a formative influence on the timing and pattern of puberty throughout the latter stages of childhood and early adolescence, with consequences for adult muscle, height, and fat mass accumulation, as well as the risk of non-communicable illnesses later in life. Nutrition has an impact on adolescent development that extends beyond orthopedic growth to respiratory health, neurodevelopment, and immunity. Adolescence constitutes a nutritionally delicate developmental period in which appropriate nutrition improves many different physiological systems (Norris et al., 2021).

21.3.4 NUTRITIONAL REQUIREMENT OF CHILDHOOD AND ADOLESCENT

Early childhood dietary habits and nutritional supplementation delivered prenatally through 2 years are linked to improved motor development and cognitive performance from infancy through preschool (DiGirolamo et al., 2020). Over-nutrition appears in adolescence as overweight and obesity, whereas under-nutrition emerges as nutrient shortage or stunting without modifying the size of the body (also referred to as hidden hunger) (Das et al., 2017). Energy requirements vary according to exercise level and are greater than for adults. A generally active adolescent female requires roughly 2300 kcal/day, while a moderately active boy requires approximately 2700 kcal/day. Obesity and disorders of eating can both be caused by an energy imbalance (Corkins et al., 2016).

1. **Physiology:** Adolescent body maturation triggered by hormonal changes results in significant changes in the composition of the body. These disparities are most obvious in sexual organ maturation, but they are also noticeable in the ratios of fat and lean body mass. Puberty can start as early as 8 years old and last up to 19 years old. Pubertal hormones such as sex hormones and growth hormones normally develop concurrently and are accountable for enhanced development of the skeleton and sexual maturation. During normal puberty, height and body weight rise (50% of the weight of an adult is gained during adolescence), bone density and strength of muscles increase, blood volume expands, and the brain, lungs, liver, heart, and kidneys all develop in size. Adolescent growth is next only to that of infancy, but it persists

for a longer time; therefore, overall nutritional needs throughout puberty are probably higher than at any other period in life (Das et al., 2017).

2. **Energy Requirement:** Adolescents require additional energy to maintain their physical development and activities. The energy requirements of men and women differ. Girls' growth rates and other hormonal features differ from males beyond the age of 11–12 years. The amount of protein, lipids, and carbohydrates needed is determined by the amount of energy required. Girls require more energy during early puberty (11–14 years), while boys demand more energy throughout middle puberty (15–18 years). In consideration of these teenage characteristics, the energy requirement for girls is around 1800–2500 calories, and for boys, it is 2500–3500 calories. Assessing development and growth is the most straightforward and appropriate method for determining the degree to which all adolescents consume adequate energy. Obesity, nutritional deficiency, delayed puberty, nutritional retardation of growth, and a lack of many nutrients can result from insufficient energy consumption. Insufficient energy intake may be associated with a restricted diet, chronic diseases, or poor socioeconomic status. In consideration of healthy dietary principles, it is proposed that cereals (rice, pasta, bread, etc.), fruits, dry legumes, and vegetables be used to meet increased energy requirements in teenagers rather than sugar and fats (Ozdemir, 2016).

   i. **Protein:** Protein requirements are necessary for maintaining body mass as well as achieving a suitable pubertal spurt and growth. A balanced diet should include 10% to 30% protein, with two-thirds coming from animal sources and one-third from highly biologically valuable sources. It is crucial to investigate the relationship between the consumption of protein and total energy intake because when energy becomes limited, the protein could be utilized as an energy substrate, reducing its availability for basic processes (Ciampo and Ciampo, 2020).

   ii. **Carbohydrates:** Carbohydrates must supply 50% to 60% of daily energy requirements. As a result, complex carbohydrates and high-fiber diets must be balanced. Sugar (10% of daily calories) must be reduced, while the consumption of complex carb-containing dry legumes like chickpeas, dry beans, lentils, and products made from whole grains and wheat must be increased. Carbohydrates are found mostly in vegetarian nutrition. Carbohydrates are present in 60–90% of grains, 10% of fruits, 10% of other vegetables, and 18% of potatoes (Karakoyun and Yagci, 2013). Furthermore, sweeteners such as fructose and sucrose should not account for more than 10% of total calories. Adolescents, on the other hand, tend to consume fewer complex carbs and fibers, as well as more basic sugars (Ozdemir, 2016).

iii. **Iron:** Iron intake is required to replace basal losses, which are mostly caused by epithelial cell sloughing, sweat, and monthly losses, but iron is also required to meet growth demands. Boys and girls up to the age of 18 require 18 mg of iron each day. Boys require 10 mg/day after the age of 19; girls, on the other hand, continue to require greater doses due to their menstruation process (Mesias et al., 2013).

21.3.5 NUTRITION FOR ADULTS

Adulthood, as you may recall, is the period beginning at the age of 19 and lasting until the age of old age. This is the stage of life when growth and development are complete. The nutrients are primarily essential for the maintenance of body structure as well as function. A good diet may assist young adults in maintaining an active lifestyle as they enter adulthood. For the majority of people, this is the moment when the bodies are in peak form. The body of an adult does not require that to devote its resources and energy to the rapid development and growth that is characteristic of youth. Childhood and adolescent feeding habits and preferences have an influence on health and fitness prolonged into adulthood.

Adult height illustrates the balance between nutritional intake and losses over time (particularly during growing phases), including losses because of physical activity, psychological stress, and illness, from conception to maturity. As a result, adult height is the result of cumulative net nutrition during the two growth phases (in combination with inheritance) and is rather consistent when contrasted with child or youth height (which may not fully represent any effects of catch-up growth). Additionally, adult height is distinct from body mass index or weight in relation to height as an index of cumulative net nutrition, which is a sign of current net nutrition and is suggestive of the immediate environment (Perkins et al., 2016).

1. **Nutritional Requirement for Adults:** Adult males should consume 2600–2800 kcal per day, and females should consume 2000–2100 kcal per day, respectively. This need varies and is greatly impacted by one's level of exercise and physical condition. Dietary imbalance causes malnutrition as well as nutrition overdose; both of these conditions are harmful to the body. The daily water requirement of the body is determined by weight, gender, age, and ambient temperature. The recommended daily intake for water is 3.7 L/day for men and 2.7 L/day for women. According to the latest research, 83% of women and 95% of men over the age of 71 did not meet the daily requirement for water (Faizan et al., 2021).

2. **Macronutrient Needs:**

    i. **Protein:** Protein is required for cell, tissue, enzyme, hormone, antibody, and transport carrier structure, maintenance, and growth. Age, weight, dietary status, and the degree of pressure imposed by illness or injury all influence daily protein requirements. Protein's DRI (Dietary Reference Intake) for healthy people is 0.8 g/kg (Kozeniecki and Fritzshall, 2015).

    ii. **Carbohydrates:** AMDR (Acceptable Macronutrient Distribution Range) refers to approximately 45 to 65% of total daily calories. Individuals of every age group need to consume less energy-dense carbohydrates, specifically refined sugar-dense ones, especially those who lead sedentary lives. Protein should make up 10 to 35% of the daily calorie requirement and can be found in lean meats, eggs, poultry, beans, peas, seeds, and almonds. According to the standards, adults should have two 4-ounce meals (or one 8-ounce dish) of fish and seafood per week.

    iii. **Lipids and Fats:** Glycerol and fatty acids are high-energy molecules that help the body develop, maintain body heat, and function as an emergency reserve. Certain essential fatty acids, such as omega-6 and omega-3, are essential for the synthesis of eicosanoids such as prostaglandins and leukotrienes and should be consumed. Fats should make up between 25 and 30% of daily calories, with saturated fats making up no more than 10%. Cholesterol can be synthesized by the body's tissues and hence does not need to be consumed. It is not recommended to exceed 300 mg per day. A high-fat diet can lead to obesity, which is also connected to an elevated risk of cardiovascular disease. Substitute red meat, deep-fried items, and fat-containing dairy products with white meat and monounsaturated fat sources such as olive oil, almonds, flaxseeds, and avocado. According to a recent study, people who ate a diet high in monounsaturated fats had a lower risk of developing cardiovascular disease, cognitive decline, and type II diabetes (Faizan et al., 2021).

21.3.6 NUTRITION DURING PREGNANCY

Women require nourishment optimally because of the unique dietary requirements related to physiological transitions such as menstruation, pregnancy, breastfeeding, and menopause. Being pregnant puts a woman's body through a lot of physiological stress as she takes care of a developing baby. Numerous physiological, biochemical, and hormonal changes in the mother's body accompany the growth of the fetus and impact the body's requirement for nutrients and how well it uses them.

Commencing in the preconception stage, diet and lifestyle preferences play a significant role in shaping the health of both the expecting mother and her children. Particularly, contemporary research highlights the significance of the first 1000 days of life (from conception up to two years of age) for avoiding the occurrence of disorders that affect adults (Adair, 2014). To ensure both the well-being of the mother and the unborn child, pregnant women need to maintain an ideal weight and dietary requirements (Stephenson et al., 2018). High birth weight, obesity, and fluctuations in the breakdown of glucose in children are all linked to certain maternal circumstances during the periconceptional time frame, including obesity and excessive weight gained during gestation, and later in life, in adults, with higher cardiovascular and metabolic risks (Berti et al., 2012).

The rate of growth during the first few months of life impacts health later in life. Breast milk is the ideal form of nutrition for infants, according to the WHO, which considers it to be a component of the reproductive process. Lactating mothers' health is also significantly impacted, with benefits ranging from decreased risk of heart disease and hip fractures after menopause to protection against certain cancers, including breast and ovarian cancer. The World Cancer Research Fund counts lactation as one of its 10 anti-cancer recommendations in this context (Marmot et al., 2016) (Table 21.2).

TABLE 21.2 Foods Preferred During Pregnancy

Food	Examples	References
Dairy Products	Milk, cottage cheese, egg, curd, yogurt, buttermilk, soy milk, tofu	De Seymour et al. (2022); Marshall et al. (2022)
Meat and Meat Products	Lean meat, chicken breast, fish (low in mercury).	
Nuts and Seeds	Almonds, walnuts, chia seeds, flaxseeds, hemp seeds.	
Fruits and Vegetables	Berries, tomatoes, bell peppers, cabbage, kale, garlic, broccoli	
Whole Grains and Legumes	Lentils, oatmeal, quinoa, bread, rice.	

21.3.6.1 NUTRITIONAL REQUIREMENTS DURING PREGNANCY

To stand by each of these alterations, getting the body prepared to undergo birth and nursing, and to guarantee the healthy development of the fetus/baby, women's nutritional demands rise throughout pregnancy and lactation. Micronutrients are crucial for numerous cellular and metabolic processes, including cell differentiation, expansion, formation of hemoglobin, oxygen transport, the formation of minerals, and others. They are mostly obtained through a balanced diet (Mensink et al., 2013).

1. **Energy Requirements:** Depending on the stage of pregnancy, dietary consumption rises gradually for fit, normal-weight women who lead moderately active lifestyles. These requirements can be met by a tiny spike in energy intake while maintaining a balanced equilibrium between macronutrients in accordance with dietary recommendations. Notably, in overweight and obese women,

an excess of calories and macronutrients during pregnancy may actually be just as harmful as an inadequate intake, increasing the risk of miscarriage, gestational diabetes, pre-eclampsia, as well as obesity and type 2 diabetes in their offspring when they reach maturity (Bruce, 2014).

2. **Protein:** When it comes to the macronutrients, protein needs raised awareness throughout pregnancy since there is a steadily rising need to aid in the fabrication of protein in order to sustain the growth of the fetus and the mother's tissues, particularly during the third trimester (Kramer and Kakuma, 2003). Consuming two or more plant meals with diverse amino acid concentrations could potentially boost the protein component's overall effectiveness.

3. **Essential Fatty Acids:** The composition of fats throughout gestation is more significant than their quantity, particularly for fetal development and neonatal growth. Consequently, it is more important to enhance the intake of docosahexaenoic acid (DHA, of the n-3 series), which is crucial for the maturation of the brain and retina, than it is to increase the relative amount of polyunsaturated fats (Sauerwald et al., 2001). The development of the fetus's brain and retina during pregnancy relies on DHA since it is the dominant polyunsaturated fatty acid found in the human brain and retinal rods. In fact, during the first few months of life, when it is provided in significant levels via breastfeeding, DHA performs crucial functions in psychomotor neurodevelopment (Innis et al., 2008). According to studies, the mother's DHA may affect the baby's verbal and visual development. During pregnancy, only 9% of the ALA that is ingested transforms to DHA and EPA. Fish and seafood are the main nutritional sources of EPA and DHA. DHA is also found in algae and egg yolks. There are currently no DRIs for EPA or DHA, and recommendations differ among groups. Adults should eat 500 mg/d of EPA and DHA daily, according to the Academy of Nutrition and Dietetics.

4. **Iron:** Due to increased blood volume, fetal growth, and the development of appendages, including the placenta, pregnant women have significantly higher iron needs (21–27 mg/day). Iron is essential for the formation of hemoglobin and for the transfer of oxygen (WHO, 2016). It should be mentioned that while tea

and coffee might decrease intestinal iron absorption (due to the presence of polyphenols), vitamin C can increase it. According to several studies, drinking tea between meals is preferable to doing so during meals. When tea is consumed one hour after an iron-rich meal, the inhibitory effects on iron absorption are lessened (Zijp et al., 2000).

5. **Iodine:** Iodine, a vital part of thyroid hormones, is necessary for the metabolism of glucose, proteins, lipids, calcium, and phosphorus, as well as thermogenesis, and for the growth, creation, and development of organs and tissues (EFSA, 2014). Iodine primarily occurs in fish and shellfish, which obtain it from the algae they consume, which draw it from seawater. Iodine, however, is also absorbed by the soil as a result of water evaporation and rain and then enters water, fruits, vegetables, milk, eggs, and then meat (to varying degrees) in relevant proportions (Novaković et al., 2013). Iodine deficiency is regarded by the WHO as the main avoidable cause of brain damage and might increase the risk of spontaneous miscarriage, perinatal death, birth abnormalities, and neurological diseases during pregnancy (Trumpff et al., 2015). Iodine shortage in the general population may be avoided by ensuring adequate intake of this mineral in the diet, for instance, by using iodized salt.

6. **Calcium:** Particularly in the third trimester, calcium plays a role in the mineralization of the fetal skeleton. Three-quarters of the 30 g of calcium that makes up the bones of a fully developed newborn are deposited during the last trimester of pregnancy. Therefore, maternal calcium requirements rise, especially beginning in the third trimester (calcium requirements range from 1000 to 1200 mg/day) (WHO, 2016). Pregnant women should take daily supplements (1.5–2.0 g of elemental calcium) to lower their risk of pre-eclampsia in populations with poor calcium consumption (O'Brien et al., 2017).

7. **Vitamin D:** There are two types of vitamin D: D2 and D3. Ergocalciferol, often known as vitamin D2, is the form present in plant-based sources. Vitamin D3 (cholecalciferol) is created by human skin and is also present in animal sources of food. Along with parathyroid hormone, its active form ensures the mineralization of

tissues (bones, cartilage, and teeth) both during and after growth. It helps to maintain calcium homeostasis (Paulson et al., 1986). A fat-soluble hormone called vitamin D is well known for its function in preserving bone health and calcium balance. The importance of vitamin D in non-skeletal processes such as glucose metabolism, angiogenesis, inflammation, and immunological function, as well as in controlling gene transcription and expression, is also well known (De-Regil et al., 2012).

8. **Vitamin A:** The word "vitamin A" refers to both free and esterified retinols found in food, their biologically active metabolites (retinol and retinoic acids) generated by the body, as well as provitamin carotenoids (β-carotene, α-carotene, and β-cryptoxanthin) (EFSN, 2015). Due to retinoic acid's function in the control of gene expression and cell development, vitamin A is required. Retinol is also necessary for vision and supports development, the immune system, and the health of mucosal epithelia, particularly that of the eye (McCauley et al., 2015).
9. **Folic Acid:** Folates are essential for a variety of metabolic processes, including the production of Deoxyribonucleic acid (DNA) and Ribonucleic acid (RNA), the conversion of homocysteine to methionine, and the metabolism of amino acids (Hoey et al., 2013). Green leafy vegetables, fruits (including oranges), cereals, and offal are the main sources of folates. The amount of anti-nutrients in food affects how bioavailable they are since they might hinder absorption (Berti et al., 2012).

The dietary requirements of a woman during pregnancy and lactation are crucial for both her health and the wellness of subsequent generations. For the first four to six months of a newborn's existence, the mother who is nursing offers the baby all the nutrition and fluids it requires to thrive. By promoting the growth and maturation of branching lactiferous ducts and lactocyte-lined alveoli, which secrete milk by producing colostrum, the body gets ready for breastfeeding throughout pregnancy. Estrogen, growth hormone, cortisol, and prolactin have been accountable for these activities. In addition, mammary alveolar clusters sprout from the ducts and enlarge towards the chest wall in response to progesterone. Breastfeeding after labor causes the production of oxytocin, which in turn prompts myoepithelial cells to expel milk from the alveoli. The newborn can then drink breast milk from the pores of the nipple (Truchet et al., 2017). Breast milk is an exceptional source of nutrition for infants (Kalantari and Haghighian, 2013) since it delivers all the nutrients needed to promote the baby's health, growth, and development (Ip et al., 2007).

KEYWORDS

- **estrogen**
- **food groups**
- **lactation**
- **lactiferous ducts**
- **lactocyte-lined alveoli**
- **life stages**
- **mammary alveolar clusters**
- **nutrition**
- **recommended dietary allowances**

REFERENCES

Abbott, S. K., Else, P. L., Atkins, T. A., & Hulbert, A. J. (2012). Fatty acid composition of membrane bilayers: Importance of diet polyunsaturated fat balance. *Biochimica et Biophysica Acta (BBA)–Biomembranes, 1818*(5), 1309–1317.

Adair, L. S. (2014). Long-term consequences of nutrition and growth in early childhood and possible preventive interventions. *Nestlé Nutrition Institute Workshop Series, 78*, 111–120.

Berti, C., Cetin, I., Agostoni, C., Desoye, G., Devlieger, R., Emmett, P. M., Ensenauer, R., Hauner, H., Herrera, E., Hoesli, I., et al. (2016). Pregnancy and infants' outcome: Nutritional and metabolic implications. *Critical Reviews in Food Science and Nutrition, 56*, 82–91.

Berti, C., Fekete, K., Dullemeijer, C., Trovato, M., Souverein, O. W., Cavelaars, A., Dhonukshe-Rutten, R., Massari, M., Decsi, I., van't Veer, P., et al. (2012). Folate intake and markers of folate status in women of reproductive age, pregnant and lactating women: A meta-analysis. *Journal of Nutrition and Metabolism, 470*, 65–69.

BourBour, F., Mirzaei Dahka, S., Gholamalizadeh, M., Akbari, M. E., Shadnoush, M., Haghighi, M., Taghvaye-Masoumi, H., Ashoori, N., & Doaei, S. (2023). Nutrients in prevention, treatment, and management of viral infections; special focus on Coronavirus. *Archives of Physiology and Biochemistry, 129*(1), 16–25.

Bray, G. A. (2011). Is dietary fat important? *The American Journal of Clinical Nutrition, 93*(3), 481–482.

Bruce, K. D. (2014). Maternal and in utero determinants of type 2 diabetes risk in the young. *Current Diabetes Reports, 14*, 446–448.

Ciampo, L. A. D., & Ciampo, I. R. L. D. (2020). Adolescent nutrition. *Austin Pediatrics, 7*(1), 1077.

Coker, S. J., Dyson, R. M., Smith-Díaz, C. C., Vissers, M. C. M., & Berry, M. J. (2023). Effects of low vitamin C intake on fertility parameters and pregnancy outcomes in guinea pigs. *Nutrients, 15*(19), 4107.

Corkins, M. R., Daniels, S. R., de Ferranti, S. D., Golden, N. H., Kim, J. H., Magge, S. N., & Schwarzenberg, S. J. (2016). Nutrition in children and adolescents. *Medical Clinics of North America, 100*(6), 1217–1235.

Dary, O., & Hurrell, R. (2006). *Guidelines on Food Fortification with Micronutrients.* World Health Organization, Food and Agricultural Organization of the United Nations.

Das, J. K., Salam, R. A., Thornburg, K. L., Prentice, A. M., Campisi, S., Lassi, Z. S., Koletzko, B., & Bhutta, Z. A. (2017). Nutrition in adolescents: Physiology, metabolism, and nutritional needs. *Annals of the New York Academy of Sciences, 1393*(1), 21–33.

De Seymour, J. V., Beck, K. L., & Conlon, C. A. (2022). Nutrition in pregnancy. *Obstetrics, Gynaecology & Reproductive Medicine, 32*(11), 253–258.

Delplanque, B., Gibson, R., Koletzko, B., Lapillonne, A., & Strandvik, B. (2015). Lipid quality in infant nutrition: Current knowledge and future opportunities. *Journal of Pediatric Gastroenterology and Nutrition, 61*(1), 8–13.

De-Regil, L. M., Palacios, C., Ansary, A., Kulier, R., & Peña-Rosas, J. P. (2012). Vitamin D supplementation for women during pregnancy. *Cochrane Database of Systematic Reviews, 2012.*

DiGirolamo, A. M., Ochaeta, L., & Flores, R. M. M. (2020). Early childhood nutrition and cognitive functioning in childhood and adolescence. *Food and Nutrition Bulletin, 41*(1), 31–40.

EFSA NDA Panel (EFSA Panel on Dietetic Products, Nutrition, and Allergies). (2014). Scientific opinion on dietary reference values for iodine. *EFSA Journal, 12*, 3660–3716.

EFSA Scientific Committee. (2015). Statement on the benefits of fish/seafood consumption compared to the risks of methylmercury in fish/seafood. *EFSA Journal, 13*, 3982–4017.

Faizan, U., & Rouster, A. S. (2022). Nutrition and hydration requirements in children and adults. *[Updated August 29, 2022].*

Grant, W. B. (2022). *Vitamins and Minerals* (2nd ed.). Elsevier.

Hoey, L., McNulty, H., Duffy, M. E., Hughes, C. F., & Strain, J. J. (2013). EURRECA—Estimating folate requirements for deriving dietary reference values. *Critical Reviews in Food Science and Nutrition, 53*, 1041–1050.

ICMR-NIN. (2020). *Revised Short Summary Report-2024, ICMR-NIN Expert Group on Nutrient Requirements for Indians, Recommended Dietary Allowances (RDA) and Estimated Average Requirements (EAR)-2020.* National Institute of Nutrition, India. Retrieved from: https://nin.res.in (accessed on 14 March 2025).

Innis, S. M., & Friesen, R. W. (2008). Essential n−3 fatty acids in pregnant women and early visual acuity maturation in term infants. *American Journal of Clinical Nutrition, 87*, 548–557.

Ip, S., Chung, M., Raman, G., Chew, P., Magula, N., DeVine, D., et al. (2007). Breastfeeding and maternal and infant health outcomes in developed countries. *Evidence Report/ Technology Assessment (Full Report), 153*, 1–186.

Jauncey, K. (2000). Nutritional requirements. In *Tilapias: Biology and Exploitation* (Vol. 42, pp. 327–375). Springer Netherlands.

Kalantari, N., & Haghighian Roudsari, A. (2013). Breastfeeding promotion in Iran: Opportunities and challenges. *Journal of Comprehensive Pediatrics, 3*(5), 165–166.

Karakoyun, & Yağcı. (2013). Recent developments in nursing and midwifery.

Kirkby, E. A. (2023). Introduction, definition, and classification of nutrients. In *Marschner's Mineral Nutrition of Plants* (pp. 3–9). Academic Press.

Kozeniecki, M., & Fritzshall, R. (2015). Enteral nutrition for adults in the hospital setting. *Nutrition in Clinical Practice, 30*(5), 634–651.

Kramer, M. S., & Kakuma, R. (2003). Energy and protein intake in pregnancy. *Cochrane Database of Systematic Reviews*.

Lokhande, T. N., Varma, K. S., Gharate, S. M., Mahajan, S. K., & Surana, K. R. (2023). Vitamins as nutraceuticals for pregnancy. In *Vitamins as Nutraceuticals: Recent Advances and Applications* (pp. 185–204).

Marmot, M., Atinmo, T., Byers, T., Chen, J., Hirohata, T., Jackson, A., & James, W. (2007). *Food, nutrition, physical activity, and the prevention of cancer: A global perspective*. Retrieved from: http://discovery.ucl.ac.uk/4841/ (accessed on 14 March 2025).

Marshall, N. E., Abrams, B., Barbour, L. A., Catalano, P., Christian, P., Friedman, J. E., Hay, W. W., et al. (2022). The importance of nutrition in pregnancy and lactation: Lifelong consequences. *American Journal of Obstetrics and Gynecology, 226*(5), 607–632.

Maurya, R., Mogra, R., & Mauriya, S. (2020). The importance of nutrition in infancy: A review. *Asian Food Science Journal*.

McCauley, M., van den Broek, N., Dou, L., & Othman, M. (2015). Vitamin A supplementation during pregnancy for maternal and newborn outcomes. *Cochrane Database of Systematic Reviews, 10*, CD008666.

Mensink, G. B. M., Fletcher, R., Gurinovic, M., Huybrechts, I., Lafay, L., Serra-Majem, L., Szponar, L., et al. (2013). Mapping low intake of micronutrients across Europe. *British Journal of Nutrition, 110*, 755–773.

Novaković, R., Cavelaars, A. E., Bekkering, G. E., Roman-Viñas, B., Ngo, J., Gurinović, M., Glibetić, M., et al. (2013). Micronutrient intake and status in Central and Eastern Europe compared with other European countries: Results from the EURRECA network. *Public Health Nutrition, 16*, 824–840.

O'Brien, E. C., Kilbane, M. T., McKenna, M. J., Segurado, R., Geraghty, A. A., & McAuliffe, F. M. (2017). Calcium intake in winter pregnancy attenuates impact of vitamin D inadequacy on urine NTX, a marker of bone resorption. *European Journal of Nutrition, 57*, 1015–1023.

Ozdemir, A. (2016). Macronutrients in adolescence. *International Journal of Caring Sciences, 9*(3), 1162.

Patel, J. K., & Rouster, A. S. (2020). Infant nutrition requirements and options.

Pathan, A. S., Jain, P. G., Mahajan, A. B., Kumawat, V. S., Ahire, E. D., Surana, K. R., Rajora, A. K., & Rajora, M. A. K. (2023). Beneficial effects of water-soluble vitamins in nutrition and health promotion. In *Vitamins as Nutraceuticals: Recent Advances and Applications* (pp. 235–251).

Paulson, S., & DeLuca, H. (1986). Vitamin D metabolism during pregnancy. *Bone, 7*, 331–336.

Perkins, J. M., Subramanian, S. V., Davey Smith, G., & Özaltin, E. (2016). Adult height, nutrition, and population health. *Nutrition Reviews, 74*(3), 149–165.

Quintaes, K. D., & Diez-Garcia, R. W. (2015). The importance of minerals in the human diet. In *Handbook of Mineral Elements in Food* (pp. 1–21).

Richter, M., Baerlocher, K., Bauer, J. M., Elmadfa, I., Heseker, H., Leschik-Bonnet, E., Stangl, G., et al. (2019). Revised reference values for the intake of protein. *Annals of Nutrition and Metabolism, 74*(3), 242–250.

Robinson, S. M. (2015). Infant nutrition and lifelong health: Current perspectives and future challenges. *Journal of Developmental Origins of Health and Disease, 6*(5), 384–389.

Sauerwald, T. U., Demmelmair, H., & Koletzko, B. (2001). Polyunsaturated fatty acid supply with human milk. *Lipids, 36*, 991–996.

Shenkin, A. (2006). The key role of micronutrients. *Clinical Nutrition, 25*(1), 1–13.

Shetty, P. S. (2002). *Nutrition Through the Life Cycle*. Royal Society of Chemistry.

Shirvani, A., Kalajian, T. A., Song, A., & Holick, M. F. (2019). Disassociation of vitamin D's calcemic activity and non-calcemic genomic activity and individual responsiveness: A randomized controlled double-blind clinical trial. *Scientific Reports, 9*, 17685.

Singh, M. (2004). Role of micronutrients for physical growth and mental development. *The Indian Journal of Pediatrics, 71*, 59–62.

Stephenson, J., Heslehurst, N., Hall, J., Schoenaker, D. A. J. M., Hutchinson, J., Cade, J. E., Poston, L., Barrett, G., Crozier, S. R., Barker, M., et al. (2018). Before the beginning: Nutrition and lifestyle in the preconception period and its importance for future health. *The Lancet, 391*, 1830–1841.

Truchet, S., & Honvo-Houéto, E. (2017). Physiology of milk secretion. *Best Practice & Research: Clinical Endocrinology & Metabolism, 31*, 367–384.

Trumpff, C., Vandevijvere, S., Moreno-Reyes, R., Vanderpas, J., Tafforeau, J., Van Oyen, H., & De Schepper, J. (2015). Neonatal thyroid-stimulating hormone level is influenced by neonatal, maternal, and pregnancy factors. *Nutrition Research, 35*, 975–981.

World Health Organization. (n.d.). *Recommendations for the Prevention and Management of Tobacco Use and Second-Hand Smoke Exposure in Pregnancy*. Retrieved from: http://apps.who.int/iris/bitstream/10665/94555/1/9789241506076_eng.pdf?ua=1 (accessed on 14 March 2025).

Zijp, I. M., Korver, O., & Tijburg, L. B. M. (2000). Effect of tea and other dietary factors on iron absorption. *Critical Reviews in Food Science and Nutrition, 40*, 371–398.

CHAPTER 22

Nourishing Wellness: Managing Diseases Through Strategic Nutrition

MAYURI RASTOGI,[1] TANNU RANA,[2] MD. SAYEED AKHTAR,[3] and ADITI RIKHARI[4,*]

[1]*Sharda School of Allied Health Sciences, Sharda University, Greater Noida, Uttar Pradesh, India*

[2]*Masters in Nutrition and Dietetics, Sharda School of Allied Health Sciences, Sharda University, Greater Noida, Uttar Pradesh, India*

[3]*Department of Clinical Pharmacy, King Khalid University, Gurager, Saudi Arabia*

[4]*Department of Nutrition and Dietetics, Sharda School of Allied Health Sciences, Sharda University, Greater Noida, Uttar Pradesh, India*

*Corresponding author

ABSTRACT

Changes in the body's structure and/or functioning are frequently linked to disease. These alterations are a part of the disease process and arise from specific irregularities in the body's metabolism of chemicals. Dietary changes can effectively cure some diseases in some cases, but in other cases, the diet only manages the condition and prevents it from getting worse. Rapid advancements in a variety of relevant scientific domains over the past few years, particularly in the amount of population-based epidemiological evidence, have made it clearer how important food is for preventing and reducing morbidity and premature death due to noncommunicable diseases. Rapid dietary and lifestyle changes brought on by industrialization, urbanization, economic growth, and market globalization

Allied Healthcare in Practice: An Introduction to Integrated Patient Care. Sally Lukose, Karuna Singh (Eds.)

DOI: 10.1201/9781998511037-25

have intensified. This transition is significantly affecting the health and nutritional status of the population. In this chapter, we will discuss the health problems arising from this transition, such as gastrointestinal diseases, liver disease, diabetes, cardiovascular disease, and their control or management through appropriate dietary therapy. The diets that are adapted or modified according to disease conditions are called therapeutic diets. Therapeutic diets are designed to maintain good health, correct deficiencies, or provide rest to specific organs while meeting daily nutrient requirements.

22.1 INTRODUCTION

Disease is often characterized by alterations in the structure and functioning of the body, which arise from specific abnormalities in how the body processes substances. Infections frequently trigger the initiation of the disease process. Diet plays an important role as a therapeutic tool in various diseases. In certain diseases, dietary interventions can lead to complete recovery, while in others, they can help manage the condition and prevent further complications. During the study of dietary management, it is important to carefully consider the challenges associated with each disease (Di Renzo et al., 2019).

Subsequently, the focus should be on how these challenges can be addressed or controlled through appropriate dietary therapy. Nutritional care of an individual is the process by which it meets the nutritional demands of the body. The type of care and diet management depends on the presence of disease, the environment, and the stage of the life cycle. Diet management for a healthy person mainly involves assessing their nutritional status, dietary patterns, and food habits, and recommending some changes to improve these. However, in the case of an ill or hospitalized individual, the nutrition care process is more complex and would involve a nutritional assessment, diet modifications, provision of enteral or parenteral nutrition if necessary, counseling, and close monitoring (Mahboub et al., 2021).

The nutritional needs of an average individual shift throughout his life cycle, from birth to childhood, adolescence, adulthood, and old age, based on the requirements of development and growth at every stage. A balanced diet at these phases minimizes the emergence of nutrient deficiency symptoms and protects against any nutritional condition or disease, as well as secondary disorders, usually infections, induced by decreased resistance due to malnourishment or undernourishment. These are treatable with good food management and nutritional care (Beam et al., 2021). Nutritional dietary management is the treatment of a disease condition by nutritional measures. Dietary management focuses on the actual administration of regular dietary habits, comprising the execution of fundamental concepts and the modification or customization of these diets to meet the unique disease situation (Lien and Vander, 2019).

22.2 OVERVIEW OF DIFFERENT TYPES OF THERAPEUTIC DIETS

Therapeutic diets refer to the use of food to treat disease. It is possible to accomplish this by modifying the patient's typical diet and making suitable dietary changes to match the requirements of any disease or injury. Doctors usually give or recommend therapeutic diets to patients in hospitals (Barazzon et al., 2020). Normal diets are used for therapeutic purposes, and they can be changed depending on the ailment or condition. Therapeutic diets are useful because:

- It maintains good nutritional status.
- Prevents any micronutrient deficiency.
- Meets the nutritional requirements in specific conditions.
- Provides a state of rest to the body.
- Managing chronic conditions.

Therapeutic diets are different for every patient, and individualized care is the utmost priority or the main goal of diet therapy. Doctors, dieticians, and nurses work in coordination to provide the best possible nutritional care to the patient (Ballesteros et al., 2020). There are various types of therapeutic diets that are most commonly used to manage specific health conditions or meet nutritional needs.

22.2.1 LIQUID DIETS

Liquid diets are of two types: clear liquid diet and full liquid diet.

22.2.2 CLEAR LIQUID DIET

Clear liquid diets are typically suggested for 1–2 days to patients in the pre- or post-operative stage. This diet is absolutely free of solids and residues, including those found in milk. Only clear drinks are provided, such as tea and coffee without cream or milk, clear soups, and so on. This diet is nutritionally deficient; however, it is only utilized for a brief length of time.

22.2.3 FULL LIQUID DIET

This diet is prescribed for individuals who are seriously unwell or who are unable to chew or swallow solid food. It contains liquid foods with solids that are easily digestible. The iron content of this diet is frequently insufficient.

22.2.4 SOFT DIET

This diet lies somewhere between a liquid diet and a regular diet. Patients recovering from surgery, gastrointestinal problems, and severe infections are served this diet. When planned based on a typical diet, it can be nutritionally adequate. The food should have a soft texture and consistency, be easy to chew, and have low roughage. This diet is designed to be simple, with easily digestible foods and no rich or very beneficial items. The diet should be high in calories and protein.

22.2.5 DIABETIC DIET

It is intended to control blood sugar levels in diabetics by restricting carbohydrate consumption and monitoring portion sizes in order to maintain stable blood glucose levels.

22.2.6 LOW-SODIUM DIET

Also known as a low-salt diet, it restricts sodium intake to manage conditions such as hypertension (high blood pressure) or heart disease. It involves minimizing the consumption of processed foods and using alternative flavoring agents.

22.2.7 RENAL DIET

Designed for individuals with kidney disease, these diets aim to reduce the workload on the kidneys by limiting protein, sodium, and phosphorus intake. They also take into account individual needs for managing electrolyte balance and fluid restrictions.

22.2.8 HIGH-FIBER DIET

Used to manage conditions like constipation, diverticulosis, or certain gastrointestinal disorders, high-fiber diets focus on consuming ample amounts of fruits, vegetables, whole grains, and legumes.

22.2.9 TUBE FEEDING FORMULAS

These specialized liquid diets are designed for individuals who are unable to consume food orally. They are administered through a feeding tube (enteral nutrition) or through IV fluids (parenteral nutrition). These are used in cases of extreme emergencies when swallowing is difficult, either due to esophageal obstruction, severe burns, gastric surgery, or similar conditions. It is also required for patients suffering from anorexia nervosa (Wu et al., 2020) (Table 22.1).

TABLE 22.1 Foods to be Included and Avoided in Different Hospital Diets

Types of Hospital Diets	Food Allowed	Food Avoided
Clear liquid diet	Mild tea or coffee without cream or milk, strained vegetables, or fruit juice. Plain gelatin, supplements like Protinules, Protinex Kernizan et al. (2020).	Milk, cream, egg, pureed vegetables or fruit sugar, butter, margarine, oil or ghee, whole-grains, legumes, poultry, fish and sweetmeats
Full liquid diet	Milk, cream, ice cream, juices, sugar, butter, strained meat broth, tea, coffee, strained soups Kernizan et al. (2020).	Whole grain cereals and pulses, vegetables such as cauliflower, onions, fish and sweetmeats, and so forth.
Soft diet	Soups, broth, and eggs (all types except fried and poached eggs) are preferred; all milk products; cooked vegetables that are soft without hard skin; butter in limited amounts; cereals should be well cooked; pulses—mung dal and mung; and meat—boiled or minced without skin Kernizan et al. (2020).	Salads, fried eggs, sweetmeats, strongly flavored vegetables like cauliflower, cabbage and fibrous. Spices and pulses like chana, chana dal, peas, and so forth. Fruits with seeds and skin and rough foods are avoided.
Normal diet	Includes all cereals, pulses, vegetables and milk products Kernizan et al. (2020).	Fried foods, pastries, processed foods

22.3 DIET IN DIFFERENT DISEASES

Our body system can be broken down into specific ways, resulting in different disease patterns and abnormalities. Some of these are discussed below, beginning with the gastrointestinal tract.

22.3.1 DIET IN GASTROINTESTINAL DISEASES

Our gastrointestinal system is made up of different organs, including the esophagus, stomach, small intestine, and large intestine. Tables 22.2 and 22.3 shows the various G.I. disorders and their dietary management.

1. **Celiac Disease:** Patients that cannot tolerate gluten, which is the protein present in wheat, are also known as having non-tropical sprue in later life or gluten-sensitive enteropathy. The remedy is to eliminate gluten from the diet by avoiding wheat, rye, barley, buckwheat, and probably oats. In India, it is possible to do this by removing wheat and wheat-based goods. It is an autoimmune disorder (Mukai et al., 2020).

   Foods that are included are rice, corn flour, soy products, skimmed milk, lean meat, fish, sugar, honey, butter, ghee, oils, all fruits and vegetables, eggs, and milk-based products. Wheat and wheat products, suji, breads, noodles, whole milk, and sweets containing maida, barley, and oats are foods to avoid (Mukai et al., 2020).

TABLE 22.2 Different Diseases of Gastrointestinal Tract

Disorder or Disease	Problem Associated	Diet Management
Disorders of esophagus and stomach indigestion (dyspepsia)	Problem in digesting food, heartburn, flatulence, epigastric pain, bloating after meals, acid regurgitation, nausea, and vomiting Feng et al. (2019).	Proper balanced diet. Give more fluids and semisolid diets in small intervals, and avoid emotional tension.
Esophagitis	Inflammation of esophageal wall and can be acute or chronic, due to gastric reflex Feng et al. (2019).	Soft and bland diet in small portions at frequent intervals; avoid trigger foods like spicy and acidic foods, chocolate, caffeine, fatty foods, and so forth. Maintain a healthy weight, as excess weight can lead to acid reflux, and drink plenty of water (which dilutes stomach acid).

TABLE 22.2 *(Continued)*

Disorder or Disease	Problem Associated	Diet Management
Hiatus hernia	Hiccupping after meals is caused by stomach protrusion via the diaphragmatic esophageal hiatus, pain in the substernal region, and herniation. Feng et al. (2019).	Weight reduction if the person is obese and provide with meals at frequent intervals in small portions
Gastritis	Inflammation of the stomach lining (mucosal lining) leads to low appetite, heartburn, and vomiting Feng et al. (2019).	Avoid trigger foods such as spicy and acidic foods, fried and fatty foods, carbonated beverages, caffeine, alcohol, and processed foods. Eat small and frequent meals. Choose cooked and easily digestible foods like steamed vegetables, soups, and so forth. Limit or avoid NSAIDs and alcohol. NSAIDs such as aspirin or ibuprofen can irritate the stomach lining. Probiotic foods like fermented foods may help alleviate gastritis symptoms and promote a healthy gut environment.
Peptic Ulcer	Defects or erosion in the gastric or duodenal mucosa in contact with the gastric juice. Epigastric pain is characterized by a gnawing or burning sensation that occurs after meals Bellini et al. (2020).	Diet low in fiber. Small, frequent meals with enough energy, protein, and fat. Avoidance of secretagogues such as spices, tea, coffee, alcohol, fruits, and nuts, as well as meat extracts, and to avoid excessive acid production.
Disorders of Small Intestine Diarrhea	Passage of loose, watery stools is a morbid evacuation of the bowels, the stools being fluid in nature, with increased frequency and foul smell, which leads to dehydration and loss of skin elasticity Bellini et al. (2020).	Oral rehydration therapy, ORS solutions to maintain electrolyte balance with small feedings at frequent intervals. Provision of fluids to compensate dehydration
Constipation	Stool that is hard and difficult to pass, lack of appetite, headache, foul breath, malaise (a general feeling of illness), and coated tongue are common among patients Jaiswal et al. (2021).	Inclusion of dietary fiber-rich foods such as whole grains, pulses, fruits, and vegetables is important. Fluids in the form of liquids or high-fluid foods like coconut water, rice water, and butter can be given. The main goal is to provide a high-fiber diet and plenty of fluids.

TABLE 22.3 Dietary Management of Different Gastrointestinal Diseases

Disorder or Disease	Problem	Diet Management
Large Intestine Ulcerative Colitis	Inflammation and ulceration of the mucosa of the large intestine or colon. Diarrhea with rectal bleeding, weight loss, dehydration, anemia, and general weakness due to severe loss of water, electrolytes, and bleeding Jaiswal et al. (2021).	5–6 small and frequent feedings. A high-calorie and high-protein diet with low residue is recommended. Tender meats, poultry, soft-boiled eggs, mildly flavored vegetables, refined cereals, custard, cottage cheese, and dehusked pulses can be given.
Hemorrhoids	Swollen veins in the lower rectum, rectal bleeding, pain or discomfort Jaiswal et al. (2021).	Consuming plenty of fruits, vegetables, and whole grains is important. Drink more fluids and liquids. Avoid trigger foods like fatty foods, spicy foods, caffeine, alcohol, and artificial sweeteners. A high-fiber diet is recommended.
Irritable Bowel Syndrome (IBS)	Abdominal pain, bloating, diarrhea and constipation Jaiswal et al. (2021).	Consuming plenty of fruits, vegetables, and whole grains is important. Drink more fluids and liquids. Avoid trigger foods like fatty foods, spicy foods, caffeine, alcohol, and artificial sweeteners. A high-fiber diet is recommended.
Diverticulitis	Inflammation or infection in the small pouches that can form in colon. Abdominal pain, fever, nausea and changes in bowel habits Jaiswal et al. (2021).	High-fiber diets should include whole grain breads and cereals, along with lots of fruits and vegetables. Aim for 20–35 grams of dietary fiber daily, along with plenty of liquids.

2. **Malabsorption Syndrome:** Malabsorption is the inability of a person to absorb nutrition. Fat is not absorbed in the body, or its absorption is impaired, resulting in a significant amount of excrement, a condition known as steatorrhea. The common feature is a variety of problems in nutrient absorption. By providing a high-energy diet and a high-protein diet while excluding specific carbohydrates, proteins, or fats that the patient does not tolerate, along with a soft or fiber-restricted diet, vitamin and mineral supplementation is required (Mukai et al., 2020).

MCTs, or medium-chain triglycerides, are particularly useful in malabsorption syndrome. MCTs are 8–10 carbon atom compounds that are rapidly digested by intestinal and pancreatic lipases. It has been found that consuming 5–7% of fat in the form of MCT is effective in reducing steatorrhea and lowering calcium, potassium, and salt losses. One such example is lactose intolerance, in which the enzyme lactase is absent, leading to lactose malabsorption in the body. It can be treated by excluding foods that are rich in lactose, such as milk and milk products, and opting for soy milk or milk derived from groundnuts. The labels should be read carefully (Mukai et al., 2020).

22.3.2 DIET IN GALLBLADDER, LIVER AND PANCREATIC DISORDERS

Disorders affecting the liver include hepatitis, cirrhosis, malabsorption syndrome, and hepatic coma (in serious conditions, the person can lead to a coma). The type of diet recommended varies for each type of disease. The major goals of dietary management in liver diseases are:

- Protection of the liver cells by a healthy diet.
- A high-carbohydrate diet to boost glycogen reserves.
- Fat restriction.
- High-quality protein for tissue regeneration and preventing fatty liver, but avoid high protein loading due to encephalopathy in cases when the liver is badly damaged.

Anorexia is a serious concern for people with liver illness, so efforts should be made to encourage patients to eat by including appealing, appetizing meals (Chang et al., 2019) (Table 22.4).

22.3.2.1 LIVER DISORDERS

1. **Hepatitis:** Hepatitis is a prevalent liver condition. The two categories encountered are viral and drug-induced. Viral hepatitis can be of two types: A and B. Type A, or infectious hepatitis, is transmitted either through fecal contamination of water or parenterally. Type A hepatitis is often mild and does not escalate to chronic hepatitis. Type B is most commonly spread through poorly sterilized surgical needles, for example. It is more severe

and has the potential to develop into a major disorder (Chang et al., 2019). Type C can be spread by blood transfusion. Drug or alcohol-induced hepatitis can occur as a result of addiction to alcohol, heroin, marijuana, or hashish, or as a result of intolerance to sulfa compounds or penicillin, or as a result of poisonous substances such as carbon tetrachloride, chloroform, and so on.

- **Symptoms:** Some of the usual symptoms in patients include stomach discomfort, anorexia, diarrhea, vomiting, fatigue, nausea, fever, and weight loss. Jaundice usually appears following these symptoms.
- **Dietary management:** A high-protein, high-carbohydrate, moderate-fat diet divided into 6–8 meals is recommended to help the patient eat well and recover quickly. It is recommended to consume one gram of high-quality protein per kilogram of body weight. Spices and condiments can be used in moderation to boost appetite. In between meals, high-protein beverages such as Protinules and Protinex in milk can be consumed.

2. **Cirrhosis:** Cirrhosis is a late-stage liver condition in which healthy liver tissue is replaced by scar tissue, causing chronic liver damage. Scar tissue obstructs blood flow through the liver, slowing its capacity to metabolize nutrients, hormones, medicines, and natural poisons. Symptoms and indicators include vomiting, discomfort, distension, jaundice, ascites, and an accumulation of fluids in the abdominal region, which can cause neurological abnormalities due to the presence of nitrogenous compounds such as ammonia in the cerebral circulation that is not mobilized by the liver. It can cause coma, and the patient may experience tiredness, restlessness, mental disorientation, and other symptoms before going into a coma (Moss, 2019).

   - **Dietary Management:** The diet can help if it is started at the right time, before the disease progresses. In infectious hepatitis, a high-carbohydrate, high-protein diet is prescribed. However, dietary protein levels should be managed in cases of hepatic coma, which is indicated by elevated levels of plasma aromatic amino acids such as phenylalanine, tyrosine, and methionine, while leucine, isoleucine, and valine levels are reduced. Dietary fat should be kept to a minimum of 10 grams. Fiber in the diet can be supplied in any amount that is tolerated. Vitamins are supplied to restore liver storage and repair tissue damage, particularly in cases of anorexia. If you have ascites and edema, you should limit your sodium intake to 500–800 mg per day. The diet's consistency should be liquid to soft, with short and frequent meals, and the diet's fiber level should be reduced (Moss, 2019).

3. **Jaundice:** Jaundice is not a disease but a symptom of liver disorders. It results in yellow discoloration of skin and body tissues. Symptoms can include fatigue, weakness, weight loss, anorexia, nausea, vomiting, fatty liver, and flatulence.
   - **Dietary Management:** Diet plays a major role, and a nutritious diet can help in reversing jaundice. A high-carbohydrate and high-protein diet is recommended. A low-fat diet with MCTs (Medium Chain Triglycerides) is recommended. Include fibers found in whole grains, fruits, and vegetables.

TABLE 22.4 Gall Bladder and Biliary System Disorders

Disease	Diet Management
Cholecystitis (inflammation in the gallbladder due to stones, which results in obstruction of bile flow, thickening of the walls of the gallbladder, and reduced function) Guo et al. (2022).	Diet includes foods that are low in residue and a low-fat diet to decrease the load on the organ. Foods like onion, turnips, radish, corn, cabbage, beans, and "rajmah" (red kidney beans) should be avoided as they can cause flatulence.
Cholelithiasis (formation of gall stones)	Weight reduction in obese or overweight individuals. Low fat diet or fat to be restricted. Surgery in case of more severe complications. High fiber diet is said to be useful. Inclusion of more fluids Guo et al. (2022).

22.3.2.2 PANCREATIC DISORDERS

- **Pancreatitis:** Pancreatitis is pancreatic inflammation that can cause aberrant pancreatic function. It can be acute (starting quickly and generally ending with the patient well recovered) or chronic (progressing slowly with ongoing, irreversible pancreatic injury) (Van den Ber et al., 2021). Dietary management of pancreatitis treatment comprises providing a diet ranging from clear liquids to semisolids to solids based on the patient's tolerance. Small, frequent meals are advised, as is a low-fat diet.

22.3.3 DIET IN CARDIOVASCULAR DISORDERS

Having high-carbohydrate, high-energy diets with a lot of fat, mostly saturated fat, cholesterol, and sodium has a negative impact on people's health and makes them more vulnerable to cardiovascular disease. Other risk factors for CVD include a sedentary lifestyle, stress, frequent smoking, and drinking. Atherosclerosis is caused by the accumulation of fatty deposits such as cholesterol and triglycerides in the artery walls and the restriction of blood flow. It is also responsible for high blood pressure, angina pectoris, cardiac failure, stroke, and chronic heart illnesses (Kris et al., 2020). High levels of lipids in the blood have been linked to cardiovascular disease in several patients. Hyperlipidemia is defined as an excess of lipid in the blood. Lipids and fibrous blood components, including calcium, quickly accumulate in the arteries and gradually clog them. Atherosclerosis is the process by which these components accumulate in the arteries. A stroke happens when the obstruction arises in the brain. Angina pectoris, myocardial infarction, or heart failure can result from complete occlusion of the heart arteries (Kris et al., 2020) (Table 22.5).

1. **Risk factors:**

- Family history hypertension, cardiovascular disease, obesity, and diabetes.
- Men are more likely than women to acquire CVD.
- Lifestyle factors like smoking, alcohol, sedentary lifestyle, tension, and a heavy workload that contribute to stress.

2. **Dietary management:**

   - Some broad suggestions for CVD dietary treatment that should be followed are:
   - The total fat should be less than or equal to 20% of the total energy intake.

- Cholesterol-raising fatty acids, like saturated fatty acids and trans-fatty acids, should be less than 7%.
- Monounsaturated Fatty Acid (MUFA) should be between 10% and 15%, and PUFA should be less than 10%.
- Carbohydrates should contribute 55%, and protein should contribute 15% of the daily energy requirement.
- Cholesterol intake must not be more than 200 milligrams a day.
- Take less refined sugars and salt in the diet.
- Engage in physical activities or encourage patients to walk daily.
- Consume foods like whole cereals, pulses, vegetables, and fruits (Kris et al., 2020).

TABLE 22.5 List of Food Items Suitable For Patients Suffering From Cardiovascular Diseases

Food to be Avoided	Food to be Included in Moderate Amounts	Food to be Allowed Liberally
• Concentrated milk preparations like burfi, processed cheese, rice puddings • Fried and oily preparations like pakodas, bhajia • Fatty read meats like organ meats, egg yolk, all types of processed meats • Alcohol and alcoholic soft drinks • Animal fats like ghee, butter, vegetable oils, palm oil, coconut oil, vanaspati and margarine • Sauces and all oil-based dressings • Nuts and oilseeds like cashewnuts, almonds, groundnuts, and so forth. • Salted foods and baked products to be avoided	• Cereals such as rice, wheat, bajra, ragi, jowar, and so forth. • Milk without cream • Root vegetables such as potato, sweet potato, yam, beetroot, pink radish, and so forth. • Lean white meat like egg white, fish, chicken • Vegetable oils, sugar, jiggery and salt	• Raw and green leafy vegetables, fruits • Clear soups, salads, sour lime, tamarind, vinegar for taste, and so forth. • Spices to taste and flavor • Coconut water • Garlic and onions

- **Hypertension:** High blood pressure is referred to as hypertension. It can be inherited, but it can also be caused by environmental variables such as salt and nutritional issues, as well as alcohol, smoking, a lack of physical activity, and stress. A low sodium diet has been shown to benefit individuals with hypertension (Table 22.6).

- **Mild restriction:** 2–3 g of salt or 2000–3000 mg. Salt can be used sparingly in cooking but not at the table. Natural fresh foods are not restricted; however, processed foods should be avoided.
- **Moderate sodium restriction:** 1 gram of salt, as well as the foregoing restrictions and some control over naturally occurring fresh foods, with no salt in cooking. Milk and meat products are used sparingly.
- **Stay away from canned vegetables and baked foods. Strict sodium limit:** 0.5 grams (500 mg). Aside from the limits listed above, meat, eggs, and milk are permitted in limited quantities, while vegetables with high salt content are prohibited.
- **Severe sodium restriction:** 0.25 grams or 250 mg of salt is used in circumstances such as cirrhosis of the liver with ascites and severe congestive heart failure (Joshi, Ettinger, and Liebman, 2020).

TABLE 22.6 Sodium Levels of Various Foods

Foods Rich in Sodium	Foods Moderate in Sodium	Foods Low in Sodium
Bread	Beetroot	Chapati
Biscuits	Carrot	Fruits
Cakes	Radish	Ghee
Pastries	Leafy vegetables	Oil
Butter	Maize	Cream
Cheese and cheese spreads	Rice flakes (puffed)	Nuts
Salted snacks	Cornflakes	Sugar
Meat extracts	Tinda	Honey
Pickles	Green tomatoes	Cabbage
Shellfish	Milk, curds	Cauliflower
Sauces	Meat	Tomato
Papads	Fish	Peas
	Poultry	Onion
		Potato

22.3.4 DIET IN RENAL DISORDERS

The kidneys are the primary organs of the body that excrete nitrogenous wastes in the form of urea. The kidneys' basic activities are endocrine, metabolic, and excretory. They keep the blood's composition and volume normal. They maintain the body's water-electrolyte equilibrium, as well as the acid-base balance, and flush away soluble pollutants (Akchurin, 2019).

1. **Acute Renal Failure (ARF):** This condition is defined by a rapid decrease in the glomerular filtration rate (GFR) within the glomerulus, resulting in urea in the circulation, a condition known as uremia. It is frequently associated with oliguria, defined as a urine flow rate of less than 15 ml per minute. The following are ARF dietary recommendations:
    - Fluid balance must be managed by ensuring that fluid intake equals primary output as well as other measurable water losses (such as drainage from fistulae, nasogastric aspirate, diarrhea, and vomiting), plus 400 ml/day. This includes water produced by metabolic reactions as well as insensible water losses via the skin and respiration.
    - Catabolism is present in the patient; weight should be reduced by 0.2 to 0.5 kg per day to avoid excessive fluid accumulation.
    - Reduce your salt, potassium, phosphorus, and magnesium consumption to avoid a build-up in your body.
    - Energy and, if possible, protein consumption should be used to meet the patient's nutritional needs. In rare cases, the standards may be more stringent than usual.
    - Limiting protein intake may also help to minimize kidney injury. Protein intake is determined by the patient's condition and whether dialysis is being conducted.
    - It may be useful to provide a liberal intake of nutrients in conjunction with dialysis for a patient who has lost a significant amount of weight.
    - A patient with almost normal urine excretion can obtain more nutrients since he or she is less likely to develop fluid and electrolyte imbalances or accumulate potentially hazardous by-products.
    - Restricting water, mineral, and amino acid consumption may lessen the requirement for dialysis in a patient with limited or no urine production and no uremia.
    - For a patient recovering from ARP, a high-calorie diet containing tiny amounts of necessary amino acids but little or no protein may be advantageous (Akchurin, 2019).

2. **Chronic Renal Failure (CRF):** There is an ongoing degradation and damage of nephrons in CRF, which leads to an ongoing decline in kidney function. In some cases, particularly in children, patients may exhibit a condition known as nephrotic syndrome, which involves a gradual deterioration of the capillary and basement membrane of the glomerulus. As this degeneration progresses, the tissue pores increase in size, allowing proteins to pass into the filtrate.

   Furthermore, as protein levels fall, cholesterol levels rise. Protein breakdown and malnutrition are other consequences of significant protein loss. Nephrotic individuals frequently appear skinny and may be deficient, including a lack of vitamin D. As a result, nephrotic individuals may suffer from a range of impairments. Nephrotic syndrome, if not treated effectively, can contribute to the onset of CRF (Saher, Aslam, and Khalid, 2019).

   Aside from hunger, weight loss, anemia, hypertension, and bone abnormalities are common clinical indicators of CRF. Because CRF care must be adjusted to individual patients, it is dependent on the degree of renal insufficiency. Energy requirements, protein content, fluid consumption, acid-base balance, and electrolyte balance should all be considered in the diet. The following factors must be considered while making dietary changes:

   - To provide adequate calories.
   - To regulate the protein content of the diet.
   - To provide sufficient amounts of electrolytes like sodium, potassium, and fluid intake.
   - To restrict phosphate and supplement the diet with calcium, iron, ascorbic acid, and B-complex vitamins.

     i. **Energy:** The calorie content of the food should be sufficient to avoid tissue loss and promote protein synthesis. A daily caloric intake of 2000–3000 kcals is adequate. Dietary options include sago, porridge, rice porridge, sago khichdi, sago vada, ice cream, rasgulla, and so on (Saher et al., 2019).

     ii. **Protein:** Patients on hemodialysis should be given 1 g/kg body weight of high-quality protein. Eggs and milk powders with biological value should meet at least 75%

of total protein requirements. Patients who do not have hemodialysis have a better nitrogen balance with 0.6 g protein per kg body weight.

iii. **Carbohydrates and fats:** PUFA are advised. The PUFA to saturated fat ratio in the diet should be at least 1:1. Carbohydrates should not exceed 60% of total calorie consumption, and cholesterol should be limited to 150–200 mg or fewer per day.

iv. **Potassium:** Hyperkalemia is found in chronic uremia. Potassium consumption for a non-dialyzed patient is limited to 1500–2000 mg. Dialysis patients can receive up to 2500 mg potassium. Because all animal proteins are high in potassium, they should be utilized with caution.

v. **Sodium:** Depending on the quantity of sodium in the urine, dietary sodium may be controlled, and serum sodium restriction may be required due to edema, hypertension, and the risk of congestive heart failure. In general, 1–2 grams is permitted.

vi. **Other minerals include:** Phosphorus intake should be limited to 600–750 mg per day. To avoid hyperparathyroidism, calcium supplements of 1.5–2.0 grams per day and vitamin D supplements of 300,000 to 600,000 International unit (IU) may be administered twice weekly.

vii. **Fluids:** Tight fluid control is required to prevent excessive retention in the body. Patients who are not dialyzed can drink 400–600 mL of fluids per day; however, dialyzed patients should drink somewhat less than one liter per day (Saher, Aslam, and Khalid, 2019).

3. **Urinary Calculi or Renal Calculi:** Kidney stones can form in the kidney, the ureter, the bladder, or the urethra. They are composed of an organic matrix with interspersed crystals of varying sizes. Different types of calculi occur under various conditions. Uric acid or urate calculi are the result of excessive metabolic synthesis of these chemicals and develop more frequently in people who have gout. Calcium oxalate calculi develop when there is an excess of oxalates in the diet, which is mostly generated from fruits and vegetables. Crystalline calcium carbonate and phosphate stones can form when the parathyroid gland is overactive, when too

much milk is ingested, or when alkalosis reduces the solubility of calcium salts. Amorphous carbonates and triple phosphates are characteristically found in calculi as a result of infection and stasis (Oswal et al., 2022).

- **Dietary Management:** However, numerous dietary factors that contribute to stone formation can be addressed by increasing fluid consumption, which dilutes the urine and decreases the concentration of the stone's contents. Doctors advise drinking at least three liters of fluid. Minerals that are important components of stones, such as calcium and oxalate, may be restricted in the diet (Oswal et al., 2022) (Table 22.7).

TABLE 22.7 Foods with High Calcium, Phosphorous and Oxalate

Foods Rich in Calcium	Foods Rich in Phosphorus	Foods Rich in Oxalates
All green leafy vegetables	Meat	Grapes
Mutton muscle	Fish	Tomato
Fish	Eggs	Cocoa
Milk	Whole grain cereals	Tea
Curds	Milk powder	Wood apple
Khoa	Cheese	Plantain flower
Milk paneer	Carrot	Gingelly seeds
Cheese	Nuts	Rhubarb stalk

22.3.5 DIET IN MUSCULOSKELETAL DISEASES

1. **Gout:** Gout is a condition characterized by the accumulation of uric acid in the blood and sodium salts of uric acid in the joints, cartilages, and kidneys. It occurs due to high levels of uric acid in the blood. There may be attacks of acute inflammatory arthritis. Severe pain in the joints and inflammation can be seen in patients. Dietary management of gout includes a low-purine diet, as purines are oxidized to uric acid in the body, so the intake should be restricted. Foods that need to be controlled include sardines, anchovies, spinach, cauliflower, dried beans, peas, lentils, mushrooms, cocoa, tea, alcoholic beverages, pork, beef, meat extracts, and so forth (Papageorgiou and Biver, 2021).

2. **Arthritis:** Arthritis is characterized by joint stiffness, and the most common forms are osteoarthritis and rheumatoid arthritis. Pain in the joints is especially noticeable when in motion or holding heavy weights. The joints of the fingers, knees, and spine are affected. Dietary management: If the patient is obese, he or she needs to decrease weight in order to reduce stress on the joints, and a low-calorie diet should be recommended to reduce obesity (Papageorgiou and Biver, 2021).

22.4 CONCLUSION

Dietary management of different diseases varies with respect to an individual's health condition. Dietary management of various diseases such as gallbladder, liver, GI tract, cardiovascular, renal, and so forth., requires careful planning of the foods to be included and avoided to reduce the chances of any further complications. In general, a fiber-restricted diet and bland diet are given in disturbances of the esophagus and stomach. MCTs are preferred in malabsorption syndrome, and a high-protein, high-carbohydrate, and low-fat diet is recommended in cardiovascular disorders. Sodium retention is necessary based on the degree of illness in heart diseases. Management of diet can help in reducing or alleviating the symptoms of these diseases.

KEYWORDS

- **cardiovascular disease**
- **diabetes**
- **dietary management**
- **fiber-restricted diet**
- **malabsorption syndrome**
- **medium-chain triglycerides)**
- **non-communicable diseases**
- **sodium retention**
- **therapeutic diets**

REFERENCES

Akchurin, M. (2019). Chronic kidney disease and dietary measures to improve outcomes. *Pediatric Clinics, 66*(1), 247–267.

Ballesteros-Pomar, M., Cherubini, A., Keller, H., Lam, P., Rolland, Y., & Simmons, S. F. (2020). Texture-modified diet for improving the management of oropharyngeal dysphagia in nursing home residents: An expert review. *The Journal of Nutrition, Health & Aging, 24*, 576–581.

Barazzoni, I. R., Bischoff, S. C., Breda, J., Wickramasinghe, K., Krznaric, Z., Nitzan, D., Pirlich, M., Singer, P., & ESPEN Expert Group. (2020). ESPEN expert statements and practical guidance for nutritional management of individuals with SARS-CoV-2 infection. *Clinical Nutrition, 39*(6), 1631–1638.

Beam, A., Clinger, E., & Hao, L. (2021). Effect of diet and dietary components on the composition of the gut microbiota. *Nutrients, 13*(8), 2795.

Bellini, M., Tonarelli, S., Nagy, A. G., Pancetti, A., Costa, F., Ricchiuti, A., De Bortoli, N., Mosca, M., Marchi, S., & Rossi, A. (2020). Low FODMAP diet: Evidence, doubts, and hopes. *Nutrients, 12*(1), 148.

Chang, C. M., Chiu, T. H., Chang, C. C., Lin, M. N., & Lin, C. L. (2019). Plant-based diet, cholesterol, and risk of gallstone disease: A prospective study. *Nutrients, 11*(2), 335.

Di Renzo, L., Gualtieri, P., Romano, L., Marrone, G., Noce, A., Pujia, A., Perrone, M. A., Aiello, V., Colica, C., & De Lorenzo, A. (2019). Role of personalized nutrition in chronic-degenerative diseases. *Nutrients, 11*(8), 1707.

Feng, C., Zhang, Y., Chong, F., Yang, M., Liu, C., Liu, L., Huang, C., Huang, C., Feng, X., Wang, X., & Chu, T. (2019). Establishment and implementation of an enhanced recovery after surgery (ERAS) pathway tailored for minimally invasive transforaminal lumbar interbody fusion surgery. *World Neurosurgery, 129*, e317–e323.

Guo, Q., Cui, M., Liu, X., Zhao, S., Liu, P., & Wang, L. (2022). Effect of epidermal growth factor in human milk and maternal diet on late-onset breast milk jaundice: A case-control study in Beijing. *Nutrients, 14*(21), 4587.

Jaiswal, F., Rai, A. K., Wal, P., Wal, A., & Singh, S. P. (2021). Peptic ulcer: A review on etiology, pathogenesis and treatment. *Asian Journal of Pharmaceutical Education and Research, 10*(4), 1.

Joshi, S., Ettinger, L., & Liebman, S. E. (2020). Plant-based diets and hypertension. *American Journal of Lifestyle Medicine, 14*(4), 397–405.

Kernizan, D., Mintz, D., Colin, M., Lee, M., Yoakam, L., Chen, Y. P., Iofel, E., Koniaris, S., & Weidner, M. (2020). Outcomes and safety of blenderized tube feedings in pediatric patients: A single center's experience. *Journal of Pediatric Gastroenterology and Nutrition, 71*(4), e124–e128.

Kris-Etherton, P. M., Petersen, K. S., Velarde, G., Barnard, N. D., Miller, M., Ros, E., O'Keefe, J. H., Williams, S. R. K., Horn, L. V., Na, M., & Shay, C. (2020). Barriers, opportunities, and challenges in addressing disparities in diet-related cardiovascular disease in the United States. *Journal of the American Heart Association, 9*(7), e014433.

Lien, E. C., & Vander Heiden, M. G. (2019). A framework for examining how diet impacts tumour metabolism. *Nature Reviews Cancer, 19*(11), 651–661.

Mahboub, N., Rizk, R., Karavetian, M., & De Vries, N. (2021). Nutritional status and eating habits of people who use drugs and/or are undergoing treatment for recovery: A narrative review. *Nutrition Reviews, 79*(6), 627–635.

Moss, O. (2019). Nutrition priorities: Diet recommendations in liver cirrhosis. *Clinical Liver Disease, 14*(4), 146.

Mukai, R., Handa, O., Naito, Y., Takayama, S., Suyama, Y., Ushiroda, C., Majima, A., Hirai, Y., Mizushima, K., Okayama, T., & Katada, K. (2020). High-fat diet causes constipation in mice via decreasing colonic mucus. *Digestive Diseases and Sciences, 65*, 2246–2253.

Oswal, M., Varghese, R., Zagade, T., Dhatrak, C., Sharma, R., & Kumar, D. (2023). Dietary supplements and medicinal plants in urolithiasis: Diet, prevention, and cure. *Journal of Pharmacy and Pharmacology, 75*(6), 719–745.

Papageorgiou, M., & Biver, E. (2021). Interactions of the microbiome with pharmacological and non-pharmacological approaches for the management of ageing-related musculoskeletal diseases. *Therapeutic Advances in Musculoskeletal Disease, 13*, 1759720X211009018.

Saher, S., Aslam, M., & Khalid, S. (2019). Dietary assessment of patients suffering from chronic renal failure with complications. *Asian Journal of Allied Health Sciences (AJAHS)*, 58–65.

Van Den Ber, G. F. F., Van Dalen, D., Hyoju, S. K., Van Santvoort, H. C., Besselink, M. G., Wiersinga, W. J., Zaborina, O., Boermeester, M. A., & Alverdy, J. (2021). Western-type diet influences mortality from necrotising pancreatitis and demonstrates a central role for butyrate. *Gut, 70*(5), 915–927.

Wu, X. S., Miles, A., & Braakhuis, A. (2020). Nutritional intake and meal composition of patients consuming texture-modified diets and thickened fluids: A systematic review and meta-analysis. *Healthcare, 8*(4), 579.

CHAPTER 23

Sight Sustenance: The Role of Nutrition in Eye Wellness

MANISH KUMAR SAH[1,*] and RUCHIKA SAH[2]

[1]*Department of Optometry, SSAHS, Sharda University, Greater Noida, Uttar Pradesh, India*

[2]*Department of Optometry, Ramlal Golchha Eye Hospital Foundation, Biratnagar, Nepal*

*Corresponding author

ABSTRACT

As a delicate organ, the eye requires a variety of essential nutrients, including vitamins, minerals, and antioxidants, to function at its peak. A diet rich in fruits, vegetables, lean meats, and good fats can help promote overall eye health. Maintaining good eye health is crucial for independence, a high quality of life, and general welfare. The three nutrients lutein, zeaxanthin, and omega-3 fatty acids are very important for preserving good vision and reducing the risk of age-related vision loss. As people become older, age-related eye conditions such as cataracts, glaucoma, and macular degeneration become more prevalent. The risk of contracting these diseases can be decreased by maintaining a healthy diet and lifestyle, even while some risk factors, such as genetics and family history, cannot be changed. In addition to examining the significance of nutrition in preventing common eye disorders such as macular degeneration, cataracts, and dry eye syndrome, the chapter emphasizes the connection between diet and age-related vision loss. A well-balanced diet rich in whole foods, healthy fats, and antioxidant-rich fruits and vegetables is recommended for fostering ideal eye health, which is another topic covered in this chapter.

Allied Healthcare in Practice: An Introduction to Integrated Patient Care. Sally Lukose, Karuna Singh (Eds.)

DOI: 10.1201/9781998511037-26

23.1 INTRODUCTION

A variety of foods are included in a balanced diet in moderation to supply the body with the vitamins, minerals, and energy it needs to function properly. In the proper proportions, a balanced diet combines macronutrients (carbohydrates, proteins, and fats) and micronutrients (vitamins and minerals) (Cena and Calder, 2020; Stipanuk and Caudill, 2018). Maintaining excellent health, preventing chronic illnesses like diabetes, heart disease, and obesity, and fostering general well-being all depend on a balanced diet (Benisi et al., 2016; Zong et al., 2016). Maintaining strong eyesight also requires a balanced, nutritious diet that includes important components. The eye is a complicated organ that needs consistent nutrition to stay healthy and perform as it should. The retina, cornea, lens, and optic nerve are just a few of the elements that make up the eye. For each of these components to work properly, it needs particular nutrients. The relationship between nutrition and eye health is a topic that is becoming more important in terms of global health. Proper food has a considerable impact on the health of different ocular structures, the avoidance of eye diseases, and the maintenance of vision over the course of a person's lifetime. The intricate relationships between diet and the eyes are thoroughly explored in this in-depth study, which also covers the architecture of the eye, crucial nutrients for eye health, commonly occurring eye disorders influenced by diet, dietary tactics for preserving eye health, and the significance of nutrition in various life phases. It is widely recognized that a healthy diet has a significant impact on overall well-being beyond just providing basic nutrition. Our dietary decisions have a big impact on our mental, emotional, and even physical health.

In order to better understand the intricate relationships between diet and eye health, we set out on a journey that demonstrates the startling ways in which our food choices can directly affect the health of our eyes. We cannot separate our eyes from the rest of our body, so the health of our eyes is intimately correlated with the nutrients we ingest. In recent years, our understanding of the critical link between diet and eye health has grown, shedding light on a compelling connection between the foods we eat and the quality of our eyesight in the future. This relationship has its origins in the intricate biological workings of the eye, where a variety of specialized tissues, from the cornea to the retina, depend on a steady stream of particular nutrients to perform at their best. We will discover the crucial role that our dietary choices have in keeping the clarity of our vision, preventing eye disorders, and sustaining ocular well-being as we set out on this journey of investigation into the junction of nutrition and eye health. This in-depth investigation will cover the wide range of nutrients, dietary practices, and foods that have an immediate bearing on the condition of our eyes. We shall delve into the world of vitamins that support the health of our retinas, as well as antioxidants, which protect us from the ravages of oxidative stress. We'll also look at the importance of omega-3 fatty acids, which are necessary for producing the tears that feed and comfort our eyes (Liu and Ji, 2014). Each of these elements is essential to the overall harmony of ocular health. We must take into account the larger context of dietary and environmental decisions that affect the health of our eyes. One of the many outside variables that might hurt our eyes is obesity. Other external factors that can affect our eyes include smoking (Kennedy et al., 2006; Latif and Naroo, 2022) and excessive UV exposure (Dishita and Pranaykumar, 2022; Lee et al., 2012). It's crucial to comprehend how these decisions will affect our eyesight if we want to keep our eyes healthy. We will also stress the importance of routine eye exams as we travel across the intersection of diet and eye health. Maintaining clear eyesight and resolving possible problems before they become incapacitating require the use of early detection and preventive techniques, which are crucial. We may take proactive efforts to protect the clarity and vibrancy of our eyesight for years to come by being knowledgeable champions for our own eye health.

A variety of dietary superheroes will be encountered as we progress through this exploration. Vitamin C, vitamin E, and beta-carotene are antioxidants that guard against oxidative stress, which can harm the delicate ocular tissues (Chen et al., 2009). Omega-3 fatty acids help to support tear formation and lower the incidence of dry eye syndrome. They are found in fatty fish and flaxseeds. Green leafy vegetables contain the carotenoids lutein and zeaxanthin (Perry et al., 2009), which help protect the retina from high-energy blue light and damaging ultraviolet (UV) light. These are only a few illustrations of the dietary miracles that help to preserve ideal eye health. Along with reviewing the helpful nutrients, we will also look at how certain eating habits, like the Mediterranean diet, can improve general health, which includes eye health. The Mediterranean diet, which is recognized for its capacity to lower the risk of chronic diseases (Romagnolo and Selmin, 2017), particularly those affecting the eyes, is distinguished by its abundance of fruits, vegetables, whole grains, and heart-healthy fats like olive oil. We may make decisions that both energize our bodies and safeguard our vision by being aware of how certain food habits affect our health.

23.2 KEY NUTRIENTS FOR EYE HEALTH

Maintaining the health of the various eye structures requires an adequate diet. This chapter examines the essential nutrients that are crucial for maintaining and promoting eye health.

23.2.1 ANTIOXIDANTS: GUARDIANS OF EYE HEALTH

Understand the foe that antioxidants fight: oxidative stress, before we go into the world of antioxidants. Our eyes, which are continually exposed to oxygen and light, are very metabolically active organs. Free radicals are a naturally occurring result of this exposure. Highly reactive chemicals called free radicals have the potential to harm the tissues and cells in the eye (Roberts, 2001). Free radicals have the amazing capacity to be neutralized by antioxidant molecules, shielding our cells from their damaging effects (Cabrera and Chihuailaf, 2011). Antioxidants are a vital part of the body's defense against oxidative stress in the context of eye health. They assist healthy eye function by lowering inflammation and preserving the integrity of the ocular tissues. Some of the most important antioxidants that are crucial for protecting our eyes include.

23.2.1.1 VITAMIN C (ASCORBIC ACID)

The aqueous humor of the eye, the clear liquid that fills the gap between the lens and the cornea, has significant amounts of this potent antioxidant. The cornea, the eye's outermost layer, is protected by vitamin C from oxidative stress and inflammation (Suh et al., 2008).

23.2.1.2 VITAMIN E (TOCOPHEROL)

The health of the cell membranes in the eyes is maintained by the fat-soluble antioxidant vitamin E (Pham-Huy et al., 2008). It aids in preventing free radical damage to the retina's sensitive photoreceptor cells.

23.2.1.3 BETA-CAROTENE

Beta-carotene is not only a potent antioxidant in and of itself, but it also functions as a precursor to vitamin A. It is crucial for protecting the retina from damage and reducing oxidative stress on the eyes (Johra et al., 2020).

23.2.1.4 ZINC

The element zinc is essential for the function of antioxidant enzymes in the eye. It contributes to the reduction of cataracts and AMD by defending against oxidative harm to the lens and retina (Newsome et al., 1996).

23.3 VITAMIN A: THE VISION VITAMIN

Retinol, retinal, and retinoic acid are three of the fat-soluble substances referred to as vitamin A. Retinol and retinal, its derivative, are primarily linked to vitamin A when discussing eye health. These substances play a crucial role in phototransduction, the process by which the eye transforms light into electrical signals that the brain perceives as visual images (Sajovic et al., 2022).

23.3.1 VITAMIN A'S FUNCTION IN PRESERVING EYE HEALTH

23.3.1.1 NIGHT VISION

Night vision depends on the generation of rhodopsin by vitamin A. Night blindness, a disease where people have trouble seeing in dim light, can result from a vitamin A deficit.

23.3.1.2 PREVENTING XEROPHTHALMIA

Dryness of the eye's surface tissues is a defining feature of the condition known as xerophthalmia, which can worsen to cause serious damage to the cornea and even blindness. Vitamin A is necessary for keeping these tissues healthy, and a lack of it is a major contributor to xerophthalmia, especially in impoverished nations (Agrawal and Agrawal, 2013; Dole and Gilbert, 2009).

23.3.1.3 PROTECTING THE CORNEA

The cornea, the clearest layer of the eye, is susceptible to harm from viruses and the environment. The cornea's structural integrity and resistance to infections are both maintained by vitamin A (Huang et al., 2018).

23.3.1.4 REDUCING THE RISK OF EYE INFECTIONS

A sufficient intake of vitamin A is associated with a lower incidence of eye infections, especially in children in regions where vitamin A deficiency (VAD) is frequent.

23.3.2 SOURCES OF VITAMIN A

It's essential to have enough vitamin A to keep your eyes healthy. The body can obtain vitamin A from food sources in two different forms:

23.3.2.1 PREFORMED VITAMIN A (RETINOL)

This kind of vitamin A is found in animal-based foods like liver, fish, dairy products, and eggs (Blaner, 2020). It can be readily absorbed by the body and used for a variety of physiological processes (Ross et al., 2020).

23.3.2.2 PROVITAMIN A CAROTENOIDS

Beta-carotene and other provitamin A carotenoids are present in many colorful fruits and vegetables (Gilbert, 2013), although they are more common in those that are orange, red, and yellow. When necessary, the body can transform these carotenoids into active vitamin A.

The following foods contain vitamin A:

- **Liver:** One of the best sources of preformed vitamin A is liver.

- **Fatty Fish:** Salmon and mackerel are two fish that contain vitamin A, particularly in the form of retinol.
- **Dairy Products:** Milk, cheese, and yogurt are dairy products that contain retinol.
- **Eggs:** Eggs are a source of vitamin A and retinol.
- **Leafy Green Vegetables:** Beta-carotene and other carotenoids are found in spinach, kale, and collard greens.
- **Colorful Fruits:** Mangoes, cantaloupes, and apricots are examples of fruits that provide beta-carotene.
- **Supplements:** Medical professionals may advise vitamin A supplements in cases of VAD or specific medical concerns.

23.3.3 VITAMIN A DEFICIENCY

In many parts of the world, VAD remains a significant public health concern, particularly in regions with limited access to a variety of healthful foods. The effects of a vitamin A shortage can be severe and harmful, partcularly for eye health (Table 23.1):

TABLE 23.1 Grade of Xerophthalmia

XN	Night blindness
X1A	Conjunctival xerosis
X1B	Bitot's spots
X2	Corneal xerosis
X3A	Corneal ulcer/ $<1/3$ cornea
X3B	Corneal ulcer/keratomalacia $\geq 1/3$
XS	Corneal scarring (from X3)
XF	Xerophthalmic fundus

Source: Mrowicka et al. (2022).

23.4 LUTEIN AND ZEAXANTHIN: EYE PROTECTION

The carotenoid family of natural pigments includes lutein and zeaxanthin. The red, orange, and yellow hues of numerous fruits and vegetables are caused by carotenoids, which are chemical molecules found in plants, algae, and some microorganisms. Although lutein and zeaxanthin cannot be produced by the human body, they are necessary for sustaining eye health and must be obtained from diet or dietary supplements. The health and functionality of the macula depend on the macular pigment, which principally consists of lutein and zeaxanthin. In the eye, lutein and zeaxanthin function as antioxidants (Nguyen et al., 2023), scavenging free radicals before they can damage the retina. By absorbing and filtering out these harmful wavelengths, these carotenoids help in the prevention of or reduction of the risk of conditions like age-related macular degeneration (ARMD) and cataracts. Reduced visual acuity, increased glare sensitivity, and decreased contrast sensitivity can all result from low amounts of lutein and zeaxanthin, compromising overall visual performance. Lutein and zeaxanthin have the ability to absorb and expel damaging high-energy photons, particularly blue light and UV rays (Narimatsu et al., 2015). These wavelengths are powerful enough to harm the retina's sensitive cells. Free radicals, which are highly reactive chemicals that can cause oxidative stress and damage to cells, including those in the retina, are produced when blue light and UV rays enter the eye.

23.5 OMEGA-3 FATTY ACIDS: NOURISHING THE RETINA

The polyunsaturated fat family, which includes omega-3 fatty acids, is distinguished by their distinct chemical makeup and crucial function in maintaining human health. The function and health of the eyes are significantly influenced by omega-3 fatty acids. These vital nutrients, which are mostly present in specific foods and supplements, have a number of advantages for the eyes. AMD, a common eye disorder, affects the macula, the central region of the retina that is responsible for providing sharp central vision (Deng et al., 2022). Docosahexaenoic acid (DHA), in particular, has been found to be an omega-3 fatty acid that may help lower the risk of AMD (Christen et al., 2011) and slow the advancement of the condition. Since omega-3s are anti-inflammatory and antioxidant, they can aid in preventing inflammation and oxidative stress on the macula. The retinal cell membranes require omega-3 fatty acids, particularly DHA, as key structural elements. These fatty acids maintain the fluidity and flexibility of the retinal cell membranes, enabling the photoreceptor cells to operate properly and transmit light signals effectively (Querques et al., 2011). Omega-3 fatty acids have been shown to contribute to maintaining the tear film's lipid layer, which lessens the signs and symptoms of dry eye syndrome (Fogt et al., 2019). This reduces tear evaporation and increases comfort for the eyes. The environment that the eyes are exposed to, including sunlight and oxygen, can cause oxidative stress and damage to the tissues of the eyes. With their antioxidant qualities, omega-3 fatty acids aid in scavenging dangerous free radicals and shielding eye cells from oxidative damage. An omega-3 fatty acid in particular, Eicosapentaenoic acid (EPA), has potent anti-inflammatory properties (Calder, 2015). Eye inflammation can cause a number of uncomfortable eye disorders. Omega-3 fatty acids contribute to better eye health by reducing inflammation in the ocular tissues.

24.6 EYE CONDITIONS INFLUENCED BY DIET

Regarding eye health, the adage "you are what you eat" is largely accurate. Our eating habits have a big influence on how well our eyes are able to see and operate. Diet has an impact on a number of eye diseases, and knowing how nutrition affects eye health can help people make better decisions to safeguard and maintain their eyesight. In this post, we will examine a number of dietary-related eye diseases, key nutrients, and dietary tactics for promoting and maintaining eye health.

23.6.1 AGE-RELATED MACULAR DEGENERATION (AMD)

- Consuming foods high in antioxidants, such as fruits and vegetables, can reduce the incidence of AMD by preventing oxidative stress in the retina. Particularly advantageous are zinc, copper, and the vitamins C and E.
- Lutein and zeaxanthin, which are found in large quantities in the macula, act as natural filters to protect the retina from harmful high-energy light waves. A diet rich in spinach, kale, corn, and egg yolks can increase lutein and zeaxanthin levels, reducing the risk of AMD.

- Omega-3 fatty acids, which are mostly present in fatty fish like salmon and mackerel, have anti-inflammatory properties that may help reduce the risk of AMD and slow its progression.
- Enough zinc and copper must be present for the retina to remain healthy. These nutrients can be found in a variety of foods, including whole grains, lean meats, fish, and nuts.
- A diet rich in low glycemic index (GI) foods can assist diabetics in managing their blood sugar levels and reduce their risk of AMD (Kaushik et al., 2008).

23.6.2 CATARACTS

- Antioxidant-rich foods, particularly those high in vitamins C and E, can help stop the oxidation of the lens. Foods including citrus fruits, berries, nuts, and seeds contain these vitamins.
- By protecting the lens from harmful light and oxidative stress, lutein and zeaxanthin are essential for avoiding AMD and may help reduce the prevalence of cataracts.
- Omega-3 fatty acids' anti-inflammatory properties may help reduce the risk of cataracts.
- It's crucial to maintain a balanced diet with a variety of vitamins and minerals. Deficits in nutrients like selenium and vitamin A have been linked to an increased incidence of cataracts.

23.6.3 DIABETIC RETINOPATHY

- For those with diabetes, monitoring and regulating carbohydrate intake is crucial for blood sugar stabilization. This objective can be accomplished by consuming complex carbohydrates with a low glycemic index.
- The anti-inflammatory properties of omega-3 fatty acids, which are present in fatty fish and supplements, may help reduce inflammation in the retinal blood vessels.
- Consuming foods high in antioxidants, such as fruits, vegetables, and whole grains, can help lower oxidative stress in the retina and possibly slow the development of diabetic retinopathy (Kang and Yang, 2020).

23.6.4 DRY EYE SYNDROME

- Omega-3 fatty acids, notably DHA and EPA, are present in fatty fish such as mackerel and salmon. These fatty acids can help maintain the lipid layer of the tear film, decreasing tear evaporation and reducing the symptoms of dry eyes.
- Vitamin A is crucial for maintaining the health of the eye's surface tissues and the generation of tears.
- Staying adequately hydrated by ingesting enough water and fluids can help prevent dry eye symptoms by ensuring the eyes receive enough moisture (Sherwin et al., 2015).

23.6.5 GLAUCOMA

- Antioxidants can aid in preventing oxidative damage to the retinal and optic nerve cells (Garcia-Medina et al., 2020). Antioxidant-rich foods, like dark berries, leafy greens, and vibrant fruits and vegetables, can be advantageous.
- Maintaining a balanced fluid intake while staying hydrated can help control intraocular pressure (IOP). However, excessive fluid intake may not be advised for some types of glaucoma; therefore, getting personalized advice from a medical professional is crucial.
- For some glaucoma sufferers, cutting back on caffeine and alcohol may help control IOP.

23.7 CONCLUSION

Diet has a big impact on how healthy eyes are generally and on different eye problems. People can support and maintain their visual health by eating a balanced diet high in antioxidants, omega-3 fatty acids, and eye-friendly minerals. Additionally, controlling particular dietary components, such as glycemic control for diabetes or hydration for dry eyes, can help prevent and treat eye disorders. The relationship between diet and eye health is apparent, and a growing body of research is demonstrating how diet affects the prevention and treatment of eye diseases. For people of all ages, it is necessary to comprehend the critical role that nutrients play in maintaining the health of ocular tissues, preventing disorders, and preserving eyesight.

People may actively protect their priceless gift of sight and preserve optimal eye health throughout their lifetimes by committing to a balanced, nutrient-rich diet, frequent eye checkups, and a healthy lifestyle.

KEYWORDS

- **age related macular degeneration**
- **antioxidants**
- **cataracts**
- **dry eye syndrome**
- **eye health**
- **eye-friendly minerals**
- **macular degeneration**
- **nutrient-rich diet**
- **nutrition**
- **ocular tissues**
- **omega-3 fatty acids**
- **zeaxanthin**

REFERENCES

Agrawal, V., & Agrawal, P. (2013). Prevalence and determinants of xerophthalmia in rural children of Uttar Pradesh, India. *Nepalese Journal of Ophthalmology, 5*(2), 226–229.

Benisi-Kohansal, S., Saneei, P., Salehi-Marzijarani, M., Larijani, B., & Esmaillzadeh, A. (2016). Whole-grain intake and mortality from all causes, cardiovascular disease, and cancer: A systematic review and dose-response meta-analysis of prospective cohort studies. *Advances in Nutrition, 7*(6), 1052–1065.

Blaner, W. S. (2020). Vitamin A and provitamin A carotenoids. In *Present Knowledge in Nutrition* (pp. 73–91). Elsevier.

Cabrera, M. P., & Chihuailaf, R. H. (2011). Antioxidants and the integrity of ocular tissues. *Veterinary Medicine International, 2011*, Article 1.

Calder, P. C. (2015). Marine omega-3 fatty acids and inflammatory processes: Effects, mechanisms, and clinical relevance. *Biochimica et Biophysica Acta (BBA)–Molecular and Cell Biology of Lipids, 1851*(4), 469–484.

Cena, H., & Calder, P. C. (2020). Defining a healthy diet: Evidence for the role of contemporary dietary patterns in health and disease. *Nutrients, 12*(2), 334.

Chen, Y., Mehta, G., & Vasiliou, V. (2009). Antioxidant defenses in the ocular surface. *The Ocular Surface, 7*(4), 176–185.

Christen, W. G., Schaumberg, D. A., Glynn, R. J., & Buring, J. E. (2011). Dietary ω-3 fatty acid and fish intake and incident age-related macular degeneration in women. *Archives of Ophthalmology, 129*(7), 921–929.

Deng, Y., Qiao, L., Du, M., Qu, C., Wan, L., Li, J., & Huang, L. (2022). Age-related macular degeneration: Epidemiology, genetics, pathophysiology, diagnosis, and targeted therapy. *Genes & Diseases, 9*(1), 62–79.

Dishita, C., & Pranaykumar, S. (2022). Effects of solar radiation on the eyes. *Cureus, 14*(10).

Dole, K., Gilbert, C., Deshpande, M., & Khandekar, R. (2009). Prevalence and determinants of xerophthalmia in preschool children in urban slums, Pune, India—A preliminary assessment. *Ophthalmic Epidemiology, 16*(1), 8–14.

Fogt, J. S., Fogt, N., King-Smith, P. E., Liu, H., & Barr, J. T. (2019). Changes in tear lipid layer thickness and symptoms following the use of artificial tears with and without omega-3 fatty acids: A randomized, double-masked, crossover study. *Clinical Ophthalmology, 2019*, 2553–2561.

Garcia-Medina, J. J., Rubio-Velazquez, E., Lopez-Bernal, M. D., Cobo-Martinez, A., Zanon-Moreno, V., Pinazo-Duran, M. D., & del-Rio-Vellosillo, M. (2020). Glaucoma and antioxidants: Review and update. *Antioxidants, 9*(11), 1031.

Gilbert, C. (2013). The eye signs of vitamin A deficiency. *Community Eye Health, 26*(84), 66.

Huang, Z., Liu, Y., Qi, G., Brand, D., & Zheng, S. G. (2018). Role of vitamin A in the immune system. *Journal of Clinical Medicine, 7*(9), 258.

Johra, F. T., Bepari, A. K., Bristy, A. T., & Reza, H. M. (2020). A mechanistic review of β-carotene, lutein, and zeaxanthin in eye health and disease. *Antioxidants, 9*(11), 1046.

Kang, Q., & Yang, C. (2020). Oxidative stress and diabetic retinopathy: Molecular mechanisms, pathogenetic role, and therapeutic implications. *Redox Biology, 37*, 101799.

Kaushik, S., Wang, J. J., Flood, V., Tan, J. S. L., Barclay, A. W., Wong, T. Y., Brand-Miller, J., & Mitchell, P. (2008). Dietary glycemic index and the risk of age-related macular degeneration. *The American Journal of Clinical Nutrition, 88*(4), 1104–1110.

Kennedy, R. D., Spafford, M. M., Parkinson, C. M., & Fong, G. T. (2011). Knowledge about the relationship between smoking and blindness in Canada, the United States, the United Kingdom, and Australia: Results from the International Tobacco Control Four-Country Project. *Optometry, 82*(5), 310–317.

Latif, N., & Naroo, S. A. (2022). Transient effects of smoking on the eye. *Contact Lens and Anterior Eye, 45*(5), 101595.

Lee, J., Kim, U. J., Lee, Y., Han, E., Ham, S., Lee, W., Choi, W. J., & Kang, S. K. (2021). Sunlight exposure and eye disorders in an economically active population: Data from the KNHANES 2008–2012. *Annals of Occupational and Environmental Medicine, 33*.

Liu, A., & Ji, J. (2014). Omega-3 essential fatty acids therapy for dry eye syndrome: A meta-analysis of randomized controlled studies. *Medical Science Monitor, 20*, 1583.

Maoka, T. (2020). Carotenoids as natural functional pigments. *Journal of Natural Medicines, 74*(1), 1–16.

Mrowicka, M., Mrowicki, J., Kucharska, E., & Majsterek, I. (2022). Lutein and zeaxanthin and their roles in age-related macular degeneration—neurodegenerative disease. *Nutrients, 14*(4), 827.

Narimatsu, T., Negishi, K., Miyake, S., Hirasawa, M., Osada, H., Kurihara, T., Tsubota, K., & Ozawa, Y. (2015). Blue light-induced inflammatory marker expression in the retinal pigment epithelium-choroid of mice and the protective effect of a yellow intraocular lens material *in vivo*. *Experimental Eye Research, 132*, 48–51.

Newsome, D. A., Miceli, M. V., Tate, D. J., Alcock, N. W., & Oliver, P. D. (1996). Zinc content of human retinal pigment epithelium decreases with age and macular degeneration, but superoxide dismutase activity increases. *The Journal of Trace Elements in Experimental Medicine, 8*(4), 193–199.

Nguyen, D., Thrimawithana, T., Piva, T. J., Grando, D., & Huynh, T. (2023). Benefits of plant carotenoids against age-related macular degeneration. *Journal of Functional Foods, 106*, 105597.

Perry, A., Rasmussen, H., & Johnson, E. J. (2009). Xanthophyll (lutein, zeaxanthin) content in fruits, vegetables, and corn and egg products. *Journal of Food Composition and Analysis, 22*(1), 9–15.

Pham-Huy, L. A., He, H., & Pham-Huy, C. (2008). Free radicals, antioxidants in disease and health. *International Journal of Biomedical Science, 4*(2), 89.

Querques, G., Forte, R., & Souied, E. H. (2011). Retina and omega-3. *Journal of Nutrition and Metabolism, 2011*, Article 1.

Roberts, J. E. (2001). Ocular phototoxicity. *Journal of Photochemistry and Photobiology B: Biology, 64*(2, 3), 136–143.

Romagnolo, D. F., & Selmin, O. I. (2017). Mediterranean diet and prevention of chronic diseases. *Nutrition Today, 52*(5), 208.

Ross, A. C., Caballero, B., Cousins, R. J., & Tucker, K. L. (2020). *Modern Nutrition in Health and Disease.* Jones & Bartlett Learning.

Sajovic, J., Meglič, A., Glavač, D., Markelj, Š., Hawlina, M., & Fakin, A. (2022). The role of vitamin A in retinal diseases. *International Journal of Molecular Sciences, 23*(3), 1014.

Sherwin, J. C., Kokavec, J., & Thornton, S. N. (2015). Hydration, fluid regulation, and the eye: In health and disease. *Clinical & Experimental Ophthalmology, 43*(8), 749–764.

Stipanuk, M. H., & Caudill, M. A. (2018). *Biochemical, Physiological, and Molecular Aspects of Human Nutrition* (E-book). Elsevier Health Sciences.

Suh, M. H., Kwon, J. W., Wee, W. R., Han, Y. K., Kim, J. H., & Lee, J. H. (2008). Protective effect of ascorbic acid against corneal damage by ultraviolet B irradiation: A pilot study. *Cornea, 27*(8), 916–922.

Zong, G., Gao, A., Hu, F. B., & Sun, Q. (2016). Whole grain intake and mortality from all causes, cardiovascular disease, and cancer: A meta-analysis of prospective cohort studies. *Circulation, 133*(24), 2370–2380.

CHAPTER 24

Detection and Management of Eye Disease

KOMAL SHARMA

Department of Optometry, School of Allied Health Sciences, Noida International University, Gautam Buddha Nagar, Greater Noida, Uttar Pradesh, India

ABSTRACT

The term "ocular disease" is used to describe any condition or problem that impairs the eye's capacity to operate normally and/or has a negative impact on the eye's visual acuity. Procedures to prevent blindness, such as surgery for the treatment of cataracts and other diseases, dietary recommendations to prevent damage from diabetic retinopathy, and long-term vision care for geriatric patients who may be at increased risk for eye disease and vision damage are all included in the management of eye diseases. Common ocular conditions leading to visual impairments are age-related macular degeneration (AMD), diabetes, cataracts, and uncorrected refractive error. The management of ocular conditions using various techniques, such as surgical and non-surgical approaches, will be covered in this chapter.

24.1 OPHTHALMOLOGY IN THE COMMUNITY

Community ophthalmology is the application of suitable techniques and strategies to lessen the impact of eye diseases within a community. Fundamental concepts – The first step in the practice of community ophthalmology is to evaluate the scope of the issue with eye disorders and

Allied Healthcare in Practice: An Introduction to Integrated Patient Care. Sally Lukose, Karuna Singh (Eds.)

DOI: 10.1201/9781998511037-27

the socioeconomic effects of blindness on the community (Feroze et al., 2023). Identifying and implementing the best eye care solutions for the particular population. These solutions include:

1. Preventive measures for the management of infectious and non-infectious eye illnesses as well as environmental health risks.
2. Promotional initiatives focusing on better diet, thorough eye health education, and improved lifestyle choices.
3. Treatment programs for common eye diseases include trachoma, cataracts, xerophthalmia, and refractive errors (Fernandez, 2018).

Common eye diseases and their management are as follows:

24.2 XEROPHTHALMIA

A lack of vitamin A leads to the degenerative eye condition known as xerophthalmia. Your tear ducts and eyes can become dry from a vitamin A deficiency (VAD). Blindness during the night or more extreme damage to your clear cornea, the topmost layer of your eye, can result from a condition called xerophthalmia, the outermost layer of the cornea that protects your eyes. Ulcers in the cornea and white spots around your eyes are two signs of this harm. Vitamin A therapy can typically reverse xerophthalmia (Feroze et al., 2023).

24.2.1 SYMPTOMS AND SIGNS OF XEROPHTHALMIA

According to the patient's age and the degree of the deficit, the following stages of xerophthalmia gradually develop (Aygün, 2020).

1. **Night Blindness (Reduced Eye Sensitivity to Light):** The inability to see in low light, potential collisions with objects, and/or decreased mobility are the early signs of xerophthalmia.

2. **Diabetic Conjunctivitis:** It is distinguished by the conjunctiva's appearance, which is thick, wrinkled, dry, and dull. Changes in the mucin (MUC) secretion that lubricates the conjunctiva cause it to develop.

3. **Bitot Marks:** It describes deposits on the conjunctiva that are white, frothy, and opaque.

4. **Corneal Xerosis:** The appearance of the cornea is foggy, dry, and dull.
5. **Keratomalacia or a Corneal Ulcer:** Ulcers and corneal weakening are frequent side effects of corneal xerosis. It can even damage and perforate the eye's cornea.
6. **Corneal Bruising:** A late-onset, severe xerophthalmia symptom is corneal scarring.
7. **Fundus Xerophthalmic:** It alludes to the structural adjustments made to the fundus, which is the interior back surface of the eye.

24.2.2 MANAGEMENT OF XEROPHTHALMIA

Since keratomalacia is a sign of extremely severe VAD, it should be handled as a medical emergency. All patients receive high-dose vitamin A, which may be administered orally or intramuscularly. The following table (Ross, 2002) lists suggested VAD treatment plans. Based on routine monitoring of the serum retinol level, the course of treatment can be changed as necessary (Table 24.1).

TABLE 24.1 Vitamin A Dosage for Different Age Groups

Age Group	Vitamin A Dosage (IU)
Young Infant (0–5 months)	50,000
Older Infant (6–11months)	100,000
Children (Male: 12 month and more; Female: 12 months to 12 years and 50 year and more)	200.000
Women (13–49years) with night blindness and/or bitot spot	100,000 every day or 24,000 every week for a least 3 months
Women (13–49years) with active corneal lesion	2000,000 on day 1.2 and 14

Patients who also have a zinc deficiency should take zinc supplements. Based on the degree of the deficiency and the provider's judgment, VAD associated with malabsorptive or other processes is treated, typically requiring daily medication. Localized ocular treatment includes intense friction, external retinoic acid, and control of fissures. Information on nutritional avenues for vitamin A and an adequate, nutrient-rich diet should be given to patients as well as their family members. Patient education is a significant part of management. If applicable, alcohol misuse needs to be addressed. Large-scale vitamin A supplementation programs exist in nations with limited resources (Sommer, 1998).

24.3 TRACHOMA

An infection of the eyes known as trachoma affects both eyes. It is the main infectious cause of blindness in the world. Trachoma is caused by a bacterium called *Chlamydia trachomatis*. The World Health Organization (WHO) reports that 1.8 million people have trachoma-related vision impairment. Of those, 450,000 are permanently blind. Trachoma first results in conjunctivitis, or pink eye. After being exposed to the bacterium for five to 12 days, the first symptoms start to emerge. These signs may manifest as moderate ocular discharge, eyelid rubbing, and itching of the eyes and eyeballs (Burton et al., 2009).

24.3.1 SYMPTOMS AND SIGNS OF TRACHOMA

If there is no secondary infection, symptoms such as the sensation of dust particles in the eyes, occasional lacrimation, stickiness of the eyelids, and sparse mucoid discharge are more prevalent. Acute mucopurulent conjunctivitis symptoms can be detected if a secondary infection is present. Together with the cornea, the conjunctiva exhibits trachoma symptoms (Figure 24.1).

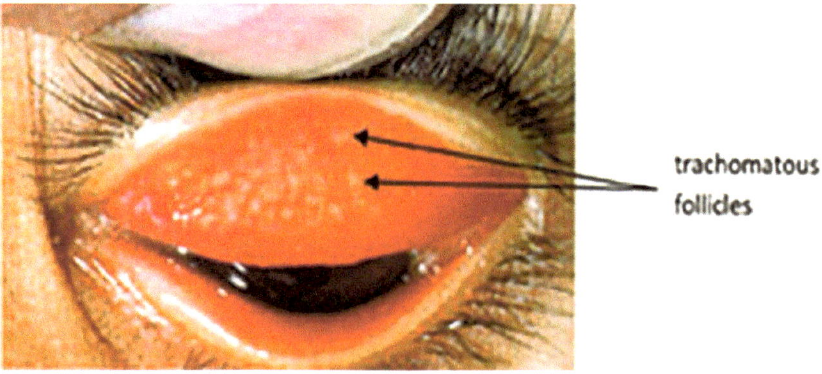

FIGURE 24.1 Trachomatous follicles.

1. **Signs in the Conjunctiva:**
    - Forniceal and upper tarsal conjunctiva are packed.
    - On the upper tarsal conjunctiva and fornix, which are also known as conjunctival follicles, follicles resembling boiled sago grain are seen.
    - Tarsal conjunctiva frequently shows papillary hyperplasia, which gives it a velvety appearance.
    - The conjunctiva becomes bruised.
    - Concretion, or hard-appearing white deposits of various sizes, is a condition that affects the upper palpebral conjunctiva.

2. **Corneal symptoms noticed:**
    - The upper corneal surface shows superficial keratitis.
    - n the limbal area, Herbert follicles are visible.
    - Vascularization, or pannus, of the cornea occurs.
    - Pannus sites have the potential to create corneal ulcers.
    - Herbert pits, which are circular pitted scars left behind after Herbert follicles have healed, are visible.
    - Corneal opacity may start in the upper portion and then spread to the lower portion, affecting the pupillary area (Figures 24.2 and 24.3).

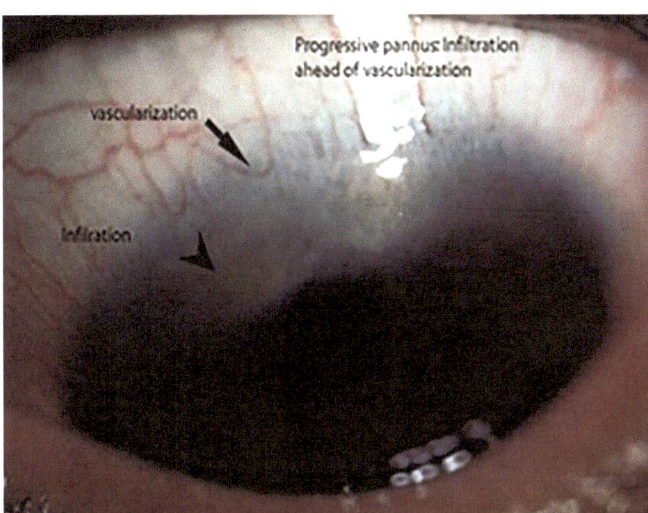

FIGURE 24.2 Progressive pannus.

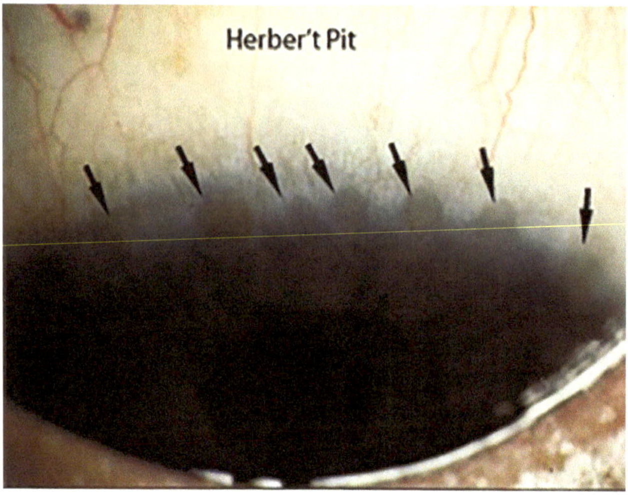

FIGURE 24.3 Herber's pit.

24.3.2 MANAGEMENT OF TRACHOMA

One of the first-line treatments for trachoma is azithromycin (Odd 240 mg x 4 days). Tetracycline is a second-line medication that should not be used on children under the age of 8. It is taken as a 1% concentration ointment four times per day for six weeks. For six weeks, sulfacetamide and tetracycline are both administered as 20% concentration eye drops three times per day. An essential step in trachoma prevention and in breaking the cycle of transmission is maintaining good oral hygiene. Environmental changes that improve sanitation and expand access to healthier water and air decrease the likelihood of coming into contact with infectious agents or vectors.

24.4 REFRACTIVE ERROR

Refractive error happens when the eye's shape causes light rays to focus in front of or behind the retina rather than directly on the retina. Refractive errors are caused by a variety of factors, including changes in the cornea's shape, aging of the lens, and eyeball length (Schiefer et al., 2016) (Figure 24.4).

24.4.1 REFRACTIVE ERROR TYPES

1. **Myopia:** It is also referred to as myopia when the eyeball is too long for the cornea and lens's refractive powers. The length of

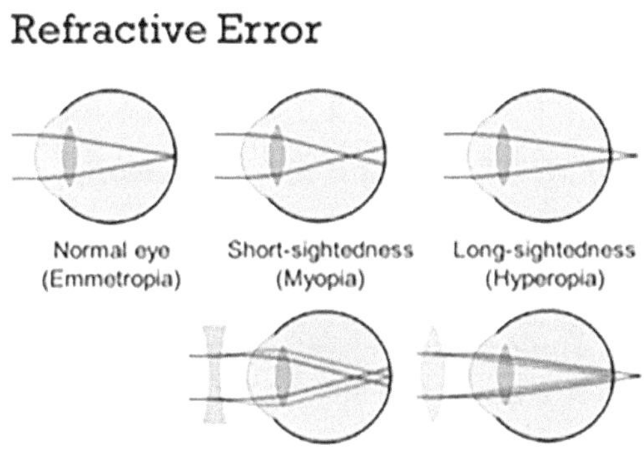

FIGURE 24.4 Refractive errors.

the retina causes the rays of light to be concentrated in front of it instead of directly upon it. A person with nearsightedness finds it difficult to see distant objects clearly.

2. **Farsightedness or Hyperopia:** This refractive defect makes it harder for affected individuals to perceive items up close. When the eyeball is too short for the cornea and lens's refractive power, it is also known as farsightedness. As a result, it is difficult to focus effectively on items that are near because the light focuses beyond the retina as it reflects.
3. **Astigmatism:** Astigmatism occurs when a lens is not completely circular. This condition inhibits the visual system from concentrating photons over the layers of the retina in an even manner, stretching and blurring objects at all distances.
4. **Presbyopia:** One can no longer focus on anything up close due to this age-related disease. The lens stiffens as people get older and can no longer easily modify its form. The eye is unable to clearly concentrate on close objects as a result.

24.4.2 SYMPTOMS AND WARNING SIGNS OF REFRACTIVE ERRORS

Blurred vision is the main sign of refractive error. Others consist of:

- Dual perception.
- Halos surrounding intense lights.
- Haziness.
- Headaches and strain on the eyes.

- Dry, itchy, and red eyes.
- Continual tear production.

24.4.3 MANAGEMENT OF REFRACTIVE ERRORS

Spectacles, Contact Lenses, Incisional Techniques, and Laser Techniques as well.

1. **Glasses:** The easiest and safest method of correcting refractive problems is with eyeglasses. To ensure that you have the clearest vision possible, your eye doctor will prescribe the appropriate eyeglass lenses.
2. **Contact Lenses:** Your eye's surface is covered with contact lenses that correct refractive faults. Your ophthalmologist will fit you for the proper lenses and demonstrate how to care for and wear them securely.
3. **Surgery:** Your cornea's shape can be altered during some procedures, such as laser eye surgery, to correct refractive problems. An ophthalmologist can advise you on whether surgery is necessary for you. Surgeries are as follows (Tran and Ryce, 2018):
    - i. **LASIK:** People who are astigmatic, nearsighted, or farsighted can benefit from LASIK, or laser *in situ* keratomileusis. To access the tissue underneath, the doctor creates a flap in the cornea's outer layer. The tissue under your cornea will then be reshaped with a laser so that it can focus light appropriately. What distinguishes LASIK from other surgeries is the flap. To create an accurate picture of your cornea for use as per orientation, the doctor might also employ a form of computer imaging known as wavefront technology.
    - ii. **PRK:** The procedure known as PRK, or photorefractive keratectomy, is used to treat mild to moderate astigmatism, nearsightedness, or farsightedness. A surgeon reshapes your cornea with a laser, unlike LASIK, which affects the tissues underneath. However, only the surface of the cornea is impacted.
    - iii. **RLE:** A crystalline lens replacement is referred to as RLE. Other names for PRELEX include clear lens extraction, clear

lens exchange, and refractive lens replacement. It is analogous to cataract surgery. A small incision is made by the doctor at the corneal border. Your native lens is removed, and it is then swapped out for an implanted plastic lens. Extreme nearsightedness or farsightedness can be treated with the technique. For those with thin corneas, dry eyes, or other mild corneal issues, it works nicely. RLE can be used in conjunction with LASIK or LASIK-related surgery to treat astigmatism.

iv. **PREFLEX:** Presbyopia, or the lack of eye flexibility, is treated using a treatment called PRELEX, which stands for presbyopic lens exchange. Your lens is taken out and replaced with a multifocal lens by the ophthalmologist.

24.5 CATARACT

An opacification on the lens due to the deposition of fats and other deposits is known as a cataract (Figure 24.5) (Table 24.2).

TABLE 24.2 Types of Cataracts

Sl. No.	Type of Cataract	Description
1	Immature Cataract	It is a treatable cause of blindness seen with a cloudy, slightly opaque area in the center of the lens.
2	Mature Cataract	Opacification is at peak in the lens and pupil appears milky white in color.
3	Hyper mature Cataract	It occurs when the opacification in the lens is left untreated and becomes pearl white in color.
4	Cortical Cataract	Are wedged-shaped opacities in the periphery of the eyes' lens.
5	Nuclear Cataract	Opacity is seen on nucleus of the lens.
6	Posterior Sub Capsular Cataract	This type of cataract is seen in the posterior part of the lens. Diabetic patients and those on steroid medication are at high risk for this type of cataract.
7	Morgagnian Cataract	It is also known as White Cataract; this stage is an extreme stage for cataract patients.
8	Secondary Cataracts	It is found in patients who have any existing diseases or are on medications for those diseases.
9	Pseudo exfoliation	It's an age-related cause due to exfoliation syndrome on lens of the eye.

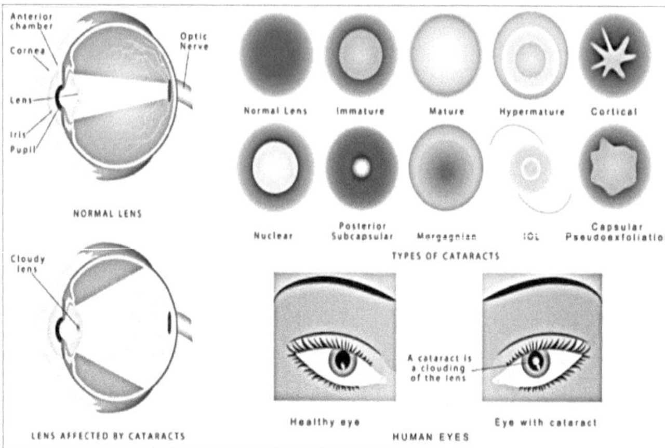

FIGURE 24.5 Types of cataracts.

24.5.1 SIGNS AND SYMPTOMS OF CATARACT

Various signs and symptoms associated with cataract are depicted in Table 24.3.

TABLE 24.3 Signs and Symptoms of Cataract

Sl. No.	Signs	Symptoms
1	Hazy or fuzzy eyesight	Brighter lighting is required for activities like devouring literature.
2	Color Vision changes,	"Halos" around lights being perceived
3	Objects are faded or seem more yellow, and double vision	Prescription for glasses or contacts changing frequently
4	Sensitivity to night time light, especially in strong sunlight,	Color fading or yellowing of Lens
5	Experiencing a halo around light sources	Monocular Double Vision

24.5.2 MANAGEMENT OF CATARACT

Management of cataract is described as medical intervention and further surgery (Dickson, 1996):

1. *Medical intervention:* Once lens opacity has taken hold, medical intervention is ineffective.

2. *Surgery:* Justification for surgery: (i) A cataract causes difficulty doing ordinary tasks because it impairs eyesight. (ii) A displaced or subluxated lens. (iii) Complications caused by lenses, such as phacomorphic glaucoma, phacoanaphylactic endophthalmitis, and photolytic uveitis.
3. *Options for Surgical Treatment Intracapsular lens extraction (ICCE):* This technique for removing ICCE, which is fast losing its use, involves rupturing the zonular ligaments in order to remove the whole lens and capsule.
4. *Extracapsular Cataracts Retraction (ECCE):* Techniques for Cataract II: (i) Customary ECCE; (ii) ECCE with SICS, a tiny incision cataract procedure; (iii) Lens removal; and (iv) Phacoemulsification.

24.6 OTHER EYE DISEASE

24.6.1 CONJUNCTIVAL DISEASE

The sclera, which is the white portion of the eyeball, and the innermost layer of the eyelid are both covered by a thin layer of tissue. Conjunctivitis is the medical term for conjunctival inflammation. It causes conjunctival hyperemia, popularly known as the redness of the eye white (Kamińska, et al., 2023).

1. *Conjunctival Chemosis:* It refers to conjunctival edema. Cold compresses, chilled artificial tears, and steroid eye drops are all effective treatments.
2. *Subconjunctival Bleeding:* Under the membrane of the conjunctiva, there is hemorrhage. Numerous tiny, delicate blood veins that often burst or tear are present throughout the membrane of the conjunctiva. Bleeding then escapes into the area between the conjunctiva and sclera when this happens.
3. *Conjunctival Xerosis:* Conjunctival scaling is the term for dryness of the eye surface brought on by a lack of tears or conjunctival secretions. It might be related to trauma, a lack of vitamin A, or an illness wherein the eyelids fail to close all the way (Feroze et al., 2023).

24.6.2 INFLAMMATORY DISEASES

Conjunctivitis, commonly referred to as "pinkeye," is caused by inflammation. These might comprise viral and bacterial conjunctivitis that is infectious. Both bacterial and viral conjunctivitis can attack one or both eyes. The discharge from bacterial conjunctivitis is frequently thicker and yellow-green in color. Both varieties may be accompanied by the common cold or by respiratory infection symptoms like throat pain. Both bacterial and viral infections spread quickly (Kamińska et al., 2023). They can spread through direct or indirect contact with an infected person's eye fluids. Both kids and adults are susceptible to these pinkeye conditions. Children have infections of the conjunctiva more frequently than adults do.

24.6.3 ALLERGIC EYE CONDITION

It affects both eyes and is a reaction to something that causes allergies, like pollen, dust, or cosmetics. Red or pink eyes are only one of the allergy signs and symptoms that can be brought on by the body's release of histamine. If you have allergic conjunctivitis, you might also sneeze a lot and have runny nasal discharge in addition to severe eye itching, tears, and inflammation.

24.6.4 IRRITABLE OR TOXIC CONJUNCTIVITIS

It is brought on by being exposed to allergens such as eye injuries, strong light (such as snow blindness), and smoke, cosmetics, unusual items, contact lens solutions, and swimming pool chlorine. It is also not communicable.

24.6.5 CORNEAL SCRATCHING

The outermost layer of the cornea is the transparent portion of the eye that covers the front portion of the eye. It shields the iris, pupil, and anterior chamber of the eye (Kamińska et al., 2023). The cornea's primary function is to refract light rays as they enter the eye. The cornea focuses the majority of light that enters the eye. In this case, the cornea could seem clean, but the patient's vision might still be incredibly fuzzy. A gouge in the cornea's surface can occur. Dust, contact lenses, or any other object might cause corneal scratching.

24.6.6 GLAUCOMA

It describes a class of eye conditions where the nerve that supplies vision is affected and begins to deteriorate. This often arises as a result of an increase in eye pressure, eventually leading to blindness and a gradual loss of vision (IOP). The range of normal intraocular pressure, which is measured by an instrument called a Schiotz tonometer (Kamińska et al., 2023). An applanation tonometer is another tool that measures IOP. It typically results from abnormally high pressure inside the eyeball. Due to optic nerve damage, the field of view is constrained in some way.

24.6.7 WATERING OF EYES

This could be caused by a foreign object or other problems, such as blocked lacrimal channels or corneal or conjunctival discomfort.

24.6.8 REDNESS OF EYE

A foreign body sensation, corneal inflammation, anterior uveitis, glaucoma, conjunctival inflammation, and so forth., is responsible for this.

24.6.9 DOUBLE VISION (DIPLOPIA OR MULTIPLE IMAGES)

Squinting, corneal edema, cataract, astigmatism, and subluxated lenses are a few possible causes.

24.6.10 PHOTOPHOBIA

This refers to the phobia of light caused by acute closure glaucoma, corneal abrasions, corneal ulcers, and anterior uveitis. It happens due to ciliary spasm that can be induced by light.

24.6.11 ITCHING

This could be an indication of conjunctivitis, allergic reactions, or dry eyes.

1. **Dry Eyes:** Dry eyes are caused by insufficient production of tears. Long-term use of mobile devices or computer work could lead to its development. When the eyes are unable to generate enough tears to keep them moisturized, it is known as dry eye syndrome. The individual suffering from this condition complains of cloudy vision (Feroze et al., 2023).
2. **Watery Eyes:** Watery eyes occur when the eyes have to deal with excessive amounts of tear production.
3. **Eye Pain:** This refers to discomfort that could arise inside or near the eye. It typically returns to normal without any treatment.
4. **Eye Emergencies:** These may occur as a result of an accident that impacts the eye's surrounding area or as a result of chemicals or an external object getting into the eye. Emergencies require urgent medical attention.
5. **Excessive Tearing:** Excessive tearing may happen as a result of poor lighting, wind, or variations in temperature. Wearing sunglasses or protective glasses to shield your eyes often resolves this issue. Tearing may also be an indication of a more serious issue such as allergies, a tear duct blockage, or the spread of infection in the eye.
6. **Issues with the Eyelids:** The eyelids defend the eye, disperse tears, and regulate how much light gets in. Eyelid problems such as drooping eyelids and inflamed exterior borders of the eyelids adjacent to the eyelashes may lead to symptoms like pain, itching, and eye watering. The options for treatment for eyelid issues usually involve surgical procedures, healthcare, or sanitation.
7. **Foreign Body Sensation in the Eye:** Any external debris that enters the eye, like dust, can cause discomfort and requires medical treatment.

8. **Blepharitis:** The swelling of the eyelash roots is known as blepharitis. However, the exact cause of this disorder is yet unknown; allergies, parasites, dandruff, and some medications can enhance the possibility of it.
9. **Eye Redness:** This condition occurs when the blood vessels in the eyes swell. Allergies, dry air, and dust are some factors. The middle layer of the eye, which is comprised of the iris, ciliary body, and choroid, is called the uvea, and uveitis is an inflammation of it. Inflammatory conditions and ocular injuries may be the root cause of this. Uveitis can also be brought on by exposure to harmful compounds used in manufacturing processes, like acids and insecticides (Kamińska et al., 2023).

KEYWORDS

- **age-related macular degeneration**
- **community ophthalmology**
- **diabetic retinopathy**
- **eye capacity**
- **geriatric patients**
- **non-surgical approach**
- **ocular diseases**
- **uncorrected refractive error**
- **visual impairments**

REFERENCES

Aygün, B. T. (2020). Xerophthalmia: From eye to fatal intestinal disease. *Beyoglu Eye Journal, 5*(2), 149. https://doi.org/10.14744/bej.2020.93063.

Burton, M. J., & Mabey, D. C. W. (2009). The global burden of trachoma: A review. *PLoS Neglected Tropical Diseases, 3*(10), e460. https://doi.org/10.1371/journal.pntd.0000460.

Dickson, R., Eastwood, A., Gill, P., Melville, A., O'Meara, S., & Sheldon, T. (1996). Management of cataract. *Quality & Safety in Health Care, 5*(3), 180–185.

Fernandez, S. (2018). Community ophthalmology: Is it still relevant in our country? *Kerala Journal of Ophthalmology, 30*(1), 2. https://doi.org/10.4103/kjo.kjo_21_18.

Feroze, K. B., & Kaufman, E. J. (2023). Xerophthalmia. *StatPearls Publishing.*

Kamińska, A., Pinkas, J., Wrześniewska-Wal, I., Ostrowski, J., & Jankowski, M. (2023). Awareness of common eye diseases and their risk factors—A nationwide cross-sectional survey among adults in Poland. *International Journal of Environmental Research and Public Health, 20*(4), 3594. https://doi.org/10.3390/ijerph20043594.

Ross, D. A. (2002). Recommendations for vitamin A supplementation. *Journal of Nutrition, 132*(9), 2902S–2906S. https://doi.org/10.1093/jn/132.9.2902s.

Schiefer, U., Kraus, C., Baumbach, P., Ungewiß, J., & Michels, R. (2016). Refractive errors. *Deutsches Ärzteblatt International, 113*(41), 693. https://doi.org/10.3238/arztebl.2016.0693.

Sommer, A. (1998). Xerophthalmia and vitamin A status. *Progress in Retinal and Eye Research, 17*(1), 9–31. https://doi.org/10.1016/s1350-9462(97)00001-3.

Tran, K., & Ryce, A. (2018). Laser refractive surgery for vision correction: A review of clinical effectiveness and cost-effectiveness. *Canadian Agency for Drugs and Technologies in Health.*

CHAPTER 25

Visual Rehabilitation

ANJALI RAWAT

Department of Optometry, Sharda School of Allied Health Sciences, Sharda University, Noida, Uttar Pradesh, India

ABSTRACT

Rehabilitation aims to promote function and independence through adaptation; it does not repair or alter the cause of harm. The term "vision rehabilitation," often known as "vision rehab," refers to a medical rehabilitation program designed to enhance vision or address low eyesight. The common ocular conditions leading to visual impairments include uncorrected refractive errors, diabetes, ARMD, and cataracts. Low vision therapy seeks to enhance daily visual functionality while also maximizing the use of residual vision in people with severe vision loss. It is the process of increasing an individual's quality of life and independence after they have lost their capacity to see due to disease or accident, while also restoring functional ability. Moreover, assisting individuals in adjusting to permanent visual loss and enhancing psychosocial functioning are goals of the visual rehabilitation process. The most effective strategy to assist patients who are blind or visually impaired is to offer them low-vision rehabilitation devices with the goal of maximizing their residual vision. The rehabilitation of vision using various techniques, such as physical approaches, mobility training, home skill training, and occupational training, will be covered in this chapter.

Allied Healthcare in Practice: An Introduction to Integrated Patient Care. Sally Lukose, Karuna Singh (Eds.)

DOI: 10.1201/9781998511037-28

25.1 INTRODUCTION

Vision plays a critical part in every phase and stage of life. It is the most dominant of the five senses and plays a very important role in every phase of our lives, helping in the communal and intellectual development of a child (Nilsson, 2013). Vision problems range from complete blindness to partial sight. More inclusive descriptive phrases like "sight loss" and "problems related to vision" have been promoted in recent years to reduce the stigma associated with visual disorders (Pumphrey, 1961). Unfortunately, many of these terms lack precise definitions, and their introduction causes uncertainty in the epidemiological community, often resulting in significantly inflated prevalence values for severe vision disorders (Kotabe et al., 2016). Near and distance visual disorders are the visual impairments that have been classified by international organizations of disease (Binns et al., 2007). In 1975, two organizations were formed to reduce blindness: the World Health Organization (WHO) and international organizations aimed at reducing the burden of global blindness. Over the following 20 years, international non-governmental organizations and WHO-PBL engaged in eye healthcare, forging a strong working partnership. To control onchocerciasis in 1994, WHO and NGOs established a combined working group to tackle the concern of increasing worldwide blindness (WHO, 2005). In 1997, the recommendations of the Task Force's work were published as "The International Campaign to Prevent the Loss of Vision." The worldwide strategy, goals, and justification are explained in the Vision 20/20 report (Thylefors et al., 1995). Trends in global vision indicate that in 1978, the first estimate of the number of blind individuals worldwide was 28 million (with corrections, vision in the working eye should be a minimum of 3/60) (Foster et al., 2005). According to Frick, if medical facilities are not improved, the world is expected to have 76 million blind individuals by 2020 as a result of population growth and a longer lifespan. Low vision (20/60 to 3/60 in the good eye) is predicted to affect three to four times as many people as blindness (Resnikoff et al., 2002). Three to four times as many persons are thought to be affected by low vision (Mariotti et al., 2009). Corneal scarring and cataract are the main causes of blindness, and the magnitude of visual loss in extremely poor nations frequently surpasses 1% (10,000+ blind persons per million people). Corneal scarring is less common in rural areas that have better nutrition, economies, and sanitation, with cataract being the most common cause. In metropolitan areas with strong financial resources and easy access to healthcare, the magnitude of vision loss due to blindness is less than 0.5%. Although cataract services are mostly available, cataract is still a cause of visual loss among the less fortunate sections of the metropolitan population, along with diabetic retinopathy and glaucoma, which are also leading causes of blindness. Even though a sizable proportion of individuals have visual loss from untreated diabetic retinopathy, age-related macular degeneration (ARMD), glaucoma, and cataract are the main causes of visual loss; cataract is not the most prevalent cause of blindness in populations with access to quality healthcare (Naipal et al., 2018).

The WHO conducted another in-depth analysis of all population-centered evaluations of blindness and low vision in 2002 by applying the data on blindness and low vision from 55 nations to the 17 WHO epidemiological sub-regions (Rustagi et al., 2012). The results show that 124 million individuals have poor vision and that roughly 37 million people are blind. The magnitude of vision loss ranges from 1% in Western Europe and North America to 1% in Africa. The 37 million visually impaired people are broken down into three age groups: 0–14 years, 15–49 years, and 50 and up. With a female-to-male impairment ratio ranging from 1.5 to 2.2, women are affected more than men. The primary causes of blindness include cataract (48%), glaucoma (12%), corneal scarring, including trachoma (9%), ARMD (9%), and diabetic retinopathy (5%). These new worldwide vision loss estimates are around 15 million lower than those previously estimated. This could be explained in part by variations in data processing, with current values derived from more survey data as well as a more rigorous epidemiological technique, which leads to more accurate estimates. However, there has been a real improvement in eye healthcare, which has reduced the number of cases of avoidable sight loss (Cugati et al., 2007).

25.2 GLOBAL MAGNITUDE OF VISUAL DISORDER

Nearly 2.1 billion partially sighted people suffer from shortsightedness or farsightedness. At least one billion of these cases—close to half—involved loss of vision that was unaddressed. One billion includes individuals with mild to significant distance sight loss or blindness due to cataract (94 million), glaucoma (7.7 million), ARMD (8 million), untreated refractive error (88.4 million), near vision impairment due to untreated presbyopia (825 million), and diabetic retinopathy (3.9 million) (Rees et al., 2007) (Figure 25.1).

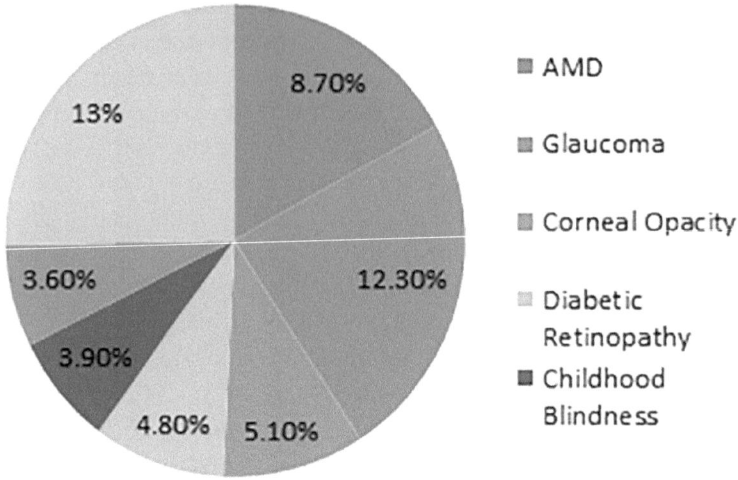

FIGURE 25.1 World-wide causes of blindness as a proportion of total blindness in 2020.

25.3 GLOBAL BURDEN OF VISUAL IMPAIRMENT

There may be ways to prevent and/or treat trachoma, juvenile blindness, cataracts, corneal opacity, onchocerciasis, glaucoma, and diabetic retinopathy. Up to 75% of blindness worldwide, according to the WHO, can be avoided. On the other hand, the prevalence of multiple types of sight loss varies widely from location to location, depending on the specifics of the local environment. Only about 50% of cases of childhood blindness can be avoided (Conrod et al., 1998).

The main factors contributing to vision impairment globally are: ARMD, uncorrected refractive error, glaucoma, cataract, and diabetic retinopathy, which are the leading causes of eyesight loss. There are considerable disparities in the reasons between and within countries, depending on the accessibility of eye care facilities, the associated expenses, and the general population's level of knowledge regarding eye care (Ackland et al., 2017). In fact, middle-income and low-income nations have a higher percentage of persons with cataracts that impair their vision compared to high-income countries. High-income nations have higher rates of diseases, including visual field disorders and ARMD. The factors that contribute to childhood visual impairment vary substantially between nations. For instance, in middle-income countries, retinal prematurity is the leading cause of eyesight loss, whereas in low-income countries, congenital cataract is more frequent. In both children and the adult population worldwide, uncorrected refractive error is the leading cause of sight loss. According to new data based on the global population of 2002, the total number of individuals who are blind due to conditions related to longer life spans has increased, while the number of people who are blind due to conditions related to infectious diseases has decreased since the estimates from the 1990s. Now there is a need to change healthcare. This new information emphasizes the requirement to alter the healthcare strategy to incorporate the treatment of the disorders that are now on the rise (Livingston et al., 1997).

25.4 RISK FACTORS OF VISUAL IMPAIRMENT

25.4.1 AGE

Age increases the possibility of a wide range of eye disorders; hence those over 55 years of age have much greater rates of blindness and moderate to severe vision impairment. Women portray this in more detail than men do. There are a total of 253 million blind persons in the world, and 80% of them are over 50 (Le et al., 2003).

25.4.2 GENDER

There are 253 million visually impaired people in the world; 139 million of them are women. There are a greater number of females who are at increased risk of acquiring an eye condition that could impair their ability to see because of the longer life expectancy of women compared to men. A few eye conditions also tend to affect women more frequently. In some countries, women may have less availability of eye care services than men do. This is the result of numerous social and cultural variables.

25.4.3 ECONOMIC AND SOCIAL STANDING

Individuals with sight loss make up about 89% of the population in low- and middle-income nations. Only 73 million people, or 51% of the entire world's population, live in South Asia, 59 million in East Asia, and 24 million in Southeast Asia, but 62% of all blind people do. On the other hand, despite housing 14% of the world's population, the five high-income regions are only home to 11% of visually impaired people (Le et al., 2003).

25.4.4 AGE PROFILE

It is difficult to compare regions if one only considers overall prevalence or numbers; this is because each region has a different age distribution, with some populations having a higher proportion of elderly individuals and fewer children than others. Comparing populations with various age profiles to one another and tracking changes over time is possible because of a method called "age standardization" (Le et al., 2003).

25.5 CURE IS VISUAL REHABILITATION

25.5.1 COUNSELING

To help visually impaired people regain self-confidence and independent living skills in order to reintegrate into the community, analyze the visual aspects of a task in order to modify the work and adjust the surroundings to the specific devices utilized. Vary components of the environment as well, such as distance from the task, lighting, contrast, color, and time permitted. Determine which sense is the most efficient for a specific task—vision, improved vision, auditory, tactual, or some combination of these senses, for example. When you have the necessary skills, you can live confidently. There are several training courses offered at the visual rehabilitation center, which include mobility training, communicating with the help of Braille, employment training, usage of low-vision devices, and how to operate different types of technologies. Training can help enhance functional vision. Many people can learn to make better use of their low vision and function effectively with little visual information. To comprehend the unique implications of low vision for everyone, it is crucial to identify the activities regularly performed by the person with low vision and other members of the same community, as well as the visual skills required to carry these out. This could be in school, the village, or the workplace. The individual should be evaluated in a location appropriate for those tasks. The functions of a good counselor include taking the history and examining the body. In order to create a rehabilitation plan, the patient's goals and diagnoses are combined with assessments of vision function and examination of low vision aids. The above information about the patient should be available to the counselor (Markowitz et al., 2006).

When vision correction surgery and other medical procedures are not used, the patient goes through expert instruction and counseling. After the patient's vision has been assessed and corrective lenses are prescribed, they must be referred to a vision expert for counseling and training. Following a low vision screening, training and counseling are the recommended solutions. After the low vision assessment and prescription, the patient must be referred for training and counseling by the low vision specialist. The goal is to reduce their reliance on others and return them to a more normal life. Educational areas, psychological aid for adjusting to life, career direction, and educational approaches are the primary areas of counseling (Stelmack, 2001). Both ensure that a person acquires the abilities and methods essential to help them achieve whatever goals they set for themselves at all stages of life. It may provide someone with the tools they need to live freely. If the patient wants to control their vision loss, travel safely, take care of their house, achieve their professional goals, and enjoy leisure activities, they may benefit from visual therapy. Even if a low vision specialist recommends methods to improve the current eyesight, there is still more that may be done. Other vision rehabilitation specialists can help with tasks that a person may no longer be able to do visually (Markowitz, 2016).

25.5.2 LOW-VISION DEVICES FOR REHABILITATION

This means that the low-vision assessment must consider everyone's specific needs. Although the doctor may guide you in the direction of resources, it is the rehabilitation counselor who makes those resources effective. Low vision devices are useful for rehabilitating the vision of visually impaired people. They include optical and non-optical devices. However, to rehabilitate vision, clinicians require non-optical devices. These help in increasing contrast and illumination and providing a comfortable ambiance for the patient. The non-optical devices have seven categories, including relative size devices, glare and contrast devices, posture and comfort maintenance devices, handwriting devices, orientation devices, and medical instrument devices that help meet the patient's needs individually (Gopalakrishnan et al., 2017). Large print books and reading materials are examples of relative image size. There are several optical and non-optical devices that help visually impaired patients restore vision.

1. **Optical Devices:** There are two types of optical devices: one for near vision and the other for distance vision. Near devices help in magnifying near objects, while distance devices are used for enlarging distant objects. In optical devices, there are several magnifying glasses with different powers, including magnifiers for reading tasks. There are handheld and stand magnifiers that help patients perform near tasks, making reading easier for them. Telescopes are also an optical option for patients who have difficulty with both near and distance vision, as they magnify both distant and near objects. These tools allow readers to read for extended periods without straining their eyes (Ager et al., 1998). A person with vision impairment can use optical equipment to read signs, recognize notes, improve their visual field, and make reading easier. These tools enable practitioners to enhance the residual vision of visually impaired individuals (Arya et al., 2010).

2. **Non-Optical Devices:** Non-optical devices include a reading light, reading guide, notex, bold-lined notepads, bold-lined books, large printed books, bold-tipped black pens, soft lead pencils in sizes 2B to 6B, and a needle threader. Different illumination levels are tested, and it is advised to use a portable floor or table light when strong illumination is needed. According to illumination mathematics, bringing the light source closer has a considerably greater impact than increasing bulb power. When placed 12 inches from the page, a 50-watt bulb shines brighter and generates less heat than a 300-watt bulb placed three feet away (Williams, 1986). The location of the light is crucial; the superior seeing eye should be on the side of the light source. Higher illumination will result from moving the lamp closer. A reading stand helps the person read comfortably. Patients should be recommended to use slant reading tables to provide an easy and comfortable posture while reading. The writing guide is a black card with horizontal rectangular cutouts spaced evenly down the card. The writer unfolds like a book, and the writing paper is positioned between them.

The patient may feel the blank cut-out gaps and write using the slots, which helps them write easily. The reading guide is a masking tool made of opaque, non-reflective black plastic or thick paper with a line carved out of it. It is a frequently used non-optical tool for glare reduction and contrast management. By reducing glare from the page and eliminating the confusion caused by lines of print above and below the line being read, this reading aid speeds up reading (Monteiro et al., 2014).

25.5.3 REFRACTIVE ERROR CORRECTION

Even though wearing spectacles to correct refractive problems is sometimes overlooked, this is the most popular and practical treatment option for patients. Patients with low vision (LV) who have recently lost their vision or have mild to severe vision loss believe it is appropriate to use glasses and want this intervention. It helps in the correction of the residual vision. Bifocal and single-vision glasses are preferred for visually impaired persons. Flattop and executive bifocals are great choices for visually impaired individuals. Along with corrective lenses, various LV devices that can improve visual functions can be mounted on the frame of eyeglasses as support (Markowitz, 2006).

25.5.4 OCCLUSION THERAPY

Before occluding any eye, the practitioner should determine the dominant eye and then occlude the weaker eye to enhance the residual vision of the person (Markowitz, 2006).

25.6 THERAPY FOR RESIDUAL SKILLS ENHANCEMENT THROUGH VISION REHABILITATION

The vision rehabilitation procedure should always consist of the training and improvement of residual vision and newly developed visual skills, which are crucial and important to any anticipated vision rehabilitation plan. It is the responsibility of an LV practitioner, ophthalmologist, or optometrist to suggest and prescribe visual rehabilitation training in order to enhance residual functional vision. In order to increase function and enhance performance for activities of daily living, occupational therapists can administer a variety of training programs aimed at developing such skills as reading and writing. Other programs help with orientation, mobility, and driving (Silver et al., 1995). For some jobs in specific age groups, visual rehabilitation training is provided in the form of focused education techniques, programs, and training drills. Prescribed courses for retraining basic visual abilities are available in cases of macular pathology (Yang, 2016). These consist of scotoma awareness exercises as well as therapy to improve fixation stability, saccades, and tracking eye movements. Occupational therapists can help older patients who commonly have both physical and visual impairments. An occupational therapist or rehabilitation teacher may need to analyze contrast, lighting, and safety hazards in the patient's home. The occupational therapists may suggest large-print versions of books, checks, playing cards, calendars, and writing paper, among other things. Other adjustments can be made, such as moving from a ballpoint pen to a bold fiber-tipped pen to improve writing legibility (Markowitz, 2006).

25.7 CONCLUSION

Dealing with the current global deficit of avoidable blindness and its expected doubling by the year 2020 is a challenge for the entire society. People who, due to their knowledge and abilities, can significantly contribute to meeting this issue have a professional and moral obligation in this regard. In the countries with the highest rates of preventable blindness, the disparity in the quantity and quality of eye care treatments available is a significant factor in poverty. A thorough LV examination should record all resolutions; recognition, contrast, and binocularity for the visual acuity are examples of aspects of the individual with residual functional vision. Residual vision should be improved by the prescription of devices, and they must keep in mind the rehabilitation activities that the patient initially chose. Meeting people's ambitions for their fundamental human right to sight is VISION 2020's goal. The WHO is in a good position to show the way forward in accomplishing this objective.

KEYWORDS

- **age related macular degeneration**
- **low vision devices**
- **mobility training**
- **rehabilitation**
- **rehabilitation training**
- **vision rehabilitation**
- **visual impairment**

REFERENCES

Ackland, P., Resnikoff, S., & Bourne, R. (2017). World blindness and visual impairment: Despite many successes, the problem is growing. *Community Eye Health, 30*(100), 71.

Agarwal, R., & Tripathi, A. (2021). Current modalities for low vision rehabilitation. *Cureus, 13*(7).

Ager, L. (1998). Optical services for visually impaired children. *Community Eye Health, 11*(27), 38.

Arya, S. K., Kalia, A., Pant, K., & Sood, S. (2010). Low vision devices. *Nepalese Journal of Ophthalmology, 2*(1), 74–77.

Aslan, U. B., Calik, B. B., & Kitiş, A. (2012). The effect of gender and level of vision on the physical activity level of children and adolescents with visual impairment. *Research in Developmental Disabilities, 33*(6), 1799–1804.

Barr, W., Hodge, S., Leeven, M., Bowen, L., & Knox, P. (2012). Emotional support and counselling for people with visual impairment: Quantitative findings from a mixed methods pilot study. *Counselling and Psychotherapy Research, 12*(4), 294–302.

Binns, A. M., Bunce, C., Dickinson, C., Harper, R., Tudor-Edwards, R., Woodhouse, M., & Margrain, T. H. (2012). How effective is low vision service provision? A systematic review. *Survey of Ophthalmology, 57*(1), 34–65.

Conrod, B. E., & Overbury, O. (1998). The effectiveness of perceptual training and psychosocial counseling in adjustment to the loss of vision. *Journal of Visual Impairment & Blindness, 92*(7), 464–482.

Corn, A. L., & Erin, J. N. (2010). *Foundations of Low Vision: Clinical and Functional Perspectives.* American Foundation for the Blind.

Cugati, S., Cumming, R. G., Smith, W., Burlutsky, G., Mitchell, P., & Wang, J. J. (2007). Visual impairment, age-related macular degeneration, cataract, and long-term mortality: The Blue Mountains Eye Study. *Archives of Ophthalmology, 125*(7), 917–924.

Dagnelie, G. (2013). Age-related psychophysical changes and low vision. *Investigative Ophthalmology & Visual Science, 54*(14), ORSF88–ORSF93.

Foster, A., & Resnikoff, S. (2005). The impact of Vision 2020 on global blindness. *Eye, 19*(10), 1133–1135.

Frick, K. D., & Foster, A. (2003). The magnitude and cost of global blindness: An increasing problem that can be alleviated. *American Journal of Ophthalmology, 135*(4), 471–476.

Gecas, V., & Schwalbe, M. L. (1983). Beyond the looking-glass self: Social structure and efficacy-based self-esteem. *Social Psychology Quarterly, 46*(2), 77–88.

Gopalakrishnan, S., Muralidharan, A., Susheel, S. C., & Raman, R. (2017). Improvement in distance and near visual acuities using low vision devices in diabetic retinopathy. *Indian Journal of Ophthalmology, 65*(10), 995.

Kotabe, H. P., Kardan, O., & Berman, M. G. (2016). The order of disorder: Deconstructing visual disorder and its effect on rule-breaking. *Journal of Experimental Psychology: General, 145*(12), 1713.

Le, A., Mukesh, B. N., McCarty, C. A., & Taylor, H. R. (2003). Risk factors associated with the incidence of open-angle glaucoma: The visual impairment project. *Investigative Ophthalmology & Visual Science, 44*(9), 3783–3789.

Liu, J. H., Cheng, C. Y., Chen, S. J., & Lee, F. L. (2001). Visual impairment in a Taiwanese population: Prevalence, causes, and socioeconomic factors. *Ophthalmic Epidemiology, 8*(5), 339–350.

Livingston, P. M., McCarty, C. A., & Taylor, H. R. (1997). Visual impairment and socioeconomic factors. *British Journal of Ophthalmology, 81*(7), 574–577.

Mariotti, S. P., Pascolini, D., & Rose-Nussbaumer, J. (2009). Trachoma: Global magnitude of a preventable cause of blindness. *British Journal of Ophthalmology, 93*(5), 563–568.

Markowitz, S. N. (2006). Principles of modern low vision rehabilitation. *Canadian Journal of Ophthalmology, 41*(3), 289–312.

Markowitz, S. N. (2016). State-of-the-art: Low vision rehabilitation. *Canadian Journal of Ophthalmology, 51*(2), 59–66.

Minto, H., & Butt, I. A. (2004). Low vision devices and training. *Community Eye Health, 17*(49), 6.

Monteiro, M. M. B., Montilha, R. D. C. I., Carvalho, K. M. M. D., & Gasparetto, M. E. R. F. (2014). Optical and nonoptical aids for reading and writing in individuals with acquired low vision. *Arquivos Brasileiros de Oftalmologia, 77*(2), 91–94.

Naipal, S., & Rampersad, N. (2018). A review of visual impairment. *African Vision and Eye Health, 77*(1), 1–4.

Nilsson, D. E. (2013). Eye evolution and its functional basis. *Visual Neuroscience, 30*(1, 2), 5–20.

Pearce, E., Crossland, M. D., & Rubin, G. S. (2011). The efficacy of low vision device training in a hospital-based low vision clinic. *British Journal of Ophthalmology, 95*(1), 105–108.

Pumphrey, R. J. (1961). Part I. Sensory organs: Vision. In *Biology and Comparative Physiology of Birds, Vol. II* (pp. 55–68). Academic Press.

Rees, G., Saw, C. L., Lamoureux, E. L., & Keeffe, J. E. (2007). Self-management programs for adults with low vision: Needs and challenges. *Patient Education and Counseling, 69*(1–3), 39–46.

Resnikoff, S., & Pararajasegaram, R. (2001). Blindness prevention programmes: Past, present, and future. *Bulletin of the World Health Organization, 79*, 222–226.

Resnikoff, S., Pascolini, D., Etya'Ale, D., Kocur, I., Pararajasegaram, R., Pokharel, G. P., & Mariotti, S. P. (2004). Global data on visual impairment in the year 2002. *Bulletin of the World Health Organization, 82*(11), 844–851.

Resnikoff, S., Pascolini, D., Mariotti, S. P., & Pokharel, G. P. (2008). Global magnitude of visual impairment caused by uncorrected refractive errors in 2004. *Bulletin of the World Health Organization, 86*(1), 63–70.

Rustagi, N., Uppal, Y., & Taneja, D. K. (2012). Screening for visual impairment: Outcome among schoolchildren in a rural area of Delhi. *Indian Journal of Ophthalmology, 60*(3), 203.

Scott, I. U., Smiddy, W. E., Schiffman, J., Feuer, W. J., & Pappas, C. J. (1999). Quality of life of low-vision patients and the impact of low-vision services. *American Journal of Ophthalmology, 128*(1), 54–62.

Silver, J., Gilbert, C. E., Spoerer, P., & Foster, A. (1995). Low vision in East African blind school students: Need for optical low vision services. *British Journal of Ophthalmology, 79*(9), 814–820.

Stelmack, J. (2001). Quality of life of low-vision patients and outcomes of low-vision rehabilitation. *Optometry and Vision Science, 78*(5), 335–342.

Thylefors, B., Negrel, A. D., Pararajasegaram, R., & Dadzie, K. Y. (1995). Global data on blindness. *Bulletin of the World Health Organization, 73*(1), 115.

Vincent, S. J. (2017). The use of contact lenses in low vision rehabilitation: Optical and therapeutic applications. *Clinical and Experimental Optometry, 100*(5), 513–521.

Williams, D. R. (1986). Non-optical aids. *Journal of the American Optometric Association, 57*(8), 608–615.

World Health Organization. (2000). *Global Initiative for The Elimination of Avoidable Blindness* (No. WHO/PBL/97.61 Rev. 2). World Health Organization.

World Health Organization. (2005). *Prevention of Blindness and Deafness*.

Wu, D. Z., Wu, L., Chang, F. X., Jin, C., & Padula, W. (1995). Visual rehabilitation in low vision patients with aging macular degeneration. *Journal of the American Optometric Association, 66*(1), 39–41.

Yang, R., & He, Y. (2016). Optically and non-optically excited thermography for composites: A review. *Infrared Physics & Technology, 75*, 26–50.

CHAPTER 26

Public Health and Optometry

MANISH KUMAR SAH[1,*] and RUCHIKA SAH[2]

[1]*Department of Optometry, SSAHS, Sharda University, Greater Noida, Uttar Pradesh, India*

[2]*Department of Optometry, Ramlal Golchha Eye Hospital Foundation, Biratnagar, Nepal*

*Corresponding author

ABSTRACT

For the purpose of reducing vision loss and preserving eye health, early diagnosis of eye illnesses is essential. Public health is one of the ways society organizes its efforts to protect, advance, and improve the health of its members. Optometrist contributions to public health are a significant issue that demands discussion. Optometrists are medical practitioners who offer basic eye care, identify and treat ocular and visual conditions, recommend corrective lenses, and offer vision therapy. A range of eye disorders, including glaucoma, cataracts, and diabetic retinopathy, require early detection and treatment by optometrists. Their skill in recommending corrective lenses to treat vision issues also enhances their patient's quality of life and productivity. Additionally, they can support legislation and initiatives that help underserved groups' access to care and eye health. They can spread awareness about the value of routine eye exams and promote eye health by taking part in community outreach programmes. The different facets of the optometrist's function in public health are explored in this chapter. The chapter also covers the role of optometrists in promoting good eye health through education and preventive care. They can advise patients on modifying their lifestyles and taking preventative actions to maintain good eye health as well as inform them on the value of wearing safety glasses.

Allied Healthcare in Practice: An Introduction to Integrated Patient Care. Sally Lukose, Karuna Singh (Eds.)

DOI: 10.1201/9781998511037-29

26.1 INTRODUCTION

Because of our eyes amazing abilities, we can feel our surroundings through sight. Our eyes have a significant influence on how we interact with the world and other people on a daily basis. Given the significance of this sensory system, it is imperative to preserve its top health and functionality. Optometrists, medical professionals with training in eye care and vision preservation, are in charge of this responsibility. The need for accurate and thorough eye care is growing, which makes optometrists' significance more and more clear. A wide variety of eye conditions and visual impairments are evaluated, managed, and treated by optometrists, medical specialists with specialised training in this field (Smith, 2002). They are typically people's first point of contact when looking for assistance with their visual health and play a critical role in providing basic eye care. Optometrists aren't like ophthalmologists, who are doctors who specialise in sophisticated eye conditions and eye surgery. The function of optometrists is more important than ever in a society when our eyes are continuously exposed to digital devices and environmental toxins. These highly skilled medical specialists are essential to maintaining the health of our eyes and vision. Optometrists are at the forefront of protecting and strengthening our most important sense, sight. They provide thorough eye exams, diagnose, and treat a variety of eye disorders.

26.1.1 COMPREHENSIVE EYE EXAMINATIONS

Conducting thorough eye exams is an optometrist's main responsibility. In addition to other vision-related characteristics, they examine visual acuity, depth perception, eye alignment, and peripheral vision (De Souza et al., 2012). Optometrists can detect refractive errors like nearsightedness, farsightedness, and astigmatism utilising state-of-the-art tools and equipment. Additionally, they examine the inside components of the eye to search for probable signs of eye issues and diseases.

26.1.2 PRESCRIBING CORRECTIVE LENSES

Refractive faults are frequently corrected by corrective lenses; such as glasses or contact lenses. Optometrists are adept at prescribing the best lenses for each patient depending on their individual needs (Dandona,

1998). They can identify the ideal lens prescription to provide clear and pleasant vision through accurate measurements and meticulous analysis, enhancing the quality of life for countless people.

26.1.3 DIAGNOSING AND MANAGING EYE CONDITIONS

Optometrists are trained to identify and treat a problems like conjunctivitis and dry eye syndrome as well as more severe disorders like glaucoma, cataracts, and diabetic retinopathy (Hau et al., 2007). Preventing further vision loss and perhaps irreparable damage requires early detection of these disorders.

26.1.4 VISION REHABILITATION AND LOW VISION CARE

Individuals with severe vision loss receive assistance from optometrists who specialise in low vision care and vision rehabilitation as they learn to live with their condition (Oam and Resnikoff, 2002). They aid patients in making the most of their remaining eyesight and regaining their independence in daily activities through the use of a variety of assistive equipment, adaptive technology, and specialised training.

In addition to diagnosing and treating eye diseases, optometrists are essential in educating patients about basic eye hygiene and preventative measures. They offer advice on proper eye care, the value of routine eye exams, and lifestyle changes that can improve eye health. Optometrists give their patients the knowledge they need so they may take charge of protecting their vision. Despite the crucial role that optometrists perform, there is still a large gap in the availability of vision care services in many parts of the world (Masnick, 2009). Optometrists are constructing eye care clinics, providing outreach programmes, and campaigning for better access to eye care services, particularly in underprivileged communities, in an effort to close this gap, along with governments and non-governmental organisations.

26.2 THE IMPORTANCE OF REGULAR EYE EXAMINATIONS

Many people may not prioritise routine eye exams because they take their vision for granted. Routine eye exams are important, though, for a number of reasons:

26.2.1 EARLY DETECTION OF EYE CONDITIONS

Some eye diseases, like glaucoma and diabetic retinopathy, may not have any symptoms at all in the beginning stages. Optometrists can detect these diseases early on thanks to routine eye exams, increasing the likelihood of effective treatment and averting vision loss.

26.2.2 UPDATES TO PRESCRIPTION

Our vision may alter as we age. Your prescription for glasses or contact lenses is kept current by routine eye exams, ensuring that you have clear and comfortable vision.

26.2.3 MONITORING EYE HEALTH

For those with certain risk factors or underlying disorders, optometrists can keep track of changes in your eye health over time.

26.2.4 PREVENTIVE CARE

Maintaining good eye health and avoiding possible problems before they worsen requires a proactive strategy, which includes routine eye exams.

26.2.5 OVERALL HEALTH INDICATOR

Sometimes, eye exams might discover underlying medical issues like diabetes or hypertension that may initially show symptoms in the eye (Liu and Swearingen, 2017).

In several nations around the world, the profession of optometry has developed in diverse ways. The primary eye care providers in the medical field nowadays are optometrists, who work all around the world. Despite the enormous obstacles they confront, they help meet the world's demands for eye health. Unquestionably, optometrists are the qualified medical personnel responsible for overseeing refractive error worldwide. The most frequent reason patients visit an optometrist is to have their refractive error determined and corrected; this includes an evaluation of their binocular vision and any necessary corrective contact or eyeglass wear. With refractive error alarmingly increasing over the past few years, particularly myopia, their service is more important than ever. According to studies, the lifestyle changes made by both children and adults in reaction to the COVID-19 epidemic are strongly related to the growth in myopia (Zhang et al., 2022). Given that 2.3 billion people have uncorrected refractive error (Thulasiraj et al., 2003) and near sightedness affects 517 million people, and farsightedness affects 153 million people (Holden et al., 2008), (Resnikoff et al., 2008), the current situation demonstrates the inherent need for optometrists to contribute to the public health problem of visual impairment. The definition of public health given by the Centres for Disease Control is "the science of protecting and improving the health of people in their communities, achieved by: promoting healthy lifestyles, researching disease and injury prevention, and detecting, preventing, and responding to infectious diseases (Binns and Low, 2015)." That definition should make it clear that public health can have many different guises. A public health endeavour is anything done to improve the health of a community (Boufford et al., 2002). Certainly, optometrists are qualified and trained to work as public health clinicians. Additionally, optometrists can help with additional illnesses that are important for the public's health, such as diabetic retinopathy, glaucoma, epidemic myopia, and binocular vision issues.

According to WHO, there are an estimated 285 million visually impaired people in the globe, of which 39 million are blind and 246 million have restricted vision (Pascolini et al., 2004), (Resnikoff et al., 2004), (Pascolini and Mariotti, 2012). The leading causes of distance vision impairment or blindness among these 1 billion people are cataract (94 million cases), refractive error (88.4 million cases), age-related macular degeneration (8 million cases), glaucoma (7.7 million cases), and diabetic retinopathy (3.9 million cases) (Steinmetz et al., 2021). Presbyopia (826 million people) is the leading disorder causing near vision impairment (Fricke et al., 2018). In India, cataracts account for 62.6% of blindness, followed by refractive errors (19.7%), glaucoma (5.8%), posterior segment pathology (4.7%), corneal opacity (0.9%), and other causes (6.2%) (Jose, Rathore and Sachdeva, 2010). Looking at the world's population, majority of the world population lose their vision due to the cataract itself (Khairallah et al., 2015). And around 90% of the visually impaired population is in developing countries (Tabbara et al., 2005). By the survey it is found that more than 17% of the world's population and an estimated 25% of the world's blind or visually impaired people reside in India (Metrics and Evaluation., 2015). With increasing prevalence of chronic conditions such as diabetes and hypertension in developing countries especially in countries such as India (Federation, 2021), the need for public health optometrists is huge for early detection of ocular complications of these conditions. Optometrists can play a significant role in educating the teams for this activity and in data management even if tele-ophthalmology as a modality for early detection is still being tested. While refractive error is one of the most frequent causes of blindness and visual impairment (Leon., 2002), it is also the easiest to 'cure'. Refractive error is easily identified, measured, and corrected, and the provision of glasses is a very affordable solution that offers quick problem rectification.

In spite of being preventable also the rate of blindness is increasing more rapidly and as well more number of population is affected by it but the main thing is people around could achieve successful vision by providing better eye care facilities in the areas. It was found that women had larger percentage of blindness due to cataract as compared to men in the world (Lou et al., 2018), (Abou-Gareeb et al., 2001). It has also been proven that half of the entire world's blindness is preventable or treatable.

26.3 OPTOMETRIST AND PUBLIC HEALTH

In an era characterized by rapidly advancing medical technologies and an aging global population, the intersection of optometry and public health has never been more crucial. A key aspect of public health is eye health, which includes a variety of plans, programmes, and initiatives aimed at enhancing and safeguarding people's and communities' visual health (Welp et al., 2016). It is impossible to overestimate the importance of eye health in the context of public health since vision has a significant impact on how people interact with their surroundings, go about their everyday lives, and uphold their general quality of life. Public health initiatives strive to prevent, identify, and manage various eye problems by addressing eye health at a societal level, thereby improving the overall health of people. The connection of healthcare and public health is more obvious than ever in today's interconnected and complicated society. One of the most important senses, vision affects almost every area of a person's life, from socialising and working to learning and engaging with the outside world (Klein et al., 1998). One's quality of life and general wellbeing can be negatively impacted by poor vision, which can have far-reaching effects. If ignored, visual impairment and eye conditions can have a negative impact on one's health, social life, and financial stability (West et al., 1997). Therefore, protecting and enhancing visual health are important public health goals.

26.4 THE ROLE OF OPTOMETRIST IN PUBLIC HEALTH

26.4.1 VISION SCREENING: THE GATEWAY TO EYE HEALTH

Community-based vision screening programmes are one of the most obvious ways that optometrists support public health. Programmes for vision screening are essential for locating people who may have vision problems (Brinks et al., 2018). These initiatives are frequently overseen by optometrists in companies, community centres, and schools. Optometrists can identify more complicated eye disorders as well as simple refractive abnormalities like myopia, hyperopia, and astigmatism through vision screening. For the purpose of preventing vision loss, early diagnosis of eye disorders is crucial. During vision exams, optometrists can spot symptoms of eye conditions such macular degeneration, diabetic retinopathy, and glaucoma (Hubley and Gilbert., 2006). The evolution of these illnesses can be stopped or at least slowed down by early intervention and referral to the proper specialists. Access to complete eye care is scarce in many places. Optometrist-led vision screening programmes offer people, particularly in underprivileged groups, fundamental eye health evaluations. By doing this, it is more likely that vision issues will be discovered early and that patients will receive the treatment they require. Programmes for vision testing offer chances for outreach and education as well. Participants are instructed by optometrists on the value of routine eye exams, good eye care, and the significance of eye health in general. These programs promote awareness and empower individuals to take control of their eye health.

26.4.2 DISEASE DETECTION: BEYOND REFRACTIVE ERROR CORRECTION

The knowledge of optometrists goes beyond recommending corrective eyewear. They have the skills necessary to identify and treat a variety of eye problems and disorders. The ability to recognise numerous disorders that could impair vision, including glaucoma, cataracts, diabetic retinopathy, and age-related macular degeneration, is a skill acquired by optometrists. Their involvement in early detection is crucial because prompt treatment can stop or halt the advancement of many illnesses, protecting patients' quality of life and vision. Optometrists provide complete eye exams that include a full assessment of the eye's health. This includes gauging intraocular pressure, examining vision fields, and evaluating retinal health. These tests are crucial for finding minute indicators of eye conditions that can go undetected during normal check-ups (Yadav and Tandon., 2019). Optometrists can manage some disorders and start treatment after making a diagnosis of an eye ailment (De Souza et al., 2012). They work together with ophthalmologists and other specialists on more complicated instances to make sure patients get the right care (Hau et al., 2007). This teamwork-based strategy improves the efficiency of healthcare delivery and maximises results. One of the main goals of public health is to prevent vision loss, and optometrists are at the forefront of these initiatives. Their capacity to identify eye conditions early and treat them successfully makes a considerable contribution to lowering the prevalence of visual impairment in the population.

26.4.3 REFRACTIVE ERROR CORRECTION: BEYOND GLASSES AND CONTACTS

One of the core functions of optometry is the correction of refractive defects such myopia, hyperopia, and astigmatism. Optometrists tackle vision correction on a case-by-case basis. Each patient's individual needs and lifestyle are carefully evaluated, taking into account things like age, employment, and interests. This guarantees that the prescription corrective eyewear gives each person the clearest eyesight possible. Optometrists are adept at solving difficult vision problems. Optometrists might recommend vision therapy and exercises to help patients with binocular vision impairments or problems like amblyopia (lazy eye) (De Souza et al., 2012). This all-encompassing strategy goes beyond only dispensing glasses or contact lenses. Safety depends on having good vision correction, especially when performing tasks like operating machinery and driving. In order to ensure that people have the vision necessary for these tasks, optometrists have a role in promoting public safety. Patients are instructed by their optometrists on the value of following their prescription for vision correction.

This includes routine follow-up visits to track any changes in eyesight as well as the correct upkeep of glasses or contact lenses.

26.4.4 LOW VISION REHABILITATION: MAXIMIZING INDEPENDENCE

Optometrists are essential in helping people with low vision make the most of their remaining eyesight and keep their independence. Optometrists prescribe and suggest a variety of assistive tools to help people with low vision carry out tasks like reading, writing, and navigating their surroundings. These tools include magnifiers, telescopes, and electronic assistance (Virgili et al., 2018). They also impart adaptive methods for enhancing independence. The goal of low vision therapy is to improve overall quality of life, not simply functional eyesight (van Nispen et al., 2020). Optometrists collaborate extensively with patients to determine their goals and create rehabilitation programmes that are tailored to their individual requirements. One of the main objectives of low vision rehabilitation is to maintain independence (Lamoureux et al., 2007), (Hinds et al., 2003). By allowing patients to carry out routine duties and participate in activities they enjoy, optometrists assist people in regaining confidence and self-esteem.

26.4.5 VISION AND PUBLIC SAFETY: BEYOND PERSONAL HEALTH

By evaluating and certifying people for the vision needs in diverse circumstances, optometrists play a crucial part in protecting public safety. Optometrists frequently evaluate people for vision-related criteria, such as those required for driving (Kobal and Hawlina, 2022), obtaining a pilot's licence, and holding particular jobs. For the sake of everyone's safety, it is essential that everyone follow these rules. Optometrists are familiar with the regulations and visual standards that apply to various activities. They contribute to the cause of effective, fact-based standards that put safety first. Optometrists help to reduce accidents by certifying people for particular vision-related jobs. For instance, ensuring that drivers have sufficient visibility lowers the possibility of accidents on the road. Optometrists evaluate and certify individuals' eyesight suitability for particular job positions in occupational contexts (Lennie and Van Hemel, 2002).

This ensures that people can carry out their tasks safely, lowering the likelihood of workplace accidents.

26.4.6 EDUCATION AND OUTREACH: EMPOWERING COMMUNITIES

To prevent eye disorders and promote eye health, effective education and outreach are essential (Welp et al., 2016). Optometrists frequently take the helm of public awareness programmes that stress the significance of regular eye exams and good eye health. These campaigns emphasise the link between eye health and general wellbeing and target a variety of demographics. Optometrists routinely go into classrooms to inform kids about the value of proper eye care habits. Children who receive early instruction are better able to appreciate the value of eye health and develop a lifelong commitment to it (Alvarez-Peregrina et al., 2020). A crucial element of public health is community engagement. Optometrists present courses and seminars about eye health in places including senior living communities, workplaces, and community centers. People can take charge of their eye health with the help of outreach and education.

26.4.7 RESEARCH AND DATA COLLECTION: ADVANCING PUBLIC HEALTH KNOWLEDGE

Optometrists actively participate in studies on vision and eye health, adding to the corpus of knowledge in the subject. Optometrists perform research to increase our knowledge of eye conditions, available therapies, and cutting-edge technologies. Their research's findings aid in the creation of novel diagnostic techniques (Sánchez-González et al.,2023),(Plainis, 2012) and therapeutic approaches. Optometrists gather critical information on the frequency of diseases and newly developing public health problems related to eye health. Evidence-based policies and initiatives are informed by this data. Optometrists frequently work with academics in a variety of disciplines, such as ophthalmology, epidemiology, and public health. These partnerships expand the reach and significance of their research projects. Optometrists are essential in converting scientific discoveries into useful therapeutic applications.

26.4.8 ADVOCACY: SHAPING PUBLIC HEALTH POLICIES

Advocates for policies and programmes that support eye health and make sure that eye care services are incorporated into public health initiatives include optometrists and their professional organisations (Prozesky et al., 2007). Optometrists support laws that place a high priority on eye health, such as laws governing eye safety standards, access to eye care services, and vision screening in schools. Funding for studies into eye health can also be obtained through advocacy. Optometrists work to make sure that research projects have the funding they require to make significant progress. To increase the effectiveness of their advocacy work, optometrists partner with other healthcare professionals and advocacy groups. These partnerships boost their power to influence public health policies (Ravilla and Ramasamy, 2012).

26.4.9 COLLABORATIVE CARE: A MULTIDISCIPLINARY APPROACH

Optometrists routinely collaborate with other medical specialists, such as ophthalmologists, family practitioners, and public health officials. Individuals obtain thorough eye treatment thanks to collaborative care. Ophthalmologists' knowledge is complemented by that of optometrists, who concentrate on primary eye care while ophthalmologists handle difficult and surgical situations (Cicinelli, Marmamula and Khanna, 2020). Collaboration facilitates the prompt interchange of information and referrals, which streamlines the delivery of healthcare. For early diagnosis and action to improve outcomes, efficiency is essential. By allowing optometrists, ophthalmologists, and other healthcare professionals to share knowledge and best practises, collaborative care promotes cross-disciplinary learning (Welp et al., 2016). Both healthcare professionals and patients gain from this ongoing education. Together, healthcare practitioners may tackle more general public health problems associated with eye health. By ensuring that eye care services are incorporated into the whole healthcare system, collaborative care promotes overall wellness.

26.5 CONCLUSION

Optometrists play a vital and complex role in the public's health. They provide preventative care, promote eye safety, serve as community educators, and work together on healthcare teams. Optometrists make a vital contribution to the health of people and communities all over the world by their dedication to promoting eye health, early disease identification, and comprehensive eye care. Their efforts not only boost people's vision but also their general quality of life, demonstrating the crucial value of their work to public health. The lives of individuals and communities are impacted by optometrists on a variety of levels, making them essential contributors to public health. Their responsibilities include disease identification through vision screening, refractive error repair, low vision rehabilitation, vision and public safety, as well as education, research, advocacy, and team-based care. Optometrists are crucial in encouraging eye health, lowering vision impairment, and improving the general well-being of people because of their knowledge and accessibility. Moving forward, it will be crucial to acknowledge and support the crucial role that optometrists play in promoting public health in order to create healthier, more welcoming communities where vision is regarded as a crucial component of wellbeing.

KEYWORDS

- **comprehensive eye care**
- **early disease identification**
- **eye health**
- **healthcare teams**
- **low vision rehabilitation**
- **optometrist**
- **public health**
- **refractive error correction**
- **vision impairment**

REFERENCES

Abou-Gareeb, I., Lewallen, S., Bassett, K., & Courtright, P. (2001). Gender and blindness: A meta-analysis of population-based prevalence surveys. *Ophthalmic Epidemiology, 8*(1), 39–56.

Alvarez-Peregrina, C., Sánchez-Tena, M. Á., Andreu-Vázquez, C., & Villa-Collar, C. (2020). Visual health and academic performance in school-aged children. *International Journal of Environmental Research and Public Health, 17*(7), 2346.

Binns, C., & Low, W. Y. (2015). What is public health? *Asia-Pacific Journal of Public Health, 27*, 5–6.

Boufford, J. I., Cassel, C., Bender, K., Berkman, L., Bigby, J., & Burke, T. (2002). *The future of the public's health in the 21st century.* Institute of Medicine of the National Academies.

Brinks, M., Zaback, T., Park, D. W., Joan, R., Cramer, S. K., & Chiang, M. F. (2018). Community-based vision health screening with on-site definitive exams: Design and outcomes. *Cogent Medicine, 5*(1), 1560641.

Cicinelli, M. V., Marmamula, S., & Khanna, R. C. (2020). Comprehensive eye care—Issues, challenges, and way forward. *Indian Journal of Ophthalmology, 68*(2), 316.

Dandona, R. (1998). Optometry and eye care in India. *Indian Journal of Ophthalmology, 46*(3), 175.

De Souza, N., Cui, Y., Looi, S., Paudel, P., Shinde, L., Kumar, K., Berwal, R., Wadhwa, R., Daniel, V., & Flanagan, J. (2012). The role of optometrists in India: An integral part of an eye health team. *Indian Journal of Ophthalmology, 60*(5), 401.

Fricke, T. R., Tahhan, N., Resnikoff, S., Papas, E., Burnett, A., Ho, S. M., Naduvilath, T., & Naidoo, K. S. (2018). Global prevalence of presbyopia and vision impairment from uncorrected presbyopia: Systematic review, meta-analysis, and modeling. *Ophthalmology, 125*(10), 1492–1499.

Hau, S., Ehrlich, D., Binstead, K., & Verma, S. (2007). An evaluation of optometrists' ability to correctly identify and manage patients with ocular disease in the accident and emergency department of an eye hospital. *British Journal of Ophthalmology, 91*(4), 437–440.

Hinds, A., Sinclair, A., Park, J., Suttie, A., Paterson, H., & Macdonald, M. (2003). Impact of an interdisciplinary low vision service on the quality of life of low vision patients. *British Journal of Ophthalmology, 87*(11), 1391–1396.

Holden, B. A., Fricke, T. R., Ho, S. M., Wong, R., Schlenther, G., Cronjé, S., Burnett, A., Papas, E., Naidoo, K. S., & Frick, K. D. (2008). Global vision impairment due to uncorrected presbyopia. *Archives of Ophthalmology, 126*(12), 1731–1739.

Hubley, J., & Gilbert, C. (2006). Eye health promotion and the prevention of blindness in developing countries: Critical issues. *British Journal of Ophthalmology, 90*(3), 279–284.

Institute for Health Metrics and Evaluation. (2015). *GBD Compare.* IHME, University of Washington.

International Diabetes Federation. (2021). *IDF Diabetes Atlas* (10th ed.).

Jose, R., Rathore, A., & Sachdeva, S. (2010). Community ophthalmology: Revisited. *Indian Journal of Community Medicine, 35*(2), 356.

Khairallah, M., Kahloun, R., Bourne, R., Limburg, H., Flaxman, S. R., Jonas, J. B., Keeffe, J., Leasher, J., Naidoo, K., & Pesudovs, K. (2015). Number of people blind or visually impaired by cataract worldwide and in world regions, 1990 to 2010. *Investigative Ophthalmology & Visual Science, 56*(11), 6762–6769.

Klein, B. E., Klein, R., Lee, K. E., & Cruickshanks, K. J. (1998). Performance-based and self-assessed measures of visual function as related to history of falls, hip fractures, and measured gait time: The Beaver Dam Eye Study. *Ophthalmology, 105*(1), 160–164.

Kobal, N., & Hawlina, M. (2022). Comparison of visual requirements and regulations for obtaining a driving license in different European countries and some open questions on their adequacy. *Frontiers in Human Neuroscience, 16*, 927712.

Lamoureux, E. L., Pallant, J. F., Pesudovs, K., Rees, G., Hassell, J. B., & Keeffe, J. E. (2007). The effectiveness of low-vision rehabilitation on participation in daily living and quality of life. *Investigative Ophthalmology & Visual Science, 48*(4), 1476–1482.

Lennie, P., & Van Hemel, S. B. (2002). *Visual Impairments: Determining Eligibility for Social Security Benefits*. National Academies Press.

Leon, B. E. (2002). Case finding in refractive error. *Community Eye Health, 15*, 43.

Liu, Y., & Swearingen, R. (2017). Diabetic eye screening: Knowledge and perspectives from providers and patients. *Current Diabetes Reports, 17*, 1–8.

Lou, L., Ye, X., Xu, P., Wang, J., Xu, Y., Jin, K., & Ye, J. (2018). Association of sex with the global burden of cataract. *JAMA Ophthalmology, 136*(2), 116–121.

Masnick, K. (2009). Narrowing the gap between eye care needs and service provision: The service-training nexus. *Human Resources for Health, 7*(1), 1–9.

Oam, B., & Resnikoff, S. (2002). The role of optometry in Vision 2020. *Community Eye Health, 15*(43), 33–36.

Pascolini, D., & Mariotti, S. P. (2012). Global estimates of visual impairment: 2010. *British Journal of Ophthalmology, 96*(5), 614–618.

Pascolini, D., Mariotti, S., Pokharel, G., Pararajasegaram, R., Etya'Ale, D., Négrel, A. D., & Resnikoff, S. (2004). 2002 global update of available data on visual impairment: A compilation of population-based prevalence studies. *Ophthalmic Epidemiology, 11*(2), 67–115.

Plainis, S. (2012). New technologies and diagnostic tools in optometry. *Journal of Optometry, 5*(3), 105.

Prozesky, D., Porter, R., Odusote, K., Morris, D. S., Francombe, J., Stevens, S., Gilbert, C., Astbury, N., Faal, H., & Khan, A. A. (2007). Advocacy for eye health. *Community Eye Health Journal, 20*(64).

Ravilla, T. D., & Ramasamy, D. (2012). Advocacy for eye care. *Indian Journal of Ophthalmology, 60*(5), 376.

Resnikoff, S., Pascolini, D., Etya'Ale, D., Kocur, I., Pararajasegaram, R., Pokharel, G. P., & Mariotti, S. P. (2004). Global data on visual impairment in the year 2002. *Bulletin of the World Health Organization, 82*(11), 844–851.

Resnikoff, S., Pascolini, D., Mariotti, S. P., & Pokharel, G. P. (2008). Global magnitude of visual impairment caused by uncorrected refractive errors in 2004. *Bulletin of the World Health Organization, 86*(1), 63–70.

Sánchez-González, J. M., Rocha-de-Lossada, C., & Cerviño, A. (2023). Exploring the cutting edge of vision science: New developments in diagnostics and treatment of ocular surface in dry eye disease. *Vision, 13*, 1584.

Smith, D. P. (2002). The 75th anniversary of the World Council of Optometry: Seventy-five years of advancing eye care by optometrists worldwide. *Optometry and Vision Science, 85*, 210–213.

Steinmetz, J. D., Bourne, R. R., Briant, P. S., Flaxman, S. R., Taylor, H. R., Jonas, J. B., Abdoli, A. A., Abrha, W. A., Abualhasan, A., & Abu-Gharbieh, E. G. (2021). Causes of blindness and vision impairment in 2020 and trends over 30 years, and prevalence of avoidable blindness in relation to VISION 2020: The Right to Sight: An analysis for the Global Burden of Disease Study. *The Lancet Global Health, 9*(2), e144–e160.

Tabbara, K. F., El-Sheikh, H. F., & Shawaf, S. S. (2005). Pattern of childhood blindness at a referral center in Saudi Arabia. *Annals of Saudi Medicine, 25*(1), 18–21.

Thulasiraj, R., Aravind, S., & Pradhan, B. (2003). Spectacles for the millions: Addressing a priority of "Vision 2020—The Right to Sight." *Journal of Community Ophthalmology, 3*(4), 19–21.

van Nispen, R. M., Virgili, G., Hoeben, M., Langelaan, M., Klevering, J., Keunen, J. E., & van Rens, G. H. (2020). Low vision rehabilitation for better quality of life in visually impaired adults. *Cochrane Database of Systematic Reviews, 2020*(1), CD006543.

Virgili, G., Acosta, R., Bentley, S. A., Giacomelli, G., Allcock, C., & Evans, J. R. (2018). Reading aids for adults with low vision. *Cochrane Database of Systematic Reviews, 2018*(4), CD003303.

Welp, A., Woodbury, R. B., McCoy, M. A., & Teutsch, S. M. (2016). *Making Eye Health a Population Health Imperative: Vision for Tomorrow.* National Academies Press.

West, S. K., Munoz, B., Rubin, G. S., Schein, O. D., Bandeen-Roche, K., Zeger, S., German, S., & Fried, L. P. (1997). Function and visual impairment in a population-based study of older adults: The SEE project (Salisbury Eye Evaluation). *Investigative Ophthalmology & Visual Science, 38*(1), 72–82.

Yadav, S., & Tandon, R. (2019). Comprehensive eye examination: What does it mean? *Community Eye Health, 32*(107), S1.

Zhang, X., Cheung, S. S., Chan, H. N., Zhang, Y., Wang, Y. M., Yip, B. H., Kam, K. W., Yu, M., Cheng, C. Y., & Young, A. L. (2022). Myopia incidence and lifestyle changes among school children during the COVID-19 pandemic: A population-based prospective study. *British Journal of Ophthalmology, 106*(12), 1772–1778.

PART IV

Safety, Quality, and Patient Care: Patient Safety and Quality Improvement

CHAPTER 27

Patient Safety and Quality Improvement in Radiology

BUSHRA KHAN

Department of Radiology, Sharda School of Allied Health Sciences, Sharda University, Greater Noida, Uttar Pradesh, India

ABSTRACT

In radiography, there are several patient safety concerns that need to be taken into account. These include safeguarding patients' physical health and preserving the best level of service delivery, preventing direct harm from the methods and technologies we employ, and safeguarding staff members so they can provide safe services. From the combined views of radiologists and radiographers, this chapter summarizes the main categories of safety concerns in the delivery of radiological services and offers resources for additional reading in all significant pertinent fields.

27.1 INTRODUCTION

Sir W. C. Roentgen confirmed the then-revolutionary discovery of X-rays in November 1895. Roentgen was completely unaware of its hazards and effects on the human body, so later radiation pioneers drew attention to the hazards of X-rays along with their medical benefits (Anderson, 1945). Ionizing radiation, such as X-rays, has a strong power to penetrate inside the human body and interact with human cells and DNA/RNA; it can change the structures of DNA, RNA, and biomolecules.

Allied Healthcare in Practice: An Introduction to Integrated Patient Care. Sally Lukose, Karuna Singh (Eds.)

DOI: 10.1201/9781998511037-31

Radioactivity and environmental factors are a few examples of natural sources of radiation, which is a phenomenon that occurs naturally. Applications for radiation and radioactive materials and their compounds are used in industry, agriculture, and medicine. It is crucial to analyze and, if necessary, control the radiation hazards that these applications could bring to the environment, workers, and people in general (Cruz Suarez et al., 2018).

In the 1950s, the scientific pioneer group established the radiation protection guidelines. It was decided that any type of radiation dose, no matter how intense or in what quantity, could bring radiation hazard effects on the patient's body. Therefore, every country has a regulatory authority and body to set the guidelines related to radiation protection, preparing laws and regulations for implementation. These guidelines are prepared in such a way that they properly ensure safety for patients, staff, and the public.

The previous classifications of different types of exposure factors into practices and actions have been substituted by the Commission's recognition of three different categories of exposure situations and types. The whole spectrum of exposure situations is intended to be explained by these three situations:

i. Preplanned exposure plans, where situations categorized as radiation hazardous practices should be well explained.
ii. Emergency radiation accidents/events, which are unanticipated events that could arise from a hostile action or during the process of a planned circumstance and require immediate care.
iii. Exposure conditions that already exist when a control presence needs to be made, such as those caused by background radiation from the Earth or natural background.

Another aspect will focus on quality improvements of medical investigations. Some rules and regulations have been established by AERB, such as the 10 Day Rule, justification of investigation (ALARA), cardinal rule, radiation measurement dosimetry and dose limits, and safety measures during procedures.

Broadly, radiation is divided into different categories. Humans and all other organisms that exist on planet Earth are exposed to radiation from natural sources. This so-called natural background emits an effective dose on a yearly average of roughly 2.5 millisieverts (mSv).

Geographically, this exposure varies significantly (from 1.5 to several tens of mSv in restricted geographic regions). Except for medicine, artificial sources only add insignificant quantities to the population (Vañó et al., 2015) (Figure 27.1).

- Environmental radiation.
- Terrestrial radiation.
- Medical radiation.
- Industrial radiation.

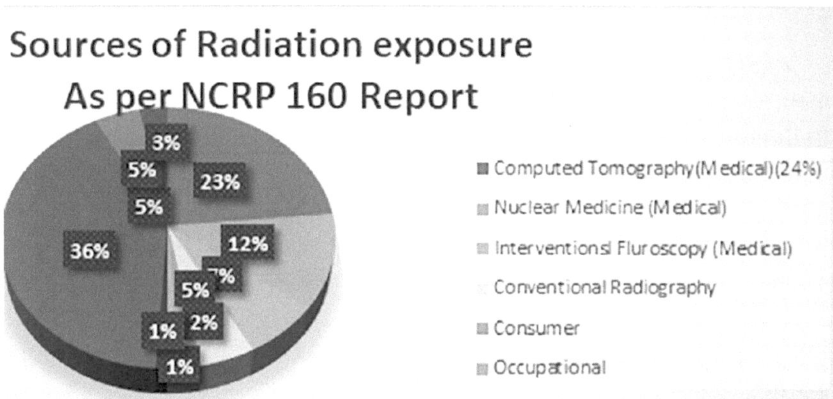

FIGURE 27.1 Radiation exposure chart about radiation contribution.

Modern diagnostic radiography provides a faster, more accurate diagnosis while making it practicable to monitor an enormous variety of disorders. According to predictions, radiographic procedures (basic screen film radiography, conventional fluoroscopy, and computed tomography) have a major effect on the time it takes to reach a diagnosis in about half of all cases, and in a significant number of those cases, they are crucial. Furthermore, a number of screening techniques, like mammography, have been developed that are advantageous for particular populations that are at relatively high risk of developing particular illnesses. The effectiveness of treating extremely serious and life-threatening disorders of the cardiovascular, CNS, and other organ systems has also been much improved by a number of interventional radiology procedures that have only been introduced in the last 10 to 20 years, such as angioplasty. Additionally, these procedures are inexpensive (Vañó et al., 2015).

The major principles of the International Commission on Radiation Protection, the United Nations Scientific Committee on the Effects of Atomic Radiation (UNSCEAR), and national organizations concerned about the radiation protection of radiation professionals and the general population in the case of radiation accidents, especially large-scale ones, briefly reduce down to the following:

- Eliminate the public's exposure to radiation's deterministic effects;
- Minimize as much as possible the stochastic effects of irradiation while also taking into consideration probable impacts on society and the economy (Ilyin, 2002).

Radiation safety is of paramount importance in a radiology department to ensure the well-being of patients, staff, and the general public. Radiology utilizes ionizing radiation in various diagnostic and therapeutic treatments and diagnoses with CT scans, X-rays, and fluoroscopy. While these procedures offer invaluable medical insights, it is essential to mitigate the potential risks linked with radiation exposure. Here are some key aspects of radiation safety in a radiology department:

27.2 CATEGORIZATION OF RADIATION

- Ionized radiation.
- Non-ionized radiation.

27.2.1 IONIZED RADIATION

Ionized radiation is an interaction of energy that can release electrons from an atom; due to atomic changes, atoms are ionized. It can take the form of electromagnetic waves, atomic and subatomic particles, or a combination. Ionizing radiation can be made up of subatomic particles, which include electrons, neutrons, and alpha particles.

27.2.1.1 IMPACT OF IONIZED RADIATION ON HEALTH

The majority of the population considers radiation to be ionizing radiation. It can harm or kill cells, cause mutations in DNA, and change molecules, and ionize atoms due to its enormous amount of energy. It may also break chemical bonds and ionize atoms. Radiation from alpha, gamma, and neutrons may turn previously non-radioactive materials radioactive and even change one element into another. Ionization generates electrical effects because it produces charged particles.

27.2.1.2 INTERACTION OF RADIATION WITH BIOLOGICAL MOLECULES

1. **Direct Reaction:** A secondary electron resulting from the absorption of an X-ray photon interacts with DNA directly by breaking the relatively weak bonds between nucleic acids to produce the effect. This results in an altered molecule that differs structurally and functionally from the original molecule.

$$\text{RH} + \text{x radiation} \rightarrow \text{Rad.} + \text{H+} + \text{e}$$

$$\text{Rad.} \rightarrow \text{X} + \text{Y}$$

$$\text{Rad.} + \text{S} \rightarrow \text{Rad S}$$

2. **Indirect Reaction:**

$$\text{X-Radiation} + H_2O \rightarrow \text{H}^{(\text{ion})\cdot} + \text{OH}^{\cdot}$$

$$\text{Rad H+OH} \rightarrow \text{Rad} + H_2O$$

$$\text{Rad H} + \text{H (ion)} \rightarrow \text{R} + H_2$$

$$\text{H (ion)}^{\cdot} + O_2 \rightarrow \text{Rad} + H_2O\ \text{(ion)}^{\cdot}$$

i. Hydroperoxyl free radicals contribute to the hydrogen peroxide in tissue

$$HO_2 + H \rightarrow H_2O_2$$

$$HO_2 + HO_2 \rightarrow O_2 + H_2O_2$$

ii. Contribution of direct and indirect effects of radiation

Direct:30 to 40%

Indirect:60 to 70%

Sparsely ionizing radiations such as X-rays or gamma rays induce damage mainly through indirect effects, while densely ionizing radiation like neutrons and alpha particles cause damage primarily through direct effects.

27.2.2 NON-IONIZED RADIATION

Non-ionized radiation is radiation that lacks the energy to ionize atoms or molecules. It does, however, contain sufficient energy for excitation, which elevates electrons to states of increased energy, for example, near-ultraviolet light, visible light, infrared radiation, microwaves, and radio waves.

27.2.2.1 EFFECTS OF NON-IONIZING RADIATION ON HEALTH

In general, the results of non-ionizing radiation heating can cause tissue damage due to excessive heating, but non-ionizing radiation at low doses is usually not harmful.

27.3 CLASSIFICATION OF BIOLOGICAL EFFECTS OF RADIATION

- Somatic and genetic effects.
- Stochastic and deterministic effects.
- Short-term and long-term effects.

1. **Deterministic Effects:** Effects that are undetectable until comparatively large dosages, such as burns on the skin. Harmful tissue responses are another term for deterministic effects. These include issues like burns on the skin and injury to the eye's lens. These effects do not show up at lower doses. Beyond this point, the impact becomes more severe with increasing dosage. Below an absorbed dosage of 100 mGy (above the natural background radiation), no deterministic effects would be predicted, and the thresholds for the majority of effects are much greater. Deterministic effects are very

uncommon; however, they may arise as a result of complicated medical procedures or disasters.

Extremely high doses given immediately may result in acute radiation sickness and even death in very rare circumstances, such as catastrophic accidents. Deterministic effects result from high-dose radiation killing cells; they appear above a threshold dose that is significantly higher than radiation doses from natural sources or from occupational exposure during normal operation. The severity of the effect is dose-dependent; at a given high dose, all exposed cells demonstrate the effect in its severe form; at higher doses, the effect cannot increase.

2. **Stochastic Effects:** Effects that are thought to carry certain risks, even at modest dosages, include cancer. Heritable effects and cancer are examples of stochastic effects. Doses greater than 100 mSv have been shown to raise the risk of cancer in reliable scientific research. Although the data is less clear below this level, it is thought that even modest doses might result in a slight increase in risk for radiological protection reasons. An additional effective dosage of about 200 mSv (beyond the natural background exposure) raises the risk of deadly cancer from approximately 25% to about 26%. Genetic effects have never been identified in humans, although they have been observed in animals. However, a small chance of heritable effects is assumed for protection's sake. The mutation effect of low-dose radiation causes stochastic effects, and the precise threshold dose is unknown. It is observed that cancer of varying locations appears above different dose ranges; the severity of the effect is independent of dose, but the frequency of the (probabilistic) effect's appearance in the exposed population group is dose-dependent and (most of the time) increases linearly with dose (Figure 27.2).

27.4 QUANTIFY THE AMOUNT OF RADIATION

There are risks, of all. The level of risk from radiation is dose-dependent, with higher doses associated with high damage. Diagnostic X-ray and nuclear medicine diagnostics provide obvious health benefits, but there

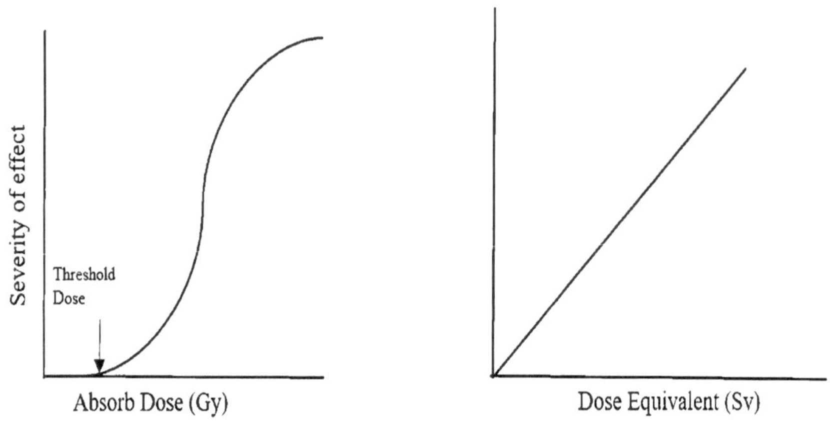

FIGURE 27.2 Deterministic and stochastic effects of radiation.

is also a relatively low chance (probability) of adverse results. When employing ionizing radiation sources for diagnosis, this fact must be considered. The risk of radiation-related side effects is considerably higher since radiation therapy requires large doses of radiation.

27.5 TRAINING AND EDUCATION

All personnel working in the radiology department should receive comprehensive training on radiation safety. This includes radiologists, radiologic technologists, nurses, and support staff. Training should cover principles of radiation physics, proper use of protective equipment, radiation monitoring, and emergency procedures. Ongoing education and updates on the latest safety guidelines should be provided to ensure everyone remains informed and vigilant.

27.6 RADIATION MONITORING

Regular monitoring of radiation levels is crucial to assess exposure levels and ensure they are within acceptable limits. Personal dosimeters should be worn by staff working in areas with potential radiation exposure. These dosimeters measure the cumulative dose received by an individual over time. Additionally, environmental monitoring devices, such as area radiation monitors, should be installed to measure radiation levels in specific areas of the department.

27.6.1 SHIELDING AND PROTECTIVE MEASURES

Radiology departments should be designed with appropriate shielding measures to reduce radiation exposure. Lead aprons, thyroid shields, and leaded eyewear are essential personal protective equipment (PPE) for staff working directly with radiation. Barriers made of lead or other radiation-absorbing materials should be in place to protect individuals in adjacent areas. It is essential to ensure that shielding equipment is regularly inspected and maintained for effectiveness.

27.6.2 OPTIMIZATION OF IMAGING TECHNIQUES

Radiologists and radiologic technologists should strive to use the lowest doses of radiation necessary to achieve medical image quality. This can be accomplished through appropriate selection of imaging protocols, exposure parameters, and equipment calibration. Regular quality assurance programs should be implemented to monitor imaging equipment and ensure optimal performance, minimizing the need for repeat examinations.

27.7 PATIENT SAFETY

Patients undergoing radiological procedures should be informed about the benefits and risks associated with radiation exposure. Imaging protocols should be tailored to individual patients, considering factors such as age, body size, and clinical indication. Radiation dose monitoring tools should be utilized to keep track of cumulative patient radiation exposure. Imaging facilities should follow established guidelines to ensure dose optimization and minimize unnecessary radiation exposure.

1. **Emergency Preparedness:** Radiology departments should have emergency procedures in place to respond to potential incidents involving radiation. This includes protocols for handling spills, equipment malfunctions, and patient emergencies. Staff should be trained in the appropriate actions to take during such situations to minimize radiation exposure and ensure the safety of all individuals involved.

2. **Regulatory Compliance:** Compliance with national and international radiation safety regulations is crucial in a radiology department. The department should have a radiation safety officer responsible for overseeing compliance with relevant guidelines and regulations. Regular audits and inspections should be conducted to assess compliance and identify areas for improvement. By adhering to these radiation safety practices, radiology departments can effectively manage and mitigate the dangers associated with ionizing radiation. Prioritizing the safety of patients and personnel ensures the continued delivery of high-quality diagnostic and therapeutic services while minimizing potential radiation-related hazards. The Atomic Energy Regulatory Board (AERB) is the authorized body in India recognized for ensuring radiation hazards, safety, and protection in various fields, including medical radiology. AERB has established comprehensive regulations and guidelines to ensure the safe use of ionizing radiation in healthcare facilities. Here are some key aspects of AERB regulations for radiation protection:

   - **Licensing and Authorization:** AERB regulations require all medical radiology facilities to obtain the necessary licenses and authorizations for operating radiation-emitting equipment. These licenses are granted based on compliance with specific safety requirements, including infrastructure, equipment specifications, and qualified personnel. With the objective to ensure that no source of exposure is unjustified in relation to its benefits or those of any other options available, the ICRP Commission recommends a dose limitation system. It further seeks to maintain any necessary radiation dose as low as is reasonably achievable, ensure that the dose equivalents received do not exceed certain limits that have been established, and allow for future development.

3. **ALARA Principle:** The short form "ALARA" stands for "As Low As Reasonably Achievable." It is a basic concept in radiation safety and protection, mostly applied to reducing ionizing radiation exposure. The goal of the principle is to limit radiation exposure to people and the general public to the lowest level that is practically possible while still allowing for the beneficial uses

of radiation in a wide range of areas, including medicine. The ALARA principle depends on the knowledge that every radiation exposure, regardless of how tiny, has some degree of risk. In order to minimize exposure levels, radiation protection methods must be optimized in relation to practical, technological, economic, and societal factors (ICRP, 1977).

Whenever conducting a cost-benefit analysis, all benefits to society are taken into account, not just those that will be received by particular individuals or groups. Benefits are occasionally evaluated, but it may be problematic to do so when the advantages go further than gratifying human objectives. Costs are viewed as the total of all detrimental effects of an operation, including monetary costs and any damage caused to the environment or to human health. Since these benefits and costs will not be distributed uniformly throughout the community as a whole, this wide process of balancing would only be valid if the harm to each individual was within an acceptable threshold. While the individual limitation of damage would be achieved through adherence to the Commission's dose-equivalent guidelines, this approach is capable of addressing ionizing radiation exposure.

- **Justification:** Benefits and potential dangers should be carefully considered before incorporating any radiation source or radiation-related practice. When the advantages outweigh the risks, radiation use should be justified.
- **Optimization:** Radiation amounts should be kept ALARA while taking into account present technology.
- **Dose Limits:** To ensure that radiation exposure remains within permissible ranges, regulatory organizations set dose limits. These limits establish a point of reference for minimizing exposure and avoiding unnecessary hazards. The Commission includes effective dose coefficients that provide reference coefficients for conditions that include prospective and retrospective dose assessments involving internal and external exposures of workers and members of the public, as well as for the administration of radiopharmaceuticals to patients.

Effective dose is determined by incorporating the other doses received during the year and the annual committed dose from internal exposures. For adults, committed dose is incorporated over a 50-year period; for young people, it is integrated up to 70 years of age when taking into account annual exposures. These are the restrictions that apply to all employees and members of the public, collectively along with the diagnostic reference levels (DRL) and limits indicated in effective dose. In addition to optimization, this provides a useful, equitable, and helpful system of protection that does not establish distinctions between people based on age, gender, or population-related variations in hazardousness per Gy.

For the purpose of maximizing worker and public protection, the average effective dose is a useful instrument. It can be used to help identify the optimal equilibrium between higher exposures for a small number of workers and lower exposures for a greater number of employees, along with the diversity of individual doses. It can be applied as an element in the optimization process for situations including planned, continuous, and emergency public doses. It has been used to compare different dose levels globally and changes in dose levels throughout the years for occupational, public, and medical exposures (Harrison et al., 2021) (Table 27.1).

TABLE 27.1 Annual Dose Limits

Tissue or Organ Dose	Radiation Employees	Member of Public
Entire body Dose	20* mSv/ yr	1 mSv/ yr
Eye lens dose	150 mSv/ yr	15 mSv / yr
skin	500 mSv / yr	50 mSv /yr
extremities	500 mSv /yr	50 mSv/ yr
After confirmation of pregnancy	2 mSv to lower trunk (I mSv to fetus)	fetus is considered too member of public

*The whole body dose limit is 20 mSv in a year while averaged over 5 yrs with a maximum of 30 mSv In any 1 year as per AERB.(ICRP, 1977).

- **Ten Days Rule:** A guideline provided by the International Commission on Radiological Protection (ICRP) Report No. 103

about females of reproductive age states that "whenever possible, one should confine the radiological examination of the lower abdomen and pelvis to the 10-day interval following the onset of menstruation," as a safety measure related to the teratogenic effect of radiation, even at the low doses usually found in medical imaging.

As of the most recent update in September 2021, the ICRP has no formal document referred to as "Publication 84." However, the ICRP has published a number of articles on pregnancy radiation protection.

This chapter explains recommendations as well as guidance on how to handle pregnant patients who might need medical imaging:

- Assessing the radiological risk for patients who are pregnant.
- Estimating the fetal dose and understanding the term "fetal dose."
- Approaches for radiation therapy and diagnostic imaging during pregnancy.
- Limitations and reference levels for fetal dosage during various medical procedures.
- Discussions of the benefits and drawbacks of medical radiation during pregnancy with patients and medical professionals.

27.8 QUALITY IMPROVEMENT IN RADIOLOGY

1. **Radiation Safety Officer (RSO):** Every medical radiology facility is required to designate a Radiation Safety Officer (RSO) responsible for overseeing radiation safety practices within the facility. The RSO ensures compliance with AERB regulations, conducts regular inspections, provides training to staff, and maintains records related to radiation safety.

2. **Equipment Requirements:** AERB sets guidelines for the safe use of radiation-emitting equipment, such as X-ray machines, CT scanners, and fluoroscopy units. The regulations specify technical parameters, equipment calibration, quality control procedures, and periodic maintenance requirements. AERB also mandates the

proper lead shielding protection measures to minimize radiation exposure to patients, staff, and the public.

3. **Diagnostic Reference Level (DRL):** The term "DRL" was first used in 1996 to refer to a type of recommendation level that was used to identify circumstances when patient exposure to medicine could qualify for increased protection (ICRP, 1996; Vañó et al., 2015).

   The Commission defines a type of radiation examination level used to maximize radiation protection in patient medical doses as a "diagnostic reference level" (DRL). The Commission suggests the adoption of two new terms: "DRL quantity" (a radiation metric that is frequently and easily measured or estimated to indicate the amount of medical imaging tasks involving ionizing radiation) and "DRL value."

   At the DRL level, a type of radiographic examination level termed a "Diagnostic Reference Level" is used to help ensure that patients are as safe as possible during medical exposure for diagnostic and interventional procedures. It is used in ionizing radiation medical imaging to show whether, under typical conditions, the radiation dose used for a specific technique is exceptionally high or low for that procedure. Radiation dose is a broad term used when referring to a specific dosimetry quantity associated with an individual's exposure to ionizing radiation.

   The DRL describes an effective method for identifying evaluations of ionizing radiation takes and requirements for maximum safety. The DRL method should be understood by everyone who is involved in exposing a patient to X-rays or ionizing radiation in order to maximize protection.

   DRL quantities need to estimate the radiation doses required to carry out a medical imaging task, be appropriate to the imaging modality for assessment, and be practical to measure or quantify. It is appropriate to set and demonstrate DRL values for both imaging modalities independently when two imaging modalities are used for the same function (e.g., CT and fluoroscopy).

4. **Local, National, and Regional DRLs:** Surveys or records are utilized to obtain the national DRL values for X-ray investigations. From a wide range of healthcare facilities, values of acceptable DRL from patient investigations are collected. The term "national DRL" refers to the median value of a DRL quantity distributed across healthcare institutions in a nation at the 75th percentile value, or "national DRL."

   National or regional DRLs should be updated every three to five years, or more frequently if new imaging procedures, major developments in technology, or improved post-processing become available.

   A thorough inquiry should be conducted to identify probable causes if a DRL result for any radiographic examination is increased. If intervention is required, a plan should be put into effect right away. DRLs are not meant to be applied to particular patients or serve as a warning sign for specific patients or investigations. DRL data are also not limitations (Vañó et al., 2015).

5. **Role of Diagnostic Reference Level (DRL) for Optimization of Radiation Protection:** To assess whether the data collected locally is significantly greater or lower than what is predictable, the appropriate DRL quantity for medical imaging procedures in a particular radiographic room or radiology department should be compared and analyzed with local, national, or regional DRL values. If a DRL value for any radiological examination is exceeded, an immediate investigation should be performed to determine the probable reasons. The DRL analysis can be applied to assess whether the doses of ionizing radiation used for radiographic examinations at and around a healthcare facility are frequently too high or too low when evaluated for an adequate number of patients for an identified clinical investigation. The DRL approach provides the identification of equipment and practices that have high radiation dose levels so that protection can be optimized.

KEYWORDS

- **CT scanners**
- **diagnostic reference level**
- **equipment calibration**
- **genetic effects**
- **heritable effects**
- **low-dose radiation**
- **medical radiology facility**
- **mutation effect**
- **radiation safety officer**
- **radiation safety records**
- **radiation-emitting equipment**
- **stochastic effects**

REFERENCES

Anderson, J. G. (1945). William Morgan and X-rays. *Transactions of the Faculty of Actuaries, 17*(January), 219–221. https://doi.org/10.1017/s0071368600003001.

Cruz Suarez, R., et al. (2018). IAEA Safety Standards for protecting people and the environment—Occupational radiation protection. *IAEA Safety Guide, 87*(6), 673–674.

Harrison, J. D., et al. (2021). ICRP Publication 147: Use of dose quantities in radiological protection. *Annals of the ICRP, 50*(1), 9–82. https://doi.org/10.1177/0146645320911864.

Ilyin, L. A. (2002). Radiation accidents: Medical effects and radiation protection experience. *International Congress Series, 1234*(C), 7–17. https://doi.org/10.1016/S0531-5131(01)00590-8.

International Commission on Radiological Protection (ICRP). (1977). Recommendations of the Radiological Protection Commission on radiological protection. *ICRP Publication 26*, 1–87. Retrieved from: https://journals.sagepub.com/doi/pdf/10.1177/ANIB_1_3 (accessed on 14 March 2025).

International Commission on Radiological Protection (ICRP). (2007). The 2007 recommendations of the International Commission on Radiological Protection. *Annals of the ICRP, 37*(2–4), 1–332. https://doi.org/10.1016/j.icrp.2007.10.003.

Vañó, E., et al. (2015). *Annals of the ICRP, Protection, International Commission on Radiological*. Retrieved from: www.icrp.org (accessed on 14 March 2025).

CHAPTER 28

An Overview of Adverse Events During Clinical Trials

MUSKAN CHADHA,[1] ANISHA ADYA,[1] HARSHITHA VERMA,[2] JANE OGOCHUKWU EZEAGAGWO,[3] WESLEYAN WENDE,[3] and ROHIT KUMAR TIWARI[3,*]

[1]*Department of Nutrition and Dietetics, Sharda School of Allied Health Sciences, Sharda University, Greater Noida, Uttar Pradesh, India*

[2]*Department of Biochemistry, Manasagangothri, University of Mysuru, Mysuru, Karnataka, India*

[3]*Department of Clinical Research, Sharda School of Allied Health Sciences, Sharda University, Greater Noida, Uttar Pradesh, India*

*Corresponding author

ABSTRACT

Clinical trials entail administering the drug, which is essential for the assessment of safety and efficacy of medical intervention on human subjects. Despite rigorous preclinical trials, unexpected adverse effects (AEs) can arise, ranging from mild discomfort to severe complications, which are further categorized based on severity, frequency, and relationship to the investigational drug or intervention. AE monitoring and reporting ensure participant safety and maintain the integrity of clinical trial data. The regulatory framework that governs AE reporting highlights the need for transparency and timely communication between investigators, sponsors, and regulatory agencies. The chapter focuses on the challenges in AE assessment, including attribution and causality determination, various types of AEs, and outcomes reported by patients. Understanding and

Allied Healthcare in Practice: An Introduction to Integrated Patient Care. Sally Lukose, Karuna Singh (Eds.)

DOI: 10.1201/9781998511037-32

managing AEs plays a pivotal role, and this overview offers insights into the strategies employed to minimize, mitigate, and appropriately respond to AEs during the conduct of clinical research.

28.1 INTRODUCTION

Adequately conducted clinical trials are indeed regarded as the gold standard for evidence-based utilization and approval of various therapeutic interventions against human ailments. This, in turn, necessitates an elaborate reporting of findings from clinical trials, which further facilitates choosing the type of treatment and subsequently provides insight into the plausible side effects of the prescribed therapeutics. Indeed, reporting the findings of a clinical trial poses a substantial risk of information loss during the translation of reports from the analyst to the investigators. During clinical trials, undesired situations may arise due to the use of investigational drugs or any other interventions. Among these, an adverse event (AE) is the occurrence of any unwarranted medical complication in a subject associated with the use of drugs in humans, whether or not considered to be drug-related. Previously, it has been shown that reporting of AEs driven by physicians is usually inferior to a complementary approach that employs physician- and patient-reported outcomes (Basch et al., 2006). The occurrence of AEs to various therapies is reported to be remarkably variable, and a few standards have been described for structured data collection, impeding the loss in reporting of AEs (Belknap et al., 2013). Furthermore, it has also been shown that peer-reviewed publications, which serve as the primary source of information to clinicians regarding the outcomes of clinical trials, report the cases of AEs sub-optimally (Ioannidis and Lau, 2001). These observations have further reported significant heterogeneity in the reporting of AEs (Ioannidis and Lau, 2001). Studies have further led to the elucidation of reporting standards for AEs during the trial. In this chapter, we focus on reviewing the actual reporting of AEs and highlighting the additional work that needs to be done in this area.

28.2 CLASSIFICATION OF ADVERSE EFFECTS

Classification of AEs is important for their appropriate review, evaluation, and monitoring; hence, AEs during clinical trials can be differentiated based on their severity, expectedness, and plausible relatedness. It is desired that the study protocols incorporate a detailed description of AEs by categorizing them into either of the classifications (Silverman et al., 2006).

28.2.1 SEVERITY OF ADVERSE EFFECTS

28.2.1.1 MILD

This relates to the awareness of signs and symptoms that are easily tolerable and may cause minor irritation, which does not restrict individuals from accomplishing day-to-day activities. Importantly, these symptoms do not require medical attention and may be transient in nature.

28.2.1.2 MODERATE

These types of AEs often lead to inconvenience of relatively lower intensity or concern among the participants. These AEs may result in some interference with the day-to-day activities of the participants. However, this type of AE can be easily managed by simple medical interventions.

28.2.1.3 SEVERE

These AEs are considered to be those that significantly affect the normal functioning of the participants during a trial and require specialized medical care and systemic therapies; they are usually incapacitating. Importantly, seriousness and severity are not synonyms. A classic example of this is the occurrence of skin rashes. A skin rash arising in a subject during a trial of a drug or therapy is not presumably a serious adverse event (SAE). Similarly, a severe headache can also not be considered an SAE during trials. However, mild chest pain in a subject may modulate the normal functioning of a subject and hence falls under the classification of SAE.

28.2.2 EXPECTEDNESS

Another important aspect of AEs during trials is their assessment for plausible expectedness of occurrence or non-occurrence. The non-occurrence of AEs may be attributed to their absence during a trial based on the protocols being followed, investigation brochures, and the label of the drug/investigational product during a clinical trial. Based on this, AEs can be further subdivided into the following categories.

28.2.2.1 UNEXPECTED

In these types of AEs, both the nature and severity of the AE are variable with reference to the study conditions, the protocol, product brochure, or the investigator brochure.

28.2.2.2 EXPECTED

These AEs are usually known to occur with a particular study condition or intervention.

28.2.3 RELATEDNESS

This may be defined as the relationship between the occurrence of an event and the intervention/participation being studied. This is usually assessed by the site investigator of the trial, and an exhaustive scale to categorize these events is discussed herewith.

28.2.3.1 DEFINITELY RELATED

AEs are conclusively dependent on the investigational product and/or procedure during a trial. Indeed, an event resulting from the administration of an intervention (drug) during a trial, which is known to occur in a sequential manner, can be categorized as a definitely related AE. These events tend to improve upon stopping the administration and tend to reappear upon exposure to a particular drug or therapy.

28.2.3.2 POSSIBLY RELATED

These events tend to follow a temporal sequence upon their administration in the subjects and are further believed to exhibit a known expected response to a particular intervention. Nevertheless, the distinguishing feature of these events is that their occurrence within the subjects can be regulated by an array of various factors.

28.2.3.3 NOT RELATED

These AEs are usually not associated with the investigational drug or therapies being administered to the subjects during a clinical trial. The probable clinical symptoms of such an event are usually irregular, and establishing a biological relationship with the interventions is implausible.

28.3 OUTCOMES REPORTED BY THE PATIENTS

Exhaustive research has led to the standardization of definitions relating to the type and severity of AEs by using the National Cancer Institute's (NCI) Common Terminology Criteria for Adverse Events (CTCAE) (Sivendran and Galsky, 2016). Reports have further outlined that physicians tend to underreport and underestimate the occurrence and severity of AEs (Di Maio et al., 2015; Fromme et al., 2004) (Figure 28.1).

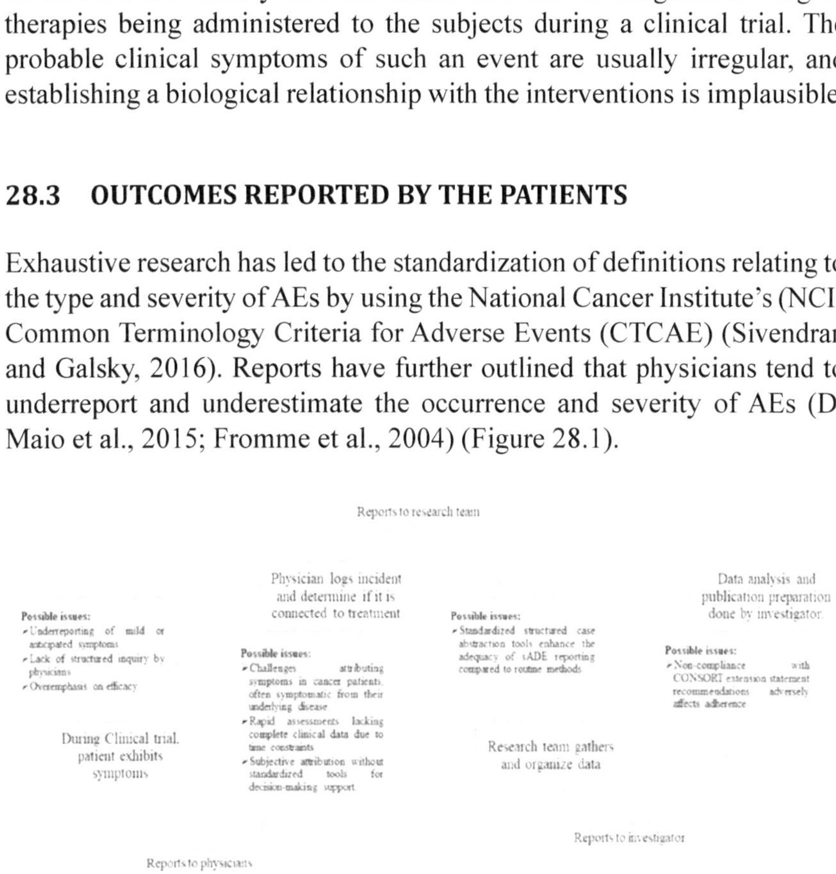

FIGURE 28.1 Adverse event reporting and patient experiences at risk due to communication.

Indeed, underreporting of symptoms by physicians is mediated by several factors, which include lesser attention towards mild and subjective toxicities. Reporting of a clinical trial is oriented towards elucidating its efficacy rather than outlining AEs and other toxicities (Di Maio et al., 2015; Montemurro et al., 2016). Importantly, other factors, including constraints of time, patient-to-physician ratio, and limited availability of data management resources, further contribute to the underreporting of AEs (Montemurro et al., 2016).

Additionally, in advanced stages of the disease, patients begin to recognize their own symptoms. It has further been shown that this, in turn, is helpful in improving the baseline symptom characterization during entry into clinical trials (Basch, 2010; Basch et al., 2009). Owing to this, the National Cancer Institute (NCI), USA, developed the Patient Reported Outcomes Version of the Common Terminology Criteria for Adverse Events (PRO-CTCAE). PRO-CTCAE is a standardized reporting of AEs through patient-centered approaches, which can be used in trials related to oncological interventions (Basch et al., 2014). Indeed, incorporating such a reporting tool would elevate comprehensive reporting of AEs during trials.

28.4 COMPREHENSIVE ANALYSIS OF THE POTENTIAL ADVANTAGES AND DISADVANTAGES OF PARTICIPANT ENGAGEMENT IN CLINICAL TRIALS

Engaging in clinical trials has both pros and cons, or potential benefits and drawbacks, which necessitate a comprehensive understanding of the consequences for all participants in their personal, medical, and ethical dimensions. These pathways are essential for research endeavors that seek to provide novel therapies or treatments to patients, enhancing patient care and increasing medical knowledge. Therefore, it is crucial to recognize the dangers and uncertainties that come along with these possible benefits.

28.4.1 POTENTIAL ADVANTAGES

28.4.1.1 ACCESS TO INNOVATIVE TREATMENTS

All clinical trials provide access to novel treatments, drugs, and procedures that may not be easily available to the general population. Phase III trials evaluate the effectiveness, impact, and safety of novel treatments, giving participants early access and the opportunity to experience future improvements in healthcare (Beauchamp et al., 2013). These advancements may provide better therapeutic results compared to traditional treatments (IOM, 2015).

28.4.1.2 CONTRIBUTION TO MEDICAL PROGRESS

Those people who participate directly contribute to the scientific information, which helps to enhance medical research and lead to the creation of novel remedies. Their participation enhances the improvement of treatment plans and a better understanding of illness through research (Mello et al., 2018).

28.4.1.3 CLOSE MEDICAL MONITORING

In-depth medical assessment and monitoring are provided to all the participants by skilled healthcare experts who frequently go above and beyond standard care. This meticulous attention to aspects has the potential to improve overall health outcomes by facilitating the early diagnosis and timely management of health concerns (Eapen et al., 2017).

28.4.2 POTENTIAL DISADVANTAGES:

28.4.2.1 RISK OF ADVERSE EVENTS

There are inherent risks associated with receiving experimental therapies, such as the possibility of unanticipated side effects or unexpected occurrences that might have a detrimental influence on the participant's health (Ioannidis, 2016).

28.4.2.2 TIME COMMITMENT AND INCONVENIENCE

Participating in clinical trials requires a significant time investment and may include inconveniences such as regular doctor visits, strict procedures, and lifestyle modifications (National Cancer Institute, 2019).

28.4.2.3 UNCERTAIN TREATMENT ASSIGNMENT

There is doubt about the true therapeutic advantages obtained from randomized controlled trials since participants may receive a placebo or an alternative therapy (FDA, 2020).

28.5 CONCLUSION

In conclusion, the effective management of AEs in oncological clinical trials requires a proactive, multidisciplinary approach, incorporating risk assessment, adaptive strategies, and continuous improvement. A commitment to participant safety, ethical conduct, and regulatory compliance is fundamental to the success of oncological clinical trials. The current landscape of identifying and managing AEs during oncological clinical trials is characterized by a commitment to precision, innovation, and patient-centricity. Being a participant in clinical trials has benefits as well as drawbacks. To guarantee the ethical conduct of clinical trials and the welfare of study subjects, it is imperative that researchers and prospective volunteers carefully consider these criteria.

KEYWORDS

- **adverse events**
- **ethical conduct criteria**
- **human ailments**
- **investigational drugs**
- **multidisciplinary approach**
- **oncological clinical trials**
- **patient-centricity**
- **proactive approach**
- **regulatory compliance**
- **therapeutic interventions**
- **treatment selection**

REFERENCES

Basch, E. (2010). The missing voice of patients in drug-safety reporting. *The New England Journal of Medicine, 362*(10), 865–869.

Basch, E., Iasonos, A., McDonough, T., Barz, A., Culkin, A., Kris, M. G., Scher, H. I., & Schrag, D. (2006). Patient versus clinician symptom reporting using the National Cancer

Institute Common Terminology Criteria for Adverse Events: Results of a questionnaire-based study. *The Lancet Oncology, 7*(11), 903–909.

Basch, E., Jia, X., Heller, G., Barz, A., Sit, L., Fruscione, M., Appawu, M., Iasonos, A., Atkinson, T., Goldfarb, S., Culkin, A., Kris, M. G., & Schrag, D. (2009). Adverse symptom event reporting by patient's vs clinicians: Relationships with clinical outcomes. *Journal of the National Cancer Institute, 101*(23), 1624–1632.

Basch, E., Reeve, B. B., Mitchell, S. A., Clauser, S. B., Minasian, L. M., Dueck, A. C., Mendoza, T. R., Hay, J., Atkinson, T. M., Abernethy, A. P., Bruner, D. W., Cleeland, C. S., Sloan, J. A., Chilukuri, R., Baumgartner, P., Denicoff, A., St Germain, D., O'Mara, A. M., Chen, A., & Schrag, D. (2014). Development of the National Cancer Institute's patient-reported outcomes version of the common terminology criteria for adverse events (PRO-CTCAE). *Journal of the National Cancer Institute, 106*(9).

Belknap, S. M., Georgopoulos, C. H., Lagman, J., Weitzman, S. A., Qualkenbush, L., Yarnold, P. R., Edwards, B. J., McKoy, J. M., Trifilio, S. M., & West, D. P. (2013). Reporting of serious adverse events during cancer clinical trials to the institutional review board: An evaluation by the research on adverse drug events and reports (RADAR) project. *Journal of Clinical Pharmacology, 53*(12), 1334–1340.

Di Maio, M., Gallo, C., Leighl, N. B., Piccirillo, M. C., Daniele, G., Nuzzo, F., Gridelli, C., Gebbia, V., Ciardiello, F., De Placido, S., Ceribelli, A., Favaretto, A. G., de Matteis, A., Feld, R., Butts, C., Bryce, J., Signoriello, S., Morabito, A., Rocco, G., & Perrone, F. (2015). Symptomatic toxicities experienced during anticancer treatment: Agreement between patient and physician reporting in three randomized trials. *Journal of Clinical Oncology, 33*(8), 910–915.

Fromme, E. K., Eilers, K. M., Mori, M., Hsieh, Y. C., & Beer, T. M. (2004). How accurate is clinician reporting of chemotherapy adverse effects? A comparison with patient-reported symptoms from the Quality-of-Life Questionnaire C30. *Journal of Clinical Oncology, 22*(17), 3485–3490.

Ioannidis, J. P., & Lau, J. (2001). Completeness of safety reporting in randomized trials: An evaluation of 7 medical areas. *JAMA, 285*(4), 437–443.

Montemurro, F., Mittica, G., Cagnazzo, C., Longo, V., Berchialla, P., Solinas, G., Culotta, P., Martinello, R., Foresto, M., Gallizioli, S., Calori, A., Grasso, B., Volpone, C., Bertola, G., Parola, G., Tealdi, G., Giuliano, P. L., Aglietta, M., & Ballari, A. M. (2016). Self-evaluation of adjuvant chemotherapy-related adverse effects by patients with breast cancer. *JAMA Oncology, 2*(4), 445–452.

Research C for DE and. (2022). Novel drug approvals for 2020. *FDA*. Retrieved from: https://www.fda.gov/drugs/new-drugs-fda-cders-new-molecular-entities-and-new-therapeutic-biological-products/novel-drug-approvals-2020 (accessed on 14 March 2025).

Silverman, D. I., Cirullo, L., DeMartinis, N. A., Damato, K., DeMeo, M., Fernandez, G. A., Glynn, L., Hegde, U., Laskay, E., Leger, R., Abu-Hasaballah, K., & Caron, J. M. (2006). Systematic identification and classification of adverse events in human research. *Contemporary Clinical Trials, 27*(3), 295–303.

Sivendran, S., & Galsky, M. D. (2016). Adverse event reporting in oncology clinical trials—Lost in translation? *Expert Opinion on Drug Safety, 15*(7), 893–896.

CHAPTER 29

Inter-Professional Collaboration in Patient Care

MAYANK SHUKLA

Department of Physiotherapy, Sharda School of Allied Health Sciences, Sharda University, Greater Noida, Uttar Pradesh, India

ABSTRACT

Population expansion and increased life expectancy worldwide, and specifically for India, in the recent decade have produced proportionate health needs. Proportions of the elderly and young ones have increased. The health care delivery system has evolved alongside knowledge expansion, technological innovations, and the evolution of newer disciplines of health care. This has further added survivors of various events who have specific rehabilitative needs and expected outcomes. Clinical care pathways and clinical reasoning formats require the involvement of many health care professionals for medicine, surgery, diagnostics, therapeutic, rehabilitative, and supportive services. Inter-professional collaboration requires collaborative clinical reasoning and treatment planning. This can be achieved through inter-professional communication, written and verbal dialogues, and pre-set codes of conduct, along with ethical practice, which forms the basis for this. The quality standards include shared decision-making and health care coordination. Shared decision-making and planning are essential components of the same, Actionable aspects include human resource planning, including their training, core education, allied education, and inter-professional education, and collaboration from the beginning may prove to be an efficient strategy for this. The application of

Allied Healthcare in Practice: An Introduction to Integrated Patient Care. Sally Lukose, Karuna Singh (Eds.)

DOI: 10.1201/9781998511037-33

IPC may also require common meetings, effective and clear documentation, referral, and technology-based advanced applications.

29.1 OVERVIEW OF INTER-PROFESSIONAL COLLABORATION IN HEALTHCARE

Population expansion, increased survival at birth and after critical events, increased life span, and knowledge explosion with advanced technologies have increased the complexity of health care. Increased complexity demands better collaboration for the desired outcomes.

29.1.1 CHANGING EPIDEMIOLOGY AND DEMOGRAPHY

The World Health Organization (WHO, 2013) defines inter-professional collaboration (IPC) as "multiple health workers from different professional backgrounds work together with families, carers, and communities to deliver the highest quality of care." WHO (2013) has also provided a framework for inter-professional collaboration, and educational settings that help to develop better inter-professional care have also been proven effective. Super-specialty and multi-specialty hospitals have large workforces of different professionals, and smooth collaboration is required among them. A single health care provider dealing with all needs may face burnout sooner rather than later (Singh, et al.; 2022, in Provider Burnout).

The world population is expanding, with 8 billion people estimated to share planet Earth, all having substantial health care requirements. India is on the verge of becoming the most populous country and is not yet categorized as a developed country, thus having unique requirements; one needs an efficient health care delivery system to cater to the population, as noted in "World Population Prospects 2022" by the United Nations (UN) population division. The life expectancy for both sexes at birth is 73.2 years, for females 75.6 years, and for males 70.8 years. It has been on the rise for a long time, which increases the elderly dependency ratio. The infant and under age 5 mortality rates have been on the decline, with infant mortality being 26.5 per 1000 live births. This further increases the youth dependency ratio.

The urban population proportion has reached 70% of the total (Chen, 2022). India has witnessed rapid urbanization, thereby burdening the healthcare system of its metros. The health care workers now cater to this increased urban and relatively younger and elderly populations through technological advancements (Thimbleby, 2013). Different demographic pictures have different demands and expectations from health care providers. Teamwork is needed to cater to this, and the team needs to communicate efficiently in real-time for collaboration towards a common goal, as seen in Figure 13.1. Therefore, it becomes clear that inter-professional collaboration at multiple levels is the new skill required to deliver healthcare for the changing epidemiology and demography of the world.

29.1.2 EXPANSION OF KNOWLEDGE BASE IN HEALTH CARE

The knowledge expansion has been significant in the field of health care; new professions are emerging to cope with this. It is not possible for one professional to manage the knowledge bank, big data, and electronic information, emerging guidelines, and higher standards demanded by modern health care. Genomics, epigenomics, and metabolomics are newer areas of omics profiling linked to health care. Therapy and allied health areas have witnessed entry-level education reaching graduation level in all fields and up to doctoral level in a few disciplines to accommodate the entire depth and scope. Interconnections of knowledge may require inter-professional dialogue and a meeting at the bedside (Cantaert et al., 2022). Limited knowledge leads to inappropriate management, diagnosis, and sub-optimal future outcomes. The gap can be filled by collaborative clinical reasoning in a case presentation. A quarterback or coordinator may facilitate the knowledge exchange (Gray et al., 2019).

Human resource educational framework for health professionals shall effectively take care of this (Tulchisky and Varavikova, 2014). Inter-professional collaboration and shared responsibilities are rooted in the classroom and practiced in hospital settings. Therefore, the collaboration and coordination of different AHPs to deliver holistic health is desirable.

29.1.3 INNOVATIVE AND TECHNOLOGICALLY ADVANCED TECHNIQUES

Regenerative medicine, transplant surgeries, and artificial prosthetic replacements have given new life to the body after one cycle. Stem cell therapies and hybrid physiological systems have produced more options for frailer bodies. Diagnostic applications include positron emission technology scans, sub-cellular investigations like electron microscopy, real-life big data of heart rate variability, and baroreflex sensitivity, and so forth. Simpler things like hand sanitization from hand washing, hand rubs to gel-based sanitizers are all newer developments, and different smaller equipment like cannulas, pacemakers, valves, and bigger additions like artificial exoskeletons and invasive procedures like deep brain stimulation are all areas demanding super specializations (Thimbleby, 2013).

29.1.4 ANCIENT, NEW AND EVOLVING HEALTH-CARE FIELDS

Inter-professional identity is essential in improving congruency and collaboration. A professional is one with a distinct set of skills and an independent knowledge bank. Interprofessional collaboration requires acceptance and recognition of different professionals in health care. A strong belief from past practices and inhibition in recognizing fellow colleagues leads to a poor fit of skills holistically for the patient. The list of different old and new health professionals is updated by the International Labor Organization (ILO); we find many including acupuncturists, naturopaths, occupational health and safety workers, physiotherapy technicians, and assistants along with others listed there (ILO, ISCO). Faith healers and village healers are seen too; yet many of these may not be found in modern hospitals. It is desirable that modern healthcare providers are aware of their work and may be able to check with them about the past treatments they provided.

29.1.5 NEED FOR PATIENT-CENTERED OUTCOMES

A team leader or quarterback is mentioned as a facilitator for patient-centered outcomes. Evidence has shown that physicians need collaborative teamwork to effectively deliver care; specialists are focused on a single area, and other professionals are required for preventive and promotive aspects of health. This improves the satisfaction of all stakeholders. To keep the patient and their outcomes at the center, the healthcare team needs to collaborate among themselves. The outcomes may include waiting time, time of stay in the intensive care unit, ward, or fatality rates from the emergency department, proportion of live births, survival rates in surgery, and so forth. These specific targets are to be met, but the big picture, as seen in Figure 29.1, shall always be in sight. The need is filled by proactive inter-professional collaboration and communication. The cost of care may become a barrier; knowledge of funding agencies and insurance companies' protocols is convenient in emergencies.

Clinical care pathways provide for the patient-centered outcome. Different guidelines and statements by professional bodies shall be taken into account. The organization must develop a framework for the care from the first step of registration to the last step of discharge and home program. Rehabilitation professionals may be considered from the beginning rather than at discharge for better outcomes. Dietary and other care providers may be consulted for optimal response from the patient; it is all the more important for deficiency diseases.

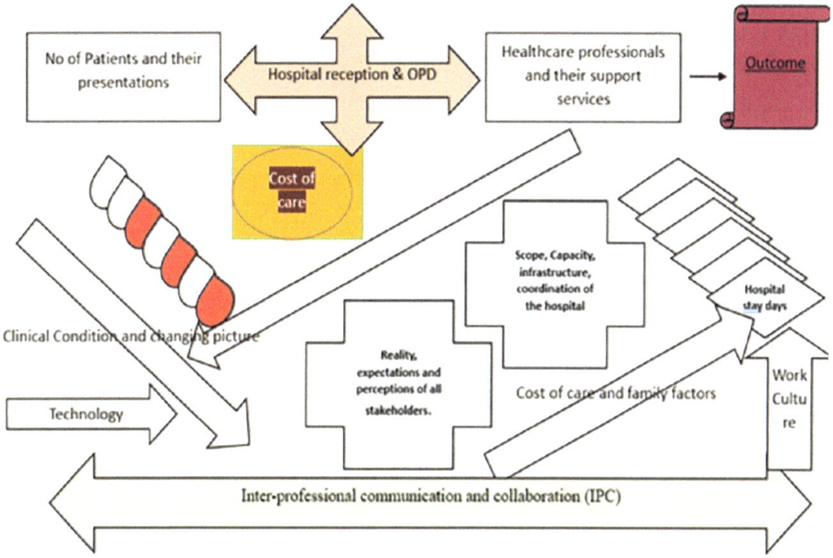

FIGURE 29.1 Role of Inter-professional communication (IPC) in clinical recovery, length of hospital stays, and cost of healthcare leading to final outcome for patients and society. IPE-Inter-professional education. Boxes are for planning; arrows are for action.

29.2 DECISION-MAKING AND CARE COORDINATION-PLANNING FOR INTER-PROFESSIONAL COMMUNICATION

Involvement of all team members brings greater knowledge and skills to the forefront. Patient ownership shall be given to the concerned healthcare professional, and policies of decentralization of large departments and horizontal expansion are needed for good collaboration and increased efficiency.

29.2.1 CLINICAL REASONING BY TEAM

The bio-psycho-social nature of presentations in patients requires collaborative clinical reasoning by the team. The technology has many positives but also a few negatives; lack of inter-professional face-to-face interaction is one. The big picture of the elephant is never clear from only one direction; therefore, the complex human body has more to reason out than can be done by just one. Clinical case presentations at the department, faculty level, or at the level of the hospital shall be undertaken to increase team reasoning for patient care (Olson et al., 2020). Most expert clinicians may be too busy to comprehensively review a case. Time management is crucial in patient care; a correct diagnosis after a long time is not desirable. Clinical reasoning as a team effort is invaluable. Thus, the role of diagnostic professionals, physiotherapists, and nurses becomes important. Additionally, how diet can affect recovery may be missed if we do not include a dietitian in our team. Staying clear about multiple facets of clinical reasoning and involving many of them improves patient outcomes. Follow-up and continuity of care are essential too.

29.2.2 MULTIDISCIPLINARY AND INTERDISCIPLINARY APPROACHES

In a multidisciplinary approach, different professionals provide their respective specialized services; however, in an interdisciplinary approach, the synthesis is done, and there is a harmonized link to the final decision. Thus, the common and coherent approach is what gives the optimal outlook. In the case of an acute intervertebral disc prolapse, if we do not give a physiotherapy (PT) trial and directly take the patient for surgery, it is not true interdisciplinary care. Even after months of PT, if the patient is not improving and we do not proceed with surgery, interdisciplinary care, where we are able to decide on the right care at the right time, is very useful (Choi and Pak, 2006). Fibromyalgia, which is a diagnosis of exclusion, is a good example of interdisciplinary care (Guisti et al., 2017).

29.2.3 COORDINATION BETWEEN DISCIPLINES

Coordination can be established by a common point of contact; in clinical settings, we have the patient as a common point of interest. The patient has to be empowered to demand combined consultation with two healthcare providers. A simple case of hypertension may require a cardiologist, nephrologist, and dietitian to start and may also involve services from yoga experts or exercise therapists. Furthermore, they may need electrophysiological studies, and all professionals have to coordinate for the patient. The patient may be at a loss and need counseling. Usually, social workers or counselors are available at the desk for this purpose. Coordination gives the idea of scope and available resources to the healthcare provider.

29.2.4 OWNERSHIP OF THE PATIENTS

Ownership of the patient is a critical aspect of interdisciplinary care. Consultants usually take ownership in a specialty care setting. General physicians may form a good point of ownership in many cases in an interdisciplinary care setting. In long-term rehabilitation cases, the ownership may be with the rehabilitation expert. Senior residents and nurses are also candidates for ownership, depending upon the case scenario. Ownership may be handed over from one professional to another. Cowley et al. (2017) have mentioned that the decision-making role fosters ownership; budding professionals specifically need to develop this attribute. Coordination and ownership shall be decided at the admission and may be handed over during the care.

29.2.5 HOSPITAL POLICIES FOR CLINICAL CARE PATHWAYS AND OUTCOME MEASURES

Hospitals can decide on their policies for the type of clinical care pathways and outcome measures to be used. Clinical care pathways may be as per the hospital manual or as per the ownership in charge of the case. Conflicts of interest shall be avoided. The outcome measures are decided by the administrator, such as admission rates, clinical outcome measures like blood pressure, or patient-reported outcome measures. Black et al. (2016)

have described patient-reported outcome measures as superior in delivering better health services. In the absence of a care pathway, usual care takes place, and it is not able to support the outcome measures. Therefore, in the case of inter-professional collaboration, a universal patient-reported outcome measure and a documented clinical care pathway must be maintained. Optimal patient outcomes for various dependent health factors, ranging from blood pressure to length of hospital stay, are positively affected by efficient IPC (Pascucci et al., 2021).

29.2.6 CORE EDUCATION, ALLIED EDUCATION, AND INTER-PROFESSIONAL EDUCATION FOR PROMOTING INTER-PROFESSIONAL COLLABORATIVE APPROACH

Inter-professional collaborative simulation for different healthcare students has been reported by Titzer et al. (2012) to foster the right attitude of collaboration among the students. Such practices can decrease the cost of care later during the professional life of the healthcare provider. This also imparts the scope and role information of different healthcare providers to each other. It is based on Interprofessional Education (IPE), where the clinical case is enacted, and different role-play techniques are used for the clarity of action pathways in an interdisciplinary team. This is part of the core and allied education of the healthcare provider. IPE models are helpful for problem-solving skills in complex cases involving multidisciplinary care. Referral and cross-consultations are part of collaborative practice.

29.3 COMMUNICATION AND TEAMWORK-APPLICATIONOF IPC

Effective collaboration requires efficient teamwork and clear communication. Impressive leadership with more horizontal expansion and well-defined verticals are essential prerequisites for this.

29.3.1 WRITTEN DOCUMENTATION

The practice of problem-oriented medical synopsis from 1966 is commonly seen. Written records have evolved into electronic databases; different formats are used for them, like SOAP – subjective, objective, assessment, and plan. This is not a very popular area for research and development, though in certain case scenarios it becomes imperative to look and relook at it, and it may speak to a lack of collaboration and coordination thereof. Patient-reported outcome measures (PROMs) are effective for this purpose. Patient-centered records are now developed, and they form the basis for electronic health records as well. Registration is done as the first step; it is added on by every department and is accessible for all, thereby increasing inter-professional collaboration and providing official documentation (Jorie et al., 2020).

29.3.2 USE OF REFERRAL CODES AS PER THE SCOPE

Medical codes allow alpha-numeric codes to be seen as diagnoses, procedures, and medical devices for a given patient. The International Classification of Diseases database provides the codes, and it has been designed by the WHO. The codes give a uniform language, remove subjectivity, and provide for the patient's diagnosis, treatment, and other services, as well as any unusual circumstances that may exist. It also helps in billing and insurance.

29.3.3 ETHICAL PRACTICE AND TEAMWORK

There are a few ethical issues in inter-professional collaboration as a team. The ownership of the patient, who decides on discharge, and so forth. Differences of opinion or lack of uniformity on a particular decision need to be tackled with the policies of the organization. Direct communication or mediation by hospital administration is a policy decision in such cases. Ethical principles can be applied at different levels – individual, professional field, inter-professional level, or at the level of the organization. A new joiner adjusts to the organization, so the organization's work culture needs to be ethically sound for the overall outcome (Clark et al., 2007).

29.3.4 VERBAL AND NON-VERBAL COMMUNICATION

Words and phrases, along with gestures like eye contact or body position, postures like crossed arms, and tone of voice with authority or request, can go a long way in successful and unsuccessful inter-professional collaboration. There are cultural differences from one place to another and differences in greetings and social distancing, where the role of leadership becomes very crucial to bridge the gap of understanding in these aspects. Differences in age, sex, background, religion, and culture make interprofessional communication a goal to achieve in perfection.

Empathy and compassion for the patient can be the thread that ties all the team members together. A patient-first approach, with less emphasis on individualism, shall be the call of the hour. Empathetic healthcare can increase patient compliance and adherence to slower therapeutic approaches like exercise therapy and hydrotherapy. Specific training interventions and simulation exercises can help healthcare providers develop these attributes. A presentable outfit and outlook, along with prompt responses, are the basis of good communication; one should always listen and understand before speaking.

29.3.5 LEADERSHIP, COMMUNICATION, AND TEAMWORK

The role of leadership shall be to bring the team together with the intention of improving outcomes; the reflective practitioner shall be able to improve on what was lacking in subsequent sessions. Common goal planning and bringing the team together require formal and informal motivation for all team members. Patients require supportive fellow humans, not science fiction heroes, to deal with them in a hospital setting.

A dedicated, slow but constant learners' team can achieve more than a single excellent professional without a team. Emotional quotient and social quotient may also be considered, along with intelligence quotient.

29.3.6 BRIEFING AND DEBRIEFING

The process of giving information prior to the procedure to all team members and after the procedure, the report is called briefing and debriefing, respectively. These are crucial aspects from the process owner to all the team members and higher-ups. This sets the ground for collaborative actions in a systematic and sequential manner and prepares the well-orchestrated conduct for the clients. They are particularly useful for surgical care, where we have preoperative, peri-operative, and postoperative procedures lined up (Stephens et al., 2016).

29.3.7 COMMUNICATION BREAKDOWN AND COLLABORATION FAILURE

Expectations, perception, and their mismatch with reality are the root causes of communication failure. Miscommunication, along with poor listening capability, is yet another cause for breakdown. A poor organizational structure with failure to plan in advance also leads to poor collaboration. Time is a key perishable asset when it comes to IPC failure. It is reported to result in 70% of adverse events in healthcare (Fewster and Velsor, 2008). There are theories that can be referred to prevent this from happening, like King's theory and Group theory.

KEYWORDS

- **clinical reasoning formats**
- **collaborative actions**
- **health-care delivery system**
- **health-care providers**
- **hospital setting**
- **increased life expectancy**
- **information sharing**
- **new health-care disciplines**
- **population expansion**
- **reflective practitioner**
- **rehabilitative needs**
- **surgery**

REFERENCES

Black, N., Burke, L., Forrest, C. B., Ravens-Sieberer, U. H., Ahmed, S., Valderas, J. M., Bartlett, S. J., & Alonso, J. (2016). Patient-reported outcomes: Pathways to better health, better services, and better societies. *Quality of Life Research, 25*, 1103–1112.

Cantaert, G. R., Pype, P., Valcke, M., & Lauwerier, E. (2022). Interprofessional identity in health and social care: Analysis and synthesis of the assumptions and conceptions in the literature. *International Journal of Environmental Research and Public Health, 19*(22), 14799. https://doi.org/10.3390/ijerph192214799.

Chen, L. K. (2022). Urbanization and population aging: Converging trends of demographic transitions in modern world. *Archives of Gerontology and Geriatrics, 101*, 104709. https://doi.org/10.1016/j.archger.2022.104709.

Choi, B. C., & Pak, A. W. (2006). Multidisciplinarity, interdisciplinarity and transdisciplinarity in health research, services, education and policy: 1. Definitions, objectives, and evidence of effectiveness. *Clinical Investigation Medicine, 29*(6), 351–364.

Clark, P. G., Cott, C., & Drinka, T. J. (2007). Theory and practice in interprofessional ethics: A framework for understanding ethical issues in health care teams. *Journal of Interprofessional Care, 21*(6), 591–603.

Cowley, D. S., Markman, J. D., Best, J. A., Greenberg, E. L., Grodesky, M. J., Murray, S. B., Corning, K. A., Levy, M. R., & Greenberg, W. E. (2017). Understanding ownership of patient care: A dual-site qualitative study of faculty and residents from medicine and psychiatry. *Perspectives on Medical Education, 6*(6), 405–412. https://doi.org/10.1007/s40037-017-0389-2.

Fewster-Thuente, L., & Velsor-Friedrich, B. (2008). Interdisciplinary collaboration for healthcare professionals. *Nursing Administration Quarterly, 32*(1), 40–48.

Giusti, E. M., Castelnuovo, G., & Molinari, E. (2017). Differences in multidisciplinary and interdisciplinary treatment programs for fibromyalgia: A mapping review. *Pain Research & Management, 2017*, 7261468. https://doi.org/10.1155/2017/7261468.

Gray, M. F., Sweeney, J., Nickel, W., Minniti, M., Coleman, K., Johnson, K., Mroz, T., Forss, B., Reid, R., Frosch, D., & Hsu, C. (2019). Function of the medical team quarterback: Patient, family, and physician perspectives on team care coordination in patient- and family-centered primary care. *The Permanente Journal, 23*, 18–147. https://doi.org/10.7812/TPP/18.147.

International Labour Organization. (2023). *Updating the International Standard Classification of Occupations (ISCO): Draft ISCO-08 Group Definitions: Occupations in Health.* Policy Integration Department Bureau of Statistics. Retrieved from: https://www.ilo.org/public/english/bureau/stat/isco/docs/health.pdf (accessed on 14 March 2025).

Jorie, M. B., Bryan, G., Lacey, L., Gayle, R., Heidi, K., Rand, R., Jennifer, H., Brenna, L., David, M., & Jonathan, N. (2020). Patient-centered care and the electronic health record: Exploring functionality and gaps. *JAMIA Open, 3*(3), 360–368. https://doi.org/10.1093/jamiaopen/ooaa044.

Olson, A. P., Durning, S. J., Fernandez Branson, C., Sick, B., Lane, K. P., & Rencic, J. J. (2020). Teamwork in clinical reasoning—Cooperative or parallel play? *Diagnosis, 7*(3), 307–312.

Pascucci, D., Sassano, M., Nurchis, M. C., Cicconi, M., Acampora, A., Park, D., Morano, C., & Damiani, G. (2021). Impact of interprofessional collaboration on chronic disease management: Findings from a systematic review of clinical trials and meta-analysis. *Health Policy, 125*(2), 191–202.

Singh, R., Volner, K., & Marlowe, D. (2022). Provider burnout. In *StatPearls Publishing*. https://www.ncbi.nlm.nih.gov/books/NBK538330/ (accessed on 14 March 2025).

Stephens, T., Hunningher, A., Mills, H., & Freeth, D. (2016). An interprofessional training course in crises and human factors for perioperative teams. *Journal of Interprofessional Care, 30*(5), 685–688.

Thimbleby, H. (2013). Technology and the future of healthcare. *Journal of Public Health Research, 2*(3), e28. https://doi.org/10.4081/jphr.2013.e28.

Titzer, J. L., Swenty, C. F., & Hoehn, W. G. (2012). An interprofessional simulation promoting collaboration and problem-solving among nursing and allied health professional students. *Clinical Simulation in Nursing, 8*(8), e325–e333.

Tulchinsky, T. H., & Varavikova, E. A. (2014). Human resources for health. In *The New Public Health* (pp. 729–770). https://doi.org/10.1016/B978-0-12-415766-8.00014-8.

United Nations Department of Economic and Social Affairs, Population Division. (2022). *World population prospects 2022: Summary of results* (UN DESA/POP/2022/TR/NO. 3). United Nations. https://www.un.org/development/desa/pd/content/world-population-prospects-2022 (accessed on 14 March 2025).

World Health Organization. (2013). *Inter-Professional Collaborative Practice in Primary Health Care: Nursing and Midwifery Perspectives*. https://apps.who.int/iris/handle/10665/120098 (accessed on 14 March 2025).

CHAPTER 30

Role of Forensic Science in Healthcare

VANDANA PRASAD,[1*] PRASHANT AGRAWAL,[2]
LALIT CHANDRAVANSHI,[2] and DAS ANAMIKA[2]

[1]School of Forensic Sciences, The West Bengal National University of Juridical Sciences, Kolkata, West Bengal, India

[2]Department of Forensic Science, School of Allied Health Sciences, Sharda University, Greater Noida, Uttar Pradesh, India

*Corresponding author

ABSTRACT

Health care is the primary issue in the current scenario. More specifically, the care of patients needs more attention after the COVID-19 phase. All the information regarding their health care, from therapy to medical confidentiality, as well as specific guidelines for health care providers while communicating with the patient, is also recommended since errors in patient treatment and diagnosis are unneglectable. Therefore, this paradigm stresses forensic science's extended role in meeting healthcare needs. Forensic science bridges individual patient health care and their rights to ensure population security. Additionally, it enhances the quality of care and preventive services. The participation of forensic science in health care might help to resolve daily healthcare issues.

30.1 INTRODUCTION

From the past to the present, health care has likely been confronted in the medical field, especially in patient care. It includes patient care from admission to discharge and the various steps of diagnosis; during this phase,

Allied Healthcare in Practice: An Introduction to Integrated Patient Care. Sally Lukose, Karuna Singh (Eds.)

DOI: 10.1201/9781998511037-34

patients require proper health diagnosis and awareness about their treatment, and so forth. However, patients suffer from various unwanted health issues due to a lack of health awareness. Furthermore, the patient database contains the most detailed patient case information. But, sometimes it is misplaced by medical professionals, leading to delays in the proper diagnosis of the patient. Introducing forensic science into the healthcare system will provide a new platform for resolving recent healthcare issues, including patient treatment, quality of care, preventive services, and database management.

These four most common healthcare issues are currently encountered in various hospitals. From diagnosis to the patient's recovery, managing patient data is vital in managing the patient's whole history. Since this step is crucial, it requires careful observation of each piece of patient information. Likewise, awareness of patients about their treatment is one of the main objectives of the healthcare system, followed by awareness of patient rights. The role of forensic science in healthcare can be explained as given in Figure 30.1.

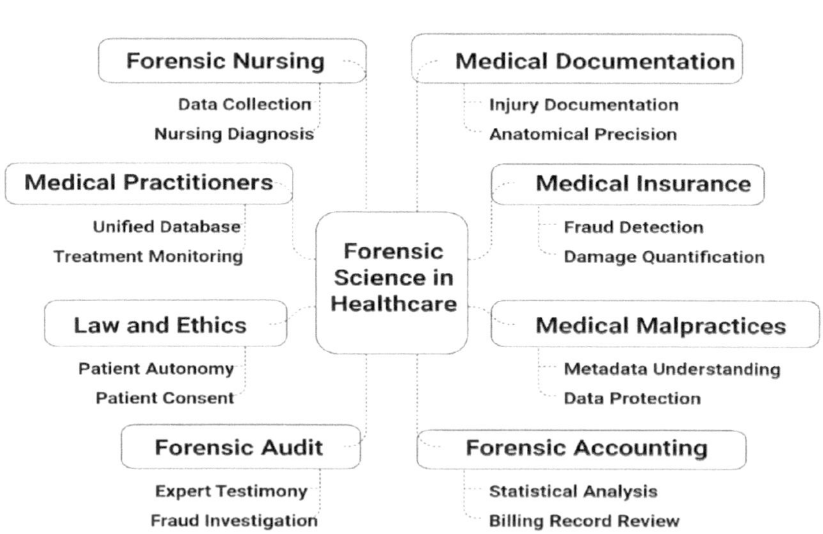
Forensic Nursing
Data Collection
Nursing Diagnosis
Medical Documentation
Injury Documentation
Anatomical Precision
Medical Practitioners
Unified Database
Treatment Monitoring
Medical Insurance
Fraud Detection
Damage Quantification
Forensic Science in Healthcare
Law and Ethics
Patient Autonomy
Patient Consent
Medical Malpractices
Metadata Understanding
Data Protection
Forensic Audit
Expert Testimony
Fraud Investigation
Forensic Accounting
Statistical Analysis
Billing Record Review

FIGURE 30.1 Represents the role of forensic science in health care system.

30.2 ROLE FORENSIC SCIENCE IN HEALTHCARE SYSTEM

30.2.1 FORENSIC SCIENCE WITH MEDICAL PRACTITIONERS

Medical professionals are the frontline workers who primarily serve patient health care. In most cases, the patient requires the immediate attention of medical professionals. However, due to the unavailability of medical professionals, the patient's health suffers from delayed treatment and poor health care. In this situation, some patients encounter poor treatment from fraudulent medical practitioners. Therefore, to assist in adequately treating a patient, cyber forensics can help by providing a unified database of the medical practitioners available during an emergency. In addition, cyber forensics can also monitor the response to the treatment provided to the patient by medical practitioners. The introduction of cyber forensics can facilitate better health outcomes for patients in their treatment and health care.

30.2.2 FORENSIC IN MEDICAL INSURANCE

Medical insurance is a product that covers the medical expenses of an insured patient. However, many companies compensate insured patients for insurance claims rather than fraudsters. The role of forensic accounting in detecting fraud shows a broad potential for estimating medical scams. It can assist the insurer in identifying fraudsters and can also quantify the damages that the policyholder pays. Overall, forensics may assist in reducing the loss for the insurer, preventing fraud, and ensuring the coverage entitled to the policyholder (Chakraborty et al., 2020).

30.2.3 COMPUTER FORENSIC IN MEDICAL MALPRACTICES

Patient medical records, specifically electronic medical records, are manipulated daily, leading to medical malpractice. This occurs when a patient requests a medical test; afterward, the details of the test results are placed in the patient's medical record or metadata. Based on medical test results, physicians prescribe medication to the patient. However, sometimes, these medical reports only show limited available metadata. Therefore, to overcome such situations, forensic computer science can help to understand the intricacies of metadata. It can also safeguard patients' medical reports from unauthorized access, destruction, or tampering. Moreover, through this metadata, which is also known as an audit log, forensic experts can identify who accessed the patient's medical record, when, where, and how. Since this record is automatically captured in the EMR system, it can lead to the successful identification of suspicious individuals (Meyer et al., 2013).

30.2.4 FORENSICS IN LAW AND ETHICS OF PATIENTS

Likewise, ethics in other fields, patient ethics is also a subset of human rights. Patient ethics refers to how patients would like to be treated with medication. Forensics can help maintain patients' ethics with appropriate documentation of the medication prescribed by medical practitioners. It includes various points, as given below (Berkman et al., 2004; Olejarczyk, 2019).

30.2.5 PATIENT AUTONOMY

This refers to the rule of living according to one's will. Additionally, it means that patients at any point can refuse treatment by medical practitioners if there is any act of beneficence. In such cases, there are chances that no paperwork between the patient and medical practitioners is done to inform the patient about the consequences of the medical proceedings. Forensics can ensure transparency between patients and medical practitioners through documentation from consultancy to medication (Berkman et al., 2004; Olejarczyk, 2019). Patient nonmaleficence states that "do not harm the patient." For example, in the process of surgery on a patient, to perform surgery, the surgeon needs to cut the patient's body and also recommend drugs for the same. In this case, the healing of the body cuts requires time. In this situation, the medical practitioner can measure the chance to minimize the harm and inform the patient about the condition for surgery. The introduction of forensics may address the issue of nonmaleficence by providing accurate, verified data on the terms and conditions of the surgical procedure to the patient and their family (Fawcett et al., 2012; Olejarczyk, 2019; Varkey, 2021).

30.2.6 PATIENT CONSENT

Patient consent is the informed consent for surgical or medical procedures. The required material for patient consent documentation includes:

- The process's benefits and risks.
- An assessment of the patient's understanding.
- Alternatives.

Forensic documentation may help the patients to be aware of all the risks and benefits of the medical or surgical procedure (Olejarczyk, 2019; Varkey, 2021).

30.2.7 FORENSIC AUDIT IN HEALTH CARE

The increased population growth leads to reliance on the health industry. Unfortunately, various issues can arise in healthcare, including healthcare businesses like fidelity claims, stocks, cybercrimes, fraud, and so forth. The application of forensic audit can provide expert testimony in lost profit claims, financial loss, and business loss (Darnell, 2018; Fawcett et al., 2012).

The forensic audit can provide healthcare services such as:

- Healthcare issues start from cyber-attacks to pandemics.
- Measuring the impact of insured loss.
- Conducting investigations into transactions of fraud.
- Providing support services in litigation and expert witness testimony.

30.2.8 FORENSIC ACCOUNTING IN HEALTH CARE

Forensic accounting comprises accounting and investigative techniques to identify financial fraud. In addition, it identifies and conducts asset recovery and establishes damage from claims. Recently, in the healthcare system, many frauds have been reported. However, forensic accounting has shown immense potential to assist in healthcare litigation matters such as billing for unnecessary health services, also seen during COVID-19, resulting in increased scams, especially in healthcare, including large amounts of data claims. Likewise, forensic accounting can assist plaintiffs' claims by statistical analysis of data, billing records, and medical records to evaluate the financial damages when a lawsuit is not feasible. This process involves designing and selecting statistical data samples of patient records or billing to assist billing activity and generalize the sample results. Furthermore, forensic accountants can assist medical providers accused of receiving overpayments from any government or private organization by reviewing and analyzing the sample utilized by the organizations. Additionally, it securitizes the sampling process of government or private organizations in the presumptions from claims or frauds (Ellouze et al., 2020; Peabody, 1927).

30.2.9 FORENSIC NURSING

Data collection is a crucial step in patient healthcare. This data assesses the individual's physiological or physical condition and formulates a nursing diagnosis. Forensic nursing incorporates legal aspects into standard nursing diagnosis to evaluate patient situations. The initial assessment includes a physical examination, review of records, and collaboration of the patient with medical staff and other healthcare providers. Once all this information is collected, it is assembled through logical thought patterns to conclude the patient's signs and symptoms. Both interpretation and evaluation are considered the next steps in developing nursing diagnoses in healthcare plans. Furthermore, the patient requires a balance of competing interests like direct care delivery versus the requirement of law and patient confidentiality against society's interests. In a traumatic situation, a patient's medical assessment is quickly done, which leads to legal consequences. However, introducing forensic nursing can render all these and provide rapid assessment and documentation (Darnell, 2018).

30.2.10 MEDICAL DOCUMENTATION

Previously, there was no patient health organization; in such scenarios, nursing documentation was not an essential part of the medical record. Often, the nurse's records were destroyed after the patient's discharge. After some decades, nurse documentation was considered part of the medical record. This step improved the overall healthcare system by providing the sequence of events and details of caregivers. Documentation of injuries is an essential step in the treatment of patients. The following types of injuries are discussed, leading to a better understanding of the injuries on the body portion record (Darnell, 2018). The precise location of the injury using the correct anatomical term.

- Mention on which side of the body was injured.
- Specify the terms, including laceration, abrasion, contusion, stab, and so forth, for different types of injuries.
- Describe and record injuries like shape, size, and color.

- Back up with sketches, diagrams, and photographs of the injuries.
- Wound description is often tricky; therefore, the body diagram can help draw them correctly.

30.3 CONCLUSION

As per previous literature, forensic science plays a vital role in the healthcare system by providing improved data collection and preservation. The combination of forensic science with medical practitioners facilitates better health for the patient in their treatment and healthcare. Likewise, forensic audit helps in the conduction of investigations of transaction fraud. In contrast, forensic nursing provides rapid assessment and documentation. Hence, introducing forensic science in the healthcare system not only leads to accurate patient care but also respects the patient's rights.

KEYWORDS

- **daily healthcare issue**
- **forensic science**
- **health care**
- **health care issues**
- **health care providers**
- **medical confidentiality**
- **medical guidelines**
- **patient treatment**
- **population security**

REFERENCES

Baryamureeba, V., & Tushabe, F. (2004). The enhanced digital investigation process model. *Digital Investigation*.

Bates, D. W. (1996). Medication errors: How common are they and what can be done to prevent them? *Drug Safety, 15*, 303–310.

Berkman, N. D., Wynia, M. K., & Churchill, L. R. (2004). Gaps, conflicts, and consensus in the ethics statements of professional associations, medical groups, and health plans. *Journal of Medical Ethics, 30*(4), 395–401.

Boyd, N. F., Pater, J. L., Ginsburg, A. D., & Myers, R. E. (1979). Observer variation in the classification of information from medical records. *Journal of Chronic Diseases, 32*, 327–332.

Centers for Disease Control and Prevention. (2003). HIPAA privacy rule and public health: Guidance from CDC and the US Department of Health and Human Services. *MMWR: Morbidity and Mortality Weekly Report, 52*, 1–7.

Chakraborty, J., Das, & Roy, I. (2020). Forensic accounting and its applications: Evidence from the Indian life insurance sector. *IUP Journal of Accounting Research & Audit Practices, 19*(2), 7–22.

CHAPTER 31

Forensic Analysis of Medical Records

ISHIKA BHARDWAJ,[1*] SALLY LUKOSE,[2] and ANJALI MALIK[1]

[1]*Department of Forensic Science, Sharda School of Allied Health Sciences, Sharda University, Uttar Pradesh, India*

[2]*Sharda School of Allied Science and Director, Ranking, Sharda University, Greater Noida, India*

*Corresponding author

ABSTRACT

Medical records are used in hospitals and healthcare facilities to assess doctors and patient care, as well as to facilitate communication among a variety of healthcare professionals. Medical records have a variety of other purposes in healthcare facilities, but today patients also value having access to these records, in addition to doctors and other healthcare professionals. This perspective naturally leads to the other requirements for a medical record, such as that it be permanent and attributable. Modern Digital Forensics and Incident Response (DFIR) can be facilitated by incorporating blockchain technology into new platforms. For instance, it is necessary to uphold many current (and new) laws and norms pertaining to authorship, auditing, and the integrity of medical records in an application field like eHealth. In this chapter, we explore the benefits and practical applications of integrating blockchain technology into contemporary DFIR systems. We show how blockchain technology benefits the use of digital forensic models and discuss why law enforcement and incident responders need to be familiar with it. Additionally, chronological recording is necessary for digital evidence to be admissible in a court of law.

Allied Healthcare in Practice: An Introduction to Integrated Patient Care. Sally Lukose, Karuna Singh (Eds.)

DOI: 10.1201/9781998511037-35

31.1 INTRODUCTION

Any study that employs pre-recorded, patient-focused data as the main source of information to address a research issue is referred to as a "medical record review" (MRR). Doctor and nurse notes, ambulance call reports, diagnostic tests (such as electrocardiograms, radiography, and laboratory tests), and records from clinics, businesses, government agencies, and/or computerized databases are some of the sources of information. The scientific record must be "capable of supplying data that are both replicable and valid," just like any other source of data used in scientific inquiry. This crucial aspect is seen to be the main drawback of MRRs (Worster et al., 2004). Medical professionals, clinic settings, and healthcare organizations stand to gain significantly from the use of medical record systems. These systems can streamline processes, enhance the standard of patient care, and increase patient safety (Bates et al., 1996; Elson, 1995; Hunt, 1998; Shea, 1996). The Institute of Medicine has named the use of information technology as one of the key strategies for raising the standard of medical treatment (Lt, 2000). Although the healthcare sector is undergoing a disruptive digital transformation, the incorporation of new technologies is not typically the cause of data breaches involving health information. According to published industry studies, there are still many confirmed data breaches as a result of loss of devices and equipment, misuse, human error, hacking, ransomware attacks, and lack of basic security precautions. Due to its inherent sensitivity, health information is one of the most desirable targets for cybercriminals, but digital investigations of incidents involving health information are frequently hampered by the lack of the necessary infrastructure for forensic readiness. Fortunately for patients and healthcare professionals, the increasing accessibility of the data generated and collected will allow for more precise and quicker clinical and biological measures, including proactive life-saving interventions (Chernyshev et al., 2019). However, it's also believed that cybercriminals find health information to be the most alluring target. A single patient's file may sell on the dark web for several hundred dollars, depending on how thorough the records are (Ryan et al., 2021).

31.1.1 DEFINITION OF HEALTH INFORMATION

Specific consideration must be given to the idea of health information. Health information, medical records, and other phrases are sometimes used virtually interchangeably. We have slightly diverse phrases and concepts that have been used across the many contexts, so there isn't a single, universal definition for health information. Considering the salient similarities between these categories, health information is viewed as:

- Handled in any way, be it digital or physical.
- Related to both physical and mental health, as well as all other facets of individual well-being.
- Associated with previous, ongoing, and upcoming interactions with healthcare providers, and gathered, sent, processed, and kept by a variety of organizations (not only healthcare providers).
- Typically connected to personally identifying information (Koo, 2003; Taylor, 2018; Yip et al., 2017).

31.1.2 A COMPREHENSIVE PATIENT CARE INFORMATION SYSTEM: THREE MODELS

The fact that the medical record is simply one part of a comprehensive patient care information system contributes in part to the assumption that it is more about what was said than what was true. A minimum of three distinct types of information, each with a unique model, will be needed for such a system:

- The information model of the medical record.
- The process model of clinical care.
- The inferred model of the patient's state.

31.2 ADDITIONAL PURPOSES FOR THE MEDICAL RECORD

Any suggested medical record model must be shown to fulfill a number of crucial purposes, which are as follows:

- Population Information for Clinical Evaluation, Research, and Health Service Management (Palmer et al., 2001).
- The requirement for population data to support research, clinical audit, and health care management has been the primary driver behind the adoption of computerized medical records. A single research effort served as the primary motivation for the development of many early record systems, including ARAMIS (Van der Lei et al., 1990).

- The second strategy involves post-hoc comparability establishment. Although there will always be challenges, establishing comparability post hoc necessitates thorough clinical data to have any chance of success. Without specific information, it will be difficult to tell whether a particular patient satisfies the case definitions, let alone if they have any additional traits that would be of interest.
- Furthermore, an analysis's foundation is frequently insufficient when it is just a list of isolated observations. Understanding the causes of an action as well as the specifics of the action is necessary for meaningful medical audit, in particular. This criterion is satisfied by the suggested two-level model, which records decision-making and reasoning as meta observations. Existing systems built on more basic concepts are unable to offer such facilities (Rector et al., 1990).

31.2.1 REASONS AND SENSITIVITY

It is crucial to understand that different levels of sensitivity are connected to health information (Collen et al., 2015). These are based on the perceived effects of the breach on the person's privacy and social well-being, as well as the various types of crimes that might be committed using various categories of health information. Although monetary gain is by far the most frequent motivation, other factors can include curiosity, resentment, and espionage (Widup et al., 2015). It is obvious why people with negative intentions are drawn to health information. Given the variety of crimes that can be committed with such information, the value of health information on the black market is at least 10 to 20 times more than the value of credit card information (Czeschik, 2018).

31.2.2 THREAT SOURCE AND RESPONSE

In contrast, physical incidents like theft and malware-related hacking would typically be attributed to foreign perpetrators. As a result, both internal and external players need to be viewed as equally important groups. Physical crimes, such as the theft of equipment and documents, have historically been a serious problem, but over the past three years, the rate of theft has dramatically decreased. Digital forensic artifacts on stolen devices, like laptops and external storage devices, may reveal whether or not health information was actually accessed by an unauthorized person. As a result, medical data found on stolen devices is presumed to have been compromised by default, and in this study, we do not further explore the digital forensic ramifications of physical threats. Similar to how breaches involving human error are not included in the discussion that follows, it is doubtful that digital investigations would frequently focus on document management, disposal, loss, and publication problems (Chernyshev, 2019; Fries et al., 1972; Langton, 2012).

31.3 INCIDENCES ON DIGITAL FORENSICS

The goal of digital forensics is to obtain evidence that can be used in court by using verified scientific techniques to analyze data on digital devices. Identification, gathering, inspection, analysis, and reporting of evidence are all standard steps in the process of digital forensic investigation. Throughout the entire process, the integrity of the evidence must be maintained in a way that can be independently verified (Baryamureeba et al., 2004). A variety of digital forensic process models (DFPM) are employed to provide structured and documented direction for digital investigations (Cohen, 2010; Kohn et al., 2013). To standardize the terminology used in the forensic process and minimize differences between the various models, the Integrated Digital Forensic Process Model (IDFPM) in particular was proposed (Tan et al., 2001). The addition of the preparation phase, which satisfies the need to develop operational and infrastructure readiness as a crucial component of the process model, is one of the fundamental components of IDFPM. We therefore contend that the healthcare sector may facilitate better results in digital investigations by aiding in the development of the crucial infrastructure-ready elements. Such preparedness would raise the value of the evidence and reduce the costs of the related investigation (Sachowski, 2019). One of the crucial aspects in the deployment of forensic readiness is knowing how to support digital artifact collection and what sources to target (Chernyshev et al., 2019). The most popular kinds of malware are:

- When it comes to misuse, privilege abuse is the biggest worry.
- The most common method employed in social engineering attacks is phishing (Jayabalan, 2017).

31.3.1 PRIVILEGE ABUSE

An organization's service handles health data that is kept in a data store. The majority of health service providers still rely on systems built using conventional client-server designs, despite the fact that emergent architectures to be adopted as part of the digital transformation of healthcare will contain a higher degree of decentralization. In particular, relational database management systems (RDBMS) that can be accessed by local or distant clients are typically used by Electronic Medical Record (EMR) systems. Although role-based access control (RBAC) policies are typically used to limit access to health information, not all EMR systems support policy definitions to the same degree of granularity, and the accuracy of these definitions frequently determines how well RBAC controls work. Additionally, some systems need particular considerations to support open access policies so that emergency situations can be handled more quickly (Jiang, 2018). Accordingly, EMR system users frequently have access to more health information than is necessary based on their role and the context of the patient, as evidenced by the number of breaches brought on by abuse or unauthorized internal access (Vargas et al., 2016).

31.3.2 PHISHING

Phishing defense requires a lot of effort and resources (Hamid et al., 2016). The ability to quickly create new infrastructure and use compromised web servers and botnets to further their campaigns is a benefit enjoyed by phishers. The techniques used to deceive targets into clicking on links and opening infected attachments are also continuously changing. There are numerous methods for identifying phishing emails, including ones that depend on the content, structure, behavior, and hybrid algorithms (Gupta BB et al., 2017). But because phishing attacks are constantly evolving, there are still a lot of problems to solve (King et al., 2017).

31.3.3 FEATURES THAT HELP TO IDENTIFY PHISHING SCAMS

Toolan and Carthy (Conklin et al., 2000) investigated the usefulness of roughly 40 such variables and assessed their efficacy using entropy and information gain. They have categorized common characteristics used for phishing email detection as:

- Features based on the email body are those that are taken from the email. Binary elements like the presence of forms, HTML, or certain words and links in the email content are included.
- Features that can be inferred from the subject of an email include whether it is a response to a prior message and the existence of terms like verify and debit.
- URL-based features: These features check things like if an IP address is used in place of a domain name, the number of images, external and internal links, the number of periods used in links, and more.
- Features that use scripting: These features examine the email for JavaScript, pop-up window code, on Click events, and so forth.
- Features that are specific to the sender, such as the distinction between the sender's address and the reply-to address.

Utilizing a blacklist is a popular method for extracting features from data parts A and B, but doing so is ineffective because blacklists are ineffective against zero-day phishing attempts (Cohen, 2010).

31.4 ELECTRONIC MEDICAL RECORD (EMR) SYSTEM ABUSE

Audit logs are anticipated to contain traces of actions taken by EMR users (or other linked services like programmatic access clients). However, since the standard doesn't have any associated implementation specifications, it can be challenging to compare the logging actions of different implementations because they typically differ.

- First, it's possible that many of the smaller healthcare service providers lack a well-established capability for information security. Additionally, there is a lack of motivation to finance and implement specific information security initiatives that concentrate on the major risks brought on by a lack of auditable activity trails.
- Second, the means to satisfy the need remains up to interpretation in the absence of a formal specification that specifies precisely what events and attributes must be logged, constituting one of the other major problems. As a result, when designing and implementing a solution, system architects must take the concept of

mandatory log events (MLEs) (forensics-enabling activities and actions) into account. Standards, resources, and heuristics-driven techniques are presented for identifying MLEs (Dhamija, 2006).

- Despite several benefits for improving privacy and digital forensics, incorporating forensically sound audit recording capabilities into the EMR system environment is a difficult challenge. There is a chance to provide intelligent solutions that can recognize MLEs based on operations of health information and can maintain the related attributes in a forensically sound manner. These problems encompass both the requirement specification and implementation issues.

31.5 CONCLUSION

The healthcare sector is still very vulnerable to breaches of sensitive health information, despite some revolutionary technical advancements. With the bulk of instances being ascribed to internal perpetrators, the dangers driving frequent healthcare data breaches constitute a distinctive pattern. Although mistakes are frequently made by people, the frequency of privilege abuse brought on by unauthorized access to health information is concerning. We have discussed the consequences for infrastructure forensic readiness with a focus on privilege abuse when it comes to the EMR systems that many healthcare service providers use to manage patient data.

KEYWORDS

- **digital forensics**
- **disease record**
- **doctor assessment**
- **electronic medical record**
- **healthcare facilities**
- **healthcare professionals**
- **incident response**
- **medical records**

REFERENCES

Chernyshev, M., Zeadally, S., & Baig, Z. (2019). Healthcare data breaches: Implications for digital forensic readiness. *Journal of Medical Systems, 43*, 1–2.

Cohen, F. B. (2010). *Digital Forensic Evidence Examination*. Fred Cohen & Associates.

Collen, M. F., & Silva, J. S. (2015). Clinical support information systems (CSISs). In *The History of Medical Informatics in the United States* (pp. 505–524).

Conklin, H. M., Curtis, C. E., Katsanis, J., & Iacono, W. G. (2000). Verbal working memory impairment in schizophrenia patients and their first-degree relatives: Evidence from the digit span task. *American Journal of Psychiatry*, 275–277.

Czeschik, C. (2018). Black market value of patient data. In *Digital Marketplaces Unleashed* (pp. 883–893).

Darnell, C. (2018). Documentation in forensic science in healthcare: Caring for patients, preserving the evidence. In *Forensic Science in Healthcare: Caring for Patients, Preserving the Evidence* (pp. 17–19). CRC Press.

Dhamija, R., Tygar, J. D., & Hearst, M. (2006). Why phishing works. *Proceedings of the SIGCHI Conference on Human Factors in Computing Systems*, 581–590.

Ellouze, N., Rekhis, S., & Boudriga, N. (2020). Forensic investigation of digital crimes in healthcare applications. In *Digital Forensics and Forensic Investigations: Breakthroughs in Research and Practice* (pp. 227–258). IGI Global.

Elson, R. B., & Connelly, D. P. (1995). Computerized patient records in primary care: Their role in mediating guideline-driven physician behavior change. *Archives of Family Medicine, 4*(8), 698–705.

Fawcett, P. J. (2012). Forensic science in healthcare: Caring for patients, preserving the evidence. *AORN Journal, 95*(3), 421–422.

Fries, J. F. (1972). Time-oriented patient records and a computer databank. *JAMA, 222*(12), 1536–1542.

Gupta, B. B., Tewari, A., Jain, A. K., & Agrawal, D. P. (2017). Fighting against phishing attacks: State of the art and future challenges. *Neural Computing and Applications, 28*(12).

Hamid, I. R. A., Samsudin, N. A., Mustapha, A., & Arbaiy, N. (2017). Dynamic trackback strategy for email-born phishing using maximum dependency algorithm (MDA). In *Recent Advances on Soft Computing and Data Mining* (pp. 37–48). Springer.

Hunt, D. L., Haynes, R. B., Hanna, S. E., & Smith, K. (1998). Effects of computer-based clinical decision support systems on physician performance and patient outcomes: A systematic review. *JAMA, 280*, 1339–1346.

Jayabalan, M., & O'Daniel, T. (2017). Continuous and transparent access control framework for electronic health records: A preliminary study. *2017 2nd International Conference on Information Technology, Information Systems and Electrical Engineering (ICITISEE)*.

Jiang, J. X., & Bai, G. (2019). Evaluation of causes of protected health information breaches. *JAMA Internal Medicine, 179*, 265–267.

King, J., Stallings, J., Riaz, M., & Williams, L. (2017). To log, or not to log: Using heuristics to identify mandatory log events—A controlled experiment. *Empirical Software Engineering, 22*(5), 1–34.

Kohn, M. D., Eloff, M. M., & Eloff, J. H. (2013). Integrated digital forensic process model. *Computers & Security, 38*, 103–115.

Langton, L. (2012). Firearms stolen during household burglaries and other property crimes, 2005–2010. *U.S. Department of Justice, Office of Justice Programs, Bureau of Justice Statistics*.

Lt, K. (2000). *To Err is Human: Building a Safer Health system*. Institute of Medicine, Committee on Quality of Health Care in America.

Meyer, J. G., Tomes, J. P., & Neubecker, L. (2013). Electronic medical records: Metadata as evidence in litigation. *Illinois Bar Journal, 101*, 422–424.

Olejarczyk, J. P., & Young, M. (2019). Patient rights and ethics. *StatPearls Publishing*.

Palmer, G. (2001). A road map for digital forensics research—Report from the first Digital Forensics Research Workshop (DFRWS). Utica, New York.

Peabody, F. W. (1927). The care of the patient. *Journal of the American Medical Association, 88*(12), 877–882.

Rector, A. L., Nowlan, W. A., & Kay, S. (1991). Foundations for an electronic medical record. *Methods of Information in Medicine*, 179–186.

Ryan, M. (2021). *Ransomware Revolution: The Rise of a Prodigious Cyber Threat*. Springer.

Sachowski, J. (2019). *Implementing Digital Forensic Readiness: From Reactive to Proactive Process*. CRC Press.

Shea, S., DuMouchel, W., & Bahamonde, L. (1996). A meta-analysis of 16 randomized controlled trials to evaluate computer-based clinical reminder systems for preventive care in the ambulatory setting. *Journal of the American Medical Informatics Association*, 399–409.

Tan, J. (2001). *Forensic Readiness*. Cambridge, MA: @ Stake.

Taylor, M. J., Dove, E. S., Laurie, G., & Townend, D. (2018). When can the child speak for herself? The limits of parental consent in data protection law for health research. *Medical Law Review, 26*, 369–391.

Vander Lei, J., Westerman, R. F., & Mosseveld, B. T. (1990). Critiquing based on automated medical records: An evaluation of HYPERCRITIC. *Medical Informatics Europe '90: Proceedings*, 369–374.

Vargas, J., Bahnsen, A. C., Villegas, S., & Ingevaldson, D. (2016). Knowing your enemies: Leveraging data analysis to expose phishing patterns against a major US financial institution. *2016 APWG Symposium on Electronic Crime Research (eCrime)*.

Varkey, B. (2021). Principles of clinical ethics and their application to practice. *Medical Principles and Practice, 30*(1), 17–28.

Widup, S., Bassett, G., Hylender, D., Rudis, B., & Spitler, M. *Protected Health Information Data Breach Report*.

Worster, A., & Haines, T. (2004). Advanced statistics: Understanding medical record review (MRR) studies. *Academic Emergency Medicine*, 187–192.

Yip, M. (2017). Personal Data Protection Act 2012: Understanding the consent obligation. *Personal Data Protection Digest, 266*.

CHAPTER 32

Legal Issues and Ethical Considerations in Forensic Science and Patient Care

ANJALI MALIK,[1,*] SALLY LUKOSE,[2] ISHIKA BHARDWAJ,[1] and KRISHNA PRASAD ACHARAYA[3]

[1]*Department of Forensic Science, Sharda School of Allied Health Sciences, Sharda University, Greater Noida, Uttar Pradesh, India*

[2]*Sharda School of Allied Science and Director, Ranking, Sharda University, Greater Noida, India*

[3]*University of Cambridge, UK*

*Corresponding author

ABSTRACT

Medical practitioners are specialized professionals bearing the skilled knowledge of medical sciences. Moreover, clinical forensic medicine is a branch of medicine that deals with the investigation of living individuals and is also associated with the assessment of medical findings in the context of the administration of justice. It primarily comprises the examination of victims and suspected perpetrators in various cases, assessment of fitness, and the illegal sharing of patients' personal data/information with the help of artificial intelligence (AI) to third parties, among many other issues. In the past few years, the area of clinical medicine has raised an alarm to seek attention towards the ethical issues encountered in regular medical practices, patient care, clinical forensic medicine, and forensic pathology. Ethics are to be understood as the obligation of a moral nature that governs medical practitioners as well as forensic examiners to follow the code of conduct. The application of sciences associated with the understanding of morality and knowledge of laws related to medical practices and patient

Allied Healthcare in Practice: An Introduction to Integrated Patient Care. Sally Lukose, Karuna Singh (Eds.)

DOI: 10.1201/9781998511037-36

care can be considered under the ethics of clinical forensic medicine. This chapter summarizes various legal considerations and ethical issues commonly encountered in clinical forensic medicine and clinical laboratories in patient care.

32.1 INTRODUCTION

A crucial component of healthcare is the provision of patient care, which is constrained not only by medical knowledge and technical proficiency but also by ethical standards and legal concerns (Beauchamp and Childree, 2019). The duty of preserving patient autonomy, fostering beneficence, and ensuring non-maleficence falls on healthcare personnel (Gillon, 2003). They also have to navigate a tricky legal environment that includes issues like patient rights, privacy, and professional responsibility (Hall et al., 2018). This is to illuminate the difficulties experienced by healthcare practitioners in striking a balance between the provision of high-quality care and ethical and legal requirements (National Institute of Justice, 2013). Moreover, forensic science plays a vital role in identifying offenders, which is highly based on modern investigative techniques to further the cause of justice (Thompson, 2008). Apart from that, there are moral and legal issues that must be taken into account in the realm of forensic science. Forensic scientists must negotiate a difficult terrain of moral dilemmas and legal responsibilities as they examine the evidence, come to conclusions, and present their analysis reports in a court of law (National Institute of Justice, 2013). This chapter examines the moral dilemmas and legal concerns that emerge in the practice of forensic science, illuminating the difficulties faced by specialists in this area.

Both patient care and forensic science depend greatly on ethical questions and legal considerations (Beauchamp and Childress, 2019). When it comes to providing patients with the finest care while respecting their autonomy, privacy, and dignity, ethical issues come into play (Hall et al., 2018). To ensure that healthcare providers follow all applicable rules and regulations while delivering treatment, legal concerns are crucial. When conducting scientific investigations to ascertain the cause and manner of death, identify criminals, and defend the rights of both the accused and the victim, ethical and legal issues come into play (Thompson, 2008). In order to ensure that people are treated accurately and impartially, ethical norms must be used in both medical care and forensic research (Beauchamp and Childress, 2019). Respect for individual liberty, beneficence, non-maleficence, and fairness are some of these ideals. Various laws, rules, and professional standards that set legal duties and give advice on ethical conduct are also applied to both areas (Hall et al., 2018). Healthcare practitioners and forensic scientists must be mindful of ethical problems and legal considerations in their work in this environment. By doing this, they may make sure that they give patients the best treatment possible, uphold the highest ethical and legal standards in their job, and keep the public's trust (Gillon, 2003).

32.2 LEGAL ISSUES IN FORENSIC SCIENCES

Employing the knowledge, techniques, and scientific principles for the purpose of crime scene investigations and legal issues is referred to as forensic science (Saks and Koehler, 2005). It plays an important role in the criminal justice system, facilitating the suspect identification, establishing guilt or innocence, and offering proof for court cases (National Research Council, 2009). To assure fairness, credibility, and accuracy, forensic evidence in courtrooms brings about a variety of legal challenges that are required to be addressed. A key element of the criminal justice system is forensic science, which offers professional testimony and scientific analysis during criminal investigations. However, forensic science is not exempt from legal problems like any other profession. The following are some typical legal problems that might develop in forensic science:

32.2.1 ADMISSIBILITY OF EVIDENCE

The morality of using scientific evidence as evidence in court is one of the major forensic science legal obstacles. Courts employ particular standards, such as the Daubert standard in the U.S., to decide whether scientific evidence is credible and pertinent (Kumho and Carmichael, 1999). If there are questions regarding the forensic expert's scientific validity, dependability, or technique, those questions may raise objections to the admissibility of the forensic evidence (Cole and Villa, 2007).

32.2.2 MISINTERPRETATION OF EVIDENCE

In order to arrive at the findings, forensic scientists must carefully analyze and examine the data (Kaye, 1993). Analysis mistakes or misinterpretations may result in false convictions or the release of guilty people.

If forensic specialists offer biased interpretations, give false testimony, or depend on antiquated or problematic methodology, legal problems may result (Cromwell, 2019).

32.2.3 CONTAMINATION OF EVIDENCE

Forensic evidence can be tainted at any point throughout the investigation, from collection to analysis (National Research Council, 2009). The integrity and dependability of evidence may be jeopardized if it is handled carelessly, kept incorrectly, or tainted with other substances. If defense counsel questions the validity of the evidence owing to alleged tampering, there may be legal repercussions (Saks and Koehler, 2005).

32.2.4 LACK OF QUALITY CONTROL AND STANDARDIZATION

For the sake of accurate and reliable findings, forensic science laboratories should follow strict quality control protocols and standardized procedures. Questions concerning the legitimacy and dependability of forensic evidence may arise due to inadequate quality control processes, a lack of standardization, or a lack of certification (National Research Council, 2009). If the defense casts doubt on the validity of the laboratory or the methods used, legal issues may arise.

32.2.5 BIAS AND SUBJECTIVITY

Forensic scientists are also humans and might be influenced by various personal reasons or subjective interpretations. The impartiality of forensic exams can be impacted by confirmation bias, which occurs when an analyst unconsciously seeks information that supports their previous view (Saks and Koehler, 2008). If bias is suspected, there may be legal repercussions, especially if it affects the validity or objectivity of the evidence (Mnookin, 2018).

32.2.6 ETHICAL CONCERNS

In their work, forensic scientists must uphold ethical standards and guidelines. If there are accusations of misbehavior, such as altering results, biased reporting, or failing to adequately disclose limitations and uncertainties, ethical issues may surface (Chisum and Turvey, 2013). Legal concerns may arise if forensic specialists' objectivity is called into doubt as a result of ethical violations. Moreover, some areas of concern also include the chain of custody and expert witness testimony. The chain of custody refers to the procedure of movement, handling, storage, and receiving of forensic evidence from the time of collection to the point at which it is to be presented in court trials as a documented record (Hall et al., 2018). The act of maintaining the chain of custody plays a vital role in ensuring the integrity and reliability of the forensic evidence to prevent tampering and contamination (Thompson, 2008); failure to do so may raise suspicion regarding the authenticity and admissibility of the evidence (Cromwell, 2019). Furthermore, an expert witness is one who possesses considerable experience and knowledge in a specific discipline. Testimony provided by such a person is termed expert witness testimony. The role of an expert witness is to provide a professional approach to a specific matter of dispute in a court of law by enlightening the facts and opinions based on their scientific expertise (Gillon, 1994). Experts should illustrate their academic qualifications, the methodology followed for the purpose of analysis, and must show the supported published reliable scientific laws and techniques as the basis of their opinions. The admissibility and weight accorded to the forensic evidence in court might be affected by challenges to the credibility or dependability of expert witness testimony (Hall et al., 2018).

32.3 ROLE OF FORENSIC SCIENTIST IN THE LEGAL SYSTEM

Forensic scientists play a vital role in court proceedings by facilitating scientific analysis and expert viewpoints to assist in criminal investigations. Moreover, they apply various scientific principles and techniques to examine and interpret physical evidence retrieved from crime scenes (National Institute of Justice, 2013). Their knowledge may assist in solving crimes by identifying suspects, establishing connections between people and crime scenes, figuring out how they died, and offering important insights (National Research Council, 2009).

32.4 ETHICAL CONSIDERATIONS IN PATIENT CARE

In the healthcare sector, moral concerns are crucial to protecting patients' rights and well-being (Beauchamp and Childress, 2019). The interactions that healthcare workers have with patients and their duties in delivering treatment are constrained by ethical considerations. Informed consent, patient privacy and confidentiality, and the need to report abuse or neglect are three crucial ethical issues in patient care that are covered in this chapter. It also looks at the ethical duties healthcare workers have to respect these standards (Creamer and Austin, 2017; Weise, 2016).

32.4.1 INFORMED CONSENT

The importance of patient autonomy and respect for their ability to make decisions is emphasized by the core ethical concept of informed consent in patient care (Beauchamp and Childress, 2001). It is the procedure through which healthcare professionals educate patients on the benefits, drawbacks, alternatives, and possible results of a particular medical intervention or therapy. This process enables patients to make well-informed choices about their healthcare (Rao, 2008). Obtaining informed consent entails numerous crucial components. First and foremost, healthcare practitioners need to provide consumers with pertinent information in an easy-to-understand way, without using typical medical jargon (Nijhawan et al., 2013). Second, patients should be given the chance to inquire about and get clarity on their available treatment options. Thirdly, patients need to be able to understand the information given and make choices in accordance with their beliefs and preferences.

Appreciating the idea of informed consent uplifts communication and builds trust between patients and healthcare providers (Jefford and Moore, 2008). It also encourages patients' autonomy and self-determination by recognizing the right of patients to diligently participate in their healthcare decisions.

32.4.2 PATIENT PRIVACY AND CONFIDENTIALITY

Confidentiality and privacy of patients are crucial ethical considerations for healthcare practitioners that safeguard patients' crucial information and develop the trust between healthcare professionals and patients (Council on Ethical and Judicial Affairs, 1994). The right of a patient to their personal information refers to the patient's privacy, and the term confidentiality concerns the commitment of healthcare professionals to maintain the privacy of patients' information obtained during treatment (Buppert, 2020). Medical health practitioners are bound to protect patients' privacy by preventing unauthorized access to patient records or information (Act A, 1996). This involves securing electronic health records, maintaining physical security in healthcare settings, and ensuring that only authorized personnel have access to patient information. Moreover, medical practitioners must obtain patient consent prior to disclosing any personal information to third parties, except in legal cases or ethical obligations to report certain information (World Medical Association, 2013).

Preserving patient confidentiality is vital for building and maintaining the privacy of sensitive health information. Healthcare experts ought to exercise caution while discussing patient cases, ensuring that conversations take place in private settings and that information is not disclosed to individuals who are not directly involved in the patient's care. Breaches of patient confidentiality can erode patient trust and compromise the therapeutic relationship, making it essential for healthcare professionals to prioritize the privacy of patient records.

32.4.3 DUTY TO REPORT ABUSE OR NEGLECT

Healthcare professionals have an ethical and legal duty to report suspected cases of abuse or neglect. This responsibility stems from the duty to protect vulnerable individuals and uphold the standards of beneficence and non-maleficence (Barsky, 2017). Abuse and neglect can take various forms, including physical, emotional, sexual, or economic mistreatment, and may arise in healthcare settings or in patients' homes (Beauchamp and Childress, 2001).

When healthcare specialists encounter signs or symptoms of abuse or neglect, they are obligated to report their concerns to the appropriate authorities, including child protective services or adult protective services, depending on the circumstances. Reporting abuse or neglect is essential in ensuring the safety and well-being of vulnerable individuals, as well as holding perpetrators accountable for their actions.

Healthcare professionals must familiarize themselves with local laws and regulations regarding the reporting of abuse or neglect, as failure to report can result in legal and ethical consequences. By fulfilling their duty to report, healthcare professionals contribute to the safety of patients and the prevention of further harm (EG, 2002).

32.5 ETHICAL RESPONSIBILITIES OF HEALTHCARE PROFESSIONALS IN PROVIDING CARE TO PATIENTS

Medical practitioners have innumerable ethical responsibilities in the process of facilitating care to patients. These responsibilities facilitate professional conduct, decision-making, and interactions with patients, families, and other healthcare professionals (Council on Ethical and Judicial Affairs, 1994). The principle of autonomy is one of the core principles of healthcare professionals, where the practitioners ensure to respect the patients' autonomy for informed decision-making regarding treatment, which may include the treatments, risks, benefits, and providing comprehensive information about diagnosis and alternative treatment options. Furthermore, beneficence and non-maleficence are key responsibilities of healthcare professionals, involving the best interests of patients while promoting their health and the norms that obligate medical practitioners to avoid harming and unnecessary harm to them, respectively (Beauchamp and Childress, 2001).

32.5.1 JUSTICE

Medical health practitioners have a responsibility to arrange the distribution of all required health resources in an adequate and equitable way without any sort of discrimination. Healthcare professionals need to ensure that the policies reformed by government agencies provide access to healthcare for all individuals, irrespective of their race, social and financial status, ethnicity, or other factors (Daniels, 1985).

32.5.2 CONFIDENTIALITY

Medical professionals have a fundamental ethical and legal commitment to maintain patients' privacy by not exposing that information without the patient's consent. Any violation of confidentiality can undermine patient confidence, jeopardize the therapeutic alliance, and perhaps lead to further legal actions (Buppert, 2015).

32.5.3 DUTY TO REPORT

In order to protect those who are vulnerable, medical professionals have an ethical and legal duty to report suspected cases/scenarios of abuse or negligence (National Association of Social Workers, 2017). Failure to report such instances may have ethical and legal repercussions.

32.5.4 PROFESSIONAL COMPETENCE AND INTEGRITY

Medical healthcare professionals must retain and regularly refresh their knowledge and abilities to ensure the delivery of effective treatment. Moreover, they must behave truthfully, transparently, and honorably while carrying out their duties morally and in an efficient manner (American Nurse Association, 2015). By adhering to these ethical responsibilities, healthcare professionals can foster trust, ensure high-quality care, and protect the rights and dignity of patients.

32.6 ETHICAL CONSIDERATIONS IN FORENSIC SCIENCE

In the criminal justice system, forensic science plays a vital role by facilitating objective and scientific analysis to aid in the investigation and resolution of criminal cases (Smith, 2017). Forensic practices also raise various ethical considerations that must be carefully addressed. This section of the chapter explores various ethical challenges related to conflicts of interest, bias, the duty to report errors or misconduct, as well as the significance of maintaining objectivity and impartiality in forensic investigations. Furthermore, it enlightens some legal and ethical considerations specific to forensic DNA analysis and forensic mental health evaluation.

32.6.1 CONFLICT OF INTEREST

While conducting analyses, investigations, and providing conclusion reports in court trials, forensic experts are bound to uphold a high level of objectivity and impartiality (Cole and Dioso-Villa, 2015). However, conflicts of interest can arise when forensic experts have personal, financial, or professional relationships with parties involved in the case, such as law enforcement agencies or attorneys. These conflicts can undermine the objectivity and credibility of the scientific evidence presented in court, leading to miscarriages of justice (National Research Council, 2009).

To address the issue of conflicts of interest, various professional organizations, like AAFS (American Academy of Forensic Sciences) and ISFG (International Society for Forensic Genetics), have established ethical guidelines that explicitly discourage forensic professionals from accepting cases where conflicts of interest may arise (AAFS, 2020). Forensic scientists are also encouraged to disclose any potential conflicts before accepting a case to ensure transparency and maintain public trust in the integrity of the forensic proceedings (Cole and Dioso, 2015).

32.6.2 BIASNESS IN FORENSIC ANALYSIS

Bias in the forensic profession can occur at various levels, such as evidence collection, examination, and interpretation (Dror and Cole, 2010). Cognitive bias, contextual bias, and confirmation bias are among the various types that may interfere with forensic examiners' judgment and lead to inaccurate or misleading conclusions (Saks and Koehler, 2005). Forensic scientists must go through extensive training and follow set procedures in order to reduce prejudice (National Research Council, 2009). They should strive to preserve objectivity and impartiality throughout their examination, and they should be mindful of the possible effects of bias on their analysis and interpretation. Any possible biases can be found and corrected with the assistance of peer review and independent findings verification (Dror and Cole, 2010).

32.6.3 DUTY TO REPORT ERRORS OR MISCONDUCT

It is the professional responsibility of forensic scientists to disclose any mistakes or unethical behavior found in their own or their colleagues' work (Kaye and Bero, 2000). For forensic evidence to be accurate and reliable, mistakes must be reported. False convictions might result from failure to report mistakes or misconduct, which would undermine the credibility of forensic science as a whole (Saks and Koehler, 2008).

The American Society of Crime Laboratory Directors (ASCLD) and the American Board of Criminalistics (ABC), two professional associations and certifying bodies, have devised processes for disclosing errors and fostering a culture of continual improvement in forensic practices (ABC, n.d.; ASCLD, n.d).

32.6.4 IMPORTANCE OF OBJECTIVITY AND IMPARTIALITY

Objectivity and impartiality are key principles in the forensic science profession. Forensic scientists should solely focus on the scientific evidence and must resist external influences, such as the need to uphold a specific theory or the need for a conviction (Kaye, 2016). Objectivity requires forensic scientists to remain unbiased and open-minded throughout the investigation and examination process (Saks and Koehler, 2008).

To promote the act of objectivity, forensic scientists must be provided with adequate resources, training, and autonomy (Saks and Koehler, 2008). Moreover, blind and double-blind testing protocols must be adopted in regular laboratory practices to avoid bias and undue influence in forensic analysis.

32.6.5 LEGAL AND ETHICAL CONSIDERATIONS IN FORENSIC DNA ANALYSIS

Out of various forensic divisions, the forensic DNA division bears the utmost importance and is considered a powerful tool for identifying suspects, exonerating the innocent, and linking perpetrators to crime scenes (Budowle et al., 2009). But along with its evident advantages, using DNA evidence also raises a number of ethical issues that need to be carefully considered in order to assure justice, privacy, and the preservation of people's rights. The following are some significant ethical issues in forensic DNA analysis:

1. **Privacy and Informed Consent:** The collection and storage of genetic material without sufficient informed permission is one of the main ethical issues in forensic DNA analysis (Greely, 2018). DNA samples are taken from crime scenes, suspects, and even people who aren't necessarily connected to a case, which raises concerns about the level of permission and awareness people have regarding the usage of their genetic data. It is vital to strike a balance between the necessity for efficient inquiry and the protection of human autonomy and privacy rights.

2. **Discrimination and Stigmatization:** Using DNA analysis to predict physical characteristics or health concerns may unintentionally result in stigmatization and prejudice. For instance, predictive DNA phenotyping makes assumptions about physical traits like eye color or facial features based on DNA data (Sankar and Cho, 2002). This might possibly have an influence on how suspects are recognized and handled, leading to racial profiling or other types of prejudice.
3. **Familial DNA Searching:** The process of finding prospective relatives of a suspect based on their genetic profiles is known as familial DNA searching (NRC, 2010). While it has the potential to be a powerful tool for solving crimes, it also raises issues about the privacy and rights of innocent family members whose genetic information may be exploited without their consent or knowledge.
4. **Data Security and Retention:** Preventing unauthorized access and potential exploitation of genetic data requires maintaining a safe and private DNA database (Kaye et al., 2016). To prevent lengthy monitoring and the possibility of data breaches, it is crucial to provide effective data retention regulations, especially for innocent people or those whose cases have been successfully concluded.
5. **Accuracy and Reliability:** When DNA evidence is viewed as infallible, it raises ethical questions and increases the possibility of erroneous convictions. To prevent injustices, it is essential to ensure the precision and dependability of DNA analysis through appropriate procedures, validation, and open reporting (Thompson, 2003).
6. **Racial and Ethical Bias:** The composition of DNA databases may not be indicative of the diversity of the community, thus leading to racial and ethnic biases in forensic analysis (Budowle et al., 2009). Due to genetic similarities, this might lead to discrepancies in identifying criminals or erroneously accusing innocent people.
7. **Unintended Consequences of DNA Evidence:** While DNA evidence can be used to identify criminals, it can also reveal unexpected facts about individuals, such as unreported paternity or health risks (NRC, 1996). This can have serious emotional,

family, and social consequences, prompting ethical concerns when dealing with such sensitive material.

8. **Transparency and Expert Testimony:** The presentation of DNA evidence in court necessitates the clear and accessible exposition of complicated scientific ideas (Thompson, 2003). Ethical issues include ensuring that expert witnesses appropriately express the limitations and uncertainties of DNA analysis in order to avoid juries from placing excessive faith in the evidence.
9. **International Collaboration and Harmonization:** Forensic DNA analysis frequently requires cross-border collaboration, each with its own legal and ethical framework (Thompson, 2003). Establishing uniform norms and processes to guarantee the appropriate and respectful use of genetic information across countries is one of the ethical issues.
10. **Continuous Education and Awareness:** Forensic DNA analysis ethics necessitate continuing education and understanding among experts, legislators, and the general public (Greely, 2018). It is critical to stay up to date on the newest advances, problems, and potential repercussions of DNA analysis in order to develop ethical practices.

In short, while forensic DNA analysis provides significant advances in criminal justice, the ethical implications of its usage must not be neglected. To ensure the competent and ethical use of DNA evidence in the pursuit of justice, it is critical to strike a balance between effective inquiry, individual rights, and societal concerns.

32.7 LEGAL AND ETHICAL CONSIDERATIONS IN FORENSIC MENTAL HEALTH EVALUATION:

Forensic mental health evaluations are frequently performed to determine a defendant's ability to stand trial, mental condition at the time of the offense, or danger of future violence (Rogers and Shuman, 2000). Evaluators must strike a balance between their duty as therapists and their legal responsibilities. When physicians are expected to deliver an opinion that corresponds with the objectives of the prosecution or defense rather than giving an impartial assessment of the defendant's mental health, ethical issues may develop (Zapf and Roesch, 2009). Evaluators must preserve their professional integrity and impartiality in such circumstances, concentrating on accurate and balanced reporting (Melton et al., 2007). To maintain the discipline's integrity and legitimacy, ethical issues are critical in forensic science. Conflicts of interest, prejudice, the obligation to report errors, and the significance of objectivity and impartiality are all important considerations for forensic scientists (Saks and Koehler, 2008). The implementation of these principles in forensic DNA analysis and forensic mental health examinations is equally important in order to guarantee justice is served, individual rights are protected, and public faith in the criminal justice system is maintained (Committee on Identifying the Needs of the Forensic Science Community et al., 2009). Professional norms and ongoing education can assist forensic specialists in maintaining the highest ethical standards and contributing to the fair administration of justice.

32.8 CONCLUSION

The intersection of medical practices, patient care, clinical forensic medicine, and forensic science emphasizes the ethical and legal obligations that these areas entail (Bach and Brown, 2010). Because of the complexities of patient care, medical practitioners must manage difficult ethical concerns such as informed consent, patient privacy, and the obligation to report abuse or neglect. These values emphasize patient autonomy, confidentiality, and the critical importance of ensuring patients' well-being and safety (Beauchamp and Childress, 2001). Healthcare workers are responsible for respecting these ethical commitments in order to create trust, provide effective treatment, and maintain the highest moral standards. Similarly, forensic science and its different subdivisions, such as clinical forensic medicine and forensic mental health assessments, operate under a complicated legal framework that creates ethical quandaries (Saks and Koehler, 2005). Forensic practitioners are concerned about conflicts of interest, prejudice, the need to report mistakes, and the maintenance of impartiality (Melton et al., 2007). The ethical use of forensic science is critical to ensuring that justice is delivered fairly, preserving public trust, and sustaining the legal system's integrity. Forensic DNA analysis, a critical component of modern criminal investigations, exemplifies the delicate balance between privacy, accuracy, and public interests. To guarantee appropriate use of genetic information, ethical considerations like privacy, possible discrimination, family DNA searches, and data security must be addressed (Budowle et al., 2009). Maintaining transparency, safeguarding expert testimony credibility, and promoting international collaboration are critical in navigating the changing world of forensic DNA analysis. By analyzing individuals' mental states and possible hazards, forensic mental health evaluations help to ensure fair legal procedures. Despite external constraints, assessors' ethical commitments to deliver unbiased evaluations emphasize the need for objectivity and impartiality in judicial proceedings. Maintaining these ethical values guarantees that people with mental illnesses are treated fairly and that their rights are protected within the legal system (Rogers and Shuman, 2000). This chapter intertwined the areas of medical practices, patient care, and forensic science with ethical and legal problems that must be handled with vigilance. While each sector has its own set of obstacles, they all have a common thread of professionalism, ethics, and patient-centered care. By adhering to these ethical values and legal norms, healthcare professionals and forensic specialists help to create a more just society by protecting individuals' rights, fostering trust, and ensuring that justice is administered impartially and fairly.

KEYWORDS

- **clinical forensic medicine**
- **credibility of forensic science**
- **forensic mental health assessments**
- **forensic practitioners**
- **forensic science**
- **forensic scientists**
- **healthcare workers**
- **patient autonomy**
- **professional responsibility**
- **scientific evidence**

REFERENCES

Act, A. (1996). *Health Insurance Portability and Accountability Act of 1996*, Public Law 104–191.

American Academy of Forensic Sciences. (n.d.). *Code of Ethics*. Retrieved from: https://www.aafs.org/ethics/code-of-ethics/ (accessed on 14 March 2025).

American Association of Nurse Practitioners. (2018). *Code of Ethics for Nurse Practitioners*. Retrieved from: https://www.aanp.org/advocacy/advocacy-resource/position-statements/code-of-ethics-for-nurse-practitioners (accessed on 14 March 2025).

American Board of Criminalistics. (n.d.). *Mission and Goals*. Retrieved from: https://abc.criminalistics.com/mission-and-goals/ (accessed on 14 March 2025).

American Nurses Association. (2015). *Code of Ethics for Nurses with Interpretive Statements*.

American Society of Crime Laboratory Directors. (n.d.). *About ASCLD*. Retrieved from: https://www.ascld.org/about-us/ (accessed on 14 March 2025).

Barsky, A. (2017). Ethics alive! The 2017 NASW code of ethics: What's new. *New Social Worker*.

Beauchamp, T. L., & Childress, J. F. (2001). *Principles of Biomedical Ethics* (5th ed.). Oxford University Press.

Beauchamp, T., & Childress, J. (2019). Principles of biomedical ethics: Marking its fortieth anniversary. *The American Journal of Bioethics, 19*(11), 9–12.

Budowle, B., Moretti, T. R., Niezgoda, S. J., & Brown, B. L. (2009). Forensic aspects of mass disasters: Strategic considerations for DNA-based human identification. *Legal Medicine, 11*(6), 283–289.

Buppert, C. (2015). *Nurse Practitioner's Business Practice and Legal Guide* (5th ed.). Jones & Bartlett.

Buppert, C. (2020). *Nurse Practitioner's Business Practice and Legal Guide*. Jones & Bartlett Learning.

Chisum, W. J., & Turvey, B. E. (n.d.). Ethical issues in forensic examination. In *Ethical Justice: Applied Issues for Criminal Justice Students and Professionals* (p. 219).

Cole, S. A., & Dioso-Villa, R. (2007). Forensic science and the *Daubert* test: The demise of the "general acceptance" standard. *EMBO Reports, 8*(4), 306–310.

Cole, S. A., & Dioso-Villa, R. (2015). Forensic science reform: Protecting the innocent. *American Criminal Law Review, 52*(3), 475–536.

Council on Ethical and Judicial Affairs. (1994). *Code of Medical Ethics: Current Opinions with Annotations*. American Medical Association.

Creamer, A. M., & Austin, W. (2017). Canadian nurse practitioner core competencies identified: An opportunity to build mental health and illness skills and knowledge. *The Journal for Nurse Practitioners, 13*(5), e231–e236.

Cromwell, P. (2019). Forensic science misconduct: Compromised forensic evidence and wrongful convictions. *Cogent Social Sciences, 5*(1), 1607616.

Daniels, N. (1985). *Just Health Care*. Cambridge University Press.

Dror, I. E., & Cole, S. A. (2010). The vision in "blind" justice: Expert perception, judgment, and visual cognition in forensic pattern recognition. *Psychonomic Bulletin & Review, 17*(2), 161–167.

Gillon, R. (1994). Medical ethics: Four principles plus attention to scope. *BMJ, 309*(6948), 184.

Gillon, R. (2003). Medical ethics: Four principles plus attention to scope. *BMJ, 326*(7384), 788–791.

Hall, M. A., Orentlicher, D., Bobinski, M. A., Bagley, N., & Cohen, I. G. (2018). *Health Care Law and Ethics*. Aspen Publishing.

Jefford, M., & Moore, R. (2008). Improvement of informed consent and the quality of consent documents. *The Lancet Oncology, 9*(5), 485–493.

K., E. G. (2002). *World Report on Violence and Health*. World Health Organization.

Kaye, D. H. (1993). *The Double-Edged Helix: Science in the Courtroom*. Harvard University Press.

Kaye, D. H. (2000). The American Law Institute's Model Penal Code: A new resource for understanding and reforming forensic science. *Wisconsin Law Review, 2000*(2), 465–552.

Kaye, D. H. (2016). The double helix and the law of evidence. *Jurimetrics, 56*(2), 165–182.

Kumho Tire Co. v. Carmichael, 526 U.S. 137 (1999).

Mnookin, J. L. (2018). The validity and admissibility of forensic evidence: The need for robust scrutiny and gatekeeping. *Annual Review of Criminology, 1*, 453–476.

National Association of Social Workers. (2017). *NASW Code of Ethics*. National Association of Social Workers.

National Institute of Justice. (2013). *Forensic Science: A Time of Transformation*. Retrieved from: https://www.ncjrs.gov/pdffiles1/nij/243296.pdf (accessed on 14 March 2025).

National Research Council. (1996). *The Evaluation of Forensic DNA Evidence*. National Academies Press.

National Research Council. (2010). *Strengthening Forensic Science in the United States: A Path Forward*. National Academies Press.

Nijhawan, L. P., Janodia, M. D., Muddukrishna, B. S., Bhat, K. M., Bairy, K. L., Udupa, N., & Musmade, P. B. (2013). Informed consent: Issues and challenges. *Journal of Advanced Pharmaceutical Technology & Research, 4*(3), 134.

Rao, K. S. (2008). Informed consent: An ethical obligation or legal compulsion. *Journal of Cutaneous and Aesthetic Surgery, 1*(1), 33.

Rogers, R., & Shuman, D. W. (2000). *Conducting Insanity Evaluations* (2nd ed.). Guilford Press.

Saks, M. J., & Koehler, J. J. (2005). The coming paradigm shift in forensic identification science. *Science, 309*(5736), 892–895.

Saks, M. J., & Koehler, J. J. (2008). The individualization fallacy in forensic science evidence. *Vanderbilt Law Review, 61*(1), 199–219.

Sankar, P., & Cho, M. K. (2002). Toward a new vocabulary of human genetic variation. *Science, 298*(5597), 1337–1338.

Smith, C. (2017). Forensic science in court: Challenges in the twenty-first century. *Legal Information Management, 17*(3), 186–193.

Thompson, W. C. (2003). DNA, forensics, and the law. *Genetics in Medicine, 5*(2), 165–167.

Thompson, W. C. (2008). Forensic science and ethical trade-offs. *Nature Education, 1*(1), 135.

Weise, M. V. (2016). Medical ethics made easy. *Professional Case Management, 21*(2), 88–94.

World Medical Association. (2013). World Medical Association Declaration of Helsinki: Ethical principles for medical research involving human subjects. *JAMA, 310*(20), 2191–2194.

CHAPTER 33

Overview of Ethical and Legal Issues in Healthcare

AMIT PRATAP SINGH CHOUHAN,[1,*] ANKUSH VERMA,[2] VANDANA SINGH,[3] KRITI SACHAN,[4] and PREETI PAL[4]

[1]*Department of Radiology, School of Allied Health Sciences, Galgotias University, Greater Noida, Uttar Pradesh, India*

[2]*Department of Radiology, Sharda School of Allied Health Sciences, Sharda University, Greater Noida, Uttar Pradesh, India*

[3]*Department of Microbiology, Sharda School of Allied Health Sciences, Sharda University, Greater Noida, Uttar Pradesh, India*

[4]*Department of Physiotherapy, Sharda School of Allied Health Sciences, Sharda University, Greater Noida, Uttar Pradesh, India*

*Corresponding author

ABSTRACT

Healthcare is a complex and evolving field that constantly grapples with a multitude of ethical and legal challenges. This chapter provides an overview of key ethical and legal issues in healthcare, shedding light on their significance and impact on patient care, healthcare professionals, and the broader healthcare system. Ethical dilemmas in healthcare are pervasive, encompassing issues such as patient autonomy, informed consent, end-of-life decision-making, and resource allocation. Balancing the rights of patients to make decisions about their own care with the duty of healthcare professionals to provide the best possible treatment can be challenging. These ethical and legal concerns have significant consequences for patient care. Failing to address them adequately can result in suboptimal care,

Allied Healthcare in Practice: An Introduction to Integrated Patient Care. Sally Lukose, Karuna Singh (Eds.)

DOI: 10.1201/9781998511037-37

patient dissatisfaction, and potential lawsuits, which can have profound implications for both patients and healthcare providers. The importance of ongoing education and training for healthcare professionals, robust institutional policies, and a comprehensive understanding of healthcare ethics and legal principles is essential to ensure the delivery of high-quality, ethical, and legally compliant care in the ever-evolving landscape of healthcare.

33.1 INTRODUCTION

In the complex and multifaceted world of healthcare, ethical and legal considerations are not just academic concepts; they are the lifeblood that sustains the profession and ensures the well-being of patients and the integrity of the healthcare system. The significance of ethical and legal issues in healthcare is profound, extending far beyond theoretical discussions into the very fabric of patient care, professional practice, and societal trust. This 1000-word exploration delves into the paramount importance of these issues, shedding light on their multifaceted significance in the contemporary healthcare landscape.

Respect for autonomy is a basic value that forms the basis of healthcare ethics. Each person has inherent value and the freedom to make informed decisions about their personal health and medical treatment, according to this idea. Patients anticipate that their independence will be honored and preserved when they entrust healthcare providers with their well-being. It is impossible to overestimate the importance of this ethical basis since it gives patients the ability to actively engage in their treatment, promoting a sense of ownership as well as authority over their health outcomes (Alus, 2016).

When the concept of beneficence—which emphasizes the duty of healthcare personnel to act in the highest possible interest of their patients—converges with the idea of autonomy, practical ethical dilemmas frequently arise. These ethical dilemmas can be gut-wrenching, such as when a patient with a terminal illness wishes to forego treatment, even if it means a shorter lifespan, in favor of a more peaceful and pain-free existence. In such cases, healthcare professionals must navigate the delicate balance between respecting the patient's autonomy and striving to maximize their well-being, highlighting the ethical tightrope they walk daily.

Furthermore, ethical considerations extend to the realm of end-of-life decision-making. The evolving field of medical technology has granted healthcare providers unprecedented power to prolong life, raising profound ethical questions about the appropriateness and futility of certain treatments. Decisions about withholding or withdrawing life-sustaining treatments, such as ventilators or artificial nutrition and hydration, are ethically fraught and require careful deliberation. In these emotionally charged situations, ethical principles guide clinicians in ensuring that patients' wishes, values, and best interests are paramount (Akdeniz et al., 2021).

Resource allocation poses yet another ethical challenge in healthcare. With limited resources, including personnel, facilities, and funds, difficult decisions must be made about how to allocate these resources equitably. Distributive justice and other ethical frameworks are essential in directing these choices and guaranteeing that resources are distributed equitably to optimize benefits for the largest number of patients. However, these choices are not without controversy, as they frequently require a delicate balancing act, setting one patient's needs against another's. Legal issues are just as important in the healthcare industry as ethical ones. Protection of patient rights, guaranteeing the standard of treatment, and holding healthcare practitioners accountable for their actions are all made possible by laws and regulations. Informed consent is a cornerstone of healthcare legislation, requiring providers to fully disclose to patients all relevant information regarding their illness, available treatments, associated risks, and potential benefits. Since informed consent gives patients the freedom to make choices based on their knowledge and moral principles, it is important as it is a fundamental component of patient autonomy (Ballard, 2003).

Healthcare legislation places a high priority on patient rights and privacy, which uphold the values of non-discrimination and confidentiality. Patients' private medical information is strongly protected under these rights, and it must be kept private and secure. This shows how important these rights are legally. In addition, rules against discrimination guarantee that everyone is treated fairly, regardless of their gender, color, disability, or other protected traits (Gray and Yousuf, 2018).

Another important aspect of healthcare law is medical malpractice, which provides a legal framework for holding medical personnel accountable for their negligent conduct when they cause injury to patients. Medical malpractice laws are important because they give harmed individuals a way to seek compensation and because they operate as a deterrent to healthcare professionals adhering to the highest levels of care (Frakes and Anupam, 2016).

Legal rules are essential to preserving the security of the healthcare system, as fraud and abuse in the medical field is a widespread issue in the sector. Overusing services, accepting bribes, and engaging in fraudulent billing can result in exorbitant expenses and jeopardize patient care. It is clear from their ability to prevent and penalize such unethical actions how important fraud and abuse regulations in healthcare are. Given how closely these two fields are related, the interaction of ethics and legislation in the healthcare industry is critical. Laws and regulations pertaining to healthcare are frequently shaped by ethical rules and concepts, which reflect the values and aspirations of society. On the other hand, laws offer a framework for upholding moral principles and ensuring they are enforced in real life. The importance of their interwoven nature is further reinforced by the fact that this symbiotic relationship forms the basis of ethical and legal issues in healthcare (Jesilow and Bryan, 2016).

Considered from the perspective of patient care, the importance of moral and legal concerns in healthcare becomes even more apparent. There are many possible outcomes, some of which can be quite serious, if these intricate concerns are not handled with care and tact. Defects in ethics have the potential to damage patient confidence, which can lower satisfaction and treatment plan adherence. Patients may experience a loss of empowerment and alienation from making their own healthcare choices when their autonomy is ignored or infringed. This emphasizes even more how important it is to follow ethical standards in patient care since it can have significant psychological and emotional effects (Pozgar, 2023).

However, there might be dire repercussions for healthcare organizations and professionals if there are legal infractions. If validated, allegations of medical malpractice may lead to significant monetary fines, harm to one's professional standing, and, in the worst situations, license suspension. The viability of healthcare institutions may be jeopardized by legal proceedings brought against them for fraud or misuse, which can result in expensive penalties and criminal prosecutions (Kroger, 2023).

Ethical and legal issues also have a big influence on the actual quality of patient treatment. Following ethical guidelines increases the likelihood that medical personnel will treat patients with patient-centered care that is in line with their values and preferences. Furthermore, moral and legal requirements place a high value on the quality of care, guaranteeing that patients receive therapies that are safe, efficient, and supported by evidence. The wider healthcare system is affected by ethical and legal challenges in addition to the care of individual patients. When it comes to the distribution of scarce resources, such as ventilator support during a global outbreak or organ transplants, ethical precepts and regulatory requirements play a significant role. These choices, which are influenced by ideas such as distributive justice, have an effect on the healthcare system's overall efficacy and equity. Healthcare policies and regulations are influenced by the ethical and legal framework of the healthcare system, which has an impact on everything from health insurance and compensation to the establishment of healthcare infrastructure. There is no denying the importance of legal and ethical issues in the healthcare industry, which affect all facets of the field as well as its larger ecosystem. Patients' autonomy is supported by ethical standards, which also serve as a framework for difficult decisions and protect people's rights and dignity. Laws and regulations pertaining to healthcare also offer a legal framework that upholds patient rights, guarantees high-quality treatment, and holds healthcare practitioners accountable for their actions. The complex relationship between ethics and legislation acts as a vital compass for medical practitioners, directing them towards the provision of exceptional patient care while preserving the integrity of the system as a whole. These concerns are not just theoretical; they are fundamental to the way healthcare is practiced every day and ultimately impact the standard of treatment patients receive as well as their level of faith in the medical community (McLean and John, 2003).

33.2 UNDERSTANDING ETHICAL ISSUES IN HEALTHCARE

Understanding ethical issues in healthcare is essential for healthcare professionals, policymakers, and patients alike. The investigation and implementation of ethical and moral standards in the framework of medical practice and decision-making is known as ethics in healthcare. It all comes down to treating patients fairly and honorably while maintaining the standards of professionalism and integrity in the healthcare system. Important ethical precepts include beneficence, which highlights the obligation to do good for patients; non-maleficence, which requires the prevention of harm; justice, which calls for a just distribution of healthcare resources; and autonomy, which upholds a patient's right to make an informed decision about their own care. The conflict between patient autonomy and safety is one of the many ethical conundrums that face the medical field.

This is particularly true when treatment alternatives are scarce or divisive. Healthcare practitioners have a difficult time navigating these complicated ethical dilemmas while upholding their duty to give their patients the best treatment possible (Luyckx et al., 2017).

33.2.1 DEFINITION OF ETHICS IN HEALTHCARE

A healthcare professional's conduct, decisions, and actions, as well as those of organizations and stakeholders in the field, are guided by a set of moral principles and ideals known as ethics. The field of ethics in question pertains to the particular ethical predicaments and obligations that arise in the healthcare industry. Fundamental ideas like respect for patient freedom, the requirement to act in good faith (beneficence), the duty to act in a way that does not harm others (non-maleficence), and the right and equal distribution of the limited resources available for healthcare (justice) are all included in these principles. The broad scope of healthcare ethics also includes topics like truth-telling, privacy for patients, informed consent, and end-of-life care, demonstrating the complexity of ethical dilemmas in this setting. Ethics in healthcare serves as a guiding framework to ensure that healthcare practices prioritize the well-being and dignity of patients while maintaining the highest standards of professionalism and integrity among healthcare providers and institutions (Aita et al., 2005).

33.3 ETHICAL PRINCIPLES AND FRAMEWORKS

Ethical principles and frameworks form the philosophical underpinnings that guide decision-making and behavior in the field of healthcare. These principles provide a structured approach to addressing complex moral dilemmas and ensuring ethical conduct. Four fundamental ethical principles widely recognized in healthcare (as shown in Figure 33.1) are autonomy, beneficence, non-maleficence, and justice.

33.3.1 AUTONOMY

Autonomy emphasizes respecting an individual's right to make informed decisions about their own medical care, ensuring that patients have the freedom to choose and control their healthcare choices.

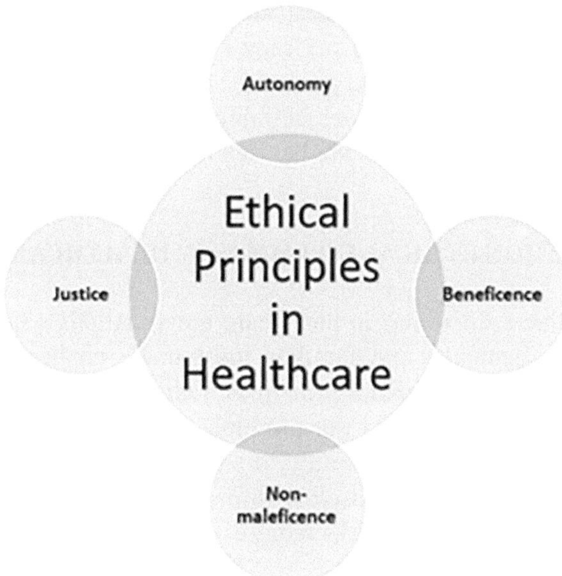

FIGURE 33.1 Showing the ethical principles in healthcare.

33.3.2 BENEFICENCE

Beneficence underscores the moral obligation to act in the best interests of patients, promoting their well-being, and striving to maximize positive outcomes in medical care.

33.3.3 NON-MALEFICENCE

Non-maleficence emphasizes the duty to do no harm and requires healthcare professionals to prioritize the avoidance of harm or minimizing potential risks to patients.

33.3.4 JUSTICE

Justice revolves around fairness and equity in healthcare resource allocation, ensuring that limited resources are distributed impartially and that all patients receive the care they need without discrimination. These ethical principles serve as a framework for healthcare professionals and organizations to navigate challenging ethical issues, make ethically sound decisions, and uphold the highest standards of ethical conduct while providing care to patients. Ethical frameworks, such as the four principles approach or virtue ethics, help guide the application of these principles to real-world healthcare scenarios, facilitating ethical decision-making in a complex and evolving healthcare landscape (Peter et al., 2020).

33.4 COMMON ETHICAL DILEMMAS IN HEALTHCARE

Common ethical dilemmas in healthcare are situations where healthcare professionals, patients, and families must make challenging decisions that involve conflicting moral principles. One such dilemma is the issue of informed consent, where the principle of patient autonomy clashes with the healthcare provider's duty to ensure the patient's best interests. Deciding when and how to disclose information about a diagnosis, treatment options, and potential risks requires a delicate balance.

1. **Informed Consent:** Informed consent is a fundamental ethical and legal concept in healthcare that ensures patients have the right to make informed decisions about their medical treatment and care. It is based on the ethical principle of autonomy, which respects an individual's right to self-determination and the freedom to choose what happens to their own body.
2. **End-of-Life Care:** End-of-life care presents another ethical challenge, particularly in situations where the patient's wishes may conflict with the desire to prolong life at all costs. The ethical principle of beneficence, which aims to promote the patient's well-being, may conflict with the patient's right to refuse life-sustaining treatment or request physician-assisted dying.
3. **Resource Allocation:** Resource allocation is a recurring ethical dilemma, especially in healthcare systems with limited resources. Decisions about who receives access to scarce resources such as organ transplants, ventilators, or critical care beds often invoke the principle of justice, as healthcare professionals must allocate resources fairly while considering the medical needs of all patients.
4. **Confidentiality:** Maintaining patient confidentiality in the digital age is an ethical concern. Striking a balance between the patient's

right to privacy and the need for electronic health records and data sharing for improved care coordination can be challenging.

5. **Truth-Telling:** Truth-telling is another ethical dilemma, particularly when delivering difficult news or disclosing errors. The ethical principle of truth-telling may conflict with the goal of minimizing harm or respecting a patient's wishes to remain unaware of certain information.

To guarantee that patients' best interests are maintained while honoring their autonomy and rights, these frequent ethical conundrums in healthcare emphasize the necessity of giving ethical principles serious thought, keeping lines of communication open, and frequently including interdisciplinary teamwork (Brown, 2020).

33.5 ROLE OF HEALTHCARE PROFESSIONALS IN ETHICAL DECISION-MAKING

Due to their position at the forefront of patient care and frequent encounters with difficult moral decisions requiring thought and judgment, healthcare workers play a critical role in ethical decision-making. These healthcare professionals, who include physicians, nurse practitioners, therapists, and other staff members, have a variety of responsibilities when it comes to maintaining moral principles, honoring patient autonomy, and providing the highest quality of care.

33.5.1 PATIENT ADVOCACY

Advocates for the rights and welfare of their patients are healthcare professionals. This advocacy also includes making sure that during the decision-making process, patients' opinions are acknowledged and their wishes are honored. They have a duty to act in their patients' best interests, putting their welfare and health first at all times.

33.5.2 INFORMED CONSENT

A fundamental duty of healthcare practitioners is to obtain patients' informed consent before administering medical treatments or performing operations. In this process, patients are given information about the treatment's nature, possible risks and benefits, available options, and how to make an independent decision. In order for patients to make educated decisions, healthcare practitioners need to ensure they comprehend the information they are given.

33.5.3 BALANCING ETHICAL PRINCIPLES

When it comes to ethical quandaries, healthcare workers often face conflicting concepts such as autonomy, beneficence, non-maleficence, and justice. For example, a doctor may have to strike a compromise between a patient's right to refuse medical intervention and their ethical obligation to act in the best interests of the individual. It takes considerable thought and frequent interaction with partners and ethics panels to navigate these ethical dilemmas.

33.5.4 CONFIDENTIALITY

One of the most important ethical obligations is to protect patient confidentiality. Unless there is a legal or ethical requirement to violate confidentiality, such as when reporting child abuse or danger to others, healthcare personnel have been provided with confidential patient information and must ensure it is not released without the patient's consent.

33.5.5 END-OF-LIFE CARE

Healthcare practitioners frequently have to make difficult moral choices while providing end-of-life care. They have to have conversations regarding DNR orders, removal of life-sustaining treatment, and palliative care. Sensitivity, effective communication, and consideration for the patient's preferences are necessary for these decisions.

33.5.6 RESOURCE ALLOCATION

Healthcare workers often have to make tough decisions regarding the distribution of resources when there aren't enough of them, such as organ transplants or ventilators during a virus outbreak. The primary factors in these decisions, which must be made impartially and in accordance with predefined criteria, ought to be fairness and overall benefit.

33.5.7 TRUTH-TELLING AND HONESTY

It is ethically required of healthcare workers to be sincere and forthright with their patients. This includes breaking bad news, talking about the prognosis, and owning up to mistakes or unfavorable outcomes. Sustaining trust and making sure patients have the information they need to make educated decisions depend on effective communication.

33.5.8 CULTURAL COMPETENCE AND SENSITIVITY

In order to make moral decisions, one must comprehend and respect cultural and religious norms and beliefs. Healthcare practitioners must possess cultural competence, acknowledging that individuals from varied origins could hold distinct viewpoints on healthcare and available treatments.

33.5.9 ADVANCE CARE PLANNING

It is ethically required to support and encourage patients to create living wills or advance directives as part of their advance care planning. By doing this, it is made possible to guarantee that patients' desires for their final care are acknowledged and honored.

33.5.10 ETHICAL DILEMMA RESOLUTION

Healthcare practitioners frequently run across moral conundrums for which there are no simple answers. In these situations, they could confer with colleagues or ask ethics committees (EC) for advice in order to make the most morally sound choice. Critical evaluation of the ethical aspects of the circumstance and multidisciplinary teamwork are required for these procedures.

33.5.11 CONTINUOUS ETHICAL EDUCATION

It's critical to stay up to date on moral precepts, legislative requirements, and industry best practices in healthcare ethics. For the purpose of improving their ability to make moral decisions and to adjust to new ethical challenges—such as those brought on by developing technology or shifting healthcare regulations—healthcare workers should pursue continual education and training.

33.5.12 SELF-REFLECTION AND MORAL INTEGRITY

To assess their own moral principles and prejudices, healthcare practitioners should practice self-reflection. In making ethical decisions, it is essential to uphold moral integrity and make sure that personal convictions do not unreasonably affect patient care.

33.5.13 PATIENT-CENTERED CARE

Making ethical decisions is intricately linked to the idea of patient-centered care. It places a strong emphasis on fostering shared decision-making, honoring each patient's autonomy and dignity, and customizing treatment to each patient's unique needs, preferences, and values.

33.5.14 REPORTING ETHICAL VIOLATIONS

It is the ethical responsibility of healthcare workers to report any unethical behavior or issues they come across in their organizations. Reporting superiors or coworkers who act unethically or implement rules that jeopardize patient care may be one way to do this.

33.5.15 ADVANCING ETHICAL POLICIES

In addition to making personal decisions, healthcare workers may help shape and enhance the ethical guidelines that are implemented in healthcare facilities. They can advocate for moral principles that put the well-being of patients and ethical integrity first, take part in ethics committee meetings, and contribute to policy debates (Louw, 2016).

It is a great burden placed on healthcare workers to successfully negotiate the complex web of ethical issues in the industry. Their duties go beyond the realm of medicine; they include advocacy, communication, and making decisions that support beneficence, autonomy, justice, and non-maleficence. Healthcare workers have a critical role to play in making sure that patients receive treatment that is not just medically sound but additionally morally and compassionately sound and patient-centered by accepting these duties (Haddad, 1998).

33.6 LEGAL FOUNDATIONS IN HEALTHCARE

33.6.1 OVERVIEW OF HEALTHCARE LAWS AND REGULATIONS

The set of laws, rules, and guidelines that control how medical professionals practice, how healthcare facilities are run, and what patients may and cannot do are known as legal foundations in the healthcare industry. In order to guarantee the ethical, high-quality, and safe provision of healthcare services, these legal underpinnings are crucial. They include state-specific healthcare rules as well as federal legislation like the Affordable Care Act (ACA) and the Health Insurance Portability and Accountability Act of 1996 (HIPAA). They also include a broad spectrum of legal concepts and regulations. Among the important areas of healthcare that these laws cover are confidentiality of patient insurance coverage, healthcare provider credentialing and licensing, and preventing fraud and abuse within the healthcare system. Protecting patient rights, maintaining the integrity of the healthcare profession, and influencing the healthcare landscape are all made possible by legal compliance, which is a basic necessity for healthcare organizations and personnel (Hodge, 2020).

33.6.2 MEDICAL NEGLIGENCE

Medical malpractice is another name for medical negligence, which is the incapacity of a healthcare provider to provide the level of care that is expected within their field of expertise or profession. It means going beyond established protocols and standard practices that other licensed medical practitioners would follow in a similar circumstance. In essence, the patient's duty of care has been breached by this.

33.6.2.1 ELEMENTS OF MEDICAL NEGLIGENCE

1. **Duty:** The patient was entitled to a duty of care from the healthcare professional. When a patient consults a healthcare provider for medical attention or care, this obligation is formed.
2. **Breach of Duty:** The medical professional violated their obligation of care by not following accepted standards of care. The determination of this violation is frequently made through expert evidence, in which other healthcare providers vouch for the quality of the treatment received.
3. **Causation:** Additionally, there needs to be a clear connection between the patient's injuries and the duty violation. Put otherwise, the damage sustained by the patient must have been directly caused by the breach.
4. **Damages:** The patient must have been harmed or incurred losses as a result of the duty violation in order to launch a medical negligence claim. Physical harm, mental anguish, monetary loss, or even death are examples of these damages (Bal, 2009).

33.6.3 MEDICAL MALPRACTICE

Medical professionals' professional behavior and the possible repercussions when their acts or inactions cause patients damage are the subject of legal concepts known as medical malpractice and negligence. Although these words are similar, they have different meanings and consequences under the law. A patient is said to have suffered an injury or harm as a result of a healthcare provider's negligent behavior, carelessness, or inability to deliver the required level of care in a scenario known as medical malpractice, which is a subset of healthcare provider negligence. Despite the fact that the phrases are sometimes used synonymously, "malpractice" denotes a more grave violation of a professional obligation. Patients who believe they have experienced injury as a result of the conduct or omissions of a healthcare professional usually file civil lawsuits to pursue allegations of medical malpractice. A monetary settlement to the aggrieved party may be awarded through settlements or jury judgments in certain circumstances. In order to shield themselves against the financial strain of defending against such allegations and to compensate patients in the event that malpractice happens, healthcare practitioners frequently carry malpractice insurance. Instances where healthcare professionals fall short of the professional standard of care and cause harm or injury to patients are referred to as medical malpractice and medical negligence. A particular kind of medical carelessness known as "medical malpractice" is the subject of civil lawsuits brought by patients who suffered as a result of the professional error or negligence of a healthcare practitioner. These legal ideas are essential for making sure that medical personnel are held responsible for their acts and that patients get the proper care and compensation when they are harmed (Oyebode, 2013).

33.6.4 PATIENT RIGHTS AND RESPONSIBILITIES

A courteous, well-balanced connection between patients and medical professionals is based on the idea that patients have rights and obligations in the constantly changing field of healthcare. This essential framework emphasizes the moral, legal, and ethical duties that both sides must fulfill in order to provide the best possible healthcare results. Patient responsibilities describe the obligations and expectations that patients should meet in exchange for receiving medical treatment, while patient rights cover a wide range of privileges intended to safeguard and enable those seeking such care. When combined, they provide a symbiotic connection that promotes cooperation, trust, and ultimately the provision of excellent healthcare services.

The basic idea that each and every person has an intrinsic right to be honored with respect, decency, and compassion throughout their whole healthcare journey is at the core of the rights of patients' movement. This includes the freedom to choose one's own doctors and encompasses the rights to privacy, confidentiality, and informed consent. The significance of ensuring that patients are fully informed about the exact nature, hazards, advantages, and alternatives of any suggested therapy or operation before providing their assent is highlighted by informed consent in particular. It gives patients the freedom to make knowledgeable decisions about their care and acts as a buffer against medical paternalism.

Secure patient data from unwanted access and disclosure is ensured by maintaining privacy and confidentiality, which are fundamental components of patient rights. Patients should know when what they provide will be utilized and which individuals will be given access to it. Additionally, they have the right to know that their private medical information will be handled with care. Conversely, autonomy goes beyond consent to include the freedom to decline medical intervention, decide how to receive care in the latter stages of life, and even select their own healthcare professionals. A person's sense of autonomy over their own health and medical course is contingent upon the preservation of these rights.

The right to impartial access to high-quality medical treatment is included in the category of patient rights. Race, ethnic background, gender, religion, handicap, sexual orientation, and financial position are just a few of the various ways that people might be discriminated against. Healthcare services must be delivered equally to all patients, and patients enjoy the right to be treated impartially and fairly. In order to remove language barriers and enable patients from a variety of backgrounds to actively participate in their treatment, these rights also frequently include the provision of interpretation and translation services.

Recognizing that patients are active participants in a joint effort to provide healthcare is equally vital in the setting of patient obligations. The dedication to giving honest and comprehensive information regarding one's medical history, present symptoms, and lifestyle decisions is at the heart of these obligations. Healthcare professionals need this information in order to diagnose patients correctly and create treatment regimens that work. To increase the likelihood of a favorable outcome, patients must also follow through on recommended medical interventions, prescription drugs, and lifestyle adjustments.

The foundation of a patient's obligations is effective communication, as it allows for candid and open discussion among patients and healthcare professionals. Asking questions, seeking clarification, and actively participating in group decision-making are all examples of this. In order to support a patient-centered approach to care, individuals ought to feel empowered to express their preferences, concerns, and aspirations. Being a knowledgeable and involved patient in this situation is not only your duty, but it's also a major factor in improving your health.

Making sensible use of available healthcare resources is another important patient duty. Patients have a responsibility to ensure that funds are used effectively, as healthcare systems throughout the world struggle with growing prices and resource shortages. Making educated judgments that weigh the possible advantages and disadvantages of medical procedures, refraining from requesting pointless testing or treatments, and following preventative measures recommendations are all part of this.

Financial obligations related to healthcare are also borne by patients. It is the responsibility of patients to be aware of their medical coverage, deductibles, and financial obligations. They should also be transparent with their healthcare professionals about any financial difficulties they may be experiencing. By using this proactive approach, unanticipated financial difficulties may be avoided, and it can be guaranteed that patients can receive the care they require without experiencing excessive difficulty.

Regarding healthcare safety, individuals are responsible for their own health and safety. They should report any concerns they may have about their care and adhere to safety protocols. Infection control procedures should be followed, fall prevention programs should be joined, and any negative occurrences or mistakes that they may see throughout their time in the medical field should be reported right away.

The delivery of high-quality medical care is contingent upon the symbiotic link between patient rights and duties. While patient duties emphasize active engagement, communication, and resource stewardship, patient rights safeguard each person's autonomy, dignity, and access to fair treatment. This approach is not only morally right, but it is also essential for fostering patient-provider trust, raising the standard of treatment, and ultimately achieving better health outcomes. The ideas of patient entitlements and responsibilities still serve as a roadmap for providing superior, more personalized treatment in an ever-more complex medical environment.

33.7 LICENSURE AND CREDENTIALING

Although licensing and credentialing are essential procedures in many different businesses and professions, they are especially important in areas like law, healthcare, and education where public safety is a concern. These procedures are designed to control and guarantee the skills, credentials, and moral character of those who wish to work in these professions. Let's examine the ideas of certification and licensing, highlighting their fundamental distinctions and examining how they function in various industries (Porcher, 2010).

33.7.1 LICENSURE

A person can only practice a certain profession or occupation after fulfilling certain educational, training, and testing criteria. This is known as licensing, which is the legal procedure through which a governmental or regulatory body authorizes someone to do so. The main goal of licensure is to safeguard the public by guaranteeing that practitioners follow accepted norms of conduct and ethics and are qualified and competent.

Doctors, nurses, chemists, and other healthcare workers must get a license in order to practice in the healthcare business. Completing an approved educational program, passing a standardized test (such as the medical board examinations), and fulfilling any extra state or federal criteria are usually required steps in the licensing process. Professionals who have obtained a license are required to abide by legal and ethical requirements and are continuously monitored (Shimberg, 1981).

33.7.2 CREDENTIALING

In contrast, credentialing is a more comprehensive procedure that extends beyond licensing and is frequently connected to professionals who work in healthcare, education, or government organizations. It involves assessing and validating a person's qualifications, experience, and background in order to determine whether or not they meet certain organizational standards and needs. Rather than being handled by government authorities, credentialing is frequently carried out by universities or credentialing groups. Credentialing is a process used in the healthcare industry to guarantee that medical professionals—including doctors, nurses, and other healthcare professionals—achieve the required levels of clinical competence, training, education, and ethical behavior. A complete examination of a candidate's qualifications, including their training, schooling, certifications, licenses, malpractice history, and references, is part of this procedure. Healthcare professionals who have earned their credentials are authorized to work in a certain type of healthcare setting, such as a medical center or hospital (Chappel et al., 2021).

33.8 APPLICATIONS IN DIFFERENT SECTORS

Outside of the medical field, certification and credentialing are important in a number of other fields: Education: To teach in public schools, teachers may need to hold a state license, and credentialing involves confirming an educator's degree and subject-specific training within a school system. Legal and Financial Services: A license from the appropriate state board may be necessary for attorneys, accounting professionals, and financial professionals. Certain legal firms and financial organizations may also have credentialing procedures in place to evaluate professionals' credentials and level of experience. Construction and Trades: State-issued licenses are frequently necessary for independent contractors, plumbers, electricians, and other tradesmen to operate lawfully, and larger construction companies may need credentials in order to work on corporate or government projects. Information Technology: Organizations such as CompTIA, Cisco, and Microsoft offer certifications that are used in the IT industry as a means of credentialing, proving one's proficiency in particular technologies or applications. The procedures of licensing and credentialing are essential to maintaining professional standards, ensuring public safety, and granting individuals the credentials they need to work in their particular industries. Unlike credentialing, which is sometimes institution-specific and focused on confirming eligibility for privileges within a certain organization or business, licensing is usually required by government authorities and is a condition for practicing a profession. In order to preserve the competence and integrity of experts in a variety of fields, both procedures are essential (Harolds Jay, 2021).

33.9 INTERSECTION OF ETHICS AND LAW IN HEALTHCARE

A complicated and multidimensional area where moral and legal concepts meet, the junction of law and ethics in healthcare frequently gives birth to difficult decisions and thought-provoking queries. Harmonizing these two crucial aspects is a difficulty faced by lawmakers, healthcare practitioners, and society at large in order to guarantee that individual rights are respected, high-quality treatment is given, and moral principles are maintained within the bounds of the law. This essay explores the intricate interplay between ethics and law in healthcare, delving into key ethical principles, legal frameworks, and real-world scenarios that highlight the challenges and opportunities that arise at this intersection (Kershner and Leslie, 2019).

33.10 FOUNDATIONS OF ETHICAL HEALTHCARE

Healthcare professionals use these principles as a moral compass as they navigate the complexities of patient care. These concepts are commonly embodied in the four pillars of biomedical ethics: autonomy, beneficence, non-maleficence, and justice.

1. **Autonomy:** The idea of autonomy holds that each person has the right to decide how they want to be treated. It highlights the need for obtaining informed consent, honoring patients' decisions, and defending their freedom to decline medical treatments or interventions. The legal notion of informed consent is intimately linked to autonomy, which is a fundamental component of patient-centered care in the healthcare industry.
2. **Beneficence:** In order to maximize patients' well-being and deliver the finest treatment possible, healthcare practitioners are obligated by virtue to act in their patients' best interests. This idea emphasizes the moral duty to advance patients' health and well-being, which frequently coincides with the legal requirement for healthcare practitioners to offer a level of care that complies with accepted standards in the industry.
3. **Non-Maleficence:** A common way to describe non-maleficence is "do no harm," which highlights the moral obligation of healthcare providers to protect their patients from harm. This idea balances beneficence and emphasizes how crucial it is to keep risks and potential harm to a minimum while implementing healthcare procedures. It conforms to the legal requirements for malpractice and negligence.
4. **Justice:** The equitable allocation of healthcare resources, benefits, and responsibilities is a matter of justice. It demands that everyone have equal opportunity for healthcare services and that unfair treatment or discrimination be prohibited on the basis of traits including gender, race, socioeconomic status, or disability. The quest for fairness in healthcare is aided by legal frameworks like anti-discrimination statutes (Candilis and Navneet, 2017).

33.11 LEGAL FRAMEWORKS IN HEALTHCARE

Legal frameworks in the healthcare industry are put in place to safeguard patient rights, regulate healthcare practitioners, and guarantee the provision of high-quality, safe treatment. These frameworks are entwined with moral precepts and frequently mirror the standards and ideals of society. Among the essential components of healthcare legal systems are:

1. **Informed Consent:** A legal obligation that is consistent with the moral precept of autonomy is informed consent. Before beginning any kind of medical care or surgery, it is required of healthcare personnel to obtain the voluntary and informed permission of the patient. Failing to do so may result in legal ramifications, such as allegations of medical malpractice.
2. **Medical Malpractice Laws:** Medical malpractice laws are designed to make healthcare practitioners legally responsible for any departures from the standard of care, which is based on ethical and professional standards. Medical malpractice claims are a means of pursuing legal action for patients who suffer injury as a result of negligence or poor treatment.
3. **Healthcare Regulations:** Governments and regulatory bodies establish and enforce healthcare regulations to safeguard public health and ensure the quality of care. These regulations encompass areas such as licensing of healthcare professionals, standards for healthcare facilities, and drug and device approvals.
4. **Patient Privacy:** Laws like the HIPAA in the United States safeguard patient privacy and the confidentiality of medical records. Protecting patient privacy aligns with ethical principles of respecting autonomy and maintaining trust between patients and healthcare providers.
5. **Anti-Discrimination Laws:** Anti-discrimination laws prohibit healthcare providers from engaging in discriminatory practices based on characteristics such as race, gender, religion, or disability. These laws reinforce the ethical principle of justice by promoting equitable access to care (Davidson et al., 2016).

33.12 CHALLENGES AT THE INTERSECTION

The intersection of ethics and law in healthcare is not always a seamless convergence of principles and regulations. Ethical dilemmas can arise when legal requirements conflict with deeply held moral beliefs or when legal standards do not fully align with ethical principles. Several challenges exemplify the complexities of this intersection:

1. **End-of-Life Care:** Decisions surrounding end-of-life care, including the withdrawal or withholding of life-sustaining treatments, can be ethically and legally fraught. While the principle of autonomy supports a patient's right to refuse life-sustaining interventions, legal frameworks vary and may require adherence to certain procedures or involve legal disputes.
2. **Reproductive Rights:** Issues related to reproductive rights, such as access to abortion and assisted reproductive technologies, involve a complex interplay of ethical beliefs and legal regulations. These debates often revolve around the ethical principles of autonomy and beneficence, but they are also heavily influenced by legal restrictions and debates over a woman's right to choose.
3. **Mental Health Care:** Legally and morally, it can be difficult to strike a balance between the requirement for treatment and the autonomy of those who suffer from mental illness. For example, when it comes to voluntary obligation and treatment, it is important to carefully evaluate ethical standards as well as legal protections to avoid any power abuses.
4. **Resource Allocation:** There may be conflicts between healthcare systems' limited resources and budgetary restrictions and the ethical values of fairness and equitable resource allocation. Resource distribution decisions might result in complex moral conundrums and even call for the creation of laws to guarantee justice.
5. **Conscientious Objection:** It is possible for medical personnel to encounter circumstances in which assisted suicide or abortion are medical therapies that go against their moral and religious views. It can be difficult to strike a compromise between patients' rights to receive morally and legally acceptable healthcare and healthcare

practitioners' rights to conscientious objection (Weerasinghe and Linda, 2003).

6. **Navigating the Intersection:** A sophisticated and careful strategy is necessary to successfully negotiate the junction of ethics and legislation in the healthcare industry. The following tactics need to be taken into account by society, legislators, and healthcare professionals:
7. **Ethical Training:** Ethics education is necessary for healthcare workers to acquire the knowledge and abilities necessary to resolve difficult moral conundrums. They may better align their behavior with moral standards and legal requirements with the aid of this training.
8. **Ethics Committees:** Ethics committees are present in many healthcare facilities and are capable of offering direction and support in resolving ethical disputes. Clinicians, legal specialists, and ethical advisors are just a few of the professionals from a variety of fields that frequently make up these committees.
9. **Legislative Reform:** Legislators have to reassess and revise healthcare legislation on a regular basis to make sure it remains current and meets new ethical requirements. Re-examining regulations pertaining to mental health, reproductive rights, and end-of-life care may be necessary to achieve this.
10. **Open Dialogue:** It is imperative that patients and healthcare professionals communicate in an honest and open manner. Healthcare practitioners must involve patients in shared decision-making wherever feasible, and patients ought to be informed about their rights and available treatments.
11. **Ethical Consultation:** Healthcare professionals can seek ethical advice from experts in the industry when they are faced with difficult ethical decisions. These consultations can help in resolving conflicts and making ethically sound decisions.
12. **Advocacy:** In order to influence healthcare legislation and regulations in a way that is consistent with moral values, advocacy groups and organizations can be extremely important. Additionally, they

can support patient rights and bring attention to ethical concerns in healthcare.

The dynamic and crucial interaction of law and ethics regarding healthcare is a feature of contemporary healthcare systems. Legal frameworks assist in safeguarding patient rights, providing high-quality treatment, and establishing accountability, while ethical standards offer a moral basis for patient care. The healthcare industry will inevitably face moral conundrums and legal obstacles along the way. Therefore, in order to achieve the best possible patient care and well-being, it is critical that legislators, healthcare professionals, and the general public engage in constant conversations and introspection about how to strike a balance between upholding the law and ethical principles (Hughes and Ayanna, 2021).

33.13 EMERGING ETHICAL AND LEGAL ISSUES IN HEALTHCARE

1. **Ethical Issues in Healthcare:** Technology breakthroughs, altering cultural standards, and changing demographics are all factors contributing to the ongoing evolution of the healthcare scene. Healthcare workers and lawmakers must continually adapt to the changing landscape and come up with answers to the ethical and legal problems that arise in the industry. This essay examines a few of the most important moral and legal dilemmas facing the healthcare industry today, emphasizing how complicated they are and how carefully they must be thought through.

i. **Affordability:** The subject of affordability and accessibility in healthcare is one of the most important ethical challenges. Marginalized groups frequently lack access to basic medical services, leading to persistent healthcare inequities in many regions of the world. With the COVID-19 epidemic exposing and exacerbating pre-existing inequities, this problem has taken on even more significance. The conflict in ethics stems from the need to balance the equitable distribution of healthcare resources under the concept of justice with the practical financial constraints associated with providing and maintaining healthcare services. In addition to managing resource limitations and financial demands, healthcare systems must contend with the ethical duty to treat everyone, regardless of their financial situation.

ii. **Accountability for AI Decisions:** The use of cutting-edge medical technology, such as genetic editing and artificial intelligence (AI), raises additional ethical questions. Even though these technologies have a lot of potential to improve patient outcomes and increase therapy options, they also present serious ethical challenges. For instance, the use of AI algorithms in medical diagnosis and treatment decisions may lead to concerns about bias and fairness, as these algorithms can inadvertently perpetuate existing healthcare disparities if not carefully designed and monitored. Genetic editing technologies like CRISPR-Cas9 have the potential to cure genetic diseases but also raise concerns about "designer babies" and unintended consequences.

iii. **Patient Autonomy:** The question of patient autonomy is at the heart of many ethical debates in healthcare. As patients gain access to more information and technology empowers them to be more involved in their healthcare decisions, the traditional paternalistic model of medicine is giving way to a model that prioritizes patient autonomy and informed consent. This shift is especially evident in end-of-life decisions, where issues like physician-assisted suicide and the use of advance directives challenge long-standing ethical norms. It can be challenging and always changing to strike a balance between patients' rights to autonomy and the responsibility of medical personnel to treat them with care.

iv. **Electronic Health Records:** The widespread use of electronic health records, or EHRs, has given rise to new moral and legal dilemmas. Data security and patient privacy are two issues that EHRs bring up, despite the fact that they have many advantages, such as better care coordination and fewer medical mistakes. Patients may suffer serious repercussions from identity theft, discrimination, or other issues if medical records are accessed or compromised without authorization. The moral conundrum is how to take advantage of EHRs' benefits while protecting patient privacy and ensuring that data is handled ethically and sensibly.

2. **Legal Issues in Healthcare:** Transitioning from moral dilemmas to legal ones, medical malpractice litigation is arguably the most notable of the many legal obstacles that the healthcare industry must overcome. Malpractice lawsuits can have serious financial and reputational repercussions for doctors and healthcare facilities, which are always the target of legal scrutiny. The evolving standard of care, informed consent, and the increasing complexity of medical procedures contribute to the growing legal risks in healthcare. Furthermore, the legal landscape for telemedicine is rapidly evolving, as healthcare providers adapt to the use of virtual platforms to deliver care. Issues related to licensure, liability, and reimbursement in telemedicine are still being defined, creating a legal gray area that needs resolution.

i. **Healthcare Fraud and Abuse:** Healthcare fraud and abuse also persist as significant legal concerns. The healthcare industry is vulnerable to fraudulent activities, such as overbilling, kickbacks, and unnecessary medical procedures. These activities not only cost the healthcare system billions of dollars but also compromise patient care and trust in the healthcare system. Legal mechanisms, such as the False Claims Act, are in place to combat fraud, but healthcare organizations must continually monitor and update their compliance programs to stay ahead of emerging schemes.

ii. **Gene Editing and Genetic Testing:** The intersection of genetics and the law poses unique legal challenges. The rise of genetic testing and personalized medicine raises questions about genetic discrimination, consent for genetic testing, and the ownership and privacy of genetic data. The Genetic Information Non-discrimination Act (GINA) in the United States provides some protection against genetic discrimination, but gaps and ambiguities in the law remain, requiring further legislative attention.

iii. **Public Health Objectives:** In the realm of public health, the tension between individual rights and the collective good is an ongoing legal and ethical debate. Vaccination mandates, quarantine measures, and contact tracing during outbreaks of infectious diseases raise questions about the balance between individual autonomy and public health objectives. This topic has gained attention recently due to incidents like the discussion over vaccination passports and mask regulations during the COVID-19 pandemic. These occurrences have also highlighted the difficulties in reaching an agreement on the proper boundaries for government involvement in healthcare.

iv. **End-of-Life Care:** There is a great deal of ethical and legal discussion around end-of-life care, including the legality of physician-assisted suicide, with opinions varying greatly by jurisdiction. A prescription for drugs that might speed up their death can be requested by terminally ill individuals in certain areas that have legalized medical assistance in dying. Supporters claim that this offers a humane solution for those in excruciating pain, while detractors point to possible misuse issues and the value of human life. The legal and ethical landscape surrounding end-of-life decisions continues to evolve as societies grapple with these complex issues. As society struggles with these difficult dilemmas, the legal and ethical framework around end-of-life decisions is still changing.

v. **Healthcare Data for Research and Innovation:** Another emerging legal issue is the use of healthcare data for research and innovation. With the growth of big data analytics and machine learning in healthcare, there are debates over who owns and controls patient data, how it can be used for research purposes, and the potential for data breaches and misuse. Regulations like the General Data Protection Regulation (GDPR) in Europe and the HIPAA in the United States attempt to strike a balance between data privacy and healthcare research needs, but the rapid pace of technological advancement continually challenges these regulations.

vi. **Medical Tourism:** The globalization of healthcare presents additional legal complexities. Medical tourism, where individuals seek medical treatment abroad, can create issues related to quality of care, patient safety, and legal recourse in the event of adverse outcomes. Furthermore, the cross-border movement of healthcare professionals and the recognition of foreign credentials raise questions about the standardization of medical qualifications and the ability of healthcare providers to practice in different countries (Baldassarre et al., 2023). The healthcare landscape is a dynamic and ever-evolving domain that continually gives rise to ethical and legal challenges. Globalization, genetics, public health initiatives, healthcare fraud, medical malpractice, access and affordability, patient autonomy, electronic medical records, healthcare fraud, and end-of-life care are just a few of the issues that need to be carefully considered by policymakers, healthcare professionals, and the general public. In order to overcome these obstacles, it will be necessary to strike a careful balance between the rights of the individual and the interests of society. Additionally, ethical standards and developing legislative frameworks that put patient welfare and healthcare system integrity first must be upheld. In order to guarantee that the core values of justice, equality, and patient-centered care continue to be at the center of the healthcare system, our ethical and legal answers must also evolve along with healthcare (Kumar et al., 2023).

33.14 CONCLUSION

The healthcare industry is a complicated, dynamic subject where legal and ethical concerns come together to influence how healthcare is administered and provided. The complexity of these concerns has been brought to light by this review, which focuses on two main points: the necessity of providing ethical healthcare services and the ongoing development of legal and ethical difficulties in the healthcare industry. It is evident that moral and legal concerns in healthcare are still evolving. As scientific research, patient empowerment, and medical technology progress, they also bring with them new legal and ethical challenges that are changing the face of healthcare. A few examples of the quickly changing issues that affect healthcare professionals, legislators, and society at large are the COVID-19 pandemic, the development of AI, the growing significance of patient autonomy, the issues of confidentiality that surround digital health records, as well as the globalization of healthcare. This growth necessitates a proactive, flexible strategy. In order to discover legal and moral solutions that are consistent with their basic beliefs and principles, healthcare providers and practitioners must be aware of newly emerging ethical and legal concerns, change their policies and practices on a regular basis, and have intelligent conversations. Ethicists, solicitors, medical professionals, and patients must collaborate in an interdisciplinary manner to successfully address these issues. It is also impossible to exaggerate the importance of providing ethical healthcare. The profession of healthcare is fundamentally founded on the values of beneficence, compassion, and the protection of human dignity. Healthcare practitioners are trusted by patients with their most personal matters and well-being, and this confidence is based on their ethical behavior and compliance with the law. Healthcare professionals must put patient-centered care first, honor informed consent, protect patient privacy, and provide treatment that is devoid of bias and discrimination in order to maintain this confidence. Medical organizations, government agencies, and the general public all have a shared duty for ensuring ethical healthcare delivery. Individual healthcare professionals are not the only ones with this obligation. In addition to promoting healthcare practices that put patients' welfare and best interests first, regulatory structures and professional standards also need to adapt to changing ethical standards. In addition, in order to enable patients to make knowledgeable decisions about their treatment and to stand up for their rights, public dialogue and training on the ethics of healthcare and legal protections are crucial.

KEYWORDS

- **artificial intelligence**
- **COVID-19 pandemic**
- **digital health records**
- **healthcare ethics**
- **healthcare industry**
- **healthcare professionals**
- **healthcare system**
- **legal issues**
- **patient autonomy**
- **patient care**
- **patient empowerment**

REFERENCES

Aita, M., & Richer, M. C. (2005). Essentials of research ethics for healthcare professionals. *Nursing & Health Sciences, 7*(2), 119–125.

Akdeniz, M., Yardımcı, B., & Kavukcu, E. (2021). Ethical considerations at the end-of-life care. *SAGE Open Medicine, 9*, 20503121211000918.

Aluaş, M. (2016). Ethical and legal considerations of healthcare informatics. *Applied Medical Informatics, 38*(3, 4), 91–98.

Bal, B. S. (2009). An introduction to medical malpractice in the United States. *Clinical Orthopaedics and Related Research, 467*, 339–347.

Baldassarre, D., Piazza, O., & McConnell, P. (2023). Emerging ethical challenges in healthcare in the 21st century. *Anaesthesia & Intensive Care Medicine.*

Ballard, K. A. (2003). Patient safety: A shared responsibility. *Online Journal of Issues in Nursing, 8*(3), 4.

Brown, J. P. (2020). Ethical dilemmas in healthcare. In *Safety Ethics* (pp. 67–82). Routledge.

Candalis, P. J., & Sindu, N. (2017). Ethics, mental health, and the law. In *Mental Health Practice and the Law.*

Chappell, K. B., Howard, M. S., Lundmark, V., & Ivory, C. (2021). Credentialing and certification: Overview, science, and impact on policy, regulation, and practice. *International Nursing Review, 68*(4), 551–556.

Davidson, G., Brophy, L., Campbell, J., Farrell, S. J., Gooding, P., & O'Brien, A. M. (2016). An international comparison of legal frameworks for supported and substitute decision-making in mental health services. *International Journal of Law and Psychiatry, 44*, 30–40.

Frakes, M., & Jena, A. B. (2016). Does medical malpractice law improve health care quality? *Journal of Public Economics, 143*, 142–158.

Gray, A., & Vawda, Y. (2018). Health legislation and policy. *South African Health Review, 2018*(1), 1–11.

Haddad, A. (1998). The future of ethical decision-making in health care. *Nursing Clinics of North America, 33*(2), 373–384.

Harolds, J. A. (2021). Quality and safety in healthcare, Part LXXII: Credentialing and privileging. *Clinical Nuclear Medicine, 46*(11), 908–910.

Hodge, J. G., Jr. (2020). Revisiting legal foundations of crisis standards of care. *The Journal of Law, Medicine & Ethics, 48*(1), 221–224.

Hughes, G. I., & Thomas, A. K. (2021). Visual category learning: Navigating the intersection of rules and similarity. *Psychonomic Bulletin & Review, 28*, 711–731.

Jesilow, P., & Burton, B. (2017). Detecting healthcare fraud and abuse in the United States. In *Oxford Research Encyclopedia of Criminology and Criminal Justice.*

Kershner, S. P., & Wolf, L. E. (2019). *The Intersection of Law, Ethics, and Public Health in the United States.* Oxford University Press.

Kröger, C., van Baarle, E., Widdershoven, G., Bal, R., & Weenink, J. W. (2022). Combining rules and dialogue: Exploring stakeholder perspectives on preventing sexual boundary violations in mental health and disability care organizations. *BMC Medical Ethics, 23*(1), 1–12.

Kumar, P., Chauhan, S., & Awasthi, L. K. (2023). Artificial intelligence in healthcare: Review, ethics, trust challenges & future research directions. *Engineering Applications of Artificial Intelligence, 120*, 105894.

Louw, B. (2016). Cultural competence and ethical decision-making for health care professionals. *Humanities and Social Sciences, 4*(2), 41.

Luyckx, V. A., Biller-Andorno, N., Saxena, A., & Tran, N. T. (2017). Health policy and systems research: Towards a better understanding and review of ethical issues. *BMJ Global Health, 2*(2), e000314.

McLean, S. A. M., & Mason, J. K. (2003). *Legal and Ethical Aspects of Healthcare.* Cambridge University Press.

Oyebode, F. (2013). Clinical errors and medical negligence. *Medical Principles and Practice, 22*(4), 323–333.

Peters, D., Vold, K., Robinson, D., & Calvo, R. A. (2020). Responsible AI—Two frameworks for ethical design practice. *IEEE Transactions on Technology and Society, 1*(1), 34–47.

Porcher, F. K. (2010). Licensure, certification, and credentialing. In *Nurse Practitioners: The Evolution and Future of Advanced Practice* (p. 415).

Pozgar, G. D. (2023). *Legal and Ethical Issues for Health Professionals.* Jones & Bartlett Learning.

Shimberg, B. (1981). Testing for licensure and certification. *American Psychologist, 36*(10), 1138.

Weerasinghe, S., & Williams, L. S. (2003). Health and the intersections of diversity: A challenge paper on selected program, policy, and research issues. In *Intersections of Diversity Seminar, Niagara Falls, Canada.*

CHAPTER 34

Patient Rights and Responsibilities

ANKUSH VERMA,[1,*] AMIT PRATAP SINGH CHOUHAN,[2] and VANDANA SINGH[3]

[1]*Department of Radiology, Sharda School of Allied Health Sciences, Sharda University, Greater Noida, Uttar Pradesh, India*

[2]*Department of Radiology, School of Allied Health Sciences, Galgotias University, Greater Noida, Uttar Pradesh, India*

[3]*Department of Microbiology, Sharda School of Allied Health Sciences, Sharda University, Greater Noida, Uttar Pradesh, India*

*Corresponding author

ABSTRACT

Patient rights and responsibilities in healthcare are fundamental, ensuring that individuals receive ethical, respectful, precise, and quality medical care. They contribute to the overall quality of care and the well-being of both patients and healthcare providers. Important components of patient rights include the availability of medical records, involvement in decisions about their treatment, and the opportunity to express complaints or concerns. Along with this, there are certain duties of patients that obligate and contribute to that individual's personal well-being as well as the efficient operation of the healthcare system. The terrain of patient rights and obligations is still being shaped by moral conundrums and legal difficulties, such as those pertaining to genetic testing, access to experimental therapies, and end-of-life counseling. This chapter discusses in detail the roles and responsibilities of patients and healthcare professionals.

Allied Healthcare in Practice: An Introduction to Integrated Patient Care. Sally Lukose, Karuna Singh (Eds.)

DOI: 10.1201/9781998511037-38

34.1 INTRODUCTION TO PATIENT RIGHTS AND RESPONSIBILITIES

Patient rights and responsibilities are the fundamental principles that govern the ethical and legal framework of healthcare (Sert and Gurkan et al., 2021). These guidelines of rights and responsibilities serve as a key role in the relationship between patients and healthcare providers, ensuring that both sides understand their roles and duties in the patient care process. Patient rights must include the fundamental principles that involve individuals expecting good quality care when seeking medical treatment, such as the right to informed consent, privacy, and access to quality care (King et al., 2014). Similarly, patient responsibilities state the importance of active participation from patients and cooperation in their own healthcare journey, including the obligation to provide accurate medical history and adhere to treatment plans. Both patient rights and responsibilities create a balanced and respectful relationship in healthcare, promoting better communication, trust, and ultimately, improved patient outcomes.

34.1.1 DEFINITION OF PATIENT RIGHTS

Patient rights in healthcare refer to the fundamental rights and privileges that ensure individuals receive ethical, respectful, precise, and quality medical care (Vahdat et al., 2014). These patients' rights include various aspects, such as the right to informed consent, which allows patients to make decisions about their treatment after being fully informed about the risks and benefits of medical treatment. Patients must have a clear understanding that they have the right to receive respectful and non-discriminatory medical treatment, regardless of their race, gender, religion, or other characteristics (Gronningsater et al., 2011). Finally, these patients have the right motive to protect the dignity, autonomy, and well-being of persons inside the medical healthcare system by building a trusting connection between patients and healthcare professionals (Delmar et al., 2011).

34.1.2 DEFINING PATIENT RESPONSIBILITIES

Patient duties in healthcare refer to the obligations and contributions that individuals have in maintaining their personal well-being as well as the efficient operation of the healthcare system. Patients must follow recommended treatment plans, medications, and follow-up visits in order to be responsible for their own health management (Muth et al., 2019). Patients should also make an effort to maintain a healthy lifestyle, which includes making wise decisions regarding their food, exercise routine, and other lifestyle practices that may have an effect on their general health. Patients must be aware to show respect and consideration for healthcare providers and staff, understanding that a collaborative and respectful relationship is vital for effective care. Additionally, it is the duty of patients to know their rights and to communicate honestly with their medical staff, raising concerns and requesting explanations when necessary. Accepting these duties contributes to improved health outcomes for all parties involved by ensuring that healthcare is a partnership between providers and patients (Batalden et al., 2016).

34.1.3 IMPORTANCE OF PATIENT RIGHTS AND RESPONSIBILITIES

Patient rights and responsibilities play a pivotal role in the healthcare system, contributing to the overall quality of care and the well-being of both patients and healthcare providers. Patient rights are essential because they safeguard individual autonomy and dignity, ensuring that every person has the right to make informed decisions about their own health and treatment. This strengthens the patient-provider bond and raises the standard of medical treatment by fostering a culture of trust and respect between patients and medical staff.

Patient duties, on the other hand, are just as important since they encourage the active participation of patients in their healthcare journey. When patients take responsibility for obtaining accurate medical information, adhering to treatment plans, and maintaining a healthy lifestyle, they are not only contributing to their own well-being but also helping to optimize the use of healthcare resources. This, in turn, reduces the burden and efforts on healthcare systems and ensures that resources are allocated more efficiently. Improved health outcomes and higher levels of patient satisfaction might result from patients knowing and carrying out their obligations (Mohammad et al., 2013). People who actively engage in their treatment are more likely to have health concerns identified and managed early on, which lessens the severity of illnesses and their related expenditures. A more cooperative and courteous interaction between patients and healthcare practitioners is also common among those who are aware of their obligations, which promotes better communication and an overall better experience with healthcare (Harris et al., 2014). Fundamentally, patient rights and duties serve as the pillars of patient-centered care, encouraging accountability, respect, and joint decision-making in the medical field. By adhering to these values, we establish a healthcare system that not only satisfies the medical requirements of patients but also respects their individuality and enables them to play an active part in their crucial health maintenance.

34.2 PATIENT RIGHTS

In the healthcare industry, patient rights are essential values and privileges that protect the honor, independence, and health of those who are receiving medical attention. These rights cover a variety of fundamental elements, such as the right to informed consent, which guarantees that patients are provided with sufficient information to make decisions about their available treatment alternatives. Patients' personal and medical privacy are preserved by the protection of sensitive medical information from unauthorized exposure through the use of privacy and confidentiality rights (Sahi et al., 2017). In addition, patients have the right to be treated with proper comfort, dignity, and without discrimination based on their traits or history. The freedom of patients to voice complaints and concerns, as well as the opportunity to view their medical records, ensures that they are informed about their present health status and that their issues are being taken seriously. Patient rights in the healthcare sector essentially serve as the keystone of moral and compassionate care, encouraging a collaborative relationship between patients and medical professionals that places importance on respect, individual autonomy, and high-quality treatment (Berenson et al., 2015).

34.2.1 RIGHT TO INFORMED CONSENT

The right to informed consent, which empowers patients to make informed decisions about their medical care, is one of the most significant ethical principles in the field of medicine. In order to enable patients to consider their options and give their voluntary and informed consent prior to any intervention, this right guarantees that they are given thorough information about the risks, advantages, contraindications, and alternatives to a planned medical procedure, diagnosis, or treatment. Healthcare professionals have a moral and legal obligation to address patients' questions and concerns by delivering relevant information in an understandable and transparent manner (Francis et al., 2013). Patient-centered care, in which individuals actively participate in making decisions about their health, is encouraged by this right. As a result, therapeutic outcomes improve, and the healthcare system as a whole becomes more ethical. It also fosters trust between patients and medical professionals.

34.2.2 RIGHT TO PRIVACY AND CONFIDENTIALITY

The ethical practice of medicine is predicated on the right to privacy and confidentiality in the healthcare sector, with the aim of safeguarding the privacy of patients' personal and medical information (Nittari et al., 2020). It ensures that individuals may trust medical practitioners with sensitive information about their health, medical history, and personal lives without fear of it being shared without their permission. Healthcare practitioners are required by law and ethics to maintain the privacy of patients, healthcare workers who are directly involved in the patient's care, and only for appropriate medical objectives. When people know that their privacy will be protected, they are more likely to seek medical attention and provide correct information. For this reason, patient confidence and the effectiveness of healthcare depend on people's ability to maintain their right to privacy and confidentiality. In the end, this right substantially supports the integrity of the doctor-patient relationship as well as the delivery of the finest care and diagnosis.

34.2.3 RIGHT TO QUALITY CARE

The right to quality care ensures that people obtain healthcare services that adhere to established standards of safety, efficacy, and professionalism. This is made possible by the core premise of the right to quality care in the healthcare system. Among the expectations associated with this right are those related to timely and sufficient medical care that is devoid of prejudice, negligence, and harm (Stoyanova et al., 2018).

High-quality care must include everything from an efficient diagnosis to evidence-based therapies, thorough follow-up, and convenient access to medical experts. The provision of patient-centered care also entails a commitment to honoring the unique needs and preferences of each patient and including them in the formulation of their treatment plans and choices. Furthermore, receiving high-quality care is crucial to helping patients achieve their desired level of health and happiness with their medical care. Prioritizing quality in healthcare administration not only increases the likelihood of recovery but also reduces medical errors and complications. Patients' confidence that their medical professionals are giving them the best care possible will increase public confidence in the healthcare system. This right involves more than simply having access to money or cutting-edge medical equipment; it also involves a dedication to delivering healthcare with empathy, dignity, and a focus on improving patients' quality of life. Striving to create a healthcare system that reliably delivers safe, efficient, and patient-centered services requires not just upholding the right to quality treatment, but also maintaining it as a moral imperative.

34.2.4 RIGHT TO ACCESS MEDICAL RECORDS

One of the most important aspects of patient empowerment and systemic openness in healthcare is the ability to access medical records. Patients have the legal right to view and obtain copies of their own medical records, which contain important data about their condition, diagnosis, course of treatment, and test findings. With the availability of these records, people can stay informed about their medical history and actively participate in the healthcare decision-making process. Medical records are made available to patients, promoting patient autonomy by allowing individuals to make informed decisions about their health, seek second opinions, and understand their conditions or diseases and treatments more thoroughly. Furthermore, it encourages open and honest communication between medical staff and patients, strengthening their relationship and developing mutual confidence as well as cooperation. Patients may review their medical records for accuracy and can update information as necessary. They can also receive a detailed picture of their medical history. This is especially useful when looking for specialty therapy or when transferring healthcare providers (Ward et al., 2015). Overall, by encouraging transparency and accountability within the healthcare system, the right to access medical information not only supports or promotes patient satisfaction and excellent healthcare, but it also encourages individual autonomy and informed decision-making.

34.2.5 RIGHT TO CHOOSE HEALTHCARE PROVIDERS

People are empowered to choose the healthcare professionals and facilities that best meet their needs and preferences in order to make informed and accurate decisions regarding their medical care. The right to make one's own decisions is a cornerstone of healthcare. This privilege acknowledges that individuals are free to select the healthcare provider who best meets their requirements, regardless of whether that provider is a hospital, general practitioner, or specialist (Pellegrino et al., 2019). It enables patients to get second opinions, investigate non-traditional treatment options, or simply build a relationship with a trustworthy healthcare professional. The freedom to select one's healthcare providers encourages competition among them, which motivates them to deliver excellent, patient-centered care in order to attract and retain patients. It also promotes a more cordial and cooperative patient-provider connection by encouraging medical staff to provide care that is in line with the patient's beliefs and preferences. Furthermore, the ability to obtain specialized treatment is contingent upon this right, especially when patients need specialized services or a certain level of expertise that may not be offered by a single institution or provider. Allowing individuals to select the healthcare providers they wish to use encourages innovation and variety in the industry, which improves patient satisfaction and healthcare outcomes in the long run. Fundamentally, one of the most important components of patient-centered care is the freedom to select the healthcare professionals who will best meet their specific requirements and preferences (Berwick et al., 2009). This allows patients to actively engage in the decision-making process regarding their treatment.

34.2.6 RIGHT TO REFUSE TREATMENT

One of the most important patient rights that emphasizes a person's autonomy and self-determination when it comes to medical care is the freedom to refuse treatment (Will et al., 2011). It guarantees that patients, even when advised to do so by healthcare professionals, have the moral and legal right to refuse any medical intervention. This right is based on the idea that people should always have the last word about what happens to their bodies and medical treatment. In regard to life-sustaining treatment options, surgical procedures, medical treatment, or any other type of healthcare intervention, it gives patients the autonomy to make decisions based on their values, beliefs, and educated judgment. A fundamental component of moral medical practice that protects individual liberties and fosters candid and open communication between patients and healthcare professionals is respecting a patient's choice to refuse treatment (Roberts et al., 2012). This right is essential to maintaining a patient's dignity and personal agency (Figure 34.1).

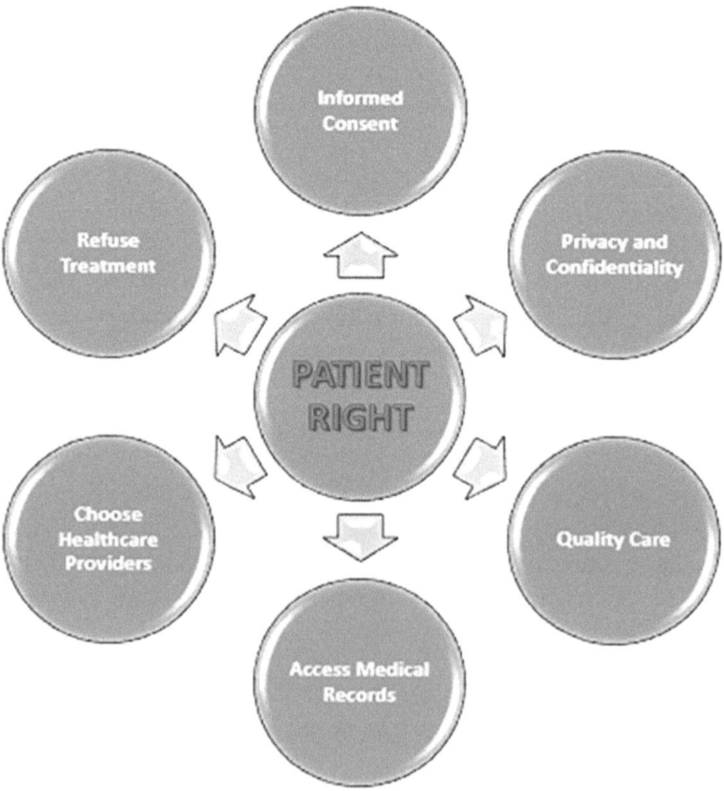

FIGURE 34.1 Showing list of various patient rights used in healthcare management.

34.3 PATIENT RESPONSIBILITIES

Patient responsibilities in healthcare refer to the duties and proactive activities that people should undertake to protect their own health and make a positive impact on the healthcare system. Providing precise and thorough medical information to healthcare practitioners, following treatment regimens, prescription drugs, and lifestyle advice, and actively engaging in their healthcare decisions are some of these duties. In addition, patients must lead a healthy lifestyle, make knowledgeable choices about their treatment, therapies, and medication, and treat staff members and medical professionals with respect (McCaffrey et al., 2017). Patients may significantly improve their own health outcomes, reduce the risk of medical mistakes, and build a cooperative, respectful relationship with their healthcare professionals by carrying out these duties, which will eventually result in more efficient and patient-centered treatment.

34.3.1 RESPONSIBILITY FOR INFORMED CONSENT

Healthcare practitioners are largely accountable for obtaining informed consent in the provision of healthcare. They have a moral and legal duty to ensure patients are informed in a clear and thorough manner about the advantages, disadvantages, options, and possible outcomes of any medical operations or treatments (Brown et al., 2004). In addition to answering patients' queries and concerns and making sure they comprehend all of the information given, healthcare professionals should encourage honest and open communication with their patients. However, patients also have a role to play in the informed consent process; they should actively participate in conversations, seek clarity, ask questions, and voice their preferences and opinions. In order to ensure that individuals may make educated decisions about their healthcare based on their beliefs and preferences, informed consent is a collaborative process involving mutual respect and communication between patients and healthcare professionals.

34.3.2 RESPONSIBILITY FOR OPEN COMMUNICATION

Patients and healthcare practitioners both have responsibilities for maintaining open lines of communication in the medical field. In order to provide a space where patients feel comfortable discussing their symptoms, medical history, and concerns, healthcare practitioners play a critical role. They have to be transparent, sympathetic, and easy to understand while providing information regarding risks, treatment alternatives, and diagnosis. On the other hand, it is the duty of patients to proactively participate in open, sincere, and truthful dialogues with their healthcare professionals, providing accurate health information and posing queries in order to get answers and clarity. Establishing trust, ensuring decisions are well-informed, avoiding medical mistakes, and providing patient-centered care that is tailored to each patient's needs and preferences all depend on open communication (Moreau et al., 2012).

34.3.3 RESPONSIBILITY FOR COMPLIANCE WITH TREATMENT PLANS

In the healthcare industry, patients have the primary responsibility for adhering to their treatment program. It is the patient's responsibility to follow a healthcare provider's recommendations after they have been made, regardless of whether they involve medication, therapy, or changes to their lifestyles. This includes adhering to prescription regimens, scheduling follow-up visits, changing one's lifestyle as needed, and taking an active role in managing one's own health (Bodenheimer et al., 2015). Following treatment plans is crucial to achieving the best possible health outcomes, avoiding complications, and ensuring that the recommended treatments work. In order to achieve good medical results and enhance overall well-being, patients must be committed to and responsible for adhering to the treatment plan, even while healthcare personnel can provide direction, support, and monitoring.

34.3.4 RESPONSIBILITY FOR HEALTH MAINTENANCE

The responsibility for health maintenance in healthcare primarily rests with the individual. It entails adopting a proactive attitude and making lifestyle adjustments meant to maintain and improve one's own health (Entwistle et al., 2015). This duty entails receiving prescribed screenings and immunizations, controlling stress, avoiding dangerous behaviors like smoking and binge drinking, and participating in regular physical exercise. It also includes keeping a balanced and healthy diet and managing stress. A person's own dedication to keeping their health is ultimately responsible, even though healthcare experts can give guidance and preventative treatment (Mackenzie et al., 2013). Assuming personal responsibility for maintaining one's health lowers the likelihood of developing chronic illnesses and other health problems. It also lessens the burden of avoidable diseases, which in turn makes the healthcare system more sustainable.

34.3.5 RESPONSIBILITY FOR TIMELY PAYMENT

The responsibility for timely payment in healthcare primarily falls on the patient or their designated payer, such as an insurance company or government program. It involves ensuring that healthcare bills, premiums, or co-payments are paid promptly and in accordance with agreed-upon terms. Timely payment is vital for sustaining the healthcare system, as it allows healthcare providers to continue offering their services, cover operational costs, and maintain access to quality care. Delays or non-payment can disrupt the healthcare ecosystem, impacting the availability of medical services and potentially burdening the broader healthcare community. Therefore, it is incumbent upon individuals and their responsible payers to fulfill their financial obligations promptly to support the integrity and accessibility of the healthcare system.

34.4 HEALTHCARE ETHICS AND PATIENT RIGHTS

Healthcare ethics and patient rights are intertwined principles that form the ethical foundation of modern healthcare. Healthcare ethics guide the moral conduct of healthcare professionals, emphasizing principles such as beneficence (doing good), non-maleficence (avoiding harm), autonomy (respecting patient choices), and justice (fair distribution of resources). These ethics underpin the respect for patient rights, ensuring that individuals receive healthcare that upholds their dignity and autonomy. Important concepts include the right to privacy and secrecy, the freedom to refuse treatment, and the right to be given informed consent, all of which are included in the category of patient rights. The aforementioned rights enable patients to make knowledgeable decisions regarding their medical treatment, safeguard their private data, and maintain their independence while making decisions about their care. In summary, patient rights and healthcare ethics work together to create a system of healthcare that is both medically and morally sound, encouraging mutual respect, trust, and the highest quality of treatment for all patients.

34.4.1 ETHICAL DILEMMAS IN PATIENT CARE

Healthcare practitioners deal with complicated and sometimes emotionally taxing ethical challenges in patient care on a daily basis. Competing ethical ideals, such as independence, kindness, impartiality, and justice, may clash and give birth to these quandaries. Examples include decisions made at the end of life, where a patient's desire for autonomy in deciding whether to refuse or stop receiving life-sustaining therapy may conflict with a healthcare provider's desire to protect life. The distribution of scarce resources, such as organ transplants, presents another frequent ethical conundrum, as it often pits the necessity to give the sickest patients priority against the ideals of justice and fairness. Healthcare professionals need to approach these difficult decisions with caution, honest dialogue, and a dedication to upholding the rights and values of their patients. Ethical decision-making is an essential aspect of providing compassionate, patient-centered care while balancing the moral obligations and responsibilities that come with healthcare practice.

34.4.2 BALANCING PATIENT RIGHTS WITH MEDICAL ETHICS

Balancing patient rights with medical ethics is a delicate and vital aspect of healthcare practice. Patient rights, including autonomy, informed consent, and privacy, are fundamental and must be upheld to ensure respect for individuals' values and preferences. Simultaneously, medical ethics, grounded in principles like beneficence (doing good), nonmaleficence (avoiding harm), and justice, guide healthcare providers to act in the best interests of patients' health. Striking this balance often involves complex decision-making when ethical principles seem to conflict. For instance, respecting a patient's right to refuse treatment while considering their well-being or safeguarding patient confidentiality when it might impact public safety. Healthcare professionals must engage in ethical deliberation, ensuring that patient rights are protected while aligning their actions with ethical obligations to provide safe, effective, and equitable care. Open communication, shared decision-making, and a deep understanding of the patient's unique circumstances are key to resolving these ethical dilemmas in a manner that honors both patient rights and medical ethics, ultimately leading to the best possible patient care.

34.5 CHALLENGES AND CONTROVERSIES

Patient rights and responsibilities in healthcare, while essential, are not without their share of challenges and controversies. One challenge lies in striking the right balance between patient autonomy and the duty to protect patients from making harmful decisions, particularly in cases where mental capacity or judgment may be compromised. Controversies can also arise when cultural or religious beliefs clash with medical recommendations, leading to ethical dilemmas. The interpretation and enforcement of patient rights and responsibilities can vary, causing discrepancies in care quality and patient experiences across different healthcare settings. Additionally, ensuring that patients are fully aware of their rights and responsibilities can be challenging, especially for vulnerable or marginalized populations. Issues related to data privacy, confidentiality, and the sharing of electronic health records raise concerns about patient information security. Despite these challenges and controversies, an ongoing commitment to open communication, ethical practice, and continuous improvement in healthcare policies and practices is crucial to address these issues and ensure that patient rights and responsibilities are respected and upheld within the healthcare system.

34.6 CONFLICTS BETWEEN PATIENT RIGHTS AND HEALTHCARE INSTITUTIONS

Conflicts between patient rights and healthcare institutions can arise due to various factors within the complex healthcare landscape. One common source of conflict is the tension between a patient's right to autonomy and a healthcare institution's commitment to safety and best practices. For instance, a patient may demand a treatment or procedure that healthcare providers believe is medically unnecessary or risky, creating a conflict between the patient's autonomy and the institution's duty to provide safe and evidence-based care. Another area of contention can be resource allocation, where limited resources such as organ transplants or expensive treatments must be distributed equitably, often raising ethical dilemmas (Gibney et al., 2023). Furthermore, conflicts may arise when patients attempt to use their right to confidentiality or refuse care in a way that contradicts the legal requirements or care standards of the institution. These disputes highlight how crucial it is to have transparent guidelines, moral standards, and lines of communication in order to resolve issues and guarantee that patients' rights are upheld while adhering to the letter and spirit of the law and maintaining the highest standard of care (Lehoux et al., 2017).

34.6.1 CONTROVERSIAL CASES AND LEGAL BATTLES

Legal disputes and contentious cases in the healthcare industry are a mirror of the many moral, legal, and societal dilemmas that can emerge in the medical sector (Backman et al., 2008). Medical decision-making for vulnerable populations, access to healthcare services, reproductive rights, and end-of-life care are just a few of the highly contentious issues addressed in these cases. Examples of historic legal disputes centered on topics such as physician-assisted death, abortion rights, and the Affordable Care Act in the United States have sparked discussions about the ethical limits of medical practice, the role of government in healthcare, and individual autonomy. Situations when medical judgments clash with religious convictions, such as disagreements over blood transfusions for Jehovah's Witnesses, can also give rise to controversial instances. Legal precedents that impact healthcare policy and practice for years to come are frequently established by such instances, which also serve as examples of the complex interplay between medical ethics, human opinions, and the law in the field of healthcare. These disputes serve as a reminder of the continuous need for strong legal frameworks and moral debate to solve difficult healthcare challenges while upholding the values and rights of both individuals and the community at large.

34.7 GLOBAL PERSPECTIVES ON PATIENT RIGHTS

The variety of healthcare systems, cultural norms, and legal frameworks among nations is reflected in the vast range of viewpoints that exist globally about patient rights in healthcare. The essential concepts of patient rights, including informed consent, privacy, and access to high-quality treatment, are widely acknowledged; nonetheless, there can be considerable variations in the degree to which these rights are respected. Patient rights are essential to the operation of the healthcare system in some nations, where they are firmly protected by law. This guarantees that patients have a role in their care and that their personal information is secured. Healthcare systems in some areas, however, could find it difficult to uphold patients' rights because of a lack of resources, cultural norms that place a premium on group decision-making, or weak legislative safeguards. International organizations such as the WHO are attempting to standardize and promote patient rights, and reaching a worldwide consensus on these rights is a continuous endeavor. Although the details may differ, the overall objective is always the same: to guarantee that patients receive high-quality, ethical, and compassionate healthcare that respects their autonomy and dignity wherever in the globe.

34.7.1 COMPARING PATIENT RIGHTS IN DIFFERENT COUNTRIES

Significant differences exist in the scope and kind of safeguards that people get within healthcare systems when patient rights in various nations are compared. Patient rights are generally protected by strong legal frameworks in many Western nations, including the U.S., Canada, and many European countries. Ensuring that patients have the ability to make healthcare decisions and that their personal information is strictly safeguarded, these nations place a strong emphasis on concepts like informed consent, privacy, and non-discrimination. On the other hand, certain nations, such as those in specific regions of Asia and Africa, may have less established legislative frameworks safeguarding patient rights because of their more centralized healthcare systems. Individual liberty may be restricted under such systems due to a possible increased focus on group decision-making or the power of the state in matters of healthcare. It is important to remember, nevertheless, that the field of patient rights is always changing, and many nations are attempting to improve the legal and moral foundations that safeguard patients. In order to further the universality of patient rights, international organizations such as the WHO offer guidelines and standards. All the same, these national differences highlight the intricate ways that legal frameworks, healthcare systems, and cultural norms interact to shape patient rights globally.

34.8 PATIENT EDUCATION

34.8.1 EDUCATING PATIENTS ABOUT THEIR RIGHTS

In order to guarantee that patients' rights and duties are respected in the healthcare system, patient education is an essential first step. Healthcare professionals enable patients to actively engage in their treatment and make educated decisions by providing them with easily available and understandable information about their rights and obligations. To properly exercise their rights, patients must be aware of them. These rights include the right to informed consent, confidentiality, and access to medical records. Additionally, teaching patients about their duties, which include adhering to treatment regimens, maintaining a healthy lifestyle, and participating in open communication with healthcare professionals, creates a sense of accountability and cooperation in the course of their medical treatment. Along with improving the patient-provider dynamic, patient education also leads to better medical outcomes, higher levels of satisfaction among patients, and an ethically sound and patient-centered healthcare system as a whole. Consequently, to ensure that patients' rights and duties are honored and maintained, healthcare organizations must place a high priority on patient education.

34.8.2 RAISING AWARENESS OF PATIENT RESPONSIBILITIES

One important step that might result in more efficient as well as patient-centered healthcare delivery is increasing awareness of patients' roles in the healthcare system. It entails informing patients of their responsibilities and roles within the healthcare system and emphasizing the value of their active involvement in their own treatment. Patients gain more empowerment to take charge of their health when duties such as providing accurate medical information, following recommended treatment programs, and choosing healthy lifestyle options are made more apparent. It also lowers healthcare expenditures and increases the effectiveness of healthcare services, all of which contribute to their overall well-being (Starfield et al., 2012). Patient satisfaction and healthcare outcomes are also enhanced when patients and healthcare professionals feel more collaborative and respectful of one another, which is fostered by increasing patient responsibility awareness (Wei et al., 2020). To ensure that patients are aware of their responsibilities and, ultimately, become a more involved and responsible patient population, healthcare organizations, experts, and advocacy organizations for patients play a crucial role in this endeavor by offering materials, educational resources, and open communication channels.

34.9 CONCLUSION

The rights and obligations of patients in the healthcare industry are always evolving due to altering cultural norms, technological breakthroughs, and the constantly changing healthcare environment. Patient rights now encompass a wider range of concerns, such as equity, cultural sensitivity, and patient-centered care, in addition to the familiar concepts of informed consent and confidentiality. With a rising focus on collaborative decision-making and patient access to their medical information, patients are becoming more recognized as active participants in their healthcare decisions. In the meantime, the role that patients have in preserving their well-being through choices about their lives, following medical procedures, and taking an active role in their care has changed as a result of all of these developments. Patient autonomy and data privacy are now more important issues to take into account with the introduction of telemedicine and digital health technology. The ongoing growth of patient rights as well as responsibilities is a dynamic and crucial component of contemporary healthcare, representing the changing demands and requirements of consumers as well as providers. This is because healthcare systems throughout the world are working to deliver more equitable and compassionate care to patients. The COVID-19 pandemic has also brought attention to the significance of public health as well as the fine line that must be drawn between individual liberties and group responsibilities. It has sparked conversations on the rights and duties of patients, including the freedom to refuse treatment and follow public health recommendations in order to protect others. The pandemic has also sped up the use of telemedicine and remote monitoring, bringing up concerns around patient consent, data security, and the extent of the patient's responsibility in maintaining their health from a distance. For these rights and obligations to remain applicable and useful in the face of new healthcare difficulties, there has to be constant discussion and adjustment at the nexus of medical ethics, technological advances, and healthcare policy. In order to promote moral, patient-centered care that respects each person's independence, dignity, and good health while addressing the complexity of contemporary healthcare, healthcare organizations, legislators, and advocacy groups are vital players in this dynamic environment. They also play a significant role in influencing the continuing evolution of individual patient rights and responsibilities.

KEYWORDS

- **digital health technology**
- **health management**
- **healthcare expenditures**
- **healthcare industry**
- **patient access**
- **patient-centered care**
- **telemedicine**
- **treatment programs**

REFERENCES

Backman, G., Hunt, P., Khosla, R., Jaramillo-Strouss, C., Fikre, B. M., Rumble, C., Pevalin, D., Páez, D. A., Pineda, M. A., Frisancho, A., & Tarco, D. (2008). Health systems and the right to health: An assessment of 194 countries. *The Lancet, 372*(9655), 2047–2085.

Batalden, M., Batalden, P., Margolis, P., Seid, M., Armstrong, G., Opipari-Arrigan, L., & Hartung, H. (2016). Coproduction of healthcare service. *BMJ Quality & Safety, 25*(7), 509–517.

Berenson, R. A., & Rice, T. (2015). Beyond measurement and reward: Methods of motivating quality improvement and accountability. *Health Services Research, 50*, 2155–2186.

Berwick, D. M. (2009). What 'patient-centered' should mean: Confessions of an extremist. *Health Affairs, 28*(Suppl1), w555–w565.

Bodenheimer, T. (2015). Helping patients improve their health-related behaviors: What system changes do we need? *Disease Management, 8*(5), 319–330.

Brown, R. F., Butow, P. N., Butt, D. G., Moore, A. R., & Tattersall, M. H. N. (2004). Developing ethical strategies to assist oncologists in seeking informed consent to cancer clinical trials. *Social Science & Medicine, 58*(2), 379–390.

Delmar, C., Alenius-Karlsson, N., & Mikkelsen, A. H. (2011). The implications of autonomy: Viewed in the light of efforts to uphold patients' dignity and integrity. *International Journal of Qualitative Studies on Health and Well-Being, 6*(2), 6045.

Entwistle, V. A., Mello, M. M., & Brennan, T. A. (2015). Advising patients about patient safety: Current initiatives risk shifting responsibility. *The Joint Commission Journal on Quality and Patient Safety, 31*(9), 483–494.

Francis, R. (2013). *Report of the Mid Staffordshire NHS Foundation Trust Public Inquiry: Executive Summary* (Vol. 947). The Stationery Office.

Gibney, B. C., & Entwistle, J. W. C. (2023). The ethics of transplantation. In *Textbook of Transplantation and Mechanical Support for End-Stage Heart and Lung Disease* (pp. 63–82).

Gronningsater, S. (2011). A patient's right to choose is not always black and white: Long-term care facility discrimination and the color of care. *JCR & Economic Development, 26*, 329.

Harris, B., Eyles, J., Penn-Kekana, L., Thomas, L., & Goudge, J. (2014). Adverse or acceptable: Negotiating access to a post-apartheid health care contract. *Globalization and Health, 10*, 1–14.

King, J. S., & Moulton, B. W. (2006). Rethinking informed consent: The case for shared medical decision-making. *American Journal of Law & Medicine, 32*(4), 429–501.

Lehoux, P., & Williams-Jones, B. (2017). Mapping the integration of social and ethical issues in health technology assessment. *International Journal of Technology Assessment in Health Care, 23*(1), 9–16.

Mackenzie, C., & Rogers, W. (2013). Autonomy, vulnerability and capacity: A philosophical appraisal of the Mental Capacity Act. *International Journal of Law in Context, 9*(1), 37–52.

McCaffrey, A. M., Pugh, G. F., & O'Connor, B. B. (2017). Understanding patient preference for integrative medical care: Results from patient focus groups. *Journal of General Internal Medicine, 22*, 1500–1505.

Moreau, A., Carol, L., Dedianne, M. C., Dupraz, C., Perdrix, C., Lainé, X., & Souweine, G. (2012). What perceptions do patients have of decision making (DM)? Toward an integrative patient-centered care model. A qualitative study using focus-group interviews. *Patient Education and Counseling, 87*(2), 206–211.

Mosadeghrad, A. M. (2013). Healthcare service quality: Towards a broad definition. *International Journal of Health Care Quality Assurance, 26*(3), 203–219.

Muth, C., Blom, J. W., Smith, S. M., Johnell, K., Gonzalez-Gonzalez, A. I., Nguyen, T. S., Brueckle, M. S., Cesari, M., Tinetti, M. E., & Valderas, J. M. (2019). Evidence supporting the best clinical management of patients with multimorbidity and polypharmacy: A systematic guideline review and expert consensus. *Journal of Internal Medicine, 285*(3), 272–288.

Nittari, G., Khuman, R., Baldoni, S., Pallotta, G., Battineni, G., Sirignano, A., Amenta, F., & Ricci, G. (2020). Telemedicine practice: Review of the current ethical and legal challenges. *Telemedicine and e-Health, 26*(12), 1427–1437.

Pellegrino, E. D. (2019). The commodification of medical and health care: The moral consequences of a paradigm shift from a professional to a market ethic. *The Journal of Medicine and Philosophy, 24*(3), 243–266.

Roberts, L. W., Geppert, C. M. A., & Bailey, R. (2012). Ethics in psychiatric practice: Essential ethics skills, informed consent, the therapeutic relationship, and confidentiality. *Journal of Psychiatric Practice, 8*(5), 290–305.

Sahi, M. A., Abbas, H., Saleem, K., Yang, X., Derhab, A., Orgun, M. A., Iqbal, W., Rashid, I., & Yaseen, A. (2017). Privacy preservation in e-healthcare environments: State of the art and future directions. *IEEE Access, 6*, 464–478.

Sert, G., & Karates, M. (2021). Human rights in health/Why patient rights. *Medicine Science, 10*(4), 1162–1167.

Starfield, B. (2012). Primary care: An increasingly important contributor to effectiveness, equity, and efficiency of health services. SESPAS report 2012. *Gaceta Sanitaria, 26*, 20–26.

Stoyanova, V. (2018). Causation between state omission and harm within the framework of positive obligations under the European Convention on Human Rights. *Human Rights Law Review, 18*(2), 309–346.

Vahdat, S., Hamzehgardeshi, L., Hessam, S., & Hamzehgardeshi, Z. (2014). Patient involvement in health care decision making: A review. *Iranian Red Crescent Medical Journal, 16*(1).

Ward, M. M., Jaana, M., & Natafgi, N. (2015). Systematic review of telemedicine applications in emergency rooms. *International Journal of Medical Informatics, 84*(9), 601–616.

Wei, H., Corbett, R. W., Ray, J., & Wei, T. L. (2020). A culture of caring: The essence of healthcare interprofessional collaboration. *Journal of Interprofessional Care, 34*(3), 324–331.

Will, J. F. (2011). A brief historical and theoretical perspective on patient autonomy and medical decision making: Part II: The autonomy model. *Chest, 139*(6), 1491–1497.

CHAPTER 35

Confidentiality and Informed Consent

SANA KANWAL

Department of Radiology, Sharda School of Allied Health Sciences, Sharda University, Greater Noida, Uttar Pradesh, India

ABSTRACT

Patient care in any medical field is a static subject. The increasing advantages of surgical procedures and ethical society have brought focused attention to patient care. This divides the main patient care steps into two categories. The first category is about the practical procedures of patient care, and the second category involves ethical steps. Ethical steps are also defined as a human duty, which is the most important step in the relationship between hospital staff and the patient. Accurate knowledge of ethical steps makes a staff worker a proper professional and the hospital a "good" hospital by maintaining the patient's willingness and confidentiality. It is said that a patient's response to any treatment is affected by his/her response to the environment. Therefore, it is important to bring a patient into the right and safe atmosphere by following the main patient care steps.

35.1 INTRODUCTION

In the medical field, confidentiality of the patient and consent are important and legalized steps defined according to the laws of the state. In all states, there is a common law, which is the duty of healthcare members to respect confidentiality steps. This means that when a patient shares his/her information, it should be kept confidential and should not be disclosed without proper legal steps and justification.

Allied Healthcare in Practice: An Introduction to Integrated Patient Care. Sally Lukose, Karuna Singh (Eds.)

DOI: 10.1201/9781998511037-39

In healthcare or medical fields, confidentiality is very important because patients tend to share secret as well as sensitive information with doctors, healthcare staff members, and physicians in hospitals. Therefore, if at any moment, the patient feels insecure that the information given to the doctor or healthcare members is not well secured and may be revealed or disclosed, then the patient might not discuss the information openly with the doctors, which also affects the patient's treatment. Therefore, the confidentiality of patient information should be kept as a top priority in all healthcare institutions.

For other lawful reasons, it is also important to have consent from the patient for the safety of the healthcare institution. The healthcare workers are the ones who obtain and maintain informed consent. This states that any information related to the patient cannot be discussed without the consent of that person.

35.2 CONFIDENTIALITY

The term "confidential" stands for the privacy concept. A patient has all the rights to make sure that the information regarding their health status or any information related to personal details is kept private until it is beneficial for him/her, as well as until there is a major harm to society if the information is not disclosed (Lillian et al., 2009). The healthcare worker should not disclose facts related to the patient's health or other information describing the patient's personal data to anyone who is not involved in the patient's treatment because confidentiality is a fiduciary or trust link between a doctor and a patient (Lillian et al., 2009). This link is based on fiduciary duty and arises when there is an honest act of the same fiduciary between the doctor and the patient. Therefore, confidentiality in the medical field is an act or behavior of doctors to keep and maintain all the information received during the patient's treatment. State or national laws, as well as hospital policies, should secure the private medical information of the patient by providing a privacy practices notice that explains the procedures for revealing and protecting patient information and also describes how a patient can receive a copy of their records, information, and care.

In 1996, the Congress recognized the requirement and importance of patient record privacy measures. Therefore, the Health Insurance

Portability and Accountability Act (HIPAA) was launched. This governmental legislation ensured that:

i. The financial details and health information of the patient will be kept private and safe, regardless of the format in which the information is recorded.
ii. The HIPAA law also protects privacy when the patient's medical details are transferred to another authority from the patient's current healthcare providers.
iii. Health-related information and the financial status of the patient will not be disclosed to any employee, facilities, or outside the medical institution without informing and obtaining written consent from the related individual.
iv. The HIPAA law also includes required measures designed to encourage electronic transactions, which save money for healthcare businesses, but this step also necessitates new measures to protect individuals' security and confidential information.

The Department of Health and Human Services (DHHS) planned laws in November 1999 to ensure patient protection and patients' rights against the misuse and disclosure of their health data. DHHS proposed the final rule in December 2000, which became active on April 14, 2001. It took about two complete years to comply with the final rules by April 14, 2003. All treatment-related reports and other patient details, whether electronic, written, or verbal, are included under the new rule (Lillian et al., 2009).

35.3 PATIENT'S RIGHTS

1. Patients have the right to have all considered ways of privacy. Treatment discussions, consultations, procedures, and diagnoses must be performed in a way that protects the privacy of the patient.
2. Patients have the right to expect that all conversations and data related to their treatment will be considered private by the care center, except in cases permitted by law, such as instances of abuse and public health hazards.
3. Patients have the right to expect that the care center or hospital will prioritize their confidentiality when releasing information to any other healthcare institution for consultation to provide better treatment.

4. Patients have the right to view their reports related to their treatment or care and to receive explanations of the information, including necessary steps, except as restricted by law.
5. Patients have the right to expect that their confidentiality will remain free from public exposure. However, the same information can be shared with the patient's legal guardian and parents if the patient is under the legal age or if the patient is not mentally stable. In such cases, the patient has the right to select the individual with whom medical information can be shared, provided they are of legal age.

Besides confidentiality or privacy laws, patients also have "tort laws," which involve any injury to the patient or property damage. This can result in receiving payment for damages from the proven party after civil litigation. It can occur either intentionally or unintentionally. According to tort laws, any misconduct by the healthcare provider can lead to:

1. **Assault:** This occurs when a patient experiences an unethical threat of touch in an injurious way without physical contact.
2. **Battery:** This involves unlawfully touching a patient without their consent. For example, if a healthcare provider performs an examination after the patient has denied consent, the provider can be charged with battery.
3. **False Imprisonment:** This refers to the unjustified restraint of a patient against their will. A patient can charge false imprisonment if they are restrained in a hospital or medical care institution without their consent. However, if there is a risk that the patient may harm themselves, restraints are legally allowed.
4. **Libel and Slander:** Healthcare members are responsible for keeping patient information confidential at all times and should not discuss a patient's confidential information without the patient's permission or written consent.
5. **Invasion of Privacy:** If a patient's information is not kept confidential by the hospital or if a patient's body is inappropriately exposed, the patient can pursue legal action against the medical institution.

The healthcare team should adhere to the aforementioned steps regarding patient confidentiality, privacy, and security of information, whether in computerized records or previous systems. The only way to comply with the law or rules is to obtain the patient's written consent when passing on confidential information.

35.4 INFORMED CONSENT

The term "consent" is an agreement between the patient and the healthcare staff, in which the patient allows the healthcare members to execute the procedure or examination. An informed consent document is an approval form for any medical examination after informing the patient of all possible unfavorable outcomes (Corti et al., 2000).

In 1958, an F.B.I. clerk named Jerry Watson Canterbury was suffering from a ruptured disk. Dr. William Spence, a famous neurosurgeon in Washington, operated on him, but after the surgery, Canterbury frequently fell from his bed while he was hospitalized and ended up with paralysis below his waist. Due to this, Canterbury charged the doctor and the hospital with malpractice and negligence. This case brought up the idea of establishing informed consent in medical examinations.

Most procedures performed in any healthcare department provide a consent form for the patient to sign, as well as for the parents or legal guardians in the case of underage or special cases. From a medical perspective, consent builds rapport with patients through multiple conversations to achieve a successful result. It is the responsibility of healthcare staff to ensure the patient signs the consent form after addressing all doubts (Manti, 2018).

Importance of the consent form:

i. Taking informed consent from the patient secures the hospital and the staff members from any legal charges.
ii. The healthcare provider connecting with the patient through effective communication lowers the patient's anxiety and also improves the results of the procedures.

An informed consent form is required for the following procedures:

i. Prior to all operative or invasive procedures like biopsy, surgical incision, paracentesis, and cystoscopy.

ii. Prior to any examination requiring sedation or anesthesia.
iii. Prior to the administration of blood.
iv. Non-surgical examinations like arteriography that may put the patient at risk.
v. An examination that uses ionizing radiation.
vi. Prior to investigational drugs or treatments.
vii. From reluctant patients.

A consent form is not considered valid if all the details of the procedure are not discussed with the patient. The must-informed information includes:

i. Explanation of the procedure.
ii. Potential risks.
iii. Benefits of the procedure.
iv. Suggested other possible options.
v. Answers to queries about the examination.
vi. Instructions to the patient that they can withdraw from the consent.

A patient should be informed of all the consequences if the recommended examination is not completed. Frequently, a patient agrees or disagrees with an examination based on the details provided by a healthcare member.

Healthcare staff should also confirm that the patient understands what steps will be taken and the various decisions available to them.

At any stage of the procedure, if the patient, parent, or legal guardian refuses the procedure information or withdraws agreement or consent, the healthcare provider should inform the patient's doctor. The examination must be stopped until the issue is sufficiently resolved (Corti et al., 2000).

35.5 VARIOUS TYPES OF INFORMED CONSENT

1. **Simple Consent:** Taking a patient's agreement to execute an examination in the absence of knowledge about the procedure. Simple consent is of two categories:

    a. Express consent, in which the patient agrees after the healthcare provider explains the suggested procedure to the patient in detail, including what they will do and suggestions of what can be done. In the express consent form, patients must express their will for the suggested procedure. However, legally, silence is not an agreement. Express consent should be obtained in the presence of an unbiased observer. The patient can express their willingness for the procedure by:

- **Gesture** – A patient could say "YES" by nodding their head. Gesture consent is risky as the doctor cannot be assured of what the patient is really saying through their movements. Therefore, the doctor should not satisfy themselves by taking gesture consent.
- **Oral** – In which a patient expresses their will through spoken words.
- **Written** – A patient expresses his/her will in writing along with their signature on the consent form presented by the hospital.

b. Implied consent is taken in emergency cases in which the healthcare provider is unable to obtain permission from the patient, and the patient's parents or legal guardians are also not available at the time. As the word "imply" suggests that the patient would give permission, the physician operates on the patient.

2. **Inadequate Consent:** If a patient is not properly informed to make an adequate decision, the patient can charge negligence against the hospital or medical institute. If the patient is injured without proper information, the battery act will be charged against the hospital. Inadequate consent is also referred to as ignorant consent.

3. **Blanket Consent:** A consent that covers all future decisions of a doctor and allows them to do what is necessary. This consent protects the surgeons from any charges because sometimes, during surgery, many unexpected developments could arise. However, it must not be used unless the second pathology is life-threatening. Blanket consent is also used when taking patient samples for future studies, as it protects a researcher from any ethical issues related to the usage of the samples. Blanket consents are also known as broad or general consent forms.

Common misunderstandings regarding a consent form:

i. A consent form is a complete process, not just a piece of paper.
ii. Partial consent is not informed consent.
iii. A form with the patient's consent is not necessarily informed consent.
iv. A patient should provide consent, not the doctor.
v. The main aim of the consent form is to ensure patient safety, not for the doctor's benefit.

KEYWORDS

- **blanket consent**
- **healthcare institutions**
- **healthcare provider**
- **ignorant consent**
- **life-threatening**
- **medical institute**
- **patient agreement**
- **patient samples**
- **patients' rights**
- **public health hazards**
- **written consent**

REFERENCES

Corti, L., Day, A., & Backhouse, G. (2000). Confidentiality and informed consent: Issues for consideration in the preservation of and provision of access to qualitative data archives. *Forum Qualitative Sozialforschung, 1*(3).

Gupta, U. C. (2013). Informed consent in clinical research: Revisiting few concepts and areas. *Perspectives in Clinical Research, 4*, 26–32.

Manti, S., & Licari, A. (2018). How to obtain informed consent for research. *Breathe (Sheff), 14*(2), 145–152.

Torres, L. S., Dutton, A. G., Watson, T. A., & Linn-Watson, T. (2009). *Patient Care in Imaging Technology* (7th ed.).

CHAPTER 36

Ethics in Laboratory Diagnostics: Perspectives and Challenges

GAURAV KAUSHIK,[1,*] RICHA VASHISHTHA,[2] and CHAITENYA VERMA[3]

[1]*School of Allied Health Sciences, Sharda University, Greater Noida, Uttar Pradesh, India*

[2]*Department of Medicine, All India Institute of Medical Sciences, New Delhi, India*

[3]*Department of Pathology, The Ohio State University Wexner Medical Center, Columbus, OH, USA*

*Corresponding author

ABSTRACT

This chapter thoroughly explores the ethical challenges associated with laboratory diagnostics, underscoring their pivotal role in maintaining the integrity and trustworthiness of medical procedures. The chapter categorizes ethical challenges within the realms of patient care, research, and professional conduct, addressing fundamental principles including beneficence, non-maleficence, autonomy, justice, fairness, honesty, and professionalism. It delves into the impact of emerging technologies such as artificial intelligence (AI), point-of-care testing, and genetic testing on ethical considerations. It also addresses national and international ethical standards, emphasizing the crucial contribution of regulatory agencies and professional associations to societal ethics. The chapter outlines various strategies for addressing ethical concerns, including interdisciplinary collaboration, ethical review panels, and initiatives for training and education. The chapter concludes with future directions and recommendations,

Allied Healthcare in Practice: An Introduction to Integrated Patient Care. Sally Lukose, Karuna Singh (Eds.)

DOI: 10.1201/9781998511037-40

offering a roadmap for understanding and navigating the intricate ethical landscape of laboratory diagnostics.

36.1 INTRODUCTION

36.1.1 DEFINITION OF LABORATORY DIAGNOSTICS

Laboratory diagnostics, commonly known as clinical diagnostics, encompasses a diverse array of tests and procedures conducted in a laboratory setting to assess and interpret biological materials. Its primary objective is to understand and manage human health effectively. This interdisciplinary field plays a crucial role in identifying diseases, monitoring treatment effectiveness, and informing medical decisions. By examining biological samples like blood, urine, tissues, and other substances, laboratory diagnostics aids healthcare professionals in diagnosing and treating a broad spectrum of medical conditions (Najjari et al., 2022). Utilizing methods such as molecular biology, immunology, biochemistry, and microbiology, this dynamic field continuously evolves to align with technological advancements and remains integral to contemporary healthcare systems worldwide (Akber, 2021).

36.1.2 IMPORTANCE OF ETHICS IN LABORATORY DIAGNOSTICS

The credibility, reliability, and societal acceptance of laboratory diagnostics hinge on a crucial element—ethics. Ethics involves employing moral standards and values to guide the conduct of professionals involved in collecting, analyzing, and interpreting patient samples. Ethics in laboratory diagnostics extends beyond the technical aspects of testing and plays a multifaceted role.

1. **Patient Confidentiality and Trust:** Ethical considerations are integral to maintaining patient trust throughout the diagnostic process. Patients must have confidence that their personal and medical information will be kept confidential at the highest level. This trust is essential for building a robust doctor-patient relationship, fostering open communication between patients and healthcare professionals.
2. **Accuracy and Reliability:** Maintaining ethical standards is crucial for ensuring the accuracy and reliability of laboratory outcomes.

This involves adhering to established protocols, implementing quality control measures, and maintaining transparency when presenting results. The dependability of diagnostic information is vital in guiding appropriate medical procedures and treatment plans.

3. **Informed Consent:** Securing informed consent before conducting diagnostic tests is a way to respect the autonomy of patients. This ensures that individuals comprehend the purpose, potential risks, and benefits of the testing, empowering them to make informed decisions about their healthcare. Informed consent forms the ethical bedrock of relationships between patients and healthcare providers.
4. **Avoidance of Conflicts of Interest:** Ethical standards in laboratory diagnostics play a crucial role in minimizing conflicts of interest that could compromise the objectivity of tests. This involves promoting transparency in financial relationships among pharmaceutical companies, healthcare providers, and laboratories to prevent undue influence on diagnostic conclusions.
5. **Equitable Access to Diagnostics:** Ethical considerations also encompass ensuring fair access to diagnostic services. Promoting justice and fairness in healthcare involves making diagnostic testing available to all societal groups, regardless of their financial circumstances.
6. **Professional Integrity:** Practitioners in laboratory diagnostics are obligated to uphold their professional integrity by demonstrating honesty, accountability, and responsibility in their work. Ethical behavior in this context is essential for maintaining public trust in the healthcare system and fostering a culture of continuous improvement.

36.2 ETHICAL PRINCIPLES IN LABORATORY DIAGNOSTICS

At the core of modern healthcare lies laboratory diagnostics, guided by a set of ethical principles that practitioners adhere to in the collection, analysis, and interpretation of patient samples. Essential for ensuring the equity, accuracy, and integrity of diagnostic processes, ethical guidelines are imperative. This section will delve into a detailed discussion of the four primary ethical principles that govern laboratory diagnostics: autonomy and informed consent, justice and fairness, integrity and professionalism, and beneficence and non-maleficence.

36.2.1 BENEFICENCE AND NON-MALEFICENCE

1. **Beneficence:** Within the realm of laboratory diagnostics, beneficence underscores the ethical obligation to enhance patients' well-being by providing timely and accurate diagnostic information. This principle emphasizes the positive impact of diagnostic testing on patient care. Professionals must strive to maximize the benefits of testing while minimizing potential risks, ensuring that the data obtained significantly contributes to improving the patient's health outcomes.
2. **Non-Maleficence:** Rooted in the principle of "do no harm," non-maleficence underscores the importance of ensuring patients' safety and preventing harm during the diagnostic process. Professionals must carefully weigh the potential risks and benefits of a diagnostic test, considering factors such as the invasiveness of the procedure, potential side effects, and the psychological impact on the patient (Ann et al., 2019).

36.2.2 AUTONOMY AND INFORMED CONSENT

1. **Autonomy:** Within laboratory diagnostics, autonomy recognizes individuals' entitlement to make informed decisions about their healthcare. This concept underscores the importance of respecting patients' autonomy and their right to determine the course of action for their bodies. Professionals are obligated to engage in honest and transparent communication with patients, providing them with the necessary information to independently decide whether to undergo diagnostic testing.

2. **Informed Consent:** In the realm of laboratory diagnostics, informed consent stands as a vital aspect of autonomy. Prior to conducting any diagnostic tests, healthcare providers must obtain the patient's voluntary and informed consent. This process involves allowing patients to ask questions, elucidating the goals of the test, outlining potential drawbacks and advantages, and presenting other available options. Informed consent ensures that patients actively participate in their healthcare decisions and are aware of the implications of diagnostic testing.

36.2.3 JUSTICE AND FAIRNESS

1. **Justice:** Within laboratory diagnostics, justice pertains to the fair distribution of the costs and benefits associated with diagnostic testing across the population. This principle advocates for equal access to diagnostic services for all individuals, regardless of their financial status, race, or other demographic factors. To ensure equitable and just treatment, healthcare systems must work to minimize disparities in access to diagnostic testing.
2. **Fairness:** Fairness extends beyond the mere availability of diagnostic tests and encompasses the fair and transparent allocation of resources within the laboratory. This involves appropriately distributing resources, prioritizing tests based on their significance, and ensuring that each patient receives timely and accurate results. Establishing equity in laboratory diagnosis is crucial for building public trust in the healthcare system.

36.2.4 INTEGRITY AND PROFESSIONALISM

1. **Integrity:** Essential to laboratory diagnosis is the adherence to principles of honesty, accuracy, and transparency. Integrity stands as a foundational ethical principle, necessitating professionals to uphold high ethical and scientific standards to ensure the precision and reliability of diagnostic information. This involves strict

adherence to established protocols, accurate documentation of results, and prompt resolution of any errors or inconsistencies.

2. **Professionalism:** Within laboratory diagnostics, professionalism encompasses a range of behaviors and qualities, including accountability, integrity, and collaborative teamwork. Professionals are tasked with fostering a culture of continuous improvement and a commitment to excellence in their work. This principle also underscores the importance of maintaining respectful relationships with colleagues, patients, and other members of the healthcare team (Talash et al., 2022).

36.3 ETHICAL CHALLENGES IN LABORATORY DIAGNOSTICS

While laboratory diagnostics provide invaluable insights into patient health, they are not devoid of ethical challenges. This section delves into the ethical dilemmas within laboratory diagnostics, categorizing them into three areas: issues related to patients, those tied to research, and those associated with professional conduct.

36.3.1 PATIENT-RELATED ISSUES

1. **Privacy and Personal Space:** Given that laboratory tests often involve sensitive patient health information, preserving privacy and confidentiality is paramount. Safeguarding patient data is essential for establishing and maintaining trust. However, the proliferation of data-sharing platforms and electronic health records has introduced new challenges. Striking a balance between patient confidentiality and accessibility for healthcare professionals remains an ongoing ethical dilemma. Mitigating these challenges requires strict access restrictions, data encryption, and adherence to ethical principles (Ethical issues in laboratory medicine, 2010).

2. **Informed Consent and Patient Autonomy:** An essential aspect of ethical medical practice is obtaining informed consent, ensuring patients have the freedom to make choices about their healthcare.

The challenge in laboratory diagnosis lies in articulating complex technical information to patients in a comprehensible manner. This is particularly pertinent in genetic testing, where results can have profound implications. Ethical professionals must navigate a delicate balance, providing patients with sufficient information to make informed decisions while avoiding overwhelming them with excessive technical details. Informed consent and ethics committee approval in laboratory medicine (Ana et al., 2018).

3. **Genetic Testing and Counseling:** Advances in genetic testing have enabled the identification of genetic predispositions and susceptibility to diseases, providing new possibilities for diagnosis. However, this progress raises ethical concerns regarding the potential psychological impact of genetic information on patients. To aid individuals in comprehending and coping with the implications of test results, genetic counseling becomes essential. Ethical obligations include ensuring comprehensive information and providing support for the psychological effects associated with genetic testing.

36.3.2 RESEARCH-RELATED CHALLENGES

1. **Inclusion of Human Subjects:** Laboratory diagnostics often involve studies that may require the participation of human subjects. Addressing ethical challenges involves ensuring that research participants are treated with respect, their rights are upheld, and their well-being is prioritized. Achieving this balance between advancing scientific knowledge and safeguarding the welfare of study subjects necessitates strict adherence to ethical standards and legal frameworks.
2. **Ethical Considerations in Clinical Trials:** The ethical complexities in laboratory diagnostics arise notably from clinical trials, which play a pivotal role in advancing medical knowledge and treatment options. Deliberate attention is required for aspects such as participant selection, study design, and evaluating potential risks and benefits. In clinical studies, where subjects often undergo experimental interventions, the significance of informed

consent becomes even more pronounced. The complexities of trial design pose a challenge for ethical practitioners aiming to uphold elevated ethical standards while ensuring comprehensive scientific investigation (Ann et al., 2019).

3. **Publication and Sharing of Data:** The ethical imperative to disseminate research findings and contribute to the knowledge base introduces challenges in navigating a delicate balance between patient privacy, safeguarding confidential information, and promoting transparency. There exists a tension between the imperative for meticulous analysis and validation and the urgency to publish results. Ethical considerations in data sharing encompass respecting the contributions of all involved parties, refraining from data manipulation, and upholding the integrity of the scientific method.

36.3.3 PROFESSIONAL CONDUCT AND ETHICAL DILEMMAS

- **Conflict of Interest:** In the realm of laboratory diagnostics, the risk of conflicts of interest is inherent, particularly with the growing prevalence of collaborations among pharmaceutical companies, laboratories, and healthcare practitioners. Such collaborations may compromise the objectivity of diagnostic decisions. Ethical practitioners prioritize patient welfare, and they are obligated to disclose any potential conflicts, managing these situations with transparency and openness.

  i. **Reporting and Communication of Test Results:** Ethical challenges arise in how test findings are communicated to both patients and medical professionals. Striking a balance between sensitivity and transparency is crucial. There is a moral obligation to convey results accurately, understandably, and compassionately, especially when these findings significantly impact the patient's health (Tarja and Helena, 2000).

  ii. **Handling Errors and Quality Control:** In the realm of laboratory diagnosis, errors, though somewhat inevitable, pose ethical challenges related to accountability and transparency.

Building and preserving trust requires disclosing errors to both patients and healthcare professionals, but it must be done with sensitivity to prevent unnecessary distress. Ethical obligations include minimizing errors through the implementation of rigorous quality control procedures. However, when errors do occur, practitioners face the ethically nuanced task of disclosure and correction.

36.4 ETHICAL GUIDELINES AND REGULATORY FRAMEWORKS

36.4.1 OVERVIEW OF INTERNATIONAL AND NATIONAL GUIDELINES

1. **International Guidelines:** Ensuring consistent and ethical laboratory diagnostic procedures is facilitated by international ethical guidelines, providing a universal framework. The World Health Organization (WHO) plays a pivotal role in shaping these recommendations. For instance, the WHO's Laboratory Quality Management System establishes standards for quality assurance, emphasizing precision, reliability, and ethical conduct in diagnostic processes. Additionally, professionals are directed to uphold the highest standards of integrity through the Code of Ethics published by the International Federation of Clinical Chemistry and Laboratory Medicine (IFCC) (Laboratory Quality Management System, 2011).
2. **National Guidelines in India:** Overseeing the regulatory landscape for laboratory diagnostics in India falls under the purview of the Central Drugs Standard Control Organization (CDSCO), a division of the Ministry of Health and Family Welfare. Ethical standards are further supported by organizations like the National Accreditation Board for Testing and Calibration Laboratories (NABL) and the Medical Council of India (MCI). The CDSCO oversees aspects like patient consent, data protection, and quality assurance to ensure that diagnostic tests meet legal requirements. The MCI establishes ethical standards for medical professionals, and NABL ensures that laboratories adhere to global quality standards (National Ethical Guidelines for Biomedical, 2017).

36.4.2 ROLE OF PROFESSIONAL ORGANIZATIONS AND REGULATORY BODIES

1. **Professional Organizations:** In India, professional associations like the Indian Society of Clinical Research (ISCR) and the Indian Association of Pathologists and Microbiologists (IAPM) play a pivotal role in shaping ethical standards. The IAPM, for example, fosters a commitment to accuracy and patient welfare by establishing codes of conduct and best practices for laboratory personnel. The ISCR contributes to the broader field of healthcare ethics by focusing on ethical guidelines within clinical research (Bhagwat and Pai, 2020).
2. **Regulatory Bodies in India:** Key regulatory bodies in India, particularly the CDSCO, play a crucial role in overseeing and enforcing ethical protocols in the laboratory diagnostics industry. They ensure the safety and efficacy of diagnostic tests by establishing guidelines for their approval. While the MCI no longer holds regulatory authority over the ethical conduct of medical practitioners, including those in laboratory diagnostics, this responsibility has been assumed by the National Medical Commission (NMC). Serving as the accrediting organization, NABL ensures that laboratories adhere to global standards and encourages a culture of continuous improvement (Gogtay et al., 2017).

36.5 IMPACT OF EMERGING TECHNOLOGIES ON ETHICS IN LABORATORY DIAGNOSTICS

36.5.1 GENETIC TESTING ADVANCEMENTS

1. **Precision Medicine and Ethical Considerations:** The advent of genetic testing, enabling the customization of therapies based on an individual's genetic profile, has ushered in the era of precision medicine. This development holds tremendous promise in addressing the diverse genetic landscape present in the Indian population. However, it introduces ethical concerns related to data

privacy, informed consent, and the potential psychological impact of genetic information. Ensuring the ethical handling of genetic data, providing appropriate counseling, and ensuring comprehensive patient understanding become moral imperatives.

2. **Genetic Counseling and Patient Autonomy:** With the increased prevalence of genetic testing, there is a growing emphasis on genetic counseling to aid individuals in comprehending and navigating the implications of test results. This focus on counseling aligns with the broader ethical principle of respecting and upholding patient autonomy in the context of genetic information. Genetic counseling assumes heightened importance in India, where cultural and socioeconomic factors significantly influence healthcare decision-making. The ethical implementation of genetic testing must prioritize the respect of patient autonomy through clear information dissemination, recognition of cultural sensitivities, and ensuring informed consent.

36.5.2 POINT-OF-CARE TESTING AND ITS IMPLICATIONS

1. **Accessibility and Timeliness:** Point-of-care testing (POCT) delivers rapid data that can immediately impact medical decisions, bringing diagnostics closer to the patient. In India, a country with a markedly disparate healthcare system, particularly in rural and underdeveloped areas, POCT has the potential to enhance accessibility. However, ethical concerns arise regarding the reliability and accuracy of such tests. Upholding ethical standards necessitates ensuring that POCT devices comply with legal requirements and providing adequate training for medical staff.

2. **Informed Decision-Making:** Point-of-care testing (POCT) often utilizes streamlined tests that can be conducted outside traditional laboratory settings. Ensuring informed decision-making involves providing patients with sufficient information about the purposes, benefits, and limitations of POCT. Given the unique challenges of decentralized testing, ethical guidelines in India should strongly emphasize the importance of offering appropriate follow-up care, obtaining informed consent, and fostering open communication channels.

36.5.3 ARTIFICIAL INTELLIGENCE AND MACHINE LEARNING IN DIAGNOSTICS

1. **Data Privacy and Security:** The integration of AI and ML with laboratory tests introduces new ethical considerations, particularly concerning the handling of extensive volumes of patient data. Ethical considerations in India must address the escalating concerns surrounding data privacy and security, encompassing issues like data security, consent for data utilization, and transparency in AI algorithms. Striking a balance between the ethical imperatives of data privacy and the diagnostic accuracy benefits offered by AI poses a significant challenge (Federico, 2023).
2. **Transparency and Accountability:** As AI algorithms become increasingly integrated into diagnostic decision-making, transparency in their operations is pivotal for maintaining trust. Ethical standards should encourage developers to disclose the rationale behind AI models, ensuring that patients and medical professionals can comprehend the basis for diagnostic recommendations. Additionally, establishing accountability mechanisms aligned with broader healthcare professional responsibility guidelines is essential to address errors or biases in AI-driven diagnostics.

36.6 STRATEGIES FOR ADDRESSING ETHICAL CHALLENGES

36.6.1 TRAINING AND EDUCATION OF LABORATORY PROFESSIONALS

1. **Foundational Education:** Addressing ethical concerns in laboratory diagnoses starts with comprehensive training and education. From the inception of their courses, laboratory personnel should be equipped with a thorough understanding of ethical standards, covering aspects such as informed consent, patient confidentiality, and professionalism. The foundational knowledge acquired forms the basis for ethical conduct throughout their professional careers.
2. **Continuing Education:** Given the dynamic nature of laboratory diagnosis and healthcare, ongoing education is imperative. Regular training programs and workshops enable professionals to stay abreast

of new technologies, evolving ethical standards, and changes in regulations. By fostering a culture of accountability and adaptability, continuous education ensures that professionals remain informed and well-equipped to navigate emerging ethical challenges.

36.6.2 *ESTABLISHING ETHICAL REVIEW COMMITTEES*

1. **Role and Composition:** Referred to as either Institutional Review Boards (IRBs) or Ethics Committees (ECs), ethical review committees (ERCs) play a crucial role in evaluating and approving research involving human participants. These committees are instrumental in overseeing the adherence of research projects in laboratory diagnostics to ethical standards. The establishment of these committees within medical institutions involves selecting a diverse group of individuals with backgrounds encompassing patient advocacy, ethics, legislation, and laboratory diagnostics (Grady 2015).
2. **Oversight of Research Protocols:** To ensure the ethical conduct of research, ERC scrutinize study designs, participant recruitment procedures, and the potential risks and benefits of the research. These committees provide oversight in laboratory diagnoses, ensuring adherence to ethical guidelines and prioritizing patient welfare in genetic testing and other diagnostic research.

36.7 COLLABORATION AND INTERDISCIPLINARY APPROACHES:

1. **Inter-Professional Collaboration:** Addressing ethical concerns in laboratory diagnoses requires the collaboration of specialists from diverse disciplines. Alongside laboratory experts, healthcare teams should include physicians, ethicists, psychologists, and legal experts. This multidisciplinary approach fosters comprehensive decision-making and facilitates a thorough understanding of ethical dilemmas.
2. **Patient Involvement:** Collaborating with patients is essential for making ethical decisions. Integrating patient perspectives throughout the development of guidelines and protocols ensures that ethical considerations align with the expectations and values

of those directly affected. Collaborative approaches facilitated by patient advocacy groups and community engagement programs prioritize patient-centered ethical practices.

36.8 FUTURE DIRECTIONS AND RECOMMENDATIONS

36.8.1 ETHICAL CONSIDERATIONS IN PERSONALIZED MEDICINE

1. **Informed Consent and Genomic Data:** As personalized medicine advances, ethical considerations must focus on ensuring that patients have a comprehensive understanding of the implications associated with genomic testing. Given the intricacies of personalized medicine, changes in informed consent procedures should acknowledge potential future uses of genomic data and their impacts on family members (Brother and Rothstein, 2015).
2. **Equitable Access to Personalized Therapies:** Addressing ethical concerns in personalized medicine requires a commitment to equal access. It is crucial to mitigate disparities in the availability of cutting-edge diagnostic and therapeutic options. Legislators and healthcare organizations should prioritize the pursuit of inclusive policies that aim for the equitable distribution of the benefits of personalized medicine.

36.8.2 INTEGRATION OF ETHICS IN LABORATORY PRACTICE

1. **Integration of Ethical Guidelines into Everyday Practice:** Moving forward, ethical considerations related to laboratory diagnostics should seamlessly integrate into routine practice. This involves updating ethical concepts in SOPs, ensuring practitioners are well-versed in ethical standards, and incorporating ethical considerations into the development and implementation of new diagnostic technologies (Dariush et al., 2021).
2. **Patient Education and Engagement:** Another dimension of embedding ethics into laboratory practice is prioritizing patient education and engagement. Offering patients information about the diagnostic process, potential implications of test results, and their right to informed consent contributes to a more ethical and patient-centered approach.

36.8.3 ETHICAL IMPLICATIONS OF EMERGING TECHNOLOGIES

1. **Artificial Intelligence (AI) and Transparent Decision-Making:** Addressing ethical challenges in the increasing integration of AI into diagnostics is crucial. Developers must prioritize transparency in AI algorithms to enable patients and medical practitioners to comprehend the decision-making process. Additionally, implementing measures to eliminate biases in AI algorithms is essential for preventing discrepancies in diagnostic results (Federico and Giuseppe, 2022; Brian et al., 2021).
2. **Data Privacy and Security in Emerging Technologies:** Ethical concerns about data security and privacy are escalating with the advent of new technologies. Future developments should include robust data protection protocols, incorporating encryption, anonymization, and stringent access controls. In the rapidly evolving landscape of technologies, establishing clear standards for the appropriate use and sharing of patient data becomes imperative (Sophie and Vanessa, 2012).

KEYWORDS

- **artificial intelligence**
- **data privacy**
- **data security**
- **diagnostic accuracy**
- **diagnostic technologies**
- **ethical challenges**
- **laboratory diagnostics**
- **machine learning**
- **medical professionals**
- **patient engagement**
- **standard operating procedures**

REFERENCES

Akber, S. S. (2021). Medical laboratory ethics. *PJE, 1*(1), 1, 2.

Bhagwat, S., & Pai, S. A. (2020). Medical ethics in laboratory medicine: A review, with an oath for pathologists. *Indian Journal of Medical Ethics.* https://doi.org/10.20529/IJME.2020.02.

Borovecki, A., Mlinarić, A., Horvat, M., & Supak Smolčić, V. (2018). Informed consent and ethics committee approval in laboratory medicine. *Biochemia Medica (Zagreb), 28*(3), 030201.

Brothers, K. B., & Rothstein, M. A. (2015). Ethical, legal, and social implications of incorporating personalized medicine into healthcare. *Personalized Medicine, 12*(1), 43–51.

Farhud, D. D., & Zokaei, S. (2021). Ethical issues of artificial intelligence in medicine and healthcare. *Iranian Journal of Public Health, 50*(11).

Gogtay, N. J., Ravi, R., & Thatte, U. M. (2017). Regulatory requirements for clinical trials in India: What academicians need to know. *Indian Journal of Anaesthesia, 61*(3), 192–199.

Grady, C. (2015). Institutional review boards: Purpose and challenges. *Chest, 148*(5), 1148–1155.

Gronowski, A. M., Budelier, M. M., & Campbell, S. M. (2019). Ethics for laboratory medicine. *Clinical Chemistry, 65*(12), 1497–1507.

Jackson, B. R., Ye, Y., Crawford, J. M., Becich, M. J., & Roy, S. (2021). The ethics of artificial intelligence in pathology and laboratory medicine: Principles and practice. *Academic Pathology, 8.*

Kapiriri, L. (2016). Medical ethics and bedside rationing in low-income countries: Challenges and opportunities. *Bioethics, 30*, 183–190.

Lenicov, F. R., & Fink, N. E. (2023). Ethical issues in the use of leftover samples and associated personal data obtained from diagnostic laboratories. *Clinica Chimica Acta, 548*, 117442.

Mathur, R., & Swaminathan, S. (2018). National ethical guidelines for biomedical & health research involving human participants, 2017: A commentary. *Indian Journal of Medical Research, 148*(3), 279–283.

Najjari, M., Karimazar, M., Ebrahimipour, M., & Budke, C. M. (2022). A review of ethical issues related to laboratory-based diagnostics. *Medical Laboratory Journal, 16*(2), 1–6.

Nyrhinen, T., & Leino-Kilpi, H. (2000). Ethics in the laboratory examination of patients. *Journal of Medical Ethics, 26*, 54–60.

Pellé, S., & Nurock, V. (2012). Of nanochips and persons: Toward an ethics of diagnostic technology in personalized medicine. *Nanoethics, 6*, 155–165.

Pennestrì, F., & Banfi, G. (2022). Artificial intelligence in laboratory medicine: Fundamental ethical issues and normative key points. *Clinical Chemistry and Laboratory Medicine, 60*(12), 1867–1874.

Talash, K., Anthias, C., & Machin, L. L. (2022). Exploring the perceived benefits of ethics education for laboratory professionals. *International Journal of Ethics Education, 7*, 201–212.

Wijeratne, N., & Benatar, S. R. (2010). Ethical issues in laboratory medicine. *Journal of Clinical Pathology, 63*, 97–98.

World Health Organization. (2011). *Laboratory Quality Management System: Handbook.*

Index

C

D

E

F

G

H

J

O

P

S

T

U

V